Transplant International

Official Journal of the European Society for Organ Transplantation

**Supplement 1
to Volume 9
1996**

Proceedings of the 7th Congress
of the European Society
for Organ Transplantation

Vienna, October 3–7, 1995

Special Editor:
F. Mühlbacher

Guest Editors:
M. Gnant
W. Klepetko
F. Längle
G. Laufer
T. Sautner
R. Steininger
P. Wamser

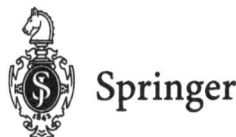 Springer

Transplant *International*

Official Journal of the European Society for Organ Transplantation

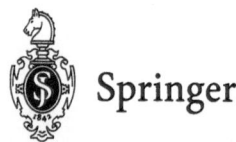

Springer

Transplant
International

Official Journal of the European Society for Organ Transplantation

Preface

This is the third supplement to *Transplant International,* which contains the Proceedings of the 7th Congress of the European Society for Organ Transplantation held in Vienna from 3–7 October 1995.

This congress was attended by a record number of 1631 participants. Some 1082 abstracts were submitted to the selection committee; 211 were selected for oral presentation and 259 for poster presentation. The overall acceptance rate was 47%. This strict selection process resulted in high-level scientific presentations and overwhelming attendance in the scientific sessions. In addition, nine invited speakers presented overview data in three plenary sessions covering the areas of organ donation, immunosuppression and late graft failure. In all, 180 authors submitted manuscripts for publication. These manuscripts were again reviewed by the editors of this supplement with emphasis on scientific content, originality and methods. Of these, 117 articles have now been accepted for publication in this supplement, which cover all topics presented at the Vienna meeting. This intensive second review process was necessary to limit publication to high-level papers only. As discussed at the Vienna meeting, liberal policies of accepting publications for the congress proceedings would jeopardize the impact factor of *Transplant International.* The editors of this book tried to find this compromise between quick publication and quality of contributions. If this attempt is successful, future ESOT congress proceedings may also be published in *Transplant International.* We encourage the readers of this book to honor this quality and to cite articles of this book in future publications.

I would like to thank the editorial and the production team for their skill and effort of reviewing, proofreading, editing and printing and hope that the readers of this book will find it a source of new, stimulating and valuable information.

Ferdinand Mühlbacher   Vienna, June 1996
Special Editor

Transplant International

International

Official Journal of the European Society for Organ Transplantation

ISBN 978-3-540-61024-3   ISBN 978-3-662-00818-8 (eBook)
DOI 10.1007/978-3-662-00818-8
Published also as Supplement 1 to Volume 9, 1996   ISSN 0934-0874

Softcover reprint of the hardcover 1st edition 1996

SPIN 10534491   24/3020-5 4 3 2 1 0 – Printed on acid-free paper.

Transplant International

Official Journal of the European Society for Organ Transplantation

Contents

Kidney

Transpl Int (1996) 9 [Suppl 1]: S3–S4
© Springer-Verlag 1996

Rat cytomegalovirus infection and chronic kidney allograft rejection

Petri K. Koskinen
Serdar Yilmaz
Erkki Kallio
Cathrien A. Bruggeman
Pekka J. Häyry
Karl Lemström

P. K. Koskinen (✉) · S. Yilmaz · E. Kallio ·
P. J. Häyry · K. Lemström
Transplantation Laboratory, University of
Helsinki and Helsinki University Central
Hospital, Helsinki, Finland

C. A. Bruggeman
Department of Medical Microbiology,
University of Limburg, Maastricht,
The Netherlands

Abstract To investigate the effect of cytomegalovirus (CMV) infection on the development of experimental chronic kidney allograft rejection, orthotopic kidney allografts from DA donors (Ag-B4, $RT1^{a1}$) to WF (Ag-B2, $RT1^u$) recipients were used. The rats received cyclosporine A (CsA) for 12 weeks. A group of recipients was infected with 10^5 plaque-forming units of rat CMV (RCMV), and another group was left non-infected and used as controls. The grafts were removed 12 weeks after transplantation. RCMV infection significantly enhanced the development of chronic kidney allograft rejection as follows: the intensity of interstitial inflammation ($P < 0.025$), particularly the degree of pyroninophilic cells in the inflammatory infiltrate ($P < 0.025$); the glomeruli mesangial matrix increase ($P < 0.05$) and capillary basement membrane thickening ($P < 0.01$); the extent of endothelial cell swelling ($P < 0.025$) and intimal proliferation ($P < 0.025$) in the graft vasculature; and the extent of tubular epithelial atrophy ($P < 0.025$). The chronic allograft damage index (CADI) was significantly increased to 4.2 ± 0.9 in RCMV-infected allografts, compared with 0.8 ± 0.4 in non-infected ($P < 0.02$). At the molecular level, RCMV infection significantly increased vascular endothelial ($P < 0.05$) and tubular epithelial ($P < 0.01$) ICAM-1 expression. Viral antigens were detected in tubular epithelial cells and in some inflammatory cells.

Key words Kidney transplantation · CMV infection · Chronic rejection · ICAM-1

Introduction

Chronic rejection, characterised by interstitial fibrosis, glomerulosclerosis, tubular atrophy and arterial narrowing, is the major reason for loss of renal allografts after the first posttransplant year [1]. Acute rejection episodes, low cyclosporine doses, and infections, especially cytomegalovirus (CMV) infection, have been recognised as most important risk factors for the development of this disorder [2].

Materials and methods

To investigate the effect of CMV infection on the development of chronic kidney allograft rejection, orthotopic kidney allografts from DA donors (Ag-B4, $RT1^{a1}$) to WF (Ag-B2, $RT1^u$) recipients were used. The kidney and 1 cm of ureter were removed en bloc, including the renal artery and the renal vein. The recipient right kidney was removed, leaving the ureter as long as possible. The donor kidney was transplanted to the recipient's abdominal aorta and inferior vena cava below the left renal artery. The rats received cyclosporine A (CsA), 5 mg/kg per day s.c. for 12 weeks. At 7 days after transplantation, left nephrectomy was performed to remove the recipient's own kidney. A group of recipients was infected with 10^5 plaque-forming units of rat CMV (RCMV) [3] 9 days after transplantation, and another group was left non-infected and used as controls. The rats were monitored twice a week for serum creat-

S4

Table 1 Effect of rat cytomegalovirus (RCMV) infection on chronic kidney allograft changes (*CADI* chronic allograft damage index, *BM* basement membrane)

	DA → WF	DA → WF + RCMV	P
CADI	4.2 ± 0.9	0.8 ± 0.4	< 0.02
Interstitium			
Inflammation	0.1 ± 0.1	0.9 ± 0.2	< 0.025
Pyroninophilic cells (%)	0 ± 0	18 ± 7	< 0.025
Glomeruli			
Mesangial matrix increase	0.4 ± 0.1	0.9 ± 0.2	< 0.05
Capillary BM thickening	0 ± 0	0.7 ± 0.1	< 0.01
Vessels			
Endothelial swelling	0 ± 0	0.6 ± 0.2	< 0.025
Intimal proliferation	0 ± 0	0.6 ± 0.2	< 0.025
Tubuli			
Epithelial atrophy	0 ± 0	0.6 ± 0.2	< 0.025
Endothelial ICAM-1	0.6 ± 0.2	1.8 ± 0.2	< 0.05
Tubular cell ICAM-1	0.2 ± 0.2	1.4 ± 0.4	< 0.01

inine and the diagnosis of acute rejection was made if there was an unexplained rise in serum creatinine > 200 µmol/l. The grafts were removed for histology 12 weeks after transplantation. The presence of RCMV early and late antigens in kidney allografts was demonstrated using a mixture of mouse monoclonal antibodies against early (#8) and late (#35) antigens of RCMV [4]. The expression of ICAM-1 was demonstrated using a mouse IgG$_1$ monoclonal antibody to rat intercellular adhesion molecule-1 (ICAM-1; CD54, 1A29, Seikagaku Co., Tokyo, Japan).

Results

RCMV significantly enhanced the chronic allograft damage index (CADI) (Table 1), which is the sum of interstitial inflammation and fibrosis, mesangial matrix increase and sclerosis of glomeruli, intimal proliferation of arteries, and tubular atrophy. The CADI was significantly increased to 4.2 ± 0.9 in RCMV-infected allografts, compared with 0.8 ± 0.4 in non-infected (P < 0.02). The vascular wall changes of RCMV infected allografts were associated with a significantly increased ICAM-1 expression in the tubular cells (P < 0.01) and in endothelial cells (P < 0.05) compared with the controls. RCMV early and late antigens could be detected in tubular epithelial cells and in some inflammatory cells of the infected allografts.

Discussion

To conclude, our results provide experimental evidence that RCMV infection is associated with enhanced chronic allograft changes reflecting the chronic kidney allograft damage index. At the molecular level, these RCMV-induced chronic changes are linked with increased vascular endothelial and tubular epithelial ICAM-1 expression. Supporting the concept that CMV is able to infect various kidney cell types, we found early and late RCMV antigen expression in tubular epithelial cells and in some interstitial inflammatory cells.

References

1. Paul LC, Häyry P, Foegh M, Dennis MJ, Mihatsch MJ, Larsson E, Fellström B (1993) Diagnostic criteria for chronic rejection/accelerated graft atherosclerosis in heart and kidney transplants: Joint proposal from the fourth Alexis Carrel conference on chronic rejection and accelerated arteriosclerosis in transplanted organs. Transplant Proc 25: 2022
2. Almond PS, Matas A, Gillingham K, Dunn DL, Payne WD, Gores P, Gruessner R, Najarian JS (1993) Risk factors for chronic rejection in renal allograft recipients. Transplantation 55: 752–757
3. Bruggeman CA, Debie WMH, Grauls G, Majoor G, van Boven CPA (1983) Infection of laboratory rats with a new cytomegalo-like virus. Arch Virol 76: 188–199
4. Bruning JH, Debie WHM, Dormans PHJ, Meyer H, Bruggeman CA (1987) The development and characterization of monoclonal antibodies against rat cytomegalovirus induced antigens. Arch Virol 94: 55–70

Transpl Int (1996) 9 [Suppl 1]: S5–S7
© Springer-Verlag 1996

KIDNEY

Helena Isoniemi
Satu Lehtonen
Kaija Salmela
Juhani Ahonen

Does delayed kidney graft function increase the risk of chronic rejection?

H. Isoniemi (✉) · S. Lehtonen ·
K. Salmela · J. Ahonen
Division of Transplantation of
IV Department of Surgery, Helsinki
University Central Hospital,
Kasarmikatu 11, 00130 Helsinki, Finland

Abstract The impact of delayed graft function (DGF) on later renal graft loss due to chronic rejection was studied in a single center using uniform protocol for organ procurement and posttransplant patient care. DGF function was observed in 34 % of 829 consecutive first cadaveric renal transplants in adults and in 47 % of 169 retransplantations ($P < 0.05$). There were no significant differences in graft survival between groups with early graft function (EGF) and DGF, either in first transplantations or retransplantations. The half-life in EGF and DGF groups of first transplants was 12.3 years and 10.5 years, respectively, and of retransplantants was 8.0 years and 6.5 years, respectively.

DGF was divided in three subgroups according to the day of onset. If graft function started during the first or second week after transplantation there were no significant differences in long-term graft survival rates compared with EGF. Only in retransplants, if graft function started later than 2 weeks postoperatively, were long-term graft survival rates significantly lower when compared with EGF and the difference persisted if other causes of graft loss except chronic rejection were censored.

Key words Chronic rejection · Delayed graft function · Graft outcome

Introduction

The reports on the impact of delayed graft function (DGF) on later graft outcome has been controversial [3, 5, 6]. Recently DGF has been shown to have an adverse effect on graft outcome at least during the first postoperative year [3, 7]. After the first year, the yearly risk of graft loss due to chronic rejection is about 4 % [4]. Several risk factors may contribute to the original injury of the endothelial cell wall in the renal allograft leading to vascular chronic rejection. Delayed graft function (DGF) can be a sign of some original injury in a renal graft. The aim of this single center study was to investigate whether DGF increases the risk of chronic rejection in cadaveric renal transplants with uniform initial immunosuppression.

Patients and methods

In Helsinki, between January 1986 and 7 December 1993, 1170 renal transplantations were performed which included 58 (5 %) transplantations in children under 16 years and 79 (6.8 %) living-related transplantations in adults. The study population consists of all 1036 consecutive cadaveric renal transplantations in adults. Two study groups were created. The possible risk of DGF was analyzed for first transplants ($n = 854$) and retransplants ($n = 182$) separately.

Graft function was defined as early (EGF) if no dialysis was needed during the first week and at the same time serum creatinine decreased spontaneously. Fifteen patients with one dialysis during the first week were included in the EGF group because serum creatinine was decreasing rapidly every day and the need for one dialysis was due to fluid overload after the operation. DGF was defined as a need for dialysis during the first week or if serum creatinine failed to decrease spontaneously. In DGF, the onset of graft function was defined as the day of first spontaneous decrease of serum creatinine. Postoperatively, serum creatinine was recorded ev-

Table 1 Graft survivals in early graft function (EGF) and delayed graft function (DGF) groups for first cadaveric renal transplants and retransplants. Furthermore, DGF is divided in subgroups according to the day of onset

	Graft survival time	EGF	DGF	Subgroups of DGF		
				1–7 days	8–14 days	> 14 days
First transplantation ($n = 829$)	3 years	82 %	75 %	73 %	75 %	74 %
	6 years	71 %	62 %	57 %	67 %	63 %
Retransplantation ($n = 169$)	3 years	77 %	75 %	86 %	72 %	71 %
	6 years	62 %	59 %	78 %	66 %	43 %

Table 2 Half-lives in years ($T^{1}/_{2}$) calculated for the EGF and DGF groups including all causes of graft losses and censoring other causes of graft loss except chronic rejection

	First transplants		Retransplants	
	$T^{1}/_{2}$	Censored $T^{1}/_{2}$	$T^{1}/_{2}$	Censored $T^{1}/_{2}$
EGF	12.3	16.2	8.0	12.1
DGF	10.5	14.8	6.5	12.9

Table 3 Half-lives in years in subgroups of DGF including all causes of graft losses and censoring other causes of graft loss except chronic rejection

DGF	First transplants		Retransplants	
	$T^{1}/_{2}$	Censored $T^{1}/_{2}$	$T^{1}/_{2}$	Censored $T^{1}/_{2}$
Onset 1–7 days	8.2	10.7	10.3	13.0
Onset 8–14 days	10.9	12.1	6.2	17.9
Onset > 14 days	13.5	16.0	3.9	5.4

ery day during the 3–4 week stay at the transplantation unit. DGF was divided in three groups according to the onset of graft function: 1–7 days, 8–14 days, and over 14 days, postoperatively. Diagnosis of chronic rejection was based on clinical criteria. Graft loss due to chronic rejection was defined as a gradual but progressive deterioration of graft function leading to dialysis in the absence of other specific causes. Biopsies were not available from all grafts, but if there was no biopsy other possible causes of late graft dysfunction were excluded by clinical investigations.

Since 1986 our immunosuppressive protocol has been the same. All cadaveric renal transplant patients have received triple therapy with cyclosporine, azathioprine, and methylprednisolone. Immunologically high risk patients (previous transplant lost due to immunological reasons and high panel-reactive antibodies) have, furthermore, received polyclonal or monoclonal antibodies for 7–10 days as induction therapy. Oral cyclosporine was started before the operation, 5 mg/kg body weight, and it continued afterwards, 10 mg/kg per day in two doses. Cyclosporine was given independently of primary graft function and the dose was adjusted to trough blood levels measured at least twice per week. All grafts were from heart-beating donors and the organs were procured according to uniform protocol.

The risk of graft loss in chronic rejection was compared between the groups of patients with EGF and DGF. The graft survival was calculated using an actuarial life-table method and the differences between groups by the log-rank method. To study the long-term effect half-life was calculated. The estimation of half-life was based on least square exponential curve fitting of survival between 1 and 6 years posttransplant. Half-life is the estimated time needed for 50 % of the grafts functioning at 1 year after transplantation to fail.

Results

The number of grafts which never function in first transplants and in retransplants were 2.9 % (25/854) and 7 % (13/182), respectively, and these grafts were excluded from the final study groups. DGF was recognised in 34 % (281/829) of first transplants and in 43 % (79/169) of retransplants ($P < 0.01$). Distribution of transplants in the three subgroups of DGF, i.e., onset of graft function during the first week, second week and after 2 weeks, were 44 % (124), 35 % (98), and 21 % of all 281 first grafts with DGF, respectively, and 29 % (23), 34 % (27), and 37 % (29) of all 79 retransplants with DGF, respectively. The 3-year and 6-year graft survival (GS) in EGF and DGF and, furthermore, in the subgroups of DGF is presented in Table 1. The difference in GS between first transplants with EGF and DGF was not significant (log-rank test, chi-squared = 4.37, $P < 0.1$) and neither in retransplants (chi-squared = 0.364, NS). In first transplants GS did not differ significantly in DGF subgroups. In retransplants GS rates decreased in DGF subgroups with increasing time of onset (Table 1), but the difference was not significant in any subgroups compared with EGF.

The calculated half-life after 1 year was slightly higher in the grafts with early function than in the grafts with DGF (Table 2), both in first and retransplants. If all other causes of graft loss but chronic rejection were censored, half-life for first grafts with DGF function was 1.4 years shorter and for retransplants with DGF half-life was 0.8 years longer compared to the grafts with early function (Table 2).

For the grafts functioning at 1 year, later graft survival rates did not differ between EGF and the DGF except GS in retransplants with EGF was significantly higher compared to the group of DGF with onset after 2 weeks (log-rank test, chi-squared = 5.67 $P < 0.05$) including all causes of graft losses and also censoring other causes except chronic rejection (chi-squared = 5.94, $P < 0.05$). Half-lives of the subgroups of DGF are presented in Table 3. In first transplants, this more close analysis showed the shortest half-life in the group of DGF with onset of function during first week. In first transplants, there was no correlation in half-lives or in GS rates after the first year including all graft losses or only graft losses due to chronic rejection. In retransplants, half-life correlated inversely with increasing time of onset including all grafts and also if other causes except chronic rejection were censored. In retransplants, GS rates after the first year were significantly lower in the group of DGF with onset after 2 weeks compared with EGF both if all causes of graft loss were included and also if other causes except chronic rejection were censored.

Discussion

In this study population, frequency of DGF (34 %–47 %) was high. EGF is usually defined as no need for dialysis. Our criteria also included the demand for spontaneously decreasing serum creatinine which increases the frequency of DGF to some extent. DGF occurred significantly more often after retransplant than after first graft which might be due to some immunological influence on graft function in retransplants.

We have shown earlier that, in our patient population, acute allograft rejection is no longer a risk for later graft outcome at least in first cadaveric renal transplants. This controversial result, compared with many other recent studies [1, 2], might be in part explained by our genetically homogenous population (all patients ethnically Finns) and low frequency of acute rejections. Furthermore, acute rejections under initial triple therapy have been mild and reversible. However, the risk of graft loss due to chronic rejection is about 4 % every year [4]. DGF can be a sign of some initial endothelial cell damage in the graft with a subsequent response to injury leading to intimal proliferation and chronic vascular rejection.

Long-term consequences of DGF, excluding the early graft losses, have seldom been investigated. Our interest was to analyze the impact of DGF on half-lives of the grafts. In first transplants, graft survival curves did not differ after the first year posttransplant in EGF and DGF groups and the half-lives did not correlate with the onset of graft function. Our results do not confirm the negative effect of DGF on later graft outcome. We found that only the subgroup of retransplants with onset of function after 2 weeks had a significantly higher risk of losing a graft compared with EGF.

Aetiology of DGF is certainly multifactorial. We can only postulate that such factors which have an impact on DGF causing the increased risk of later graft loss are minimised in our program. In our center many possible causes of DGF are minimised. HLA matching is used for donor selection. The quality of organs is optimized with strict donor criteria and the same transplant team is responsible in the whole country for the organ harvesting program. Moreover, it is interesting that although we started the cyclosporine before kidney transplantation and it was continued irrespective of early graft function, there were no significant differences in long-term graft survival rates or in the half-lives between EGF and DGF groups in first transplants. What the consequence of our cyclosporine policy is to the low acute rejection frequency is not known.

In conclusion, we could not confirm the impact of DGF on later graft outcome on first transplants. Retransplants had more DGF compared with first transplants. Only retransplants with the onset of graft function later than 2 weeks postoperatively showed poorer outcome compared with EGF.

References

1. Almond PS, Matas AJ, Gillingham KJ, et al (1993) Risk factors for chronic rejection in renal allograft recipients. Transplantation 55: 752–757
2. Gulanikar AC, MacDonald AS, Sugurtekin U, Belitsky P (1992) The incidence and impact of early rejection episodes on graft outcome in recipients of first cadaver kidney transplants. Transplantation 53: 323–328
3. Halloran PF, Aprile MA, Farewell V, Ludwin D, Smith K, Tsai SY, Bear RA, Cole EH, Fenton SS, Cattran DC (1988) Early function as the principal correlate of graft survival. Transplantation 46: 223–228
4. Isoniemi H, Kyllönen L, Eklund B, Höckerstedt K, Salmela K, Willebrand v E, Ahonen J (1995) Acute rejection under triple immunosuppressive therapy does not increase the risk of late first cadaveric renal allograft loss. Transplant Proc 27: 875–877
5. Miwa H, van Loenen M, Vanderwerf BA (1989) The long-term effect of delayed graft function on cadaveric renal transplants treated with low dose cyclosporine. In: P Terasaki (ed) Clinical transplants 1989. UCLA Tissue Typing laboratory, Los Angeles, pp 275–278
6. Sanfilippo F, Vaughn, WK, Spees EK, Lucas BA (1985) The effects of delayed graft function on renal transplantation. Transplant Proc 17: 13–15
7. Troppmann C, Gillingham KJ, Benedetti E, Almond PS, Gruessner R, Najarian JS, Matas AJ (1995) Delayed graft function, acute rejection, and outcome after cadaver renal transplantation. Transplantation 59: 962–968

Transpl Int (1996) 9 [Suppl 1]: S8–S10
© Springer-Verlag 1996

T. Wujciak
G. Opelz

Evaluation of the permissible mismatch concept

T. Wujciak (✉) · G. Opelz
Institute of Immunology, University of
Heidelberg, Im Neuenheimer Feld 305,
D-69115 Heidelberg, Germany

Abstract Maruya et al. described a method of separating one HLA-A+B+DR mismatched transplants into permissible and immunogenic categories (published in Clinical Transplants 1993). For the permissible subgroup, they observed an outcome similar to that of zero-A+B+DR mismatched transplants. The classification was based on the HLA type combination of donor and recipient. We evaluated this concept with the data of the Collaborative Transplant Study (CTS). We did not obtain significant differences between the outcome of immunogenic and permissible mismatched transplants. The pairwise p-values for the comparison of zero-mismatched with permissible mismatched transplants are significant for cadaver transplants. The indifferent results obtained in our analysis do not support the concept of permissible mismatches. A more restrictive definition of the permissible mismatches might be helpful. The current method appears to be of insufficient reliability due to the relatively small numbers of transplants in the individual subgroups used to identify permissible combinations.

Key words HLA compatibility · Permissible mismatch

Introduction

There have been extensive discussions recently concerning the report by the University of California at Los Angeles (UCLA) registry that, depending on the recipient's human lymphocyte antigen (HLA) profile, certain HLA mismatches may be *permissible* and thus not have a negative impact on graft survival [1]. It was proposed that this concept could be transformed into an improved algorithm for the allocation of cadaver kidneys. We re-examined the attractive UCLA concept based on an analysis of the larger Collaborative Transplant Study (CTS) data base in order to determine whether such an approach would indeed allow an identification of HLA mismatches that could safely be ignored. The implications, of course, are important, because it would be easier to find tissue-compatible donor-recipient combinations.

Methods

A total of 15915 cadaver and 4470 living related donor transplants performed in North America and 40333 cadaver and 2397 living related donor transplants performed in Europe were analyzed. We followed the exact specifications for the identification of *permissible* and *immunogenic* mismatches published by the UCLA group [1]. Actuarial rates of graft survival were computed according to the method of Kaplan and Meier.

Results

The original UCLA study in which *permissible* profiles were identified was based on an analysis of related donor transplants. Indeed, when the CTS data for related transplants reported from North America were analyzed, a confirmatory trend was observed. Transplants with one HLA mismatch that were categorized as *permissible* did as well as zero-mismatch transplants, and

Table 1 Graft survival rates with the permissible mismatch concept. (*HLA* Human lymphocyte antigen)

HLA mismatches	Graft survival in North America		Graft survival in Europe	
	Related (1 year/3 years)	Cadaver (1 year/3 years)	Related (1 year/3 years)	Cadaver (1 year/3 years)
Zero A + B + DR	95 %/91 % (*n* = 1269)	91 %/83 % (*n* = 719)	93 %/87 % (*n* = 422)	86 %/79 % (*n* = 2137)
One permissible	98 %/90 % (*n* = 112)	83 %/74 % (*n* = 157)	90 %/78 % (*n* = 78)	84 %/74 % (*n* = 1403)
One immunogenic	91 %/86 % (*n* = 252)	84 %/73 % (*n* = 397)	90 %/86 % (*n* = 167)	83 %/74 % (*n* = 2101)

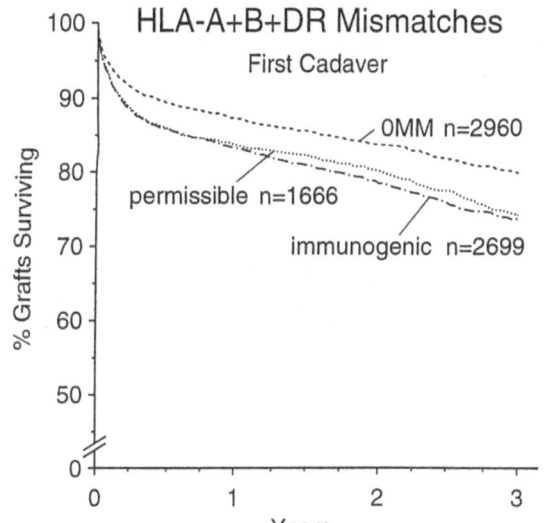

Fig. 1 Graft survival analysis of first cadaver kidney transplants according to whether grafts had no mismatches on the human lymphocyte antigen (HLA)-A, HLA-B and HLA-DR loci *(0 MM)*, or whether one mismatch was present which was defined as *permissible* or *immunogenic*. The numbers of patients studied are indicated. The one-mismatch grafts had significantly lower survival rates than the zero-mismatch grafts, regardless of whether the mismatch was *permissible* or *immunogenic*

better than transplants with one HLA mismatch categorized as *immunogenic* (Table 1).

When the same type of analysis was performed on related donor transplants reported from Europe, however, the improved outcome of grafts with one *permissible* mismatch could not be confirmed. Because the number of related grafts available for analysis from North America was much larger than that from Europe, this result was not considered too disturbing. More critical was the following analysis of cadaver donor transplants, since the UCLA inference was that cadaver organs could be allocated better by considering certain HLA mismatches as *permissible*.

Among first cadaver transplants done in North America, grafts with one HLA mismatch did worse than zero-mismatch grafts, regardless of whether the one mismatch was *permissible* or *immunogenic* (*P* < 0.02). When the same type of analysis was performed for European cadaver transplants, there was no differ-

ence at all between the survival rates of *permissible* and *immunogenic* mismatches. The outcome of both one-mismatch groups was significantly inferior to that of true zero-mismatch grafts (*P* < 0.006). An analysis of the total CTS file, including transplants from all geographical regions of the world, also failed to show an advantage of transplants with permissible mismatches. True zero-mismatch transplants did significantly better (*P* < 0.0001) than either the permissible or the immunogenic one-mismatch groups (Fig. 1).

Discussion

It is evident from this analysis that the permissible mismatch concept cannot be confirmed, at least not as proposed by the UCLA group. Of course, the concept itself, of identifying certain HLA mismatches as non-deleterious, remains attractive. Most of us have observed that some poorly matched transplants function very well. However, the likelihood of good graft outcome is much greater for a good match than for a poor match, especially when long-term survival is considered.

When the UCLA group analyzed the influence on overall graft survival, the results of the conventional and the current UCLA method were better than those obtained with the permissible matching scheme [2, 3]. Even a refinement of this concept was not considered as satisfactory by the authors [4].

At present, we know of no reliable method that would allow a prediction of good graft survival in the presence of several HLA mismatches. Unfortunately, the permissible mismatch concept, as currently proposed, does not appear to hold its promise in this respect.

Acknowledgements The contribution of data by centers participating in the Collaborative Transplant Study is gratefully acknowledged. This work was supported by a grant from Deutsche Stiftung Organtransplantation, Neu Isenburg, Germany.

References

1. Maruya E, Takemoto S, Terasaki PI (1994) HLA matching: identification of permissible HLA mismatches. In: Terasaki PI, Cecka JM (eds) Clinical transplants 1993. UCLA Tissue Typing Laboratory, Los Angeles, pp 511–520

2. Takemoto S, Gjertson DW, Terasaki PI (1994) HLA matching: maximizing the number of compatible transplants. In: Terasaki PI, Cecka JM (eds) Clinical transplants 1993. UCLA Tissue Typing Laboratory, Los Angeles, pp 521–531

3. Takemoto S, Terasaki PI, Gjertson DW, Cecka JM (1994) Equitable allocation of HLA-compatible kidneys for local pools and for minorities. N Engl J Med 331: 760–764

4. Takemoto S, Terasaki PI (1995) Refinement of permissible HLA mismatches. In: Terasaki PI, Cecka JM (eds) Clinical transplants 1994. UCLA Tissue Typing Laboratory, Los Angeles, pp 451–466

Transpl Int (1996) 9 [Suppl 1]: S11–S15
© Springer-Verlag 1996

The significant effect of HLA-DRB1 matching on acute rejection in kidney transplants

Michio Nojima
Hideari Ihara
Masahiro Kyo
Mitsuo Hashimoto
Kiichiro Ito
Seiji Kunikata
Tatsuya Nakatani
Ryosuke Hayashi
Haruhiko Ueda
Yasuji Ichikawa
Fumihiko Ikoma

M. Nojima (✉) · H. Ihara · F. Ikoma
Department of Urology, Hyogo College of
Medicine, 1-1 Mukogawa-cho,
Nishinomiya, Hyogo 663, Japan

M. Kyo · M. Hashimoto · Y. Ichikawa
Department of Urology and Renal
Transplantation Center, Hyogo Prefectural
Nishinomiya Hospital, 13-6 Rokutanji-cho,
Nishinomiya, Hyogo 662, Japan

K. Ito
Department of Urology, Osaka Prefectural
Hospital, 3-1-56 Mandai-higashi,
Sumiyoshi, Osaka 558, Japan

S. Kunikata
Department of Urology, Kinki University,
377-2 Onohigashi, Sayama, Osaka 589,
Japan

T. Nakatani
Department of Urology, Osaka City
University, 1-5-7 Asahicho, Abeno,
Osaka 545, Japan

R. Hayashi
Takahashi Clinic, 1-1-6 Shonainishi-machi,
Toyonaka, Osaka 561, Japan

H. Ueda
Department of Urology, Osaka Medical
College, 2-7 Daigakucho, Takatsuki,
Osaka 569, Japan

Abstract The object of the present study was to confirm the HLA-DRB1 matching effect on rejection crisis, its severity, and kidney graft survival based on genotyping. Ninety-four renal allografts were included in this study. DNA typing of HLA-DRB1 was performed by the polymerase chain reaction sequence-specific oligonucleotide method. The incidence of acute rejection within 6 months following transplantation, the frequency of OKT3 administration for steroid-resistant rejection, histopathological findings, and graft survival rate were compared between the DRB1-matched (n = 23) and DRB1-mismatched (n = 71) groups. Four acute rejections occurred in the DRB1-matched group (incidence; 17 %) and 40 in the DRB1-mismatched group (56 %). In the DRB1-matched group, the incidence of acute rejection was significantly less frequent than that of the DRB1-mismatched group ($P < 0.005$). In the DRB1-matched group, only one patient received OKT3 administration (4 %), in contrast to 16 of 71 patients in the DRB1-mismatched group (23 %). The use of OKT3 was significantly less frequent in the DRB1-matched group ($P < 0.05$). Histopathological findings from biopsy specimens showed no constant distribution of pathological grades of acute rejection according to DRB1 matching in the present study. The graft survival rate in the two groups did not differ significantly, but the graft survival rate in the DRB1-mismatched group had a tendency to decrease as the grafts survived longer. In conclusion, the results of the present study confirm that HLA-DRB1 matching has marked beneficial effects on kidney transplants through reduction of the acute rejection rate and decrease of the severity of rejection, and suggest that improvement of graft survival will be obtained through kidney allocation to a DRB1-matched recipient.

Key words Kidney transplantation · HLA-DRB1 matching · Acute rejection

Introduction

Rejection is the most serious factor affecting kidney graft survival. Gulanikar et al. [3] reported that acute rejection affected long-term kidney graft survival. On the other hand, Nankivell et al. [15] demonstrated that HLA-DR mismatch and the presence of vascular rejection were the most important predictors of the severity of rejection. Some reports have shown a significantly lower incidence of acute rejection in HLA-DRB1-compatible grafts than in DRB1-incompatible grafts, both in living-related and cadaver cases [11, 12, 20]. Our previous reports showed that linkage disequilibria between HLA-B and DRB1 were so strong that HLA-DRB1 could be inferred in Japanese donor-recipient pairs according to the two locus associations [5, 10]. The inferred HLA-DRB1 matching had a critical effect on long-term kidney graft outcome [6–8]. The results revealed no difference in kidney graft survival between HLA-identical siblings and zero-mismatch for HLA-DRB1 in living-related and cadaver donor transplants [6, 7]. These suggested that the 4-antigen and 6-antigen match effects as a result of the locus associations within HLA alleles.

The object of the present study was to confirm the HLA-DRB1 matching effect on rejection crisis, its severity, and kidney graft survival based on genotyping.

Materials and methods

HLA typing

In all of the recipients and donors included in this study, HLA class II typing was performed by two methods, serotyping and genotyping. Conventional serological typing was performed with a complement-dependent microcytotoxicity test using well-standardized alloantisera. DNA typing of HLA-DRB1 was performed by polymerase chain reaction with the sequence-specific oligonucleotide (PCR-SSO) method. Reference protocols were as reported previously [4, 5]. A brief protocol of procedures for this study is presented here.

DNA was extracted and precipitated after the lysis of the tissue cellular component. Genomic DNA was amplified with Taq DNA polymerase and primers in a DNA thermal cycler. The amplified DNA was spotted and hybridized with digoxigenin-11-dUTP-labelled SSO probes, which were determined at the 11th International HLA Workshop [1]. Thirty-one HLA-DRB1 alleles were found in the previous study on 916 Japanese individuals [5].

Patient and immunosuppression

Ninety-four renal allografts performed at Hyogo College of Medicine and Hyogo Prefectural Nishinomiya Hospital were included in this study. Fifty-eight were engrafted from living-related donors and 36 were from cadaver donors. There were 46 males and 48 females. The mean age was 33.5 ± 1.4 ($\pm$ SE) years. The mean age of the donors was 49.4 ± 1.7 ($\pm$ SE) years. The mean follow-up period after transplantation was 59.7 ± 6.0 months. Cyclosporine-based immunosuppression was conducted in 71 patients, and azathioprine-based immunosuppression and tacrolimus (FK506)-based immunosuppression were conducted in 11 and 12 patients, respectively. Steroid was given to all patients.

According to the genotyped DRB1 matching, 94 patients were divided into two groups, zero mismatch for DRB1 (n = 23) and 1 or 2 mismatches for DRB1 (n = 71). Age and gender of the recipients, age of the donors, posttransplant follow-up period, and immunosuppressive regimens were compared between the two groups. Characteristics of each group are summarized in Table 1.

Diagnosis and treatment of acute rejection

A diagnosis of acute rejection was confirmed from both the clinical and histopathological findings. The clinical parameters were as follows; 25 % reduction in renal function, graft tenderness or swelling, fever, proteinuria, increase in urine-FDP or in -NAG, decrease of urine volume. Core needle biopsy was performed in 37 cases, espe-

cially in the case to whom OKT3 was administered. Other non-immunological events causing renal dysfunction, such as drug nephrotoxicity, infection, or surgical complications, were ruled out by the histopathological, radiological, and/or microbiological findings. Acute rejection was ruled out in 9 cases by histopathological diagnosis: 5 with nephrotoxicity from FK506, 1 with nephrotoxicity from cyclosporine, 1 with acute tubular necrosis, 1 with glomerulonephritis, and 1 with hemolytic uremic syndrome, respectively. The severity of acute rejection was classified by histopathology and the kinds of anti-rejection therapies. Histopathologically, acute rejections were classified as follows: mild interstitial acute cellular rejection (grade I AR), moderate interstitial acute cellular rejection (grade IIA AR), moderate interstitial acute cellular rejection with vascular component (grade IIB AR), and severe vascular rejection (grade III AR) according to the Banff working classification [21].

Intravenous high doses of pulse steroids and OKT3 were administered as anti-rejection therapies. Pulse steroids were used initially in patients at their first acute rejection, whereas OKT3 was used in patients with more severe and steroid-resistant acute rejection. The incidence of acute rejection during the first 6 months following transplantation and the time from transplantation to the onset of the first acute rejection were compared between the DRB1-matched and DRB1-mismatched groups in this study. Cases with severe rejection in whom OKT3 had been administered were also compared. Histopathological analysis of the grade of acute rejection was carried out. Statistical significance was evaluated by the chi-squared test.

Graft survival rate

The graft survival rate was calculated on 31 August 1995 by Kaplan-Meier's method. Patient death or return to hemodialysis was regarded as a graft failure. The Cox-Mantel test was used to evaluate the statistical significance.

Results

Characteristics of patients according to matching or mismatching are shown in Table 1. The groups were compatible in recipient age, donor age, gender distribution, the rate of living-related donors, and the posttransplant follow-up period, with the exception of the frequency of cyclosporine use. In the DRB1-matched group, the use of cyclosporine was less frequent ($P <$ 0.05): 13 of 23 patients received cyclosporine, in contrast to 58 of 71 in the DRB1-mismatched group.

Acute rejection

Table 2 shows the incidence of acute rejection and the use of OKT3 in each group. Intravenous pulse steroids were given initially to all patients with acute rejection. Forty-four acute rejection episodes were observed in 94 patients. There were four acute rejection episodes in the DRB1-matched group (17 %) and 40 in the DRB1-mismatched group (56 %). In the DRB1-matched group, the incidence of acute rejection was significantly less frequent than that of the DRB1-mismatched group

Table 1 Characteristics of the groups with and without HLA-DRB1 matching

	Group		*P*
	DRB1-matched (n = 23)	DRB1-mismatched (n = 71)	
Recipient age (years)[a]	33.4 ± 2.0	33.5 ± 1.2	NS
Donor age (years)[a]	47.5 ± 2.0	50.0 ± 1.7	NS
Male	11 (48 %)	35 (49 %)	NS
Living-related grafts	15 (65 %)	43 (61 %)	NS
Follow-up months[a]	62.3 ± 9.8	58.9 ± 4.8	NS
Main immunosuppressant			
Azathioprine	5 (22 %)	6 (8 %)	NS
Cyclosporine	13 (57 %)	58 (82 %)	< 0.05
FK506	5 (22 %)	7 (10 %)	NS

[a] Mean ± SE

Table 2 Incidence, severity, and timing of acute rejection according to DRB1 matching

	Group		*P*
	DRB1-matched (n = 23)	DRB1-mismatched (n = 71)	
Patients with acute rejection	4 (17 %)	40 (56 %)	< 0.03
OKT3 administration	1 (4 %)	16 (23 %)	< 0.05
Days from transplant to rejection[a]	37.3 ± 12.3	38.7 ± 6.8	NS

[a] Mean ± SE

Table 3 Histopathological diagnosis of acute rejection, classified according to Banff working classification

	Group	
	DRB1-matched (n = 2)	DRB1-mismatched (n = 25)
Grade I (mild interstitial rejection)	0	16
Grade IIA (moderate interstitial rejection)	1	8
Grade IIB (moderate interstitial rejection with vascular component)	1	1

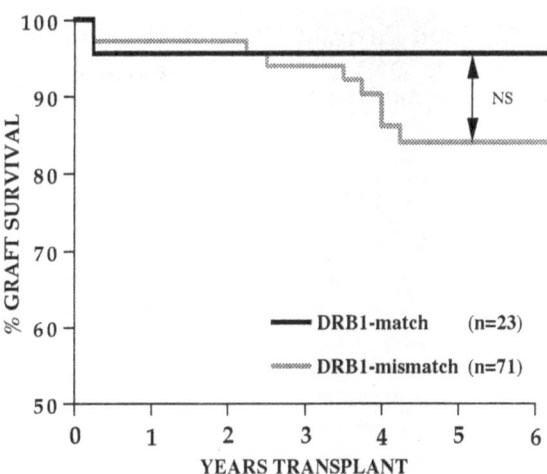

Fig. 1 Graft survival rate in years after transplantation is shown according to genotyped HLA-DRB1 compatibility

ceived OKT3 administration (4 %), in contrast to 16 of 71 patients in the DRB1-mismatched group (23 %). The use of OKT3 was significantly less frequent in the DRB1-matched group than in the DRB1-mismatched group (*P* < 0.05).

Histopathological diagnosis

A biopsy specimen was taken in 37 of 94 patients. Twenty-seven of these 37 biopsies were included in this study. The histopathological diagnoses of the patients with acute rejection are shown in Table 3. In the DRB1-matched group, 2 biopsy specimens were diagnosed as acute rejection, 1 as moderate interstitial cellular rejection (grade IIA AR) and 1 as moderate interstitial cellular rejection with vascular component (grade IIB AR). On the other hand, 25 cases were diagnosed as acute rejection in the DRB1-mismatched group. There were 16 cases of mild interstitial cellular rejection (grade I AR) observed in the DRB1-mismatched group. More severe acute rejection was found in 9 of the DRB1-mismatched patients, 8 cases were grade IIA AR and 1 was grade IIB AR. No severe vascular rejection (grade III AR) was observed in either group.

Graft survival rate

The overall graft survival rate is shown in Fig. 1. The graft survival rate at 3 years was almost the same in the two groups: 96 % in the DRB1-matched group and 94 % in the DRB1-mismatched group. Patients with a DRB1-matched graft had a 12 % higher survival rate at 5 years than patients with a DRB1-mismatched graft (96 % vs 84 %). Although there was no significant differ-

(*P* < 0.005). Mean time from transplantation to onset of the first acute rejection episode was 38.4 ± 6.2 days (Table 2). Acute rejection occurred at 37.3 ± 12.3 days after transplantation on average in the DRB1-matched group and 38.7 ± 6.8 days in the DRB1-mismatched group. There was no significant difference in the time between the two groups.

OKT3 treatment

Seventeen of 94 patients (18 %) received OKT3 as rescue therapy for steroid-resistant acute rejection (Table 2). In the DRB1-matched group, only 1 patient re-

ence in the graft survival between the two groups, the difference in the graft survival rate between the DRB1-matched group and DRB1-mismatched group gradually increased.

Discussion

Acute rejection is an important cause of graft dysfunction in the early posttransplant period and has been correlated with permanent graft impairment, graft loss, and decreased graft survival [2, 9, 13, 23]. In the serological study, the severity of acute rejection was associated with the matching grade of HLA-DR [15]. It has been reported that the incidence of acute rejection in HLA-DRB1-matched patients was less than that in DRB1-mismatched patients [11, 12, 20]. The significance of DRB1 matching in renal transplantation has been discussed because of its precision and specificity [17, 22]. To assess the effect of DRB1 matching on long-term kidney graft outcome, we previously reported that DRB1 alleles could be inferred from the linkage disequilibrium between HLA-B antigens and DRB1 alleles [5, 10]. In the inference study, the graft survival rate of HLA-DRB1-matched patients was almost the same as in HLA-identical siblings and was significantly higher than that of HLA-DRB1-mismatched cases. In contrast, the HLA-DRB1-mismatched group had nearly the same success rate as the serologically HLA-DR mismatched group. In our analysis of 511 kidney transplants, the 5-year graft success rate was 94 % in the DRB1-matched group, compared to 73 % in the DRB1-mismatched group [6–8]. These results are supported by the fact that the number of genomic HLA-DR mismatches in long-term survivors were significantly less than in recent transplants [19]. A retrospective study on the effect of genotyped DRB1 matching on graft survival has also been reported [16]. This benefit of DRB1 matching has been attributed to a lower rejection rate than occurs with DRB1-mismatched grafts [11, 12, 20]. In the present study, the incidence and the time of onset of acute rejection, the frequency of OKT3 administration which was used to treat severe and steroid-resistant acute rejection, the severity of rejection according to the histopathological diagnosis, and the graft survival rate were compared between the DRB1-matched and DRB1-mismatched groups. Our study has revealed that the incidence of acute rejection episodes was significantly less in the DRB1-matched group than in the DRB1-mismatched group ($P < 0.005$). Furthermore, the frequency of use of OKT3, which has been used only as rescue treatment for steroid-resistant acute rejection in our institute, was also significantly less in the DRB1-matched transplants ($P < 0.05$). These results demonstrate that DRB1 matching has beneficial effects not only in decreasing the incidence of acute rejection, but also in decreasing severe rejection. Nankivell et al. [15] reported that the increase in the rate of acute rejection and the greater severity of renal dysfunction with each acute rejection episode were effects derived from increased HLA-DR mismatch. Our data support the notion that this correlation of HLA-DR matching and acute rejection could be emphasized in an HLA-DR genotyped study.

On the other hand, histopathological findings from biopsy specimens showed no constant distribution of pathological grades of acute rejection according to DRB1 matching in the present study. The lack of correlation between HLA-DR mismatch and the degree of cellular infiltration on biopsy during rejection was seen in other studies [14, 15]. Although a larger number of cases is required to draw a conclusion on the correlation between DRB1 matching and histopathological characteristics, it is noteworthy that a few moderately interstitial rejections were observed even in the DRB1-matched transplants.

Graft survival rate in the DRB1-matched group and the DRB1-mismatched group did not differ significantly, but the graft survival rate in the DRB1-mismatched group had a tendency to decrease as the grafts survived longer. The reason why the result of the genotyped study was less clear compared with that in the inferred study may be that about two-thirds of the cases were genotyped retrospectively, so that patients losing grafts in the early posttransplant period were not included in the analysis. Many of these patients, were assumed to be mismatched for DRB1 based on their serology. A recent report indicates that the genotyped HLA-DR antigen matching has significant effect on graft survival, but no more effect than with further split-typing of HLA-DR in genomic DNA typing [18]. Our study suggests that the benefit of compatibility for HLA class II at the DNA level can be derived from HLA-DRB1 typing because of its specificity and precision.

In conclusion, the results of the present study confirm that HLA-DRB1 matching has marked beneficial effects on kidney transplants through the reduction of the acute rejection rate and the decrease of the severity of rejection, and suggest that improvement of graft survival will be obtained through kidney allocation to a DRB1-matched recipient.

Acknowledgements This work was partly supported by the Grant-in-Aid for Scientific Research (No. 07671758) from the Ministry of Education, Japan.

References

1. Bodmer JG, Marsh SGE, Albert ED, Bodmer WF, Dupont B, Erlich HA, Mach B, Mayr WR, Parham P, Sasazuki T, Schreuder GMTh, Strominger JL, Svejgaard A, Terasaki PI (1992) Nomenclature for factors of the HLA system, 1991. Tissue Antigens 39: 161–173

2. Ferguson R (1994) Acute rejection episodes – Best predictor of long-term primary cadaveric renal transplantation. Clin Transplant 8: 328–331

3. Gulanikar AC, MacDonald AS, Sungurtekin U, Belitsky P (1992) The incidence and impact of early rejection episodes on graft outcome in recipients of first cadaver kidney transplants. Transplantation 53: 323–328

4. Hashimoto M, Kaneshige T, Kinoshita T, Murayama A, Asai S, Yamasaki M, Nojima M, Ichikawa Y, Fukunishi T (1994) A new DR-14-related DRB1 allele, DRB1*1412, which differs from DRB1*1403 only at codon 86. Tissue Antigen 43: 133–135

5. Hashimoto M, Kinoshita T, Yamasaki M, Tanaka H, Imanishi T, Ihara H, Ichikawa Y, Fukunishi T (1994) Gene frequencies and haplotypic associations within the HLA region in 916 unrelated Japanese individuals. Tissue Antigens 44: 166–173

6. Ichikawa Y, Hashimoto M, Nojima M, Sata M, Fujimoto N, Kyo M, Ishibashi M, Ohshima S, Amomiya H, Fukunishi T, Nagano S, Sonoda T (1993) The significant effect of HLA-DRB1 matching on long-term kidney outcome. Transplantation 56: 1368–1371

7. Ichikawa Y, Hashimoto M, Kinoshita T, Yamasaki M, Ihara H, Sata M, Hanafusa T, Fujimoto N, Kyo M, Takahara S, Ohshima S, Fukunishi T, Amemiya HP, Nagano S (1994) Long-term graft survival rate of zero-mismatch kidney transplants for HLA-DRB1. Transplant Int 7: S281–S285

8. Ichikawa Y, Hashimoto M, Hanafusa T, Kyo M, Fujimoto N, Matsuura O (1995) Delayed graft function dose not have impact for long-term outcome in cadaver donor kidney transplant without mismatch for HLA-DRB1. Transplant Int (in press)

9. Kerman RH, Kimball PM, Lindholm A, Van Buren CT, Katz SM, Lewis RM, McClain J, Podbielski J, Williams J, Kahan BD (1993) Influence of HLA-matching on rejections and short- and long-term primary cadaveric allograft survival. Transplantation 56: 1242–1247

10. Kinoshita T, Hashimoto M, Yamasaki M, Ihara H, Ichikawa Y, Fukunishi T (1994) Striking conservation of three extended HLA-DR13 haplotypes in Japanese population. Tissue Antigens 44: 294–299

11. Kobayashi T, Yokoyama I, Uchida K, Tominaga Y, Inoko H, Tsuji K, Takagi H (1992) The significance of HLA-DRB1 matching in clinical renal transplantation. Transplantation 54: 238–241

12. Kobayashi T, Yokoyama I, Uchida K, Orihara A, Takagi H (1993) HLA-DRB1 matching as a recipient selection criterion in cadaver renal transplantation. Transplantation 55: 1294–1297

13. Lindholm A, Ohlman S, Abrechtsen D, Tufveson G, Persson H, Persson NH (1993) The impact of acute rejection episodes on long-term graft function and outcome in 1347 primary renal transplants treated by 3 cyclosporine regimens. Transplantation 56: 307–315

14. McWhinnie DL, Fuggle SV, Thompson JF, Wood RF, Morris PJ (1987) The influence of HLA-A, B and -DR matching on leucocyte infiltration in renal allografts. Tissue Antigens 29: 214–223

15. Nankivell BJ, Allen RDM, O'Connell PJ, Chapman JR (1995) Renal dysfunction in acute rejection: effect of HLA typing, therapy and histology. Transplantation 60: 28–36

16. Nojima M, Ichikawa Y, Ihara H, Ishibashi M, Ohshima S, Ikoma F (1994) Long-term kidney graft outcome based on HLA-DRB1 matching. Transplant Proc 26: 1884–1886

17. Opelz G, Mytilineos J, Wujciak T, Schwarz V, Back D (1992) Current status of HLA matching in renal transplantation. The collaborative study. Clin Invest 70: 767–772

18. Opelz G, Mytilineos J, Scherer S, Dunkley H, Trejaut J, Chapman J, Fischer G, Fae I, Middleton D, Savage D, Bignon JD, Bensa JC, Norren H, Albert E, Albrecht G, Schwarz V (1993) Analysis of HLA-DR matching in DNA-typed cadaver kidney transplants. Transplantation 55: 782–785

19. Poli F, Scalanogna M, Mascaretti L, Tarantino A, Pappalettera M, Nocco A, Sirchia G (1993) Genomic HLA-DR compatibility in long-term surviving recipients of cadaver kidney transplants. Transplantation 56: 97–100

20. Poli F, Mascaretti L, Pappalettera M, Scalamogna M, Bernardi L, Sirchia G (1995) HLA-DRB1 compatibility in cadaver kidney transplantation: correlation with graft survival and function. Transplant Int 8: 91–95

21. Solez K, Axelsen RA, Benediktsson H, Burdick JF, Cohen AH, Colvin RB, Croker BP, Droz D, Dunnill MS, Halloran PF, Häyry P, Jennette JC, Keown PA, Marcussen N, Mihatsch MJ, Morozumi K, Myers BD, Nast CC, Olsen S, Racusen LC, Ramos EL, Rosen S, Sachs DH, Salomon DR, Sanfilippo F, verani R, Willebrand EV, Yamaguchi Y (1993) International standardization of criteria for the histologic diagnosis of renal allograft rejection: The Banff working classification of kidney transplant pathology. Kidney Int 44: 411–422

22. Tercy JM, Goumaz C, Mach B, Jeannet M (1991) Application of HLA-DR oligotyping to 110 kidney transplant patients with doubtful serological typing. Transplantation 51: 1110–1114

23. Vereerstraeten P, Dupont E, Andrien M, Pauw LD, Abramowicz D, Goldman M, Kinnaert P (1995) Influence of donor-recipient HLA-DR mismatches and OKT3 prophylaxis on cadaver kidney graft survival. Transplantation 60: 253–258

Transpl Int (1996) 9 [Suppl 1]: S16–S19
© Springer-Verlag 1996

Gerhard Opelz
for the Collaborative
Transplant Study

Five-year results of renal transplantation in highly sensitized recipients

G. Opelz (✉) for the Collaborative
Transplant Study
Department of Transplantation
Immunology, Institute of Immunology,
University of Heidelberg,
Im Neuenheimer Feld 305,
D-69120 Heidelberg, Germany

Abstract A special program for the priority allocation of cadaver donor kidneys to highly sensitized patients was initiated 10 years ago. During the period from 1985 to 1994, 329 transplants were performed at 35 transplant centers. Five-year graft survival rates were: $59 \pm 4\%$ for 156 first grafts, $52 \pm 5\%$ for 133 second grafts, and $18 \pm 7\%$ for 40 third or fourth grafts. The success rates of first and second grafts were comparable with the corresponding success rates of first and second cadaver transplants in non-sensitized recipients reported to the Collaborative Transplant Study. There was a highly significant impact of HLA matching on graft survival. Among first and second grafts, 35 transplants with no mismatches for HLA-B+DR had a $76 \pm 8\%$ success rate at 5 years, compared with a $55 \pm 4\%$ rate for 208 grafts with one or two mismatches and a $37 \pm 8\%$ rate for 46 grafts with three or four mismatches (weighted regression $P < 0.001$).

Key words Presensitization · Highly immunized patients · HLA matching

Introduction

Patients with highly reactive preformed lymphocytotoxic antibodies have an impaired graft success rate and experience prolonged waiting times for transplantation. A special program (called HIT for „Highly Immunized Tray") was initiated in 1985 as a substudy of the Collaborative Transplant Study (CTS) to provide these patients with cross-match-negative kidneys. Patient sera were exchanged every 2 months among 35 transplant centers and cross-match-negative kidneys were allocated with priority to patients participating in the HIT program. Preliminary short-term success rates of these transplants were reported in two previous publications [1, 2]. We now report on a 5-year analysis of 329 transplants performed from 1985 to 1994.

Patients and methods

A description of the technical procedures followed in this program was provided previously [1]. Briefly, patient sera were sent every 2 months to the study center in Heidelberg, Germany, and distributed onto tissue-typing trays. The trays were sent to the tissue-typing laboratories of the participating transplant centers and cross-matches were performed with lymphocytes of local cadaver donors. A second cross-match was performed prior to transplantation in the laboratory of the recipient center. Only patients with a serum reactivity of > 80 % in at least two consecutive screenings 2–3 months apart were accepted for the program. The patients had to have a negative autologous cross-match. During the first 3 years of operation, the HLA match was disregarded. In 1988, a recommendation was made to transplant kidneys with no more than one mismatch on each of the HLA loci HLA-A, HLA-B, and HLA-DR. In 1993, the recommendation was changed to a request for no more than one mismatch on the HLA-B locus and no more than one mismatch on the HLA-DR locus.

The transplants were performed at the following centers: Aachen, Barcelona, Basel, Bern, Berlin, Brussels, Cologne, Düsseldorf, Essen, Frankfurt, Freiburg, Geneva, Gent, Gothenburg, Hannover, Heidelberg, Helsinki, Innsbruck, Kaiserslautern, Lausanne, Leuven, Lübeck, Lund-Malmö, Madrid, Marburg, Milan,

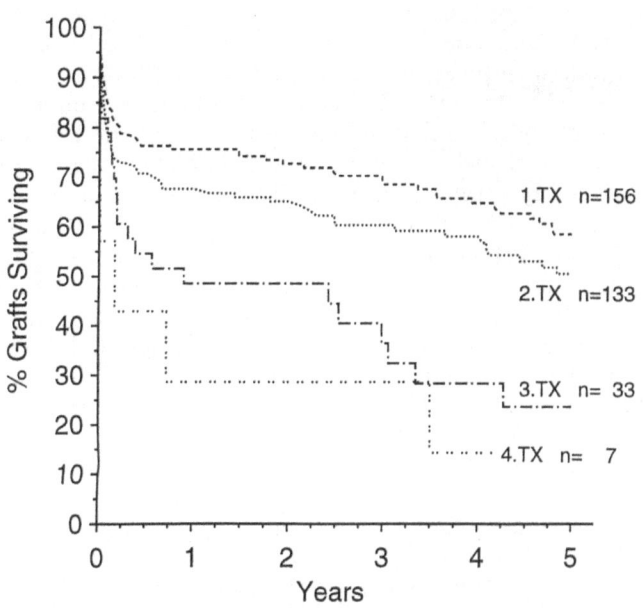

Fig. 1 Graft survival rates in highly immunized cadaver kidney recipients (*1. TX* first transplants, *2. TX* second transplants, *3. TX* third transplants, *4. TX* fourth transplants). The number of patients studied is indicated for each curve

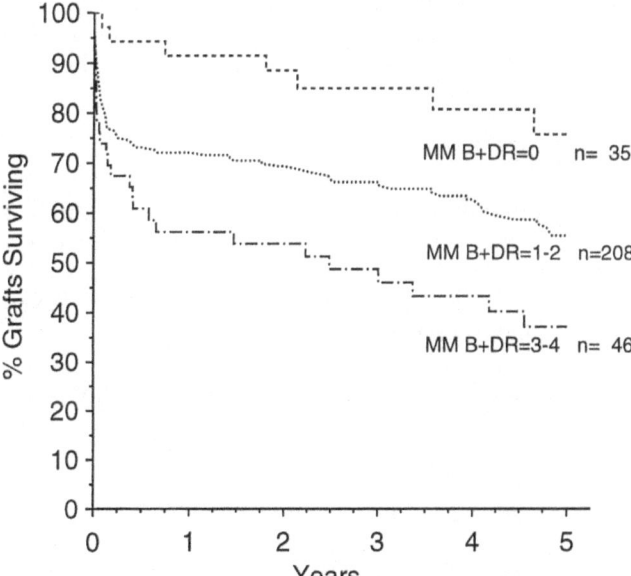

Fig. 2 Influence of matching for the HLA-B and HLA-DR antigens on graft outcome in highly immunized recipients of first or second cadaver transplants. The combined number of mismatched HLA-B and HLA-DR antigens was analyzed (*MM* mismatches). The influence of matching was statistically significant (*P* regression < 0.001)

Munich, Münster, Prague, Rostock, Tübingen, Vienna, Warsaw, and Zürich.

Graft survival rates were computed by the Kaplan-Meier method. One transplant was excluded because the repeat cross-match was positive but the transplant operation had been carried out

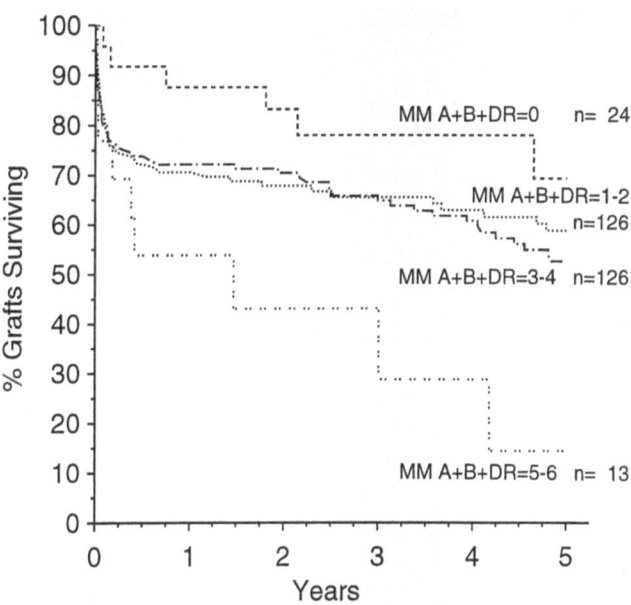

Fig. 3 Influence of HLA-A, HLA-B, and HLA-DR mismatches on graft outcome in highly sensitized patients. Number of mismatched antigens and number of patients studied are indicated (*P* regression < 0.01)

without awaiting the cross-match result. No other exclusions were made. Patients who died with functioning grafts were counted as graft failures.

Results

The 5-year graft survival rates of first, second, third, and fourth cadaver transplants in highly immunized recipients are illustrated in Fig. 1. Remarkably, the $59 \pm 4\%$ 5-year success rate of first grafts is only 1 % lower than the success rate of cadaver transplants in all non-sensitized recipients reported to the CTS (P = ns), and it was more than 10 % higher than the 5-year success rate in all 1085 CTS-registered recipients with a preformed antibody reactivity of > 80 % ($47 \pm 2\%$). The $52 \pm 5\%$ 5-year success rate of second grafts was similar to that of all 821 CTS-registered second transplants into patients with > 80 % antibody reactivity ($47 \pm 2\%$). The results of third and fourth transplants, although not significantly different from other third and fourth transplants in highly sensitized recipients reported to the CTS, must be considered unsatisfactory.

The effect of HLA matching on graft survival was analyzed in first and second transplants. Mismatches at the HLA-A and HLA-B loci tended to decrease graft survival, although this did not reach statistical significance. At 5 years, 45 grafts with no mismatches survived at a rate of $66 \pm 8\%$, 196 grafts with one or two mismatches at a rate of $54 \pm 4\%$, and 48 grafts with three or four mismatches at a $47 \pm 8\%$ rate (P = ns). When the HLA-DR locus was analyzed, 92 transplants with no

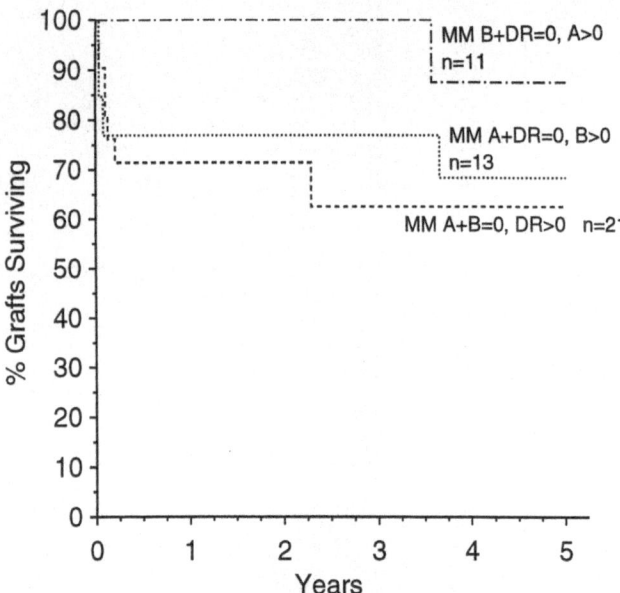

Fig. 4 Survival rates of transplants that were matched at two of the three HLA loci and mismatched at the third locus. Mismatches at the HLA-A locus appeared to be the least harmful

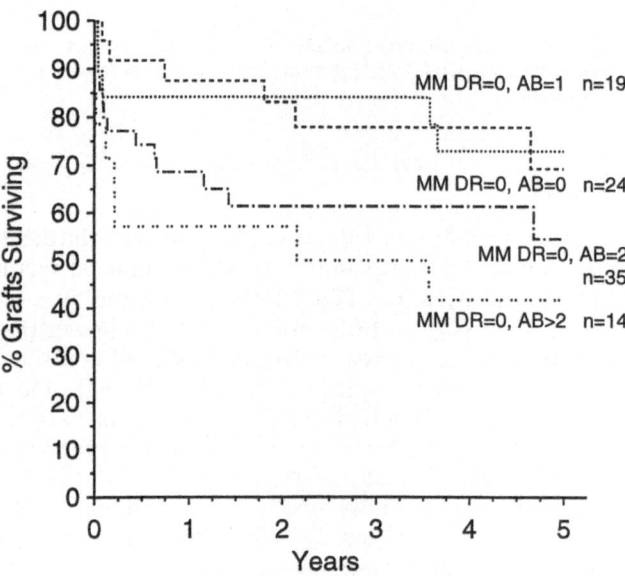

Fig. 5 Analysis of HLA-A+B mismatches in transplants with no HLA-DR mismatches (P regression = 0.06)

mismatches and 167 with one mismatch had similar 5-year survival rates of $60 \pm 6\%$ and $58 \pm 4\%$, respectively. Thirty grafts with two HLA-DR mismatches survived at a poor $19 \pm 8\%$ rate, significantly lower than the none or one mismatch groups (log-rank $P < 0.001$).

A highly significant impact of HLA matching was found when the combination of HLA-B+DR mismatches was analyzed. Five-year graft survival rates were $77 \pm 8\%$ for grafts with no mismatches, $55 \pm 4\%$ for

grafts with one or two mismatches, and $37 \pm 8\%$ for grafts with three or four mismatches (weighted regression $P < 0.001$) (Fig. 2). As shown in Fig. 3, the effect of matching was similar when mismatches at the HLA-A locus were included in the analysis (weighted regression $P < 0.01$). Grafts with five or six mismatches did extremely poorly, but there were only 13 transplants in this group. Further evidence that HLA-A locus mismatches had only a weak influence is shown in Fig. 4. Grafts which were matched at two HLA loci and had mismatches only at the third locus did exceedingly well if the mismatch was at the HLA-A locus. Because of the small numbers of transplants available for analysis, this result must be treated with caution.

An important result is shown in Fig. 5. When grafts with no mismatch at the HLA-DR locus were further separated according to mismatches for HLA-A+B, a deleterious effect of A+B mismatches was apparent (weighted regression $P = 0.06$). Thus, even in the absence of HLA-DR mismatches, mismatches at the HLA-A and HLA-B loci cannot be ignored.

Because there were only 40 third and fourth transplants in the analysis, it was unlikely that a significant effect of HLA matching would be obtained. However, it was disappointing that not even a trend for improved graft outcome was found when mismatches for HLA-DR, B+DR, or A+B were analyzed (data not shown).

Discussion

It is gratifying to see that the encouraging preliminary short-term results of the HIT program which were reported earlier [1, 2] have been sustained in this analysis of a larger patient series with a longer follow-up. Several lessons have been learned:

1. Excellent results can be obtained in highly immunized patients receiving first or second transplants. The outcome of third and fourth transplants, however, has been consistently poor.
2. A negative cross-match alone is an insufficient indicator of a patient's chance of success.
3. HLA matching has a significant influence on graft outcome in highly sensitized recipients of first or second transplants. Since it is not realistic to wait for perfectly HLA-compatible kidneys for all patients, our current policy of accepting donor kidneys with no more than one HLA-DR mismatch and one HLA-B mismatch seems a reasonable compromise.
4. Third and fourth transplants into highly sensitized patients do poorly and there is no evidence so far that better HLA matching improves the results in this group of patients.
5. The efforts involved in the bimonthly serum exchange, tray preparation, and performance of cross-

matches appears amply justified in the light of the very good transplant results obtained. The efficiency of the program would benefit from an increase in the number of potential donors whose lymphocytes are tested on the special cross-match trays. This could be accomplished best by increasing the number of centers participating in the program.

Acknowledgements We thank tissue-typing laboratories at the centers participating in the HIT program and the staff at Eurotransplant for their support. Excellent technical assistance was provided by Martina Rausch and Miriam Benger. This project was supported by a grant from Deutsche Stiftung Organtransplantation, Neu-Isenburg, Germany.

References

1. Opelz G for the Collaborative Transplant Study (1988) Priority allocation of cadaver kidneys to highly presensitized transplant recipients. Transplant Int 1: 2–5

2. Opelz G for the Collaborative Transplant Study (1992) Success rate and impact of HLA matching on kidney graft survival in highly immunized recipients. Transplant Int 5 (1): S601–603

Transpl Int (1996) 9 [Suppl 1]: S20–S24
© Springer-Verlag 1996

D. J. Bevan
B. S. Carey
R. W. Vaughan
A. N. Hillis
M. Fallon
R. M. Higgins
M. Bewick
B. M. Hendry

Anticipation of highly sensitised renal patients' immunoadsorption requirements by prescreening using protein A minicolumns

D. J. Bevan (✉) · B. S. Carey ·
R. W. Vaughan
South Thames Regional Tissue Typing
Laboratory, Guy's Hospital,
London SE1 9RT, UK
Fax + 44 171 407 6370

A. N. Hillis · M. Fallon · R. M. Higgins ·
B. M. Hendry · M. Bewick
Renal Unit, King's Healthcare, Dulwich
Hospital, London SE22 8PT, UK

Abstract We are able to subdivide highly sensitised renal patients who wish to enter our immunoadsorption programme into two groups; those who will require acute pretransplant immunoadsorption only and those requiring regular immunoadsorption prior to transplantation. This division of patients is based on the results obtained from laboratory assessment using protein A minicolumns. Patient's plasma is passed down a minicolumn for 6×10 min cycles, a sample of plasma is kept after each cycle for analysis by cell flow cytometric cross-match (FCXM). The samples are screened against cells from two normal volunteers, one expressing a previously mismatched Class I HLA antigen (MMA) to which the patient has raised persistent IgG antibodies, the other, whilst not expressing any MMAs, should express a cross-reactive HLA Class I antigen (XRA) to which the patient has formed persistent IgG antibodies. Patients are allocated into the acute pretransplant immunoadsorption group if, after 6 minicolumn cycles, the T cell FCXM vs XRA and MMA is reduced to less than 1 Log median fluorescence intensity shift above the negative control and that both these values have been reduced by at least 15 % from the preimmunoadsorption figure. If these criteria are not met, regular immunoadsorption is required under cover of cyclophosphamide. Eleven patients who have been allocated by these criteria have subsequently been transplanted without any incidence of hyperacute rejection.

Key words Renal transplantation · Immunoadsorption · Minicolumn · Cross-match

Introduction

Dialysis-dependent patients in end-stage renal failure with high levels of anti-HLA panel-reactive antibodies (PRA) owing to previous blood transfusions, pregnancy or previous failed organ transplants have a greatly reduced likelihood of obtaining a graft which does not carry the HLA antigens to which they have raised antibodies. These antibodies may be removed and their resynthesis reduced by immunoadsorption (IA) and the administration of cyclophosphamide, respectively. IA has proved to be well tolerated and is efficient at lowering PRA levels and anti-HLA titres against specific antigens [1, 5]. However, there is some resynthesis of anti-HLA antibodies despite cyclophosphamide cover [2, 3]. Previously, patients with only narrow ranges of anti-HLA specificities have been immunoadsorbed and transplanted in our region [6]. In our current programme, patients with a broad range of anti-HLA antibody specificities are offered treatment, thus making immunoadsorption available to most highly sensitised patients.

IA to remove anti-HLA antibodies from sensitised renal patients is often carried out over several sessions before a potential donor has been identified [3, 4]. If a donor is not found during, or within a short period after, the schedule of IA treatments then the patient's anti-

HLA antibodies will often 'rebound' to, or beyond their pre-IA levels [3, 6]. It was felt that sensitised patients who would require only one or two acute IA sessions immediately pretransplant, to remove sufficient quantities of their anti-HLA antibodies in order to achieve a negative cross-match against a suitable donor, could be identified. These patients would be considered for acute IA only prior to transplantation without the necessity of their undergoing a series of IA sessions, with concomitant immunosuppression, in the hope of a suitable donor becoming available within this period.

The aim of this study was to develop a predictive laboratory test capable of distinguishing between those patients requiring acute pretransplant IA only and those requiring repeated IA sessions over several weeks in order to obtain a negative cross-match prior to transplantation.

Patients and methods

Patients

Between August 1993 and August 1995, 11 patients (5 males, 6 females; age range 11–54 years) in total renal failure with high titre anti-HLA antibodies were studied. The major reactivity of these patients' anti-HLA antibodies was to Class I antigens, demonstrated by a high T cell PRA value. However, 2 of the patients with low PRA values (18 % and 45 %) did in fact have high titre, broadly reactive antibodies to HLA Class II antigens. The anti-HLA antibodies present in all but 1 of the patients had primarily been induced by previous renal allografts.

Protein A minicolumn assessment

A protein A minicolumn (Excorim, Lund, Sweden) was set up in circuit with a flow cell spectrophotometer set to read at 280 nm and a pump set at a flow rate of 1.8 ml/min. The column was washed through with 25 ml of phosphate-buffered saline (PBS), pH 7.2. Patient's plasma (13 ml) was centrifuged at 750 g for 10 min to remove any debris, and then 12 ml was applied to the column and 1 ml was reserved for cross-match (XM) analysis. The PBS eluted from the column was discarded. The plasma was continuously circulated through the column for 10 min before being recovered and 100 μl was removed for XM analysis. Unbound protein was washed from the column with PBS until the absorbance measured in the UV flow cell had returned to baseline. Glycine-HCl buffer, 0.1 M pH 2.5, was added to the column in order to elute the bound IgG from the column. The addition of buffer was continued until all the bound immunoglobulin had been eluted (absorbance returned to baseline). The column was rinsed with PBS until the pH of the eluate had reached 7.2. The collected plasma was reapplied to the column and the cycle of protein binding/elution repeated for a minimum of 6 cycles, ensuring that 100 μl of plasma was stored from each cycle.

Extracorporeal immunoadsorption

All patients except one received a 'trial' long (> 6 hours) extracorporeal immunoadsorption session after their minicolumn assessment to check the veracity of the minicolumn results. Subsequent-

ly, all patients underwent IA treatments in accordance with their minicolumn results. Extracorporeal immunoadsorption was performed using a Citem 10 system (Excorim, Lund, Sweden). The system consisted of a parallel arrangement of two Immunosorba 62.5 ml staphylococcal protein A columns. The patient's blood, anticoagulated with heparin, was separated by a Gambro PF2000 filter into plasma and cellular fractions. Acid citrate dextrose was also used at 10 % of flow rate as additional anticoagulation and also to prevent complement activation. The protein A columns were perfused alternately with 200–400 ml of plasma per 10 min cycle. The columns were regenerated using an acidic buffer followed by washing with buffered saline. The treated plasma was recombined with the other blood constituents and returned to the patient. An IA session was usually of at least 7 h duration. Aliquots of serum were collected before, at hourly intervals during, and also after the IA procedure. Samples from the 'trial' IA sessions were stored at −20 °C prior to screening for their cytotoxic antibodies (CAB) by CXM and also for CAB/non-cytotoxic IgG anti-HLA antibodies by TFCXM and BFCXM against two normal lymphocyte donors carrying MMA and XRA, respectively. Samples from the immediate pretransplant IA sessions were snap-frozen before being screened against donor spleen and auto peripheral blood T and B cells by CXM and FCXM.

Normal volunteer and patients' autologous lymphocytes

Peripheral blood lymphocytes (PBL) were separated from the blood of two normal volunteers and also from the patient being screened by density gradient centrifugation. The volunteers were selected so that one of them expressed at least one previously mismatched Class I HLA antigen to which the patient being screened had raised IgG antibodies. The second volunteer, who did not express any previously mismatched HLA antigens, expressed at least one cross-reactive antigen to which the patient had formed IgG antibody. The two lymphocyte populations were each resuspended (separately) in two separate aliquots for CXM and FCXM screening.

Cytotoxic cross-match (CXM)

Screening against MMAs and XRAs

The lymphocyte populations from the normal volunteers and the patient (to check for the presence of autoantibodies) were resuspended (separately) at 2×10^6/ml in RPMI 1640 medium. A standard NIH microcytotoxicity assay was used (false positive CXMs owing to autoantibodies were excluded by the addition of DTT or by setting up a CXM using autologous PBL). Briefly, 1 μl aliquots of the normal donor cells were incubated with 1 μl aliquots of the patient's serum (double diluted in RPMI 1640 from 1:1 to 1:512) at 22 °C for 30 min in Terasaki plates. Rabbit complement (5 μl) was added to each well followed by 60 min incubation at 22 °C. The percentage of cells killed was assessed by the addition of an EB/AO mix. The plates were viewed using an inverted UV microscope.

Screening against potential donors

Single cell suspensions of donor spleen cells were separated by density-gradient centrifugation, with the mononuclear cell layer being harvested. The CXMs were set up as detailed above.

T and B cell flow cytometric cross-match (T & B FCXM)

Screening against MMAs and XRAs

The normal donor cells and the patient's own lymphocytes were resuspended at between 2 and 4×10^7/ml in PBS – 0.1 % bovine serum albumin – 0.1 % sodium azide (PBA). Duplicate 20 μl aliquots of the stored serum samples were each added to 30 μl of each of the donor cells, normal AB serum was used as a negative control. The cells and serum were incubated for 30 min at 22 °C. PBA (2 ml) was added to each tube which were then centrifuged for 5 min at 150 g. The supernatant was decanted and the cell pellet resuspended in the residual liquid. This 'washing' process was repeated. Normal mouse serum (5 μl) was added to each tube which was then mixed and incubated at RT for 10 min. Mouse anti-CD3-phycoerythrin (4 μl) (Dako Ltd.) was added to one set of each of the XRA and MMA cells, mouse anti-CD19-phycoerythrin was added to the second set. Rabbit anti-human IgG-fluorescein isothiocyanate (4 μl) (Dako Ltd., non-crossreacting with mouse IgG) was added simultaneously to all of the cell pellets in the tubes, followed by gentle mixing and 20 min incubation at 4 °C. The cells were washed twice in PBA and then resuspended in approximately 300 μl of PBA. Ten thousand events from each tube were acquired using a live lymphocyte gate, set on forward and side scatter, on a 'Facscan' flow cytometer. Lysis II data management software was used for the analysis. Using a dot plot, a gate was set to include all the CD3-PE$^+$ cells in the positive and negative controls. This defined the T cell gate. Histograms were generated of the FITC fluorescence intensity for the T cells in the test samples and the data was analysed by overlaying the FITC histograms. The peak to peak distances for each of the histograms from the AB negative control were measured. This gave the median fluorescence intensity for each sample, as a measure of the amount of binding of the patient's IgG on the T cells. Fluorescence intensity was measured on a Log scale, a shift in fluorescence intensity of greater than 0.5 of a Log above the AB control was considered to be positive. The analysis was repeated using a B cell gate which was set on the positive and negative controls to which CD19-PE had been added.

Some patients exhibit an 'unmasking' of non-cytotoxic IgG autoantibodies during IA. This has also been demonstrated using the minicolumns. These autoantibodies would affect a FCXM, therefore, an autoFCXM was also set up when a patient was being screened. Any positive values obtained from the autoFCXM were subtracted from the FCXM values obtained against the MMA and XRA volunteer cells.

Screening against potential donor cells

The density-gradient separated spleen lymphocytes were resuspended in PBA at between $1–1.5 \times 10^7$/ml. The FCXMs were set up as detailed above, including an autoFCXM.

Immunosuppression and transplantation

Patients undergoing acute IA only prior to transplantation commenced their associated immunotherapy immediately prior to the IA treatment (oral cyclophosphamide 2 mg/kg per day and prednisolone 0.5 mg/kg per day). Other patients undergoing a regular programme of IA received the same immunosuppression commencing 3 days prior to the first IA treatment, the cyclophosphamide dose was adjusted according to the neutrophil counts. Following transplantation, all patients received a 10-day course of antithymocyte globulin (ATG, Fresenius, FRG or Merieux at the manufacturers' recommended dose) in addition to triple therapy (cyclos-

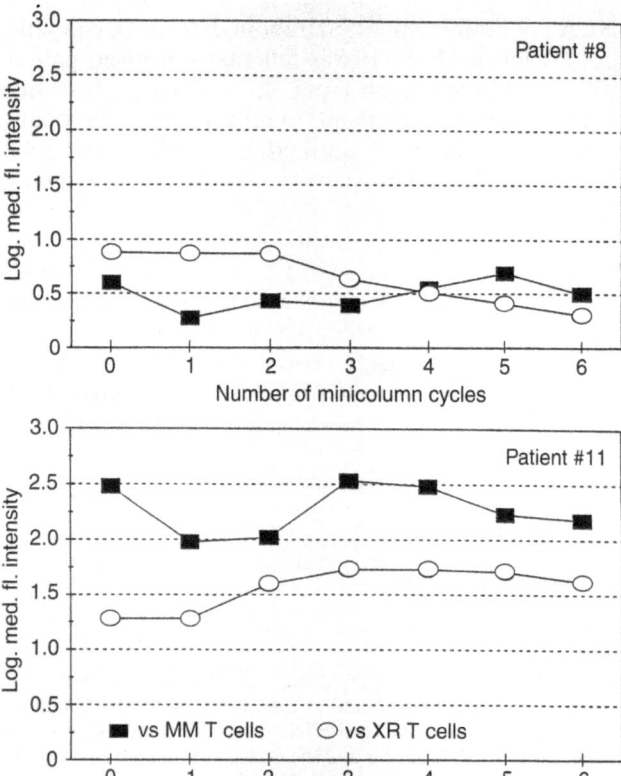

Fig. 1 Minicolumn analysis

porin A was given to achieve whole blood trough levels of 200–300 ng/ml, prednisolone at 20 mg/day and cyclophosphamide). Three months posttransplantation, azathioprine at 50–100 mg/day was substituted for the cyclophosphamide.

Rejection was diagnosed on the basis of a rising creatinine level (when there was urine output) confirmed by renal biopsy.

Results

Statistical analysis

Graft loss was considered to be at the time of nephrectomy or return to dialysis. Graft survival figures excluded death with a viable graft. Transplant survival figures included death with a viable graft.

Minicolumns

All patients in this study underwent a minicolumn analysis prior to extracorporeal IA. Figure 1 shows the TFCXMs obtained from two patient's minicolumn analysis. The upper panel shows the results from patient # 8 who was assigned to the acute IA group. The lower panel of Fig. 1 is patient # 11's results who was assigned to scheduled IA. Of the 11 patients studied, 5 fulfilled

Table 1 Patient data prior to transplantation (*Tx* transplantation, *PRA* panel-reactive antibodies, *IA* immunoadsorption, *CXM* cytotoxic cross-match, *XM* cross-match)

Patient	Sex	Age at Tx (years)	Number positive XMs prior to Tx	Minicolumn result	% PRA pre-IA	% PRA post-IA	CXM titre pre-IA/pre-Tx	CXM titre post-IA/pre-Tx
1	M	50	27 (42 months)	Scheduled IA	18	16	1:256	0
2	F	54	4 (29 months)	Acute IA	98	76	1:8	0
3	F	45	76 (98 months)	Scheduled IA	88	20	1:32	0
4	M	11	55 (72 months)	Scheduled IA	100	51	> 1:512	0
5	F	45	9 (28 months)	Acute IA	45	11	1:2	0
6	M	36	100+ (156 months)	Acute IA	64	19	0	0
7	M	25	61 (88 months)	Scheduled IA	100	36	1:4	0
8	F	32	30 (23 months)	Acute IA	82	7	1:2	0
9	M	43	92 (94 months)	Scheduled IA	90	58	0	0
10	F	38	84 (58 months)	Acute IA	95	13	1:4	0
11	F	40	31 (67 months)	Scheduled IA	100	13	1:16	0

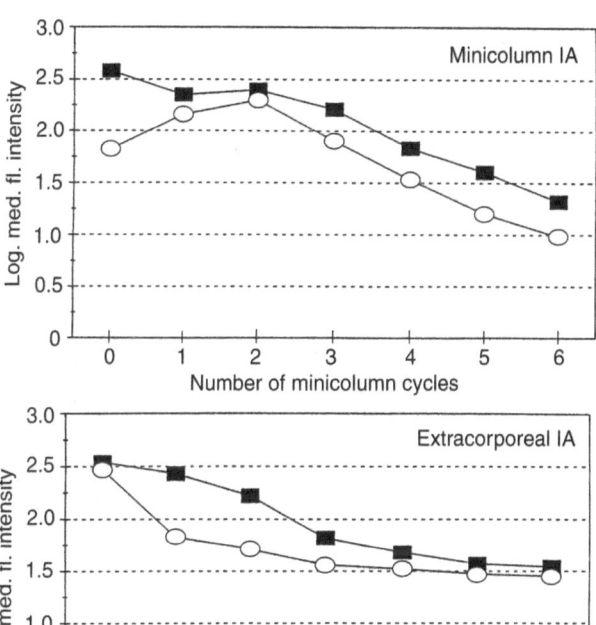

Fig. 2 T cell flow cytometric cross-match results (patient # 7)

Table 2 HLA matching and graft function (*MM* mismatch, *ATG* antithymocyte globulin)

Patient	Donor MM A/B/DR	Current plasma creatinine (µm/l)	Outcome
1	00/01/11	Not applicable	Non-immunol-related death
2	01/01/01	167	Function
3	01/01/01	264	Function
4	11/11/11	200	Function
5	11/11/11	186	Function
6	11/01/11	147	Function
7	11/11/11	1007	Rejected (ATG withdrawn)
8	11/01/11	1459	Technical failure
9	01/01/01	285	Function
10	01/01/00	827	Technical failure
11	00/11/11	250	Function

the criteria for acute pretransplant IA only whilst the remainder, who did not, were assigned to a schedule of IA sessions (Table 1). Figure 2 shows the T cell flow cytometric cross-match results (TFCXM) of the minicolumn and also the first extracorporeal IA samples for patient # 7. It can be seen that the results obtained from the minicolumn are very similar to those of the extracorporeal IA.

The mean PRA of the 'acute' group prior to extracorporeal IA was 77 % (± 9.8 SEM), this was reduced to a mean of 25 % (± 22.6 SEM) by the acute pretransplant immunoadsorption. The mean PRA of the 'scheduled' group was 83 % (± 13.1 SEM), reducing to a mean of 32 % (± 18 SEM) after the schedule of immunoadsorptions had been carried out. There was no significant difference in PRA reduction between the groups. The average of the fall in the % PRA for each group was 52 % (acute IA) and 51 % (scheduled IA) (Table 1).

The one year graft survival for all patients is 75 % (n = 8), with 13 % (n = 1) being lost to rejection within this period and the one year transplant survival is lower at 64 % (n = 7), as shown in Table 2. The functioning grafts, all of which are continuing to show a gradual reduction of plasma creatinine levels with time, have a range of plasma creatinine values from 147 to 285 µM/l (Table 2). Three of the patients were completely mismatched at the A, B and DR loci; the other patients had some degree of HLA matching (Table 2).

Discussion

The present single centre study indicates that we are able successfully to identify, using the formula devised, the pretransplant IA requirements of sensitised patients in order to render them cross-match negative once a potentially suitable donor kidney has been identified. The level of reduction in the %PRA for each patient group following their prescribed programme of immunoadsorption was essentially the same, indicating that the desired 'windows of opportunity' regarding the removal of cross-reactive anti-HLA antibodies had been attained for both groups. Following IA and transplantation, the 1-year graft survival figures for these patients is only slightly lower (75 %) than for the equivalent period for regrafted patients in UKTSSA-participating centres (77 %, average for all regrafts). Our transplant survival figure of 63 % is, however, lower than the national figure of 74 % for regrafted individuals [7]. The small de-gree of HLA matching that occurred in this study was entirely fortuitous as a compatible blood group with a negative cross-match against the donor were the only selection criteria used. This lack of matching does not appear to have compromised the graft survival figures when compared to the national average obtained for sensitised renal patients within the same period [7].

The results obtained from this small study would seem to indicate that the patients were assigned to the correct treatment groups. The preassessment of patients by minicolumn analysis prior to entering our immunoadsorption programme allows us to maximise resources and to avoid patients undergoing unnecessary treatments. These results should ideally be further tested in a multicentre study.

Acknowledgements We would like to thank Excorim (Lund, Sweden) for the gift of the protein A minicolumns.

References

1. Brocard JF, Farahmand H, Fassi S, Plaisant B, Fries E, Cantarovich M, Bismuth A, Lambert T, Hiesse C, Lantz O, Fries D, Charpentier B (1989) Attempt at depletion of anti-HLA antibodies in sensitized patients awaiting transplantation using extracorporeal immunoadsorption, polyclonal IgG, and immunosuppressive drugs. Transplant Proc 21: 733–734
2. Charpentier BM, Hiesse C, Kriaa F, Rousseau P, Farahmand H, Bismuth A, Fries D (1992) How to deal with the hyperimmunized potential recipients. Kidney Int (suppl) 38: S176–S181
3. Esnault V, Bignon JD, Testa A, Preud'homme JL, Vergracht A, Soulillou JP (1990) Effect of protein A immunoadsorption on panel lymphocyte reactivity in hyperimmunized patients awaiting a kidney graft. Transplantation 50: 449–453
4. Gil-Vernet S, Griñó JM, Martorell J, Castelao AM, Serón D, Díaz C, Andrés E, Gonzalez-Castellanos L, Alsina J (1990) Anti-HLA antibody removal by immunoadsorption. Transplant Proc 22: 1904–1905
5. Palmer A, Taube D, Welsh K, Brynger H, Delin K, Gjörstrup P, Konar J, Söderström T (1987) Extracorporeal immunoadsorption of anti-HLA antibodies: Preliminary clinical experience. Transplant Proc 19: 3750–3751
6. Palmer A, Welsh K, Gjorstrup P, Taube D, Bewick M, Thick M (1989) Removal of anti-HLA antibodies by extracorporeal immunoadsorption to enable renal transplantation. Lancet 1: 10
7. United Kingdom Transplant Support Service Authority (1995) Renal transplant audit 1984–1993

Transpl Int (1996) 9 [Suppl 1]: S25–S27
© Springer-Verlag 1996

I. Koyama
Y. Taguchi
S. Sugahara
N. Akimoto
R. Omoto

Weak expression of blood type B antigen in kidney tissue and successful B-incompatible kidney transplantation without special treatments

I. Koyama (✉) · Y. Taguchi · S. Sugahara ·
N. Akimoto · R. Omoto
Department of Surgery, Saitama Medical
School, 38 Morohongo, Moroyama,
Iruma-gun, Saitama, Japan 350-04

Abstract Much attention has been paid to only natural antibody titer of the recipients in ABO-incompatible kidney transplantation. In this study, we looked at the distribution of blood type antigens in the kidney tissue. Thirty-seven biopsy specimens from patients with nephritis or transplanted kidneys were recruited. Fifteen were type A, 14 were type B, and 8 were type AB. Kidney tissues were stained with anti-A or anti-B antibody using immunohistological staining. The stained dots in each section were regarded as the area and were measured by image analyzer. B antigen was expressed very weakly both in the glomeruli and in interstitium as compared with A antigen. In type AB, B antigen was less expressed than A antigen. Based on these results, we performed B-incompatible kidney transplantation. No rejection was seen without preoperative depletion of natural antibody and splenectomy. These results may suggest that type B-incompatible kidney transplantation might possibly be performed without preoperative depletion of natural antibodies.

Key words ABO-incompatible kidney transplantation · Blood type antigen · Anti-B antibody · B-incompatibility

Introduction

Since Alexandre et al. [1] reported the first series of successful scheduled ABO-incompatible kidney transplants, many experiences of these cases have accumulated. Removal of the anti-A or anti-B antibodies of the recipients by plasmapheresis or immunoadsorption has become an essential treatment for kidney transplantation across the ABO barrier [2–4]. As a result, graft and patient survival are nearly equal to those of ABO-compatible transplantation [9]. However, discussions have been focused on only the anti-A or anti-B antibody titer of the recipient, and quantitative evaluation of ABO antigens in the kidney tissue of the donor has been neglected. This study was undertaken to clarify the characteristics of expression of AB antigens in kidney tissue. We applied the above results to ABO-incompatible kidney transplantation clinically. We will report here a successful B-incompatible transplantation without special treatment such as plasmapheresis or splenectomy.

Materials and methods

Thirty seven kidney specimens taken as biopsies from patients who had nephritis or a transplanted kidney were analyzed in this study. Fifteen were blood type A, 14 were type B, and 8 were type AB. The specimens were stained with anti-A or anti-B antibody (monoclonal antibody, Nichirei) using the ABC method of immunohistopathology. The stained dots in each section were regarded as the area and were analyzed by an image analyzer (IP-100 apparatus, Asahi Corp.) to measure the amount of antigens. The amount of blood antigen was expressed as a percent area per field.

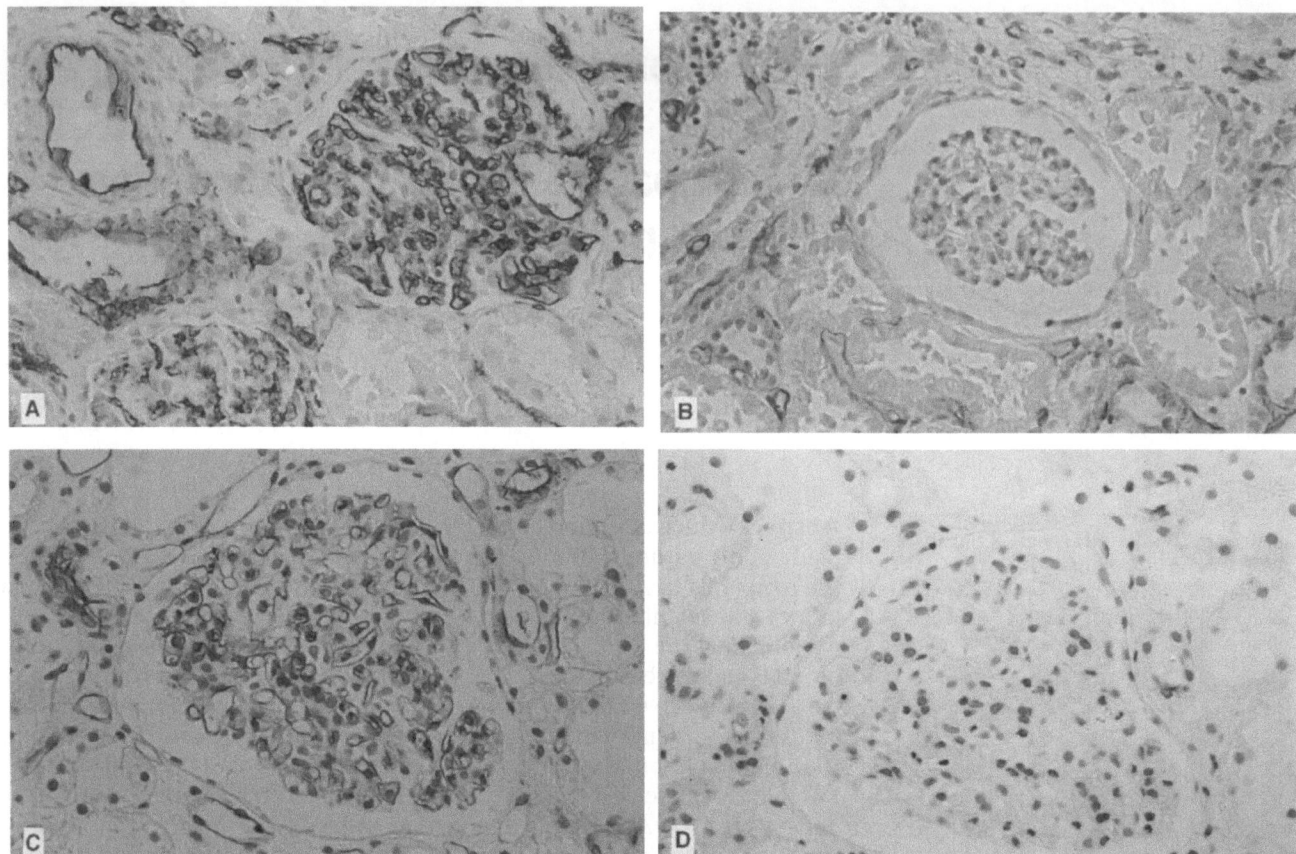

Fig.1 A–D Immunohistological stainings for blood type antigens with anti-A or anti-B antibody (ABC method) × 400. **A** A antigen in blood type A. **B** B antigen in blood type B. **C** A antigen in type AB. **D** B antigen in type AB

Results

Antigen expression

Type A or B antigen was mainly expressed on vascular endothelium in the glomeruli and interstitium, and not in tubular cells or mesangial cells. In type A kidneys, type A antigen was expressed $9.2 \pm 2.7\%$ in the glomeruli and $5.6 \pm 2.1\%$ in the interstitium. In type B kidneys, B antigen was distributed only $0.7 \pm 1.4\%$ in the glomeruli and $1.8 \pm 1.4\%$ in the interstitium. In type AB, B antigen was expressed only $1.4 \pm 2.7\%$ in the glomeruli and $0.99 \pm 1.0\%$ in the interstitium, while type A antigen was shown to be $9.3 \pm 4.1\%$ in the glomeruli and $4.5 \pm 2.7\%$ in the interstitium (Figs. 1–3).

Clinical application

On the basis of the above results, we performed a B-incompatible kidney transplantation. The patient was 43-year-old man whose blood type was O. He had been given insulin for 23 years, due to juvenile diabetes, and had been on dialysis for 4 years. He received the kidney from his 70-year-old mother whose blood type was B. The IgM titer of anti-B antibody of the recipient was 128, and the IgG titer was 512. No depletion of antibodies was planned before transplantation. Combination therapy of cyclosporine, azathioprine, and prednisolone was administered as a maintenance immunosuppression. Deoxyspergualin (5 mg/kg i.v.) was added for 7 days after transplantation. Following the transplantation, the titer of IgM dropped, remarkably, to 2 and slightly increased to 4 in the 2nd week. Thereafter, the titer was maintained at the level of 2 and no rejection developed. The graft is functioning well after 16 months.

Discussion

Before the introduction of plasmapheresis or immunoadsorption to remove anti-A or anti-B natural antibody, kidney transplantation across the ABO barrier usually resulted in irreversible rejection of the graft. However, some B-incompatible grafts were reported to function well. Since Alexandre et al. [1] recommended a combination therapy of the preoperative removal of

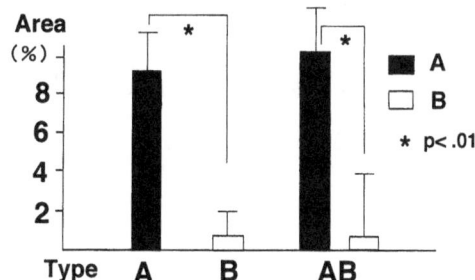

Fig. 2 Amount of blood type antigens in glomeruli

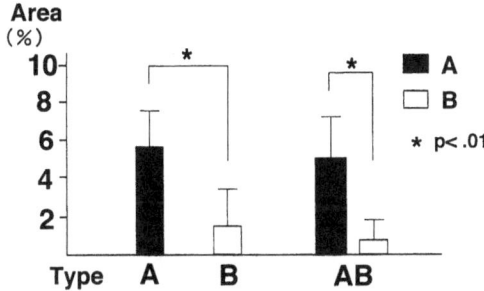

Fig. 3 Amount of blood type antigens in interstitium

anti-A or anti-B antibody and splenectomy, this strategy has become essential for incompatible kidney transplantation. Since then, attention has been paid only to the natural antibody titer of the recipients. It is likely that the lower the antibody titer, the less hyperacute rejection was seen after transplantation [7].

Blood type antigens in the graft, however, have often been overlooked. Breimer et al. [6] studied blood type A antigens in A_2 type human kidneys, biochemically, and demonstrated the lack of certain blood type A structures together with a low number of A determinants in A_2 kidneys. These findings were helpful for understanding the mechanism under which successful kidney transplantation from blood type A_2 kidneys to O recipients can be carrier out. Breimer et al. [5] also showed that the major blood type ABH carrier of kidney tissue is the globo-series. Our study suggests that the blood type B antigens are expressed very weakly in kidney tissue, compared with type A antigens. Very few data are available concerning the presence of globo-B antigen in kidney tissue [8]. Further study will be needed for a better knowledge about the distribution of ABH antigens in kidney tissue.

In our reported case, the preoperative depletion of natural antibody and splenectomy were intentionally avoided. Ota et al. [9] reported the results of 51 cases and recommended a reduction of antibody titers below 16 at the time of transplantation for a successful outcome. Although this patient showed a high titer of natural antibody against B antigen before transplantation, the titer dropped just after transplantation and maintained at low level thereafter. Deoxyspergualin administered soon after transplantation might play a role in inhibiting B cell activation.

We conclude that not only the anti-blood type antigen titer but also the blood type antigen in the graft should be considered for ABO incompatible transplantation. Moreover, it is likely that B-incompatible transplantation could be successfully performed without the depletion of natural antibodies.

References

1. Alexandre GPJ, Squiflet JP, Bruyere MD, Latinne R, Reding R, Gianello P, Carlier M, Pirdon Y (1987) Present experiences in a series of 26 ABO-incompatible living donor renal allografts. Transplant Proc 19: 4538–4542
2. Bannett AD, Bensinger WI, Raja R, Baquero A, McAlack RF (1987) Immunoadsorption and renal transplant in two patients with a major ABO incompability. Transplantation 43: 909–911
3. Bannett AD, McAlack RF, Raja R, Baquero A, Morris M (1987) Experiences with known ABO-mismatched renal transplants. Transplant Proc 19: 4543–4546
4. Bensinger WI, Baker DA, Buckner CD, Clift RA, Thomas ED (1981) Immunoadsorption for removal of A and B blood-group antibodies. N Engl J Med 304: 160–162
5. Breimer ME, Jovall PÅ (1985) Structural characterization of a blood group A heptaglycosylceramide with globo-series structure. The major glycolipid based blood group A antigen of human kidney. FEBS Lett 179: 165–172
6. Breimer ME, Brynger H, Rydberg L, Samuelsson BE (1985) Transplantation of blood group A2 kidneys to O recipients. Biochemical and immunological studies of blood group A antigens in human kidneys. Transplant Proc 17: 2640–2643
7. Chopek MW, Simmons RL, Platt JL (1987) ABO-incompatible kidney transplantation: Initial immunopathologic evaluation. Transplant Proc 19: 4553–4557
8. Clausen H, Hakomori S (1989) ABH and related histo-blood group antigens; Immunochemical differences in carrier isotopes and their distribution. Vox Sang 56: 1–20
9. Ota K, Takahashi K, Agishi T, Sonoda T, Oka T, Ueda S, Amemiya H, Shiramizu T, Okazaki H, Akiyama N, Hasegawa A, Kawamura T, Takagi H, Ueno A (1992) Multicentre trial of ABO-incompatible kidney transplantation. Transplant Int 5 [1]: S40–S43

Transpl Int (1996) 9 [Suppl 1]: S28–S31
© Springer-Verlag 1996

A. Rodrigues
T. Morgado
A. Castro Henriques
A. Morais Sarmento
M. Pereira
S. Guimarãcs

Outcome of renal graft recipients with hepatitis C virus infection

A. Rodrigues (✉) · T. Morgado · A. Castro
Henriques · A. Morais Sarmento ·
M. Pereira · S. Guimarãcs
Department of Nephrology and Renal
Transplant Unit, Hospital Geral Santo
António, Largo Professor Abel Salazar,
P-4000 Porto, Portugal

Abstract Hepatitis C virus (HCV) is a major cause of posttransplantation chronic liver disease. The aim of this study was to evaluate the prevalence of HCV in renal transplant recipients and to investigate risk and prognostic factors. Of 427 renal transplants carried out between July 1983 and January 1993, we retrospectively studied 66 (15.5 %) HBsAg-negative patients with anti-HCV detected by enzyme-linked immunosorbent assay (ELISA) and recombinant immunoblot assay (RIBA). Patient and graft survivals were estimated. Anti-HCV positive patients had more time on hemodialysis and pretransplant blood transfusions ($P = 0.0001$) than did the seronegative population. In a mean follow-up of 52.3 ± 27.7 months, 36 patients (54 %) had biochemical evidence of liver disease, predominantly with a persistently high pattern of serum alanine aminotransferase (ALT). Pretransplantation ALT elevation was associated ($P = 0.004$) with chronic liver disease (CLD) in the graft recipient. None of the other variables studied predicted posttransplantation CLD. Liver failure occurred in two (3 %) and was the cause of death in one of the patients. Death occurred in eight significantly more aged ($P = 0.0001$) patients, at 45.5 ± 28.8 months posttransplant. In 50 % of the cases, death was ascribed to sepsis. The biochemical pattern of HCV showed no predictive value for prognosis. The disease had no significant effect on the number of rejections or graft survival. The study revealed lower actuarial survival ($P = 0.004$) for HCV-positive patients in comparison with the seronegative population.

Key words Hepatitis C ·
Kidney transplantation

Introduction

Hepatitis C virus (HCV) is the major cause of liver disease in patients on dialysis and awaiting renal transplantation [1–3]. The renal recipient is at increased risk of reactivation of the disease or infection acquired from blood products at the time of transplantation or from the graft [4]. The prevalence and the severity of HCV infection in this high risk population is underestimated with the current biochemical and serologic tests [4–7]. Liver failure is the cause of death in 8–28 % of long-term survivors after renal transplantation [4]. However, the impact of hepatitis C in patient and graft survival remains controversial. The current study evaluates the prevalence, the clinical expression, and the prognosis of hepatitis C in renal allograft recipients.

Patients and methods

This study included 427 renal transplant recipients who were managed at Santo António General Hospital between July 1983 and January 1993. We have carried out a retrospective analysis of 66 HBsAg-negative patients, who were anti-HCV-positive on at

Table 1 Characteristics of the anti-hepatitis C virus-positive *(anti-HCV⁺)* patients: comparison with the seronegative *(HCV⁻)* population. *(NS* Not significant)

Characteristic	HCV⁺	HCV⁻	P value
Sex (male/female)	43/23	151/127	NS
Age (years)	38.3 ± 11.8	35.1 ± 13.3	NS
Timeonhemodialysis (months)	76.3 ± 45	40.2 ± 35	0.0001
Transfusion (units)	11.5 ± 12.9	4.7 ± 6.5	0.0001
Follow-up (months)	52.3 ± 27.7	55.3 ± 28	NS

Table 2 Chronic liver disease *(CLD)*. *(ATG* Anti-thymocyte globulin, *HLA* human leukocyte antigen, *NS* not significant)

Characteristic	CLD (n = 36)	No CLD (n = 30)	P value
Sex (male/female)	25/11	18/12	NS
Age (years)	40.7 ± 11.9	38.9 ± 9.8	NS
Hemodialysis (months)	89.5 ± 72.5	72.8 ± 62,8	NS
Transfusions (units)	12.4 ± 13.4	10.3 ± 12.5	NS
Clinical hepatitis	6	2	NS
Immunosuppression with ATG	14	13	NS
HLA compatibility (< 3, = 3, > 3)	22; 8; 6	17; 9; 4	NS
Second graft	5	4	NS
Follow-up (months)	56.7 ± 27.3	47.1 ± 27.9	NS

Table 3 Pattern of serum transaminase levels: correlation with posttransplantation CLD. *(NS* Not significant)

Pretransplantation profile	CLD (n = 36)	No CLD (n = 30)	P
Abnormal	29	11	0.004
Fluctuating	11	0	0.004
Occasional elevation	10	6	NS

least one occasion, detected by enzyme-linked immunosorbent assay II and confirmed by recombinant immunoblot assay II (Ortho Diagnostics). Not until 1991 were the clinicians of this hospital able to have access to these serological tests.

There were 43 men and 23 women with HCV infection. The mean age of the patients was 38.3 ± 11.8 years and time on hemodialysis averaged 76 ± 45 months (Table 1). We evaluated the clinical history and the pretransplantation chemical profile. The immunosuppression included azathioprine and prednisolone in 4 (6 %) patients; cyclosporine and prednisolone in 32 (48.5 %) patients; cyclosporine, azathioprine, and prednisolone in 3 (4.5 %) patients; anti-thymocyte globulin (ATG), cyclosporine, and prednisolone in 11 (16.7 %) patients; ATG, cyclosporine, azathioprine, and prednisolone in 16 (24.3 %) patients.

Chronic liver disease (CLD) was defined by fluctuating or persistently elevated transaminases (ALT) for at least 6 months. Any value above normal, as defined by the local laboratory, was considered elevated. Liver failure was diagnosed by prothrombin activity > 70 %; hypoalbuminemia < 3 g/l; portal hypertension. The follow-up was of 52.3 ± 27.7 months. We evaluated the prevalence and the impact of hepatitis C in patient and graft survival.

Statistical analysis was performed using the chi-square test to determine the statistical differences between proportions by entered 2 × 2 contingency tables; Student's *t*-test was used to evaluate the differences between normally distributed continuous variables. Graft and patient actuarial survivals were calculated with the

STAT (Statistics for Windows) software program. Results are expressed as mean ± SD. *P* < 0.05 was considered significant.

Results

HCV serology was unknown in 134 (31 %) patients; 227 patients were seronegative. We verified a prevalence of HCV infection of 22.5 %.

Anti-HCV-positive patients had significantly more time on hemodialysis and pretransplant blood transfusions (*P* = 0.0001) than did the seronegative population (Table 1). Three infected patients have never been transfused. The lack of stored serum from the donors precluded us from implicating the role of donor organ transmission of HCV in this study.

Forty-one (60.6 %) patients had pretransplantation ALT elevation: 11 with a fluctuating profile; 16 with an occasional elevation; 12 with elevated ALT only detected at transplantation day; 2 with an unknown pretransplantation profile of elevated ALT. Eight (12 %) of these had clinical hepatitis. In 69.1 % of the patients the diagnosis of infection was done after transplantation, so we could not study the influence of immunosuppression on the sensitivity of serological tests for hepatitis C.

Thirty-six patients had posttransplantation fluctuating (41.7 %) or persistently elevated (58.3 %) ALT. Thirty maintained normal enzyme levels. None of the patients with pretransplantation CLD showed biochemical normalization under immunosuppression. Six renal allograft recipients who had never had elevated ALT showed at an average of 1 year (max. 2 years; min. 3 months) post-transplantation, a persistently elevated profile of ALT. One of these had liver disease and died of sepsis. All of these had perioperative transfusions. The HCV statuses of the donors are unknown.

None of the variables studied was associated with posttransplantation CLD (Table 2). Pretransplantation, however, abnormal ALT levels were correlated with CLD in the renal graft recipients (Table 3).

Two patients (3 %) had liver failure. Eight patients, significantly more aged (*P* = 0.0001), died at 45.5 ± 28.8 months posttransplantation. They did not differ from the HCV-positive survivors in time on hemodialysis, number of transfusions of follow-up (Fig. 1). Four patients died with functioning grafts. In four (50 %) of the cases, death was ascribed to sepsis; two patients died of cardiovascular accident, one had fatal liver failure, and one died at home, of unknown cause.

We verified no significant differences in the number of rejection episodes [17/66 (25 %) in HCV-positive patients versus 92/275 (33 %) in seronegatives] or graft actuarial survival in the HCV-positive group. HCV-positive patients with CLD had a similar actuarial survival when compared with the infected patients who main-

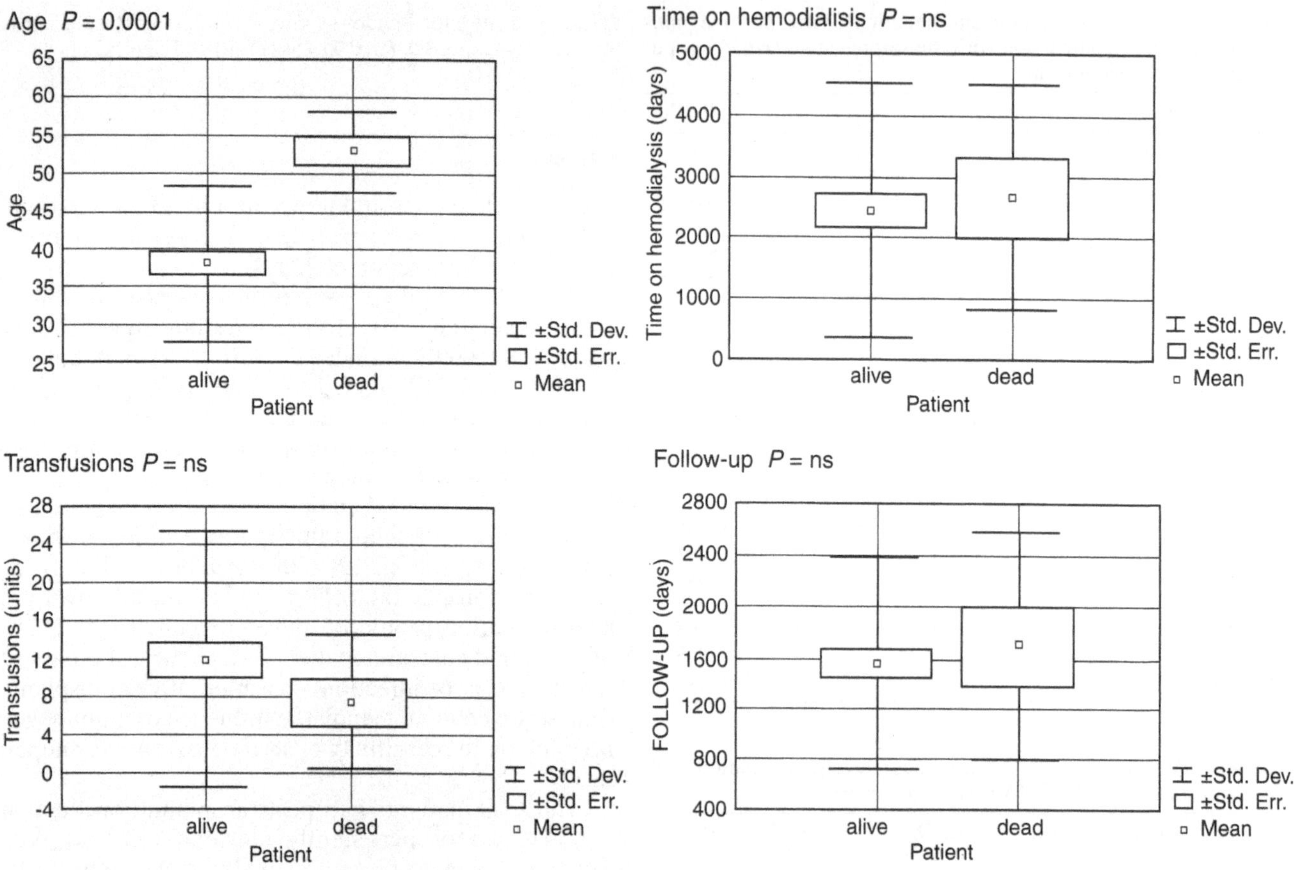

Age *P* = 0.0001

Time on hemodialysis *P* = ns

Transfusions *P* = ns

Follow-up *P* = ns

Fig. 1 Mortality (*n* = 8) in the hepatitis C virus-positive (HCV⁺) group. Comparison with the HCV⁺ survivors

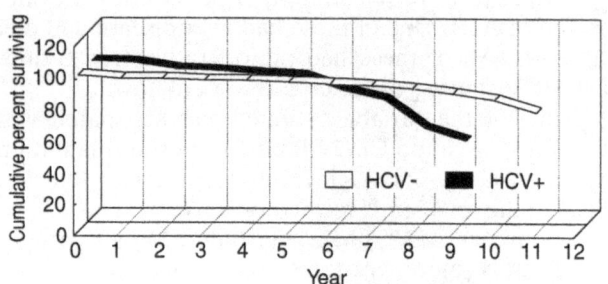

Fig. 2 Impact of HCV infection on patient survival (log rank *P* = 0.004)

tained normal enzyme levels. The actuarial HCV-positive patient survival differed significantly from that of the seronegative group. The results were: 99 %, 91 %, 58 % and 98 %, 96 %, 92 % at 1, 5, and 8 years, respectively, for HCV-positive and -negative groups (log-rank test *P* = 0.004, Fig. 2).

Discussion

The prevalence of HCV infection in our renal transplant population is similar to those of other series [2–7]. Time on hemodialysis and number of transfusions were risk factors for acquisition of the infection. Because of the lack of stored serum from the donors, we could not verify the role of the graft in the HCV transmission [4, 8–15]. The majority of the patients had CLD following renal transplantation, with no correlation with the type of immunosuppression. We found a poorer survival rate of the HCV-positive group. In agreement with several other published series, Morales et al. [2] and Pereira et al. [4] had suggested that HCV hepatitis is more aggressive in renal allograft recipients [16–19]. In a previous study of mortality in our renal transplant population [20] cardiovascular disease was the main cause of death. In this HCV-positive group, 50 % died of sepsis. In fact, hepatitis C has been incriminated in increasing the risk of infectious death [21].

Although hepatitis C is said to contribute to the long-term morbidity and mortality of renal transplant recipients, many studies were unable to demonstrate any significantly adverse effect on patient and graft survival [22–25]. The prognosis of these patients depends on the histological severity of hepatitis [17]. Those who died in our series had probably had a long-term infection. More severe liver disease, with a higher Knodell index, is said to exist as a function of time [26]. These patients were also more aged at transplantation day and hepatitis under immunosuppression may be more aggressive in the aged.

The prognostic importance of HCV genotypes is currently under investigation. From the several isolated strains, type 1, principally type 1 b, seems to be associated with a worse prognosis [27]. Coinfection of 1 b-HCV virus with other HCV strains is said to occur frequently in the hemodialyzed, which may justify a more aggressive pattern of disease. This may correlate with the severity of liver disease, cirrhosis in particular. Furthermore, HCV infection is associated with persistent viremia in the immunosuppressed renal allograft recipients [4].

We did not find more rejection episodes or worse graft survival in the HCV-positive patients. The infection may immunologically protect the graft, although recent results are contradictory [21]. The understanding of the natural history of hepatitis C in renal allograft recipients will grow with longer follow-up of these patients. The prevalence of infection is underdiagnosed by clinical and serological parameters, therefore, the detection of HCV by the polymerase chain reaction (PCR) is important for diagnosis [28–30]. Neither viremia nor the serological and biochemical profiles can accurately predict the severity of liver disease [26], although persistent elevations in alanine aminotransferase may be associated with more severe liver histology [31]. Liver biopsy is needed for definitive diagnosis of hepatitis in pretransplantation evaluation [21, 26, 32]. Milder histological abnormalities such as chronic persistent hepatitis are associated with a minor risk of mortality or morbidity in renal transplant recipients. Those with chronic active hepatitis and liver fibrosis often progress to micronodular cirrhosis, which may be a contraindication for isolated renal transplantation [17, 32]. Older patients are at an increased risk [17]. The better quality of life of the transplant patient should be weighed against the low but definite risk of development of chronic liver failure.

The results of this study emphasize that HCV hepatitis is a frequent complication that may have an adverse impact in morbidity and mortality of renal transplant recipients. It was associated with death from sepsis in 50 % of cases. The infection did not affect the number of rejection episodes or graft actuarial survival. It is important to obtain histological data to better understand the natural progression of hepatitis in the immunosuppressed host. Liver biopsy should be incorporated into the pretransplantation evaluation of hepatitis C.

References

1. Dubois DB, Gretch D, et al (1994) Am J Kidney Dis 24: 795–801
2. Morales M, Campo C, Castellano G, Colina F, et al (1992) Transplant Proc 24: 78–80
3. Ponz E, Campistol JM, Barrera JM, et al (1991) Transplant Proc 23: 1371–1372
4. Pereira BJG (1993) Curr Opin Nephrol Hypertens 2: 912–922
5. Oliveras A, Lloveras J, Puig JM, et al (1991) Transplant Proc 23: 2636–2637
6. Chan TM, Lok ASF, Cheng IKP (1991) Transplantation 52: 810–813
7. Druwe PM, Michielsen PP, Ramon AM, De Broe ME (1994) Nephrol Dial Transplant 9: 230–237
8. Gomez E, Aguado S, Gago E, et al (1991) Transplant Proc 23: 2654–2655
9. Tesi Raymond J, Waller K, Morgan CJ, et al (1994) Transplantation 57: 826–831
10. Pereira BJG, Milford EL, Kirman RL, et al (1993) Transplant Proc 25: 1458–1459
11. Morales JM, Andres A (1993) N Engl J Med 328: 511
12. Miller J, Roth D, Schiff ER (1993) N Engl J Med 328: 512
13. Candinas D, Joller Jemelka HI, Largiader F (1993) N Engl J Med 328: 512
14. Pereira BJG, Levey AS (1993) N Engl Med 328: 513
15. Vincenti F, Weber P, Kuo G, et al (1991) Transplant Proc 23: 2651–2652
16. Morales JM, Munoz MA, Castellano G, et al (1993) Transplant Proc 25: 1450–1453
17. Rao KV, et al (1993) Am J Med 94: 241–250
18. Ihara H, Ikoma F (1994) Transplant Proc March: 781
19. Boyce NW, et al (1988) Am J Kidney Dis 11: 307–312
20. Lobato L, et al (1994) Rev Port Nefrol Hipert 8: 113–121
21. Roth D, et al (1994) Kidney Int 45: 238–244
22. Fernandez JA, Roth D, et al (1991) Transplant Proc 23: 444–445
23. Goffin E, Pirson Y, Cornu C, et al (1994) Kidney Int 45: 551–555
24. Orloff SL, Stempel CA, Wright TL, et al (1995) Clin Transpl 9: 119–124
25. Pol S (1994) Actualités néphrologiques. Flammarion Medecine-Sciences, Paris
26. Caramelo C, et al (1993) Am J Kidney Dis 22: 822–828
27. Dusheiko G, et al (1994) Hepatology January: 13–18
28. Arita S, et al (1992) Transplant Proc 24: 1538–1540
29. Brunson ME, et al (1993) Transplantation 56: 1364–1367
30. Pereira BJG, et al (1992) N Engl J Med 24: 910–915
31. Chan T, et al (1994) Transplantation 58: 996–1000
32. Roth D (1995) Am J Kidney Dis 25: 3–16

Transpl Int (1996) 9 [Suppl 1]: S 32–S 33
© Springer-Verlag 1996

Pharmacokinetics and immunodynamics of chimeric IL-2 receptor monoclonal antibody SDZ CHI 621 in renal allograft recipients

J. M. Kovarik
E. Rawlings
P. Sweny
O. Fernando
R. Moore
P. J. Griffin
P. Fauchald
D. Albrechtsen
G. Sodal
K. Nordal
P. L. Amlot

J. M. Kovarik (✉)
Clinical Pharmacology,
Sandoz Pharma Ltd., CH-4002 Basel,
Switzerland

E. Rawlings · P. Sweny · O. Fernando ·
P. L. Amlot
Departments of Immunology and
Nephrology, Royal Free Hospital School of
Medicine, London NW3 14D, UK

R. Moore · P. J. Griffin
Cardiff Royal Infirmary, Cardiff, UK

P. Fauchald · D. Albrechtsen · G. Sodal ·
K. Nordal
Rikshospitalet, Oslo, Norway

Abstract SDZ CHI 621 is a murine-human chimeric monoclonal antibody (mAb) to the interleukin-2 (IL-2) receptor (CD25) intended for prophylactic immunosuppression against acute rejection in the first several weeks following kidney transplantation. A multicentre, prospective, dose-finding study was conducted in 37 primary, mismatched cadaver kidney transplant patients to assess its tolerability, pharmacokinetics and immunodynamics. Successive cohorts of patients were stratified to receive total doses of 20, 30, 40 or 60 mg ($n = 4$, 4, 14, 15, respectively) administered as 15- or 20-mg intravenous infusions with the first dose given preoperatively and subsequent doses within the first 10 days posttransplant. Daily mAb serum concentrations were analysed by a radioimmunoassay method and the percentage of peripheral T-lymphocytes expressing CD25 from serial blood samples was determined by FACScan. Intravenous administrations were well tolerated. mAb concentration profiles exhibited a biphasic decline with an initial $t_{1/2}$ of 14.4 ± 14.2 h, terminal $t_{1/2}$ of 13.4 ± 6.0 days, distribution volume (V_{ss}) of 6.9 ± 3.3 l and clearance of 17.4 ± 7.8 ml/h. The concentration-effect (mAb-CD25) relationship indicated that mAb concentrations exceeding a threshold of about 0.7 µg/ml corresponded to complete suppression of CD25 ($\leq 3\%$ CD25$^+$ T-cells). The threshold mAb concentration was exceeded at all dose levels, whereas the duration above the threshold (and thus of CD25 suppression) rose with increasing dose: 20 mg, 20 ± 7 days; 30 mg, 32 ± 6 days; 40 mg, 37 ± 10 days; and 60 mg, 53 ± 17 days. As mAb concentrations declined below the threshold following the last dose, CD25 expression returned to baseline (18–44% CD25$^+$ T-cells) within a few days.

Key words Immunosuppression · Monoclonal antibodies · Renal transplantation · Pharmacokinetics · Pharmacodynamics

Introduction

The development of antibody therapy in the prophylaxis against acute rejection in transplantation has progressed from aspecific polyclonal antisera to increasingly selective monoclonal antibodies, which have the potential to regulate specific immunological responses via functional receptors. In this context, rat and mouse mono- clonal antibodies to the interleukin-2 receptor (IL-2R) have shown promise in preventing acute rejection in renal allograft recipients [1, 2]. However, their clinical use has been limited by the rapid development of neutralising antibodies. In an attempt to reduce immunogenicity, a chimeric mouse-human anti-IL-2R monoclonal antibody has been developed. SDZ CHI 621 contains a murine variable region (RFT5) and a human constant region (IgG1$\varkappa$) and demonstrates high affinity for the CD25 activation antigen on the IL-2Rα chain. An investigation was designed to characterise the pharmacokinetics and immunodynamics of SDZ CHI 621 in renal allograft recipients.

Methods

A multicentre, open-label dose-finding study was undertaken in recipients of primary, mismatched cadaver kidneys. Successive cohorts of patients were stratified to receive total SDZ CHI 621 doses of 20, 30, 40 or 60 mg. Total doses were administered as 15- or 20-mg intravenous infusions delivered over 30 min. The first infusion was given prior to transplant surgery, with subsequent administrations within the first 10 postoperative days. Blood samples were collected daily for the determination of serum SDZ CHI 621 concentrations by a radioimmunoassay (RIA) method. For pharmacokinetic analysis, concentration-time data were fitted to a two-compartment, open model with first-order elimination from the central compartment. Blood samples were obtained twice weekly over the study duration for pharmacodynamic measurements. Specifically, lymphocyte subpopulations were analysed by FACScan flow cytometry (Becton-Dickinson) and the percentage of CD25A$^+$ T-cells was quantified.

Results and discussion

Patient population and clinical observations

Thirty-nine patients were enrolled in this investigation; data from the 37 who provided evaluable pharmacokinetic profiles are presented. There were 23 men and 14 women aged 48 ± 14 years (range 18–71 years) and weighing 74 ± 16 kg (range 46–103 kg). They were stratified as follows among the dose levels: 4 (20 mg), 4 (30 mg), 14 (40 mg), 15 (60 mg). The infusions of SDZ CHI 621 were safe and well-tolerated and no cytokine-release syndrome or hypersensitivity reactions were observed.

Pharmacokinetics

Peak serum SDZ CHI 621 concentrations at the end of the infusion ranged between 5 and 10 µg/ml; the distribution volume (V_{ss}) was 6.9 ± 3.3 l. Concentrations subsequently declined in a biphasic manner with a prolonged terminal disposition half-life of 13.4 ± 6.0 days. The total body clearance was 17.4 ± 7.8 ml/h; the between-subject variability in clearance was not influenced by body weight, supporting dosing on a milligram basis in adults.

Immunodynamics

The baseline percentage of CD25A$^+$ T-cells from pretreatment blood samples ranged from 18 % to 44 %. In the presence of SDZ CHI 621, CD25A was continuously suppressed, with the percentage of T-cells expressing this activation marker below 3 %. Clinically relevant suppression was maintained until SDZ CHI 621 concentrations declined to a threshold region around 0.7–1.0 µg/ml (as determined by RIA) following the last administration. At this point, CD25A counts returned to baseline within a few days. The concentration-effect relationship was also explored by plotting the paired determinations of SDZ CHI 621 concentration versus the percentage of CD25A$^+$ T-cells, pooling the data pairs from all study patients. Again, concentrations exceeding approximately 0.7–1.0 µg/ml were associated with CD25A suppression (≤ 3 % CD25A expression), while concentrations below this threshold region were associated with the pre- and post-treatment baseline values (> 3 % CD25A expression). All cumulative dose levels assessed in this investigation yielded CD25A suppression; however, the duration of suppression increased with increasing total dose. Specifically, at total doses of 20, 30, 40 and 60 mg, the duration was 20 ± 7, 32 ± 6, 37 ± 10 and 53 ± 17 days, respectively. These data were used as a basis for dose selection in the indication of immunosuppressive prophylaxis following kidney transplantation.

References

1. Kirkman RL, Shapiro ME, Carpenter CB, et al (1991) A randomized prospective trial of anti-Tac monoclonal antibody in human renal transplantation. Transplantation 51: 107

2. Soulillou JP, Cantarovich D, Le Mauff B, et al (1990) Randomised controlled trial of a monoclonal antibody against the interleukin 2 receptor (33B3.1) as compared with rabbit antithymocyte globulin for prophylaxis against rejection of renal allografts. New Engl J Med 322: 1175

Transpl Int (1996) 9 [Suppl 1]: S34–S37
© Springer-Verlag 1996

KIDNEY

Ursula Jacobs
Detlef Niese
Wulf-Dietrich Miersch
Hans-Ulrich Klehr

Acute rejection relapses posttransplant: definition of risk group and evaluation of potent therapeutic regimens

U. Jacobs (✉) · D. Niese · H.-U. Klehr
Department of General Internal Medicine,
University Hospital,
Rheinische Friedrich-Wilhelms-Universität
Bonn, Sigmund-Freud-Straße 25,
D-53105 Bonn, Germany
Tel. +49-228-230389;
Fax +49-228-2874323

W.-D. Miersch
Department of Urology,
University Hospital Bonn, Germany

Abstract A group of 113 patients were investigated after allogenic cadaver renal transplantation to analyse whether the small number of patients presenting acute rejection relapses could be defined by risk factors and whether there is an efficacious regimen for the safe therapy of recurrent rejection episodes. According to these results we are aware of a group of "highly reactive rejectors" especially within the younger recipients and there are further characteristics which can be identified as being associated with an elevated risk of recurrent acute rejection. By adequate antirejection therapy we can achieve a favourable transplant survival rate of 97 % in the critical first year. An additional benefit may result from ALG consolidation related to suppression of the remaining CD8-positive human natural killer cells.

Key words Acute rejection relapses · Risk factors · Transplant outcome · ALG

Introduction

Despite potent and intense antirejection therapy with repeated triple combinations of cyclosporine A (CsA), cortisone and antithymocyte globulin, (ATG), and consecutive CD3 monoclonal antibodies (OKT3) in acute rejection, there still remain transplant recipients presenting acute rejection (AR) relapses. In a group of patients after allogenic transplantation, we investigated whether a recipient group could be defined by risk factors and if there is an efficacious regimen for the safe therapy of recurrent rejection episodes.

Patients and methods

In a group of 113 patients after allogenic cadaver renal transplantation (Tx), we analysed pre- and posttransplant risk factors for the recurrence of > 2 AR episodes and evaluated short-term efficacy of the antirejection regimen. Simultaneously, we analysed lymphocyte subsets before and weekly after Tx and while on antirejection treatment. We compared patients with ≤ 2 ($n = 95$; 84 %) with patients with 3 or 4 ($n = 18$; 16 %) AR episodes. Rejec-

tion was diagnosed uniformly by one referential pathologist using the histological triple technique.

Therapeutic regimen

All patients received CsA, cortisone and ATG for 7 days. In patients at risk of rejection this was followed by CsA, cortisone and azathioprine. In acute clinical rejection, cortisone pulses were given (500 mg, 3 days). AR diagnosed histologically could be classified as interstitial or vascular. Patients with interstitial AR were treated with OKT3 and plasmapheresis (6 ×). If patients responded to OKT3, a second course was given, but if they did not respond (13 patients) the ATG therapy was given. Antilymphocyte globulin (ALG) (5 ml/kg per day) consolidation was given for a 5-day period to patients at risk of recurrent AR episodes.

Cytomegalovirus (CMV) monitoring

Simultaneously, patients were monitored for cytomegalovirus (CMV) disease [weekly CMV IgM titre (ELISA), virus culture from urine and throat swabs, pp-65-CMV-early antigen (+PCR)] in order that virustatic therapy with ganciclovir could be instituted prophylactically.

Cytoimmunological monitoring

The following lymphocyte subsets were analysed by a flourescent-activated cell sorter (FACS): CD2 (T11, SRBC-rec), CD3 (T3, T-cell antigen), CD4 (helper inducer T-cells), CD8 (suppressor T-cells), CD25 (interleucin-2 receptor), CD57 (human natural killer cells), CD56 (natural killer, LGL cells), CD20 (B-cells, B1), HLA-DR+ (monocytes, B-, activated T-cells), CD11b (monocytes, granulocytes, CR3), CD8+/HLA-DR+ (activated T-cells), CD3+/CD25+ (interleucin-2+ T-cells), HLA-DR+ monocytes, HLA-DR/CD11b (monocytes), CD8+/HNK-1+ (CD8-Subset) and CD8+/NKH-1+ (CD8-Subset).

Bioimmunological monitoring

The following were monitored: circulating immunocomplexes C1q, circulating immunocomplexes IgG, IgM and IgA, immunoglobulins IgG, IgM, IgA and IgE, C3 and C4 complement, C-reactive protein quantitative, and β-2-microglobulin.

Clinical variables

The pre- and posttransplant variables that were analysed are detailed in Table 1.

Statistical analysis

Data were analysed by Student's t-test, the Mantel-Haenszel procedure and the chi-squared test.

Results

The occurrence of AR episodes was as follows: none in 19 patients (17 %), one in 45 patients (40 %), two in 31 patients (27 %), three in 11 patients (10 %) and four in 7 patients (6 %) (Fig. 1). The mean number of AR episodes was 1.5 ± 1. Statistically significant clinical and immunological risk factors associated with the occurrence of more than two AR episodes are as follows (see also Table 2): younger recicipient age ($P < 0.0001$), elder donor age ($P = 0.0264$), duration of preceding haemodialysis ($P = 0.0265$), transfusions before Tx ($P = 0.0179$, negative CC), cytotoxic antibodies ($P = 0.0327$), body weight index before Tx ($P = 0.05$), CD8+/HLA-DR+ after Tx ($P = 0.00039$), CD8+/HNK+ after Tx ($P = 0.0324$), C4 complement after Tx ($P < 0.0001$, negative CK) and β-2-microglobulin after Tx ($P = 0.0094$) (Fig. 2). The number of HLA-B matches (negative CC), the number of HLA mismatches and the number of transfusions after only showed a statistical trend. Differences of cold ischemia time or histocompatibility could be excluded.

With our therapeutic regimen 1-year graft survival improved up to 97 %. In all except 1 patient the severe recurrent AR was finally overcome and transplant (TP) function stabilised after ALG consolidation with

Table 1 Clinical variables analysed to define risk factors associated with acute rejection episode relapses

Pretransplant	Posttransplant
Recipient age	–
Donor age	–
Histocompatibility	–
Cytotoxic antibodies	Cytotoxic antibodies
Cold ischemia time	Acute renal failure
CMV status donor/recipient	CMV disease
Blood transfusions	Blood transfusions
Duration of dialysis	Duration of dialysis
Renal disease	Urinary tract infection
Blood group	–
Sex	–
Body weight index	–

Table 2 Clinical and immunological risk factors associated with recurrence of acute rejection after renal allografting

1. Younger recipient age	$P < 0.0001$
2. Elder donor age	$P = 0.0264$
3. Duration of preceding dialysis	$P = 0.0265$
4. Transfusions before Tx	$P = 0.0179$ (negative CC)
5. Cytotoxic antibodies	$P = 0.0327$
6. Body weight index before Tx	$P = 0.05$
7. CD8+/HLA-DR+ after Tx	$P = 0.0003$
8. CD8+/HNK+ after Tx	$P = 0.0324$
9. C4-complement after Tx	$P < 0.0001$ (negative CK)
10. β-2-microglobulin after Tx	$P = 0.0094$
Number HLY-B matches	statistical trend (negative CC)
Number of HLA mismatches	statistical trend
Transfusions after Tx	statistical trend

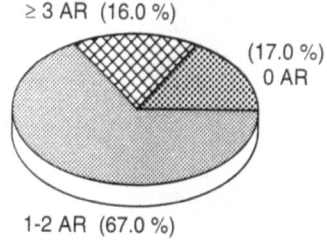

Fig. 1 Prevalence of acute rejection episodes in a group of 113 patients analysed after renal allotransplantation

a resulting serum creatinine level of 1.74 ± 0.77 mg/dl (> 2 AR episodes) vs 1.38 ± 0.48 mg/dl (< 2 AR episodes) (follow-up 2.7 ± 1.2 years). Cytoimmunologically, the risk group was characterised by an enhanced expression of CD8+HLA-DR+ (activated T-cells) and CD8/HNK+ (CD8 positive human natural killer cells) that finally could be significantly reduced only by ALG ($P = 0.0155$). An additional immunological effect of ALG consolidation after > 3 AR episodes was observed in patients characterised by a significant increase of CD8+/HLA-DR+ ($P = 0.0095$), in patients with vascular AR without decrease of CD3 after OKT3 plus in-

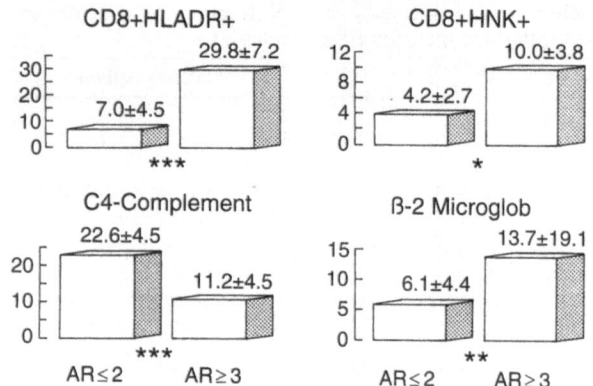

Fig. 2 Immunological differences between the group with ≤ 2 acute rejection (AR) episodes vs the group with ≥ 3 AR episodes. (Mean values post Tx during recurrence of rejection)

crease of HLA-DR+ ($P = 0.0450$) prior to ALG. In 3 patients severe AR was complicated by TP rupture, all could be revised operatively. OKT3-enhanced incidence of CMV disease, defined as the manifestation of one virologic parameter plus organ deterioration, was up to 50 % vs 31 % for the entire study group but early treatment with ganciclovir (+ hyperimmunoglobulins) was safe and without any remaining complications. There were no lymphoproliferative disorders in the highly immunosuppressed group. In patients with > 2 AR episodes the survival rate was 100 %. In a follow-up we evaluated our results with regard to long-term TP function. After 2.7 ± 1.2 years there was only a difference in actual serum creatinine as a parameter of long-term TP function (1.74 ± 0.77 vs 1.38 ± 0.48 mg/

dl), but no difference in TP survival comparing the two groups (Table 3).

Discussion

According to these results and especially within the younger recipient group, we have to be aware of "highly reactive rejectors". Further factors can be identified as being associated with a significantly elevated risk of recurrent acute rejections. The adequate antirejection therapy results in a very high transplant survival rate of 97 % in the critical first year. Our immunological data conceivably elucidate a beneficial effect of ALG consolidation upon suppression of the remaining CD8-positive human natural killer cells even after OKT3. In patients with AR relapses after OKT3 we should focus on the cells referred to as non-T- and non-B-cells and they probably respond neither to ATG nor to CD3 antibodies but more likely to ALG as was demonstrated by our data. It is also noteworthy that in patients with vascular rejection treated with OKT3 plus plasmapheresis, there may remain a risk group characterised by an insufficient reduction of CD3 cells after OKT3 in whom finally ALG could succeed in lowering the expression of these cells. Thus this agent turned out to be of additional therapeutic and consolidating value in a small group of patients presenting acute rejection episodes not responding sufficiently to so-called OKT3 rescue as do most of the patients with < 2 AR. These unanticipated immunological results may elucidate observations with undefined ALG effect noticed by others [1]. As expected, OKT3 results in an enhanced risk profile of symptom-

Table 3 Summary of patients' characteristics (*AR* acute rejection episode, *TP* transplant)		Patients with ≥ 3 AR (*n* = 18)	Patients with ≤ 2 AR (*n* = 95)
Pretransplant status			
Recipient age	***	35 ± 11 years	42 ± 13 years
Donor age	*	42 ± 14 years	34 ± 13 years
HLA mismatches	n. s.	4 ± 1	4 ± 2
Cold ischemia	n. s.	19.3 ± 6.6 h	17.5 ± 5.7 h
Duration of dialysis	*	4.5 ± 4.4 years	3.9 ± 4.4 years
Transfusion	*	2.8 ± 2.7	5 ± 7
Posttransplant status			
Number of acute rejections		2.5 ± 1	1.5 ± 1
TP rupture		2 patients	1 patient
OKT3 incidence		18 patients	25 patients
ALG incidence		13 patients	None
Patients' survival		100 %	100 %
Transplant lost		1	2
After 2.7 ± 1.2 years follow-up			
Actual serum creatinine	*	1.74 ± 0.77	1.38 ± 0.48 mg/dl
Actual proteinuria		0.54 ± 0.62	0.39 ± 0.55 g/day
CMV disease		23 %	34 %
Malignancies		1 patient	3 patients

Statistics: Student's *t*-test; * $P < 0.05$; *** $P < 0.001$; n. s. = non significant

atic CMV infection justifying ganciclovir prophylaxis in the CMV-risk group according to serostatus donor/recipient. As is known from the literature, the number of AR episodes affects long-term TP outcome with regard to the increased risk of so-called "chronic rejection": in renal TP we could demonstrate the same effect in patient groups studied [2–5]. Besides overall improvements in the results of cadaveric renal transplantation, the literature still focuses on high-risk renal TP recipients who experience excessive graft loss [6–8]. Our immunosuppressive antirejection regimen provides a highly effective therapy yielding favourable success rates even in these patients. Long-term results of this regimen including neoplastic potentiation addressed at a follow-up of 2.7 ± 1.2 years do not show differences between the two groups studied.

References

1. Dennis MJ, Foster MC, Ryan JJ, Burden RP, Morgan AG et al (1989) The increasing importance of chronic rejection as a cause of renal allograft failure. Transpl Int 2: 214–217
2. Matas A (1994) Chronic rejection in renal transplant recipients – risk factors and correlates. Clin Transplant 8: 332–335
3. Shaikewitz ST, Chan L (1994) Chronic renal transplant rejection. Am J Kidney Dis 23: 884–893
4. Sharples LD, Scott JP, Denis C, Higenbottam TW, Stewart S et al (1994) Risk factors for survival following combined heart-lung transplantation. The first 100 patients. Transplantation 57: 218–223
5. Yilmaz S, Häyry P (1993) The impact of acute episodes of rejection on the generation of chronic rejection in rat renal allografts. Transplantation 56: 1153–1156
6. Addonizio LJ, Hsu DT, Douglas JF, Kichuk MR, Michler RE et al (1993) Decreasing incidence of coronary disease in pediatric cadaveric transplant recipients using increased immunosuppression. Circulation 88: II 224–229
7. Pirsch JD, D'Alessandro AM, Sollinger HW, Hoffmann RM, Roecker E et al (1992) The effect of donor age, recipient age, and HLA match on immunologic graft survival in cadaver renal transplant recipients. Transplantation 53: 55–59
8. Sugimoto H, Akiyama N, Otsubo O, Tomikawa S, Mita K et al (1989) Clinical studies on 228 renal transplants. Nippon Geka Gakkai Zasshi 90: 120–126

Transpl Int (1996) 9 [Suppl 1]: S 38–S 40
© Springer-Verlag 1996

KIDNEY

Michael Olausson
Lars Mjörnstedt
Hans Brynger
Ingemar Blohmé

Steroid-resistant rejection in kidney-transplanted patients: is ATG treatment for three or ten days preferable?

M. Olausson (✉) · L. Mjörnstedt ·
H. Brynger · I. Blohmé
Department of Surgery, Division of
Transplantation, Liver and Vascular
Surgery, Sahlgrenska University Hospital,
S-413 45 Göteborg, Sweden

Abstract We carried out a randomized prospective trial to compare a 3-day with a 10-day course of antithymocyte globulin (ATG)- (Fresenius) for treatment of steroid-resistant rejection after renal transplantation. The aim was to study whether a short 3-day course was as safe and effective as the longer 10-day treatment. Thirty patients over a 3-year period were included. Patients that did not respond to treatment after 3 days received additional ATG from day 5 to day 10. The graft survival and the proportion of rejections reversed with the treatment were compared. Fifty percent responded promptly in the 3-day group and a further 29 % after additional treatment. In the 10-day group, 62 % reponded to the treatment. There was no significant difference between the groups. We, therefore, suggest that the standard antirejection treatment with ATG could be shortened without an increased risk of graft failure.

Key words ATG · Steroid-resistant rejection · Kidney transplantation

Introduction

Antithymocyte globulin (ATG) has been used in clinical practice for more than 20 years as a potent drug for prophylaxis against allograft rejection as well as in the treatment of steroid-resistant rejection [1–5]. The recommended duration of the treatment usually varies between 7 and 14 days. The standard antirejection treatment with steroids after transplantation usually includes 3 or 4 days with methylprednisolone bolus injections. An extended time of ATG treatment is expensive, possibly harmful [4], and might not be necessary. The present study aimed to investigate whether a 3-day ATG course was sufficient as treatment for steroid-resistant allograft rejection in kidney-transplanted recipients, or if a standard 10-day course was required.

Materials and methods

Study design

The study was designed as a randomized, prospective, open study. Patients were not stratified according to immunological risk factors. All patients with steroid-resistant rejection and a clinical decision to commence ATG treatment were included.

Patients and immunosuppressive therapy

For 3 years, 30 patients undergoing kidney transplantation were studied. All recipients received standard triple-drug treatment with prednisolone, azathioprine, and cyclosporine. Prednisolone was started on the day of surgery at a dose of 100 mg, followed by a reducing dose over 2 weeks down to 20 mg. Azathioprine was given preoperatively (2 mg/kg per day) and then adjusted according to daily levels of white blood cells. Oral cyclosporine (8 mg/kg per day) was started as soon as the kidney began to function, usually the day after transplantation. The cyclosporine dose was adjusted to levels of cyclosporine in whole blood (monoclonal RIA assays) corresponding to 150–200 ng/ml).

Table 1 Demographic data and graft survival (*M/F* male/female, *LD* live donor, *ReTx* retransplantation, *PRA* + panel-reacting antibodies in pretransplant sera, *PrDia* pretransplant dialysis, *Rev* number of patients with reversed rejection (A vs B n.s.)

Group	Number	Mean age (95 % confidence)	M/F	LD	ReTx	PRA+	PrDia	Rev
A	14	34.5 ± 4.6	9/5	7	2	6	10	11
B	13	43.1 ± 8.0	9/4	3	0	5	12	8

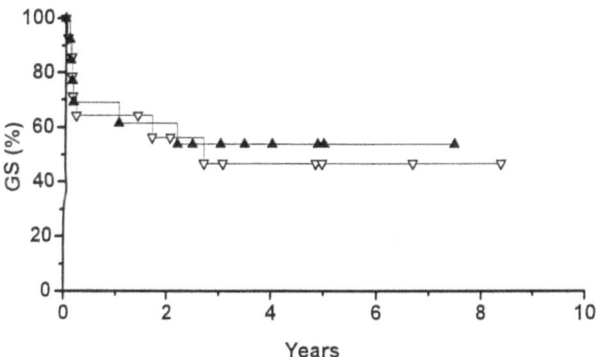

Fig.1 Actuarial graft survival in patients treated with 3 or 10 days of antithymocyte globulin (ATG) for steroid-resistant rejection (—▽— ATG 3 days, —▲— ATG 10 days)

Diagnosis and treatment of rejection

Rejection was diagnosed clinically and verified with a core needle biopsy. All patients with allograft rejection received standard antirejection treatment consisting of a bolus dose of methylprednisolone i.v. for 4 consecutive days (500 + 250 + 250 + 250 mg). Recipients not responding with improved kidney function on the fifth day of the steroid treatment were defined as having a steroid-resistant rejection.

Randomization and treatment protocol

After a steroid-resistant rejection had been defined and the decision taken to commence ATG therapy, patients were randomized to either a 3-day (group A) or a 10-day (group B) ATG (Fresenius AG) course. ATG was given i.v. at a dose rate corresponding to 3 mg/kg body weight daily. Patients in the 3-day treatment group were evaluated on day 4. If the creatinine had leveled off or decreased, no further ATG was given. If on the other hand the creatinine level continued to rise on the fourth day, ATG was continued from day 5 to day 10. All recipients were evaluated after 10 days to establish whether the treatment had been effective in reversing the rejection episode. The number of grafts rejected after 3 months were registered and the graft survival was calculated.

Statistical analysis

Categorical data were analyzed using Fisher's exact test for two-by-two tables. The Kaplan-Meir method with the Cox-Mantel logrank test was used to calculate graft actuarial survival rates.

Results

All patients that completed at least 3 days of ATG therapy were eligible for analysis. One patient in group A lost his graft on day 2 after starting ATG and was, therefore, excluded. One patient in group B was excluded due to early graft failure (day 2) during the ATG therapy and another patient in the same group received only one dose of ATG due to severe thrombocytopenia and was, therefore, excluded as well. Demographic data and graft survival of the remaining 27 patients eligible for analysis are presented in Table 1. Seven patients in group A (50 %) responded primarily to the 3-day course and an additional 4 responded after prolonged therapy, resulting in 11/14 patients (79 %) in total, responding in group A. In group B, 8 patients (62 %) responded to treatment. There was no statistically significant difference between the two groups with respect to the ability to reverse allograft rejection. The actuarial graft survival of groups A and B were compared. No statistically significant difference could be seen. The follow-up was 5–8 years.

Discussion

Since the first clinical application of antilymphocyte globulin in 1967 by Starzl, many investigators have confirmed the powerful effect of this and other antithymocyte drugs in suppressing T-cell activation as well as their ability to prevent and reverse allograft rejection [1–5]. It is also known that, although a high dose of ATG is effective in preventing or reversing allograft rejection, it is at the cost of many undesirable side effects such as a high incidence of viral and bacterial infections [4]. One way to reduce the total immunosuppressive load on the patient is to reduce the ATG dose after T-cell monitoring using flow cytometry, as shown by Abouna and co-workers [4]. A reduction both in treatment costs and number of infections was seen with a lower ATG dose [5]. Another way to reduce the amount of ATG given would be to shorten the length of the treatment period.

In the present study we have demonstrated that both short- and long-term results measured as rejected grafts at 3 months and actuarial graft survivals were similar, irrespective of the length of treatment. Although not all of the patients receiving an initial 3-day ATG course reversed, it was possible and safe to commence ATG treatment again on day 5. No graft was lost due to too short a treatment period with ATG. We, therefore, suggest that the standard antirejection treatment with ATG could be short. A prolonged course could be initiated in cases not responding promptly.

Acknowledgements This study was supported by grants from the Professor L-E Gelin Memorial Foundation, Fresenius AG, Federal Republic of Germany, Riksförbundet för Njursjuka.

References

1. Neuhaus P, Bechstein WO, Blumhardt G, Wiens M, Lemmens P, Langrehr JM, Lohmann R, Steffen R, Schlag H, Slama K-J, Lobeck H (1993) Comparison of quadruple immunosuppression after liver transplantation with ATG or IL-2 receptor antibody. Transplantation 55: 1320–1327
2. Steininger R, Mühlbacher F, Hamilton G, Längle F, Gnant M, Popow T, Sautner T, Götzinger P, Wamser P, Stockenhuber F, Mirza D, Piza F (1991) Comparison of CyA, OKT3, and ATG immunoprophylaxis in human liver transplantation. Transplant Proc 23: 2269–2271
3. Birkeland SA (1975) A controlled clinical trial of treatment with ALG on established rejection of renal allografts. Acta Med Scand 198: 489
4. Abouna GM, Al-Abdullah IH, Kelly-Sullivan D, Kumar MSA, Loose J, Phillips K, Yost S, Seirka D (1995) Randomized clinical trial of antithymocyte globulin induction in renal transplantation comparing a fixed daily dose with dose adjustment according to T cell monitoring. Transplantation 59: 1564–1568
5. Bock HA, Gallati H, Zürcher RM, Bachofen M, Mihatsch MJ, Landman J, Thiel G (1995) A randomized prospective trial of prophylactic immunosuppression with ATG-Fresenius versus OKT3 after renal transplantation. Transplantation 59: 830–840

Transpl Int (1996) 9 [Suppl 1]: S41–S44
© Springer-Verlag 1996

KIDNEY

L. B. Hilbrands
J. Rischen-Vos
R. Hené
W. Weimar
K. Assmann
A. J. Hoitsma

Randomized trial of misoprostol in patients with chronic renal transplant rejection

L. B. Hilbrands (✉) · K. Assmann ·
A. J. Hoitsma
Academic Hospital St. Radboud,
G. Grooteplein 10, NL-6525 GA Nijmegen,
The Netherlands

J. Rischen-Vos · W. Weimar
Academic Hospital Dijkzigt,
Dr. Molewaterplein 40,
NL-3015 GD Rotterdam, The Netherlands

R. Hené
Academic Hospital Utrecht,
Heidelberglaan 100,
NL-3584 CX Utrecht, The Netherlands

Abstract Chronic vascular rejection is a major cause of long-term graft failure after renal transplantation. We investigated the effect of the addition of misoprostol (200 μg four times daily) to standard immunosuppressive therapy on the outcome of chronic rejection in a double-blind, placebo-controlled trial. Patients had to fulfill predefined histological and clinical criteria. After an entry of 40 patients into the study (22 misoprostol, 18 placebo), the inclusion of additional patients was terminated because of a high incidence of withdrawal due to adverse effects. Of the patients who used their study medication for at least 3 months (16 misoprostol, 15 placebo), graft function deterio-rated in all but 5 misoprostol-treated and all but 2 placebo-treated patients. There was no difference in dialysis-free survival. Withdrawal because of adverse effects (mainly gastrointestinal complaints) occurred in 3 cases in the placebo group and in 11 cases in the misoprostol group ($P < 0.05$). In conclusion, we found no evidence for a beneficial effect of misoprostol on the course of chronic renal allograft rejection, while use of the drug was accompanied by a high incidence of side effects.

Key words Renal transplantation · Chronic rejection · Misoprostol

Introduction

Short-term graft survival rates after renal transplantation have significantly improved in recent decades. However, chronic rejection continues to result in a steady number of late allograft failures. When graft loss due to patient death is excluded, chronic rejection is the leading cause of late allograft loss in renal transplant patients [4, 11]. The pathophysiological mechanisms leading to chronic rejection are not clear. There is ample evidence that the immunological response plays an important role, at least in the initiation of vascular injury that ultimately results in luminal obliteration [6, 12]. In recent years, non-immunological factors such as ischemia-reperfusion injury, reduced nephron mass, cyclosporine nephrotoxicity, hypertension, and hyperlipidemia have increasingly been implicated in the course of chronic allograft dysfunction [1, 12]. Currently, there is no effective treatment for patients with chronic rejection. Misoprostol is a synthetic prostaglandin E_1 analogue with high oral bioavailability. In animal models [3, 13] and human renal transplantation [7], misoprostol has been demonstrated to possess immunosuppressive properties. In addition, misoprostol was shown to protect against ischemic and toxic renal injury [8, 9] and to improve renal allograft function [7]. On the basis of these results, we initiated a randomized prospective trial to investigate the efficacy of misoprostol for the treatment of chronic rejection in renal transplant recipients.

Table 1 Clinical characteristics of patients at entry into the study. Numerical data are given as medians with ranges (*M/F* male/female, *CsA* cyclosporine A, *Aza* azathioprine, *Pred* prednisone)

		Misoprostol ($n = 22$)	Placebo ($n = 18$)
Sex (M/F)		17/5	10/8
Age (years)		43 (26–61)	45 (18–68)
First/second graft		17/5	12/6
Time after transplantation (months)		41 (13–194)	62 (12–147)
Baseline immunosuppressive therapy:	CsA + Pred	8	5
	CsA + Aza	1	0
	CsA + Aza + Pred	3	2
	Aza + Pred	10	11
Creatinine clearance (ml/min)		34 (10–60)	30 (11–68)
Proteinuria (g/l)		1.9 (0–7.4)	2.6 (0.1–8.8)
Mean arterial pressure (mm Hg)		113 (100–143)	116 (92–147)
Number of antihypertensive drugs		2 (0–3)	2 (0–3)

Patients and methods

Patient population

Forty adult renal tansplant patients with chronic rejection were recruited from three Dutch transplantation centers between December 1991 and February 1994. Patients were eligible for this study if a graft biopsy showed the presence of arterial intimal fibrosis and/or chronic transplant glomerulopathy. All biopsies were examined by one pathologist (K. A.). Moreover, one or both of the following clinical criteria had to be met for inclusion into the study: (a) an increase of serum creatinine by more than 15 % during the last 6 months and (b) the presence of proteinuria of at least 1 g/l for at least 2 months. Other reasons for an increase in serum creatinine, such as ureteral obstruction, cyclosporine nephrotoxicity, or changes in medication, had to be ruled out as much as possible. Patients with histological signs of a recurrence of the original kidney disease in the graft or with signs of acute rejection were excluded. Additional exclusion criteria were diabetes mellitus, pregnancy, prior malignancy, signs of cerebrovascular insufficiency, and angina pectoris or myocardial infarction during the preceding 6 months.

Study design

After they had given informed consent, patients were randomized to receive 200 µg misoprostol or matching placebo tablets four times daily, at meal times and before bedtime. The study was carried out in a double-blind fashion. Treatment was continued for 2 years or until the start of renal replacement therapy if this preceded the end of the treatment period. The reasons for premature withdrawal of a patient from the study were intractable side effects supposed to be caused by the study medication, changes in baseline immunosuppressive therapy (other than changes in dosage), start of an ACE inhibitor, and the occurrence of angina pectoris, myocardial infarction, or cerebrovascular insufficiency. The study protocol was approved by the ethics committees of the participating hospitals.

Analysis

Clinical and laboratory examinations were carried out as part of routine posttransplant patient care. Creatinine clearance was estimated according to the formula of Cockcroft and Gault. In patients with a duration of treatment exceeding 3 months, impairment of renal function was defined as a decrease in creatinine clearance of at least 5 % at the end of the follow-up, whereas an increase in proteinuria was defined as a rise in proteinuria of at least 0.5 g/day or 0.2 g/l. Based on the assumption that with misoprostol the frequency of impairment of renal function and/or increase of proteinuria would be reduced by 15 % or more, 100 patients should be enrolled to have an 80 % chance of detecting a difference between the study groups. However, patient enrolment appeared to lag expectations. Moreover, many patients had to be withdrawn from the study because of adverse effects. We, therefore, decided to end patient recruitment after inclusion of 40 patients and to analyze the data after a minimum duration of follow-up of the remaining patients of 1 year.

Results are given as medians with ranges. Between group comparisons of numerical data were carried out with Wilcoxon's rank-sum test. Proportions were compared by chi-squared analysis. Probabilities of survival were calculated by the Kaplan-Meier product-limit method and for comparison of survival curves the log-rank test was used. A P value less than 0.05 was considered statistically significant.

Results

Of the 40 study participants, 7 were included because of a rise in serum creatinine, 12 because of proteinuria, and 21 patients fulfilled both clinical inclusion criteria. There were no significant differences in clinical characteristics of the patients in the misoprostol and placebo group (Table 1). Median duration of treatment with study medication was 3.5 months (1–21) and 6.5 months (0–24) in the misoprostol and placebo group, respectively (NS). The tendency to a shorter duration of treatment in the misoprostol group was related to a higher frequency of withdrawal due to adverse effects (Table 2). In 6 of the 11 patients in whom misoprostol was discontinued because of adverse effects, treatment with a lower dosage had also appeared to be unsuccessful. The incidences of patient death, start of dialysis, impairment of renal function, and increase in proteinuria did not differ between the groups (Table 3). Estimated dial-

Table 2 Reasons for premature withdrawal from the study

	Misoprostol	Placebo	P
Intractable side effects	11 (50 %)	3 (17 %)	0.03
Change in base-line immunosuppression	1 (5 %)	1 (6 %)	NS
Start of an ACE inhibitor	0	2 (11 %)	NS
Patient ends cooperation	2 (9 %)	2 (11 %)	NS

Table 3 Patient survival, graft function, and proteinuria

	Misoprostol ($n = 22$)	Placebo ($n = 18$)
Patient death	1 (5 %)	3 (17 %)
Graft failure	5 (23 %)	6 (33 %)
Impairment of renal function (including graft failure)[a]	11/16 (69 %)	13/15 (87 %)
Increase of proteinuria[a,b]	6/15 (40 %)	6/12 (50 %)

[a] In patients receiving study medication for at least 3 months
[b] Insufficient data in 4 patients

ysis-free survival at 1 year after the start of treatment was 60 % in the misoprostol group and 84 % in the placebo-treated patients (Fig. 1, NS). Sixteen misoprostol-treated patients and 7 patients receiving the placebo experienced one or more adverse effects ($P = 0.03$). The incidence of all side effects is given in Table 4.

Discussion

Our data do not indicate a favorable effect of misoprostol on the course of chronic rejection after renal transplantation. We recognize, however, that the small numbers of subjects and the short duration of follow-up do not allow for firm conclusions. This study was initiated after the promising results of Moran et al. [7] had been published. Since then, other trials have not confirmed the beneficial effect of misoprostol on acute rejection incidence and renal function after renal transplantation [2, 10, 14]. Taken together, there is no strong evidence for additive immunosuppressive efficacy of misoprostol in renal transplant recipients.

The high incidence of adverse effects, mostly of the gastrointestinal tract, was responsible for a substantial

Table 4 Adverse effects (The figure in brackets indicates the number of cases in which the particular side effect was the main reason for discontinuation of study medication)

	Misoprostol ($n = 22$)	Placebo ($n = 18$)
Diarrhea	10 (5)	4 (1)
Dyspepsia/nausea	10 (2)	5 (2)
Abdominal pain	4 (1)	2
Hypermenorrhoe	2 (2)	–
Infections necessitating hospitalization	1	2
Other	2 (1)	2

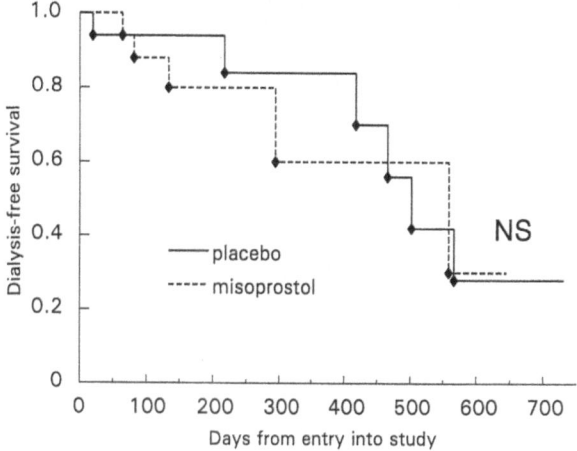

Fig. 1 Proportion of patients free of dialysis

drop-out rate in the misoprostol group. Similar frequencies of side effects have been observed in other studies applying the same dosage of 800 µg/day [7, 14]. Although the side effects of misoprostol appear to be dose dependent [5], many of our patients who had to discontinue the drug did not tolerate a lower dosage either (data not shown). Based on the questionable immunosuppressive efficacy and the high rate of complications, we believe that further studies on the potential of misoprostol to influence the course of chronic rejection are not warranted.

Acknowledgements Searle Nederland B. V., Maarssen, The Netherlands, is gratefully acknowledged for providing the study medication.

References

1. Bia MJ (1995) Nonimmunologic causes of late renal graft loss. Kidney Int 47: 1470–1480

2. Curtis LD, Anwar N, Briggs JD, Buckels JA, Jones M, Karim MS, Koffman G, McGregor E, Neild G, Riad HN (1993) Misoprostol in renal transplantation. Transplant Proc 25: 602

3. Duffie GP, Romanelli RR, Ellis NK, Young MR, Wepsic HT (1988) The effects of E series prostaglandins on blastogenic responses in vitro and graft vs. host responses in vivo. Immunopharmacol Immunotoxicol 10: 597–615

4. Dunn J, Golden D, Van Buren CT, Lewis RM, Lawen J, Kahan BD (1990) Causes of graft loss beyond two years in the cyclosporine era. Transplantation 49: 349–353

5. Garris RE, Kirkwood CF (1989) Misoprostol: a prostaglandin E1 analogue. Clin Pharm 8: 627–644

6. Hostetter TH (1994) Chronic transplant rejection. Kidney Int 46: 266–279

7. Moran M, Mozes MF, Maddux MS, Veremis S, Bartkus C, Ketel B, Pollak R, Wallemark C, Jonasson O (1990) Prevention of acute graft rejection by the prostaglandin E1 analogue misoprostol in renal-transplant recipients treated with cyclosporine and prednisone. N Engl J Med 322: 1183–1188

8. Paller MS (1988) Effects of the prostaglandin E1 analog misoprostol on cyclosporine nephrotoxicity. Transplantation 45: 1126–1131

9. Paller MS, Manivel JC (1992) Prostaglandins protect kidneys against ischemic and toxic injury by a cellular effect. Kidney Int 42: 1345–1354

10. Pouteil Noble C, Chapuis F, Berra N, Hadj Aissa A, Lacavalerie B, Lefrancois N, Martin X, Touraine JL (1994) Misoprostol in renal transplant recipients: a prospective, randomized, controlled study on the prevention of acute rejection episodes and cyclosporin A nephrotoxicity. Nephrol Dial Transplant 9: 552–555

11. Schweitzer EJ, Matas AJ, Gillingham KJ, Payne WD, Gores PF, Dunn DL, Sutherland DE, Najarian JS (1991) Causes of renal allograft loss. Progress in the 1980s, challenges for the 1990s. Ann Surg 214: 679–688

12. Tullius SG, Tilney NL (1995) Both alloantigen-dependent and -independent factors influence chronic allograft rejection. Transplantation 59: 313–318

13. Wiederkehr JC, Dumble L, Pollak R, Moran M (1990) Immunosuppressive effect of misoprostol: a new synthetic prostaglandin E1 analogue. Aust N Z J Surg 60: 121–124

14. Wilkie ME, Beer JC, Newman D, Raftery MJ, Marsh FP (1992) Evidence that the risks of misoprostol outweigh its benefits in stable cyclosporine-treated renal allograft recipients. Transplantation 54: 565–567

Transpl Int (1996) 9 [Suppl 1]: S45–S48
© Springer-Verlag 1996

S. Tanabe
M. Ueda
Y.-S. Han
T. Nakatani
T. Kishimoto
S. Suzuki
H. Amemiya

Increased tenascin expression is an early feature of the development of transplant renal arteriopathy in humans

S. Tanabe · Y.-S. Han · T. Nakatani ·
T. Kishimoto
Department of Urology, Osaka City
University Medical School, Osaka, Japan

M. Ueda (✉)
Department of Pathology, Osaka City
University Medical School, 1-4-54,
Asahi-machi, Abeno-ku, Osaka, Japan
Tel. +81 66 45 20 41; Fax 46 30 93

S. Suzuki · H. Amemiya
National Children's Medical Research
Center, Tokyo, Japan

Abstract Transplant renal arteriopathy (TRA) is a major obstacle to the long-term survival of human renal allografts. Tenascin (TN) is an extracellular matrix glycoprotein associated with cell growth and differentiation. We investigated TN expression in intrarenal arteries with TRA, in association with cellular components, with phenotypic expression of smooth muscle cells (SMC) and with fibronectin expression. Ten renal allografts that had been removed due to rejection were available. Monoclonal antibodies against SMC, macrophages, T cells, B cells, fibronectin, and TN were used. In the early stages, medial SMC showed a de-differentiated phenotype and the neointima consisted largely of T cells and macrophages. At these stages, increased expression of TN was observed in the media. In later stages, the neointima consisted almost entirely of SMC of a differentiated phenotype and no TN expression was found. Up-regulation of TN may play a role in the migration and phenotypic modulation of SMC at an early stage of TRA in humans.

Key words Tenascin · Transplant renal arteriopathy · Smooth muscle cell · Phenotype · Fibronectin

Introduction

Transplant renal arteriopathy (TRA) is a major obstacle to the long-term survival of human renal allografts. TRA has been characterized histologically by concentric intimal thickening that induces severe luminal narrowing [1]. Our previous studies using immunocytochemical techniques have shown that the thickened intima of TRA basically consists of macrophages, T cells, and smooth muscle cells, although a change in the cellular composition occurs during the evolution of TRA [2, 3]. Recently, we have also revealed that enhanced expression of fibronectin, which is one of the major extracellular matrix glycoproteins, is associated with the development of TRA in human renal allografts [3].

Tenascin is a more recently isolated extracellular matrix glycoprotein associated with remodeling events during embryogenesis and pathological processes [4–7]. Experimental studies have shown that tenascin may play a role in the migration and proliferation of vascular smooth muscle cells [8, 9]. Thus far, however, little is known about tenascin expression in the development of TRA in humans. Therefore, we have focused on the expression of tenascin in intrarenal arteries with TRA, in association with a change in the cellular composition, and with phenotypic expression of smooth muscle cells related to the interval after transplantation. In addition, we have also investigated a difference in the expression between fibronectin and tenascin during the evolution of TRA in human renal allografts.

Materials and methods

This study is based on ten renal allografts that were removed due to rejection. In these patients, intervals between transplantation and removal of the allografts ranged from 1 month to 4 years. Table 1 gives the relevant clinical data of the patients. Arteries in ten normal renal tissues were also examined as controls.

After fixation in methanol-Carnoy's fixative (60 % methanol, 30 % chloroform, and 10 % glacial acetic acid), tissue blocks were

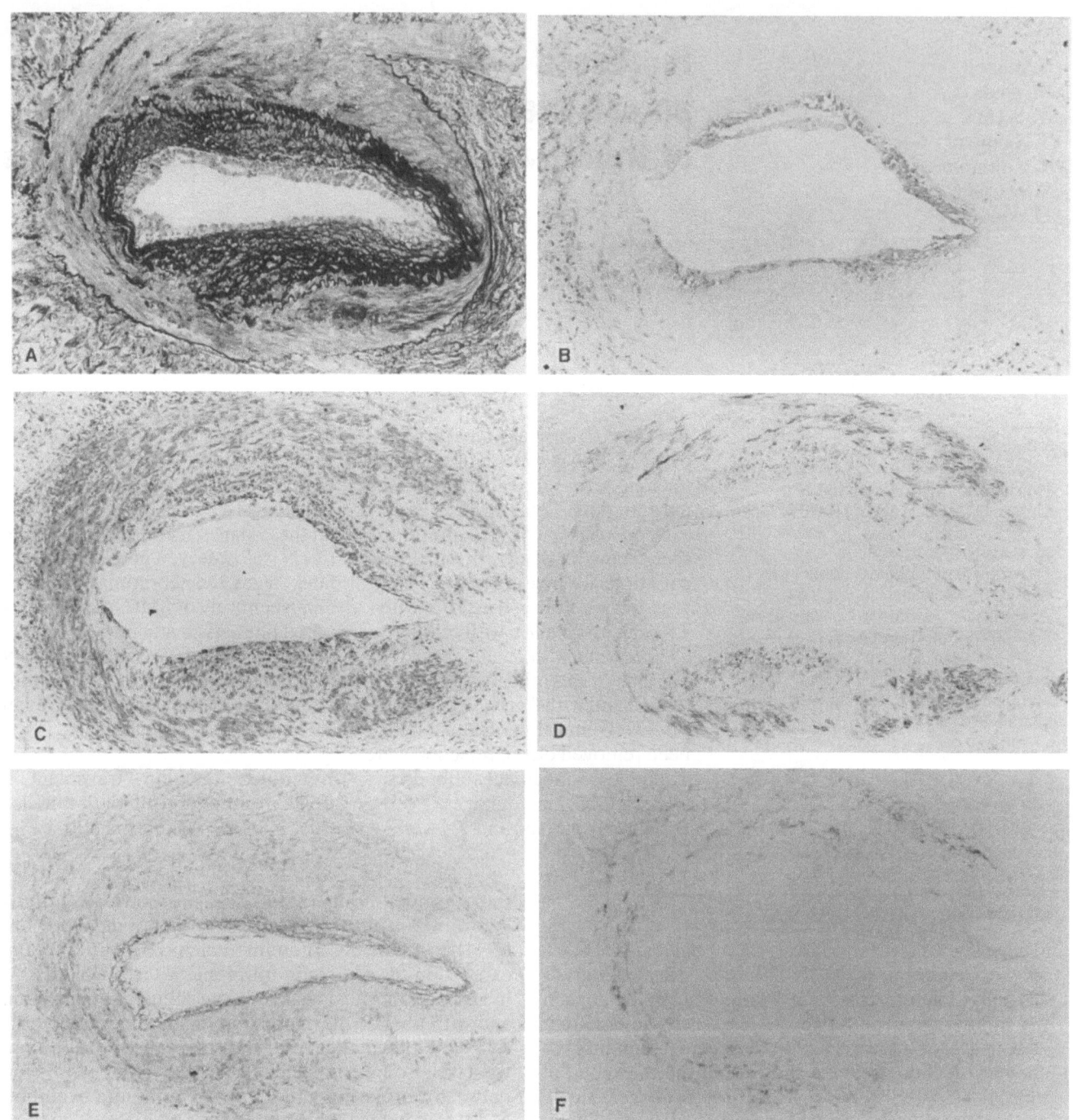

Fig. 1 A–F Intrarenal artery with transplant renal arteriopathy (TRA), 1 month after transplantation. **A** Weigert's elastic van Gieson' stain. **B** Anti-macrophage antibody, HAM 56. **C** Anti-vi-mentin antibody. **D** Anti-smooth muscle cell actin antibody, CGA-7. **E** Anti-fibronectin antibody. **F** Anti-tenascin antibody

obtained from each transplanted or normal kidney and embedded in paraffin. Thirty serial sections, 5 μm thick, were cut from each block. Every first, second, and third section was stained with hema-toxylin and eosin, Weigert's elastic van Gieson's, and periodic acid-Schiff stain, respectively. The other sections were used for immu-nohistochemical staining.

The monoclonal antibodies used were as follows: anti-smooth muscle cell actin antibody, CGA-7; anti-vimentin anti-body; anti-macrophage antibody, HAM 56; anti-T cell antibody, UCHL1; anti-B cell antibody, L26; anti-fibronectin antibody; and anti-tenascin antibody. The labeled streptavidin-biotin com-plex system with nickel chloride color modification was per-

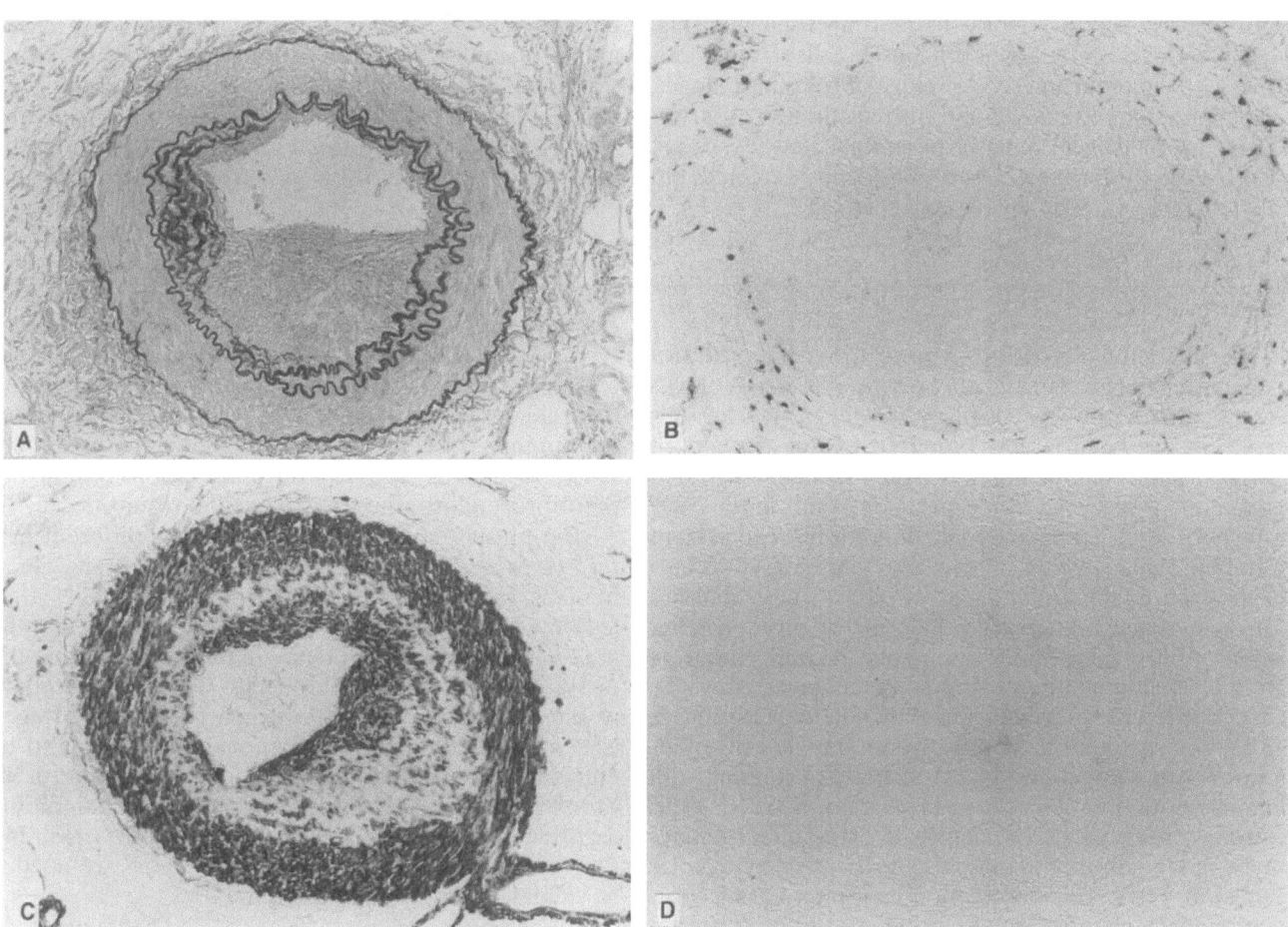

Fig. 2 A–D Intrarenal artery with TRA, 5 months after transplantation. **A** Weigert's elastic van Gieson's stain. **B** Anti-macrophage antibody, HAM 56. **C** Anti-smooth muscle cell actin antibody, CGA-7. **D** Anti-tenascin antibody

Table 1 Relevant clinical data

Case number	Age (years)	Sex	Interval between transplant and hemodialysis (months)	Interval between transplant and nephrectomy (months)
1	37	M	–	1
2	43	F	–	2
3	37	F	–	2
4	27	F	3	4
5	37	F	3	4
6	17	F	2	5
7	49	F	18	31
8	41	M	27	39
9	43	M	28	40
10	32	F	53	54

formed in all instances. Sections were counterstained with methyl green.

Results

In the arteries of the normal kidneys, medial smooth muscle cells stained positive with both vimentin and CGA-7. In these arteries, no expression of fibronectin and tenascin was observed. In transplanted kidneys, TRA was found in all instances, frequently in the interlobular and arcuate arteries. In the early stages of TRA, 1 or 2 months after transplantation, medial smooth muscle cells of intrarenal arteries with TRA showed a marked loss in staining with anti-smooth muscle cell actin marker, CGA-7 (Fig. 1 A–D). The neointima consisted largely of T cells and macrophages, intermixed with some spindle-shaped cells (Fig. 1 B,C). These spindle-shaped cells stained positive with vimentin, but negative with CGA-7 (Fig. 1 C, D). At these stages, the media and preexistent intima showed increased expression of both fibronectin and tenascin (Fig. 1 E, F). In contrast, the neointima stained positive with fibronectin, but negative with tenascin (Fig. 1 E, F).

In later stages of TRA, from 4 months onward, the staining density with CGA-7 in the media of intrarenal arteries was almost restored (Fig. 2 A-C). The neointima consisted almost entirely of smooth muscle cells, intermixed with only a few T cells and macrophages (Fig. 2 B, C). The neointimal smooth muscle cells stained positive with vimentin and CGA-7 (Fig. 2 C). At these stages, no expression of tenascin and fibronectin was observed in the media (Fig. 2 D). In the neointima, however, weak expression of fibronectin was occasionally detected, but no tenascin expression was found (Fig. 2 D).

Discussion

The extracellular matrix is known to be important in regulating the growth and phenotypic expression of vascular smooth muscle cells [8, 9]. However, thus far, this concept has been largely based on findings in experimental animals. Our previous study has demonstrated that enhanced fibronectin expression occurs in the early stages of TRA in human renal allografts [3]. The present study provides further information that tenascin is also expressed in the early stages of TRA. These findings strongly suggest that extracellular matrix glycoproteins, at least fibronectin and tenascin, play an important role in the development of neointima in human arteries.

The present study documents that, in the early stages after transplantation, medial smooth muscle cells of arteries with TRA showed a distinct loss in staining with anti-smooth muscle cell actin marker, CGA-7. This strongly suggests that a change in cytoskeletal phenotype of medial smooth muscle cells occurred at an early stage of TRA. This observation is of interest since our immunocytochemical study, using the same anti-actin marker CGA-7, on human coronary arteries after angioplasty injury has demonstrated that de-differentiation of medial smooth muscle cells, as revealed by a marked loss in staining with CGA-7, is a fundamental change preceding neointimal formation in humans [10]. The present findings show that a similar phenomenon occurs during the development of TRA in human renal allografts. Furthermore, the present study also demonstrated that an increased expression of both fibronectin and tenascin in the media in the early stages of TRA is closely related to the change in the cytoskeletal phenotype of medial smooth muscle cells. Experimental studies have reported that the expression of fibronectin and tenascin by vascular smooth muscle cells is a marker for the immature, or de-differentiated state, of smooth muscle cells [8, 9, 11, 12]. Our observations in humans, therefore, endorse these experimental results.

The present study, moreover, shows a different pattern of expression between fibronectin and tenascin in humans. In arteries with TRA in the early stages after transplantation, tenascin was distinctly expressed in the media, but there was no tenascin expression within the neointima. In contrast, fibronectin was expressed both in the media and in the neointima in the early stages. The interpretation of this phenomenon remains to be elucidated, but could relate to different roles of fibronectin and tenascin in cell attachment and migration, as previously shown in experimental studies [13, 14]. Obviously, further studies with more cases are needed to validate the present observations.

References

1. Hume DM, Merrill JP, Miller BF, Thorn GW (1955) Experiences with renal homotransplantation in the human: Report of nine cases. J Clin Invest 34: 327–382
2. Han Y-S, Ueda M, Tanabe S, Nakatani T, Kishimoto T, Suzuki S, Amemiya H (1994) Immunocytochemical analysis of obliterative arteriopathy of human renal allografts. Transplant Proc 26: 931–934
3. Tanabe S, Ueda M, Han Y-S, Nakatani T, Kishimoto T, Suzuki S, Amemiya H (1995) Enhanced fibronectin expression is associated with the development of graft arteriosclerosis in human renal allografts. Transplant Proc 27: 1078–1081
4. Chiquet M, Fambrough DM (1984 a) Chick myotendinous antigen. I. A monoclonal antibody as a marker for tendon and muscle morphogenesis. J Cell Biol 98: 1926–1936
5. Chiquet M, Fambrough DM (1984 b) Chick myotendinous antigen. II. A novel extracellular glycoprotein complex consisting of large disulfide-linked subunits. J Cell Biol 98: 1937–1946
6. Chiquet-Ehrismann R, Mackie EJ, Pearson CA, Sakakura T (1986) Tenascin: an extracellular matrix protein involved in tissue interactions during fetal development and oncogenesis. Cell 47: 131–139
7. Mackie EJ, Halfter W, Liverani D (1988) Induction of tenascin in healing wounds. J Cell Biol 107: 2757–2767
8. Hedin U, Holm J, Hansson GK (1991) Induction of tenascin in rat arterial injury: Relationship to altered smooth muscle cell. Am J Pathol 139: 649–656
9. Mackie EJ, Scott-Burden T, Hahn AWA, Kern F, Bernhardt J, Regenass S, Weller A, Bühler FR (1992) Expression of tenascin by vascular smooth muscle cells. Am J Pathol 141: 377–388
10. Ueda M, Becker AE, Naruko T, Kojima A (1995) Smooth muscle cell de-differentiation is a fundamental change preceding wound healing after percutaneous transluminal coronary angioplasty in humans. Coron Artery Dis 6: 71–81
11. Hedin U, Thyberg J (1987) Plasma fibronectin promotes modulation of arterial smooth-muscle cells from contractile to synthetic phenotype. Differentiation 33: 239–246
12. Hedin U, Sjölund M, Hultgardh-Nilsson A, Thyberg J (1990) Changes in expression and organization of smooth-muscle-specific α-actin during fibronectin-mediated modulation of arterial smooth muscle cell phenotype. Differentiation 44: 222–231
13. Chiquet-Ehrismann R, Kalla P, Pearson CA, Beck K, Chiquet M (1988) Tenascin interferes with fibronectin action. Cell 53: 383–390
14. Chiquet-Ehrismann R (1990) What distinguishes tenascin from fibronectin? FASEB J 4: 2598–2604

Transpl Int (1996) 9 [Suppl 1]: S 49–S 53
© Springer-Verlag 1996

A. Bersztel
J. Wadström
G. Tufveson
G. Gannedahl
M. Bengtsson
C. Bergström
L. Frödin
K. Claesson
B. Wikström
J. Wahlberg

Is kidney transplantation in sensitized recipients justified?

A. Bersztel (✉) · J. Wadström · G. Tufveson
G. Gannedahl · C. Bergström · L. Frödin ·
K. Claesson · J. Wahlberg
Department of Transplantation Surgery,
University Hospital, S-751 85 Uppsala,
Sweden

M. Bengtsson
Department of Clinical Immunology,
University Hospital, Uppsala, Sweden

B. Wikström
Department of Nephrology,
University Hospital, Uppsala, Sweden

Abstract The objective of the study was to determine if it is justified to use the scarce resources of cadaveric kidneys on HLA-sensitized patients, by reviewing the initial and long-term outcome of cadaveric renal transplantation at Uppsala University Hospital, Sweden. Between January 1988 and December 1994, 402 renal transplantations were performed. The patients were divided into one group of sensitized recipients (peak panel antibody reactivity $\geq 25\%$; $n = 84$) and a second of non-sensitized recipients (panel reactive antibodies $< 25\%$; $n = 318$). The groups were comparable in terms of recipient and donor age, gender, HLA-A, -B and -DR mismatches and numbers of diabetics. None of the sensitized patients received a six-antigen-matched kidney. For the non-sensitized group, life table analysis showed a 1-year actuarial graft survival (GS) of 91.8 % and a 4-year GS of 84.4 %. The corresponding GSs for the sensitized group were 79.9 % and 68.7 %, respectively ($P < 0.01$). The statistical significance vanished if patients with primary non-function were excluded. When excluding donors above 55 years of age, kidneys with cold ischemia time above 20 h, and two-antigen (HLA-DR) mismatches, there was no detectable difference between the non-sensitized and sensitized groups at 1-year or 4-year GS. Although there is a statistical significance in GS between non-sensitized and sensitized recipients of a kidney transplant, this does not differ from other risk groups such as diabetics, rheumatoid disease sufferers or elderly recipients. We therefore conclude that the sensitized patient should be accepted on the waiting list for a kidney transplant and that it is worthwhile to do the utmost to transplant this category of patients. Our data indicate that kidney GS in sensitized recipients is more affected by negative risk factors such as older donors, long cold ischemia time and two-antigen HLA-DR mismatch, than the non-sensitized recipient. To improve the outcome, those negative factors should be avoided or reduced.

Key words Kidney transplantation · Graft survival · Immunization

Introduction

With the increasing shortage of cadaveric kidneys, the accumulation of patients on the waiting list for kidney transplantation is becoming a critical problem. One possibility of reducing this problem would be to limit the opportunity of a transplant to any individual that stands an increased risk of a reduced graft survival. A group that could be targeted by such a policy is sensitized patients, with panel reactive antibodies (PRA), who are steadily increasing in numbers on waiting lists for kidney transplantation in Europe and North America [2].

Table 1 Demographic data, expressed as mean with standard deviation when appropriate or percentage of population. (*PRA* Panel reactive antibodies, *NS* not significant)

	Peak PRA < 25 %	Peak PRA ≥ 25 %	P
n	318	84	
Time on waiting list (months)	8.8 ± 6.1	11.7 ± 7.8	< 0.01
Gender			
Female	40.3 %	44.0 %	NS
Male	59.7 %	56.0 %	NS
Age (years)	48.2 ± 12.7	44.3 ± 12.8	NS
Retransplant	8.5 %	59.2 %	< 0.01
Cold ischemia time (min)	1030 ± 366	1119 ± 302	< 0.05
Donor age (years)	44.5 ± 16.5	44.1 ± 17.1	NS
Mismatch HLA-A, -B, -DR	4.3 ± 1.4	4.2 ± 1.3	NS
Mismatch HLA-DR	1.4 ± 0.7	1.4 ± 0.7	NS
Six-antigen matched	2.2 %	0 %	
Two-DR antigen matched	11.3 %	13.1 %	NS
Diabetes	25.2 %	19.0 %	NS
Number of blood transfusions prior to transplant	4.3 ± 10.8	11.6 ± 17.9	< 0.01

A decision to exclude a group of patients from the potential benefit of a kidney transplantation due to any level of PRA would be highly controversial. The influence on graft survival of an increase in PRA levels has not been fully determined. Both inferior and equal results compared with the outcome for non-sensitized recipients have been reported [7, 8, 10, 15]. However, it is undisputed that sensitized recipients pose a problem in finding a suitable cross-matched negative donor [9, 10], which prolongs their time on the waiting list.

At our unit we have always had a positive and aggressive policy of accepting sensitized patients on the waiting list for a kidney transplant. The controversial question mentioned earlier has also been raised at our centre, and therefore we were interested in a retrospective evaluation of our present policy, in particular, bearing in mind that we are facing a decline in the frequency of cadaveric donors.

In this paper we have defined the sensitized group as having a historical or current PRA value of 25 % or higher, since this group was found to have a prolonged time on the waiting list.

Materials and methods

Between January 1988 and December 1994, a total of 402 cadaveric renal transplantations were performed. Recipients were divided into two groups: the sensitized group, with peak PRA reacting to at least 25 % of the cells, consisted of 84 patients, and the other consisted of 318 patients who were considered to be non-sensitized. The PRA reactivity was measured by testing the recipient serum against a panel of lymphocytes from 24 different blood donors. This panel was selected to cover the most common HLA anti-

gens. A panel cell was considered positive if a cytotoxic activity could be detected by the NIH technique.

Most of the kidneys were harvested locally. A few were obtained through the kidney exchange program from other centres in Scandinavia, allocated by Scandiatransplant [5]. However, none of the sensitized patients received a six-antigen-matched kidney.

All patients were treated with a cyclosporine-based immunosuppressive protocol and had a negative current serum cytotoxic T-cell cross-match. Twenty patients, who where either considered as highly sensitized (PRA > 50 %) or had had a prolonged time on the waiting list, were included in a pretransplant program consisting of plasmapheresis aimed at decreasing their PRA levels [1]. In patients with delayed onset of graft function, the cyclosporine treatment was temporarily halted and substituted with anti-lymphocyte globulin (ALG). Rejections were initially treated with Solu-Medrol and, if resistant, with anti-thymocyte globulin (ATG) or OKT-3.

The two groups were comparable in terms of recipient and donor age, recipient and donor gender, HLA-A, -B and -DR mismatches, and whether the kidney was harvested locally or shipped. The sensitized group had a significantly longer time on the waiting list, longer cold ischemia time, a higher proportion of retransplants, and more blood transfusion before transplantation (Table 1). Actuarial graft survival was computed using the Kaplan-Meyer life table method, where patient death was handled as lost to follow-up. For comparison, an overall graft survival was calculated in the same manner but managing patient death as graft loss instead. In reality, none of the patients were actually recorded as lost to follow-up. Statistical analysis was performed using the Student *t*-test for comparison of groups and the Cox-Mantel log-rank test for evaluation of Kaplan-Meyer survival tables, utilizing the Winstat software package.

Table 2 Results, expressed as mean with standard deviation when appropriate or percentage of population

	Peak PRA < 25 %	Peak PRA ≥ 25 %	P
n	318	84	
Number of rejections	1.1 ± 1.1	1.0 ± 1.3	NS
Free from rejections	40.9 %	46.4 %	NS
First rejection within 1 month	44.5 %	34.5 %	NS
No onset	2.5 %	8.3 %	< 0.05
Graft lost within 1 month (no-onset excluded)	6.3 %	7.2 %	NS
Delayed onset (no-onset excluded)	19.0 %	28.6 %	NS
Actuarial graft survival, 1 year	91.8 %	79.9 %	
Actuarial graft survival, 4 years	84.4 %	68.7 %	
Overall graft survival, 1 year	82.0 %	70.1 %	
Overall graft survival, 4 years	65.9 %	54.2 %	
Creatinine at 1 year	160 ± 74 (n = 216)	162 ± 82 (n = 48)	NS
Creatinine at 4 years	153 ± 63 (n = 97)	120 ± 38 (n = 27)	< 0.05

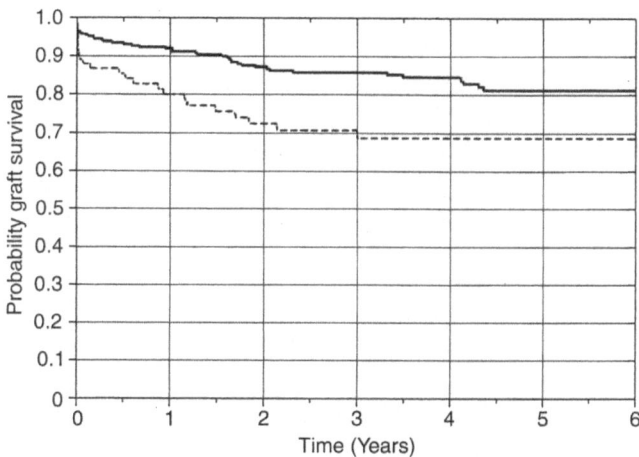

Fig. 1 Actuarial graft survival. (*Solid line* non-sensitized, *dotted line* sensitized, $P < 0.01$)

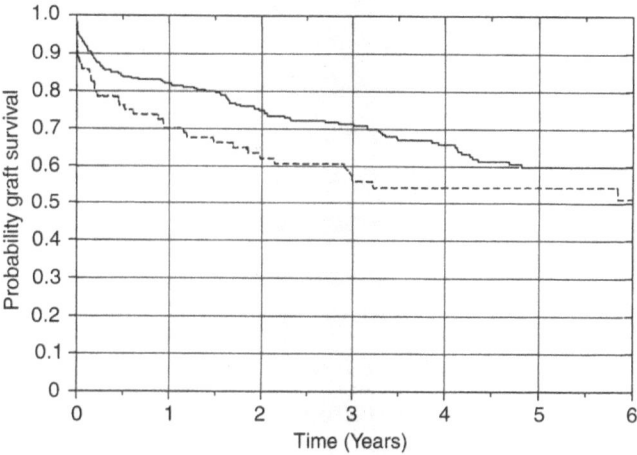

Fig. 2 The overall graft survival for cadaveric grafts. (*Solid line* non-sensitized, *dotted line* sensitized, $P = 0.06$)

Results

The non-sensitized group had significantly higher actuarial 1-year and 4-year graft survivals than did the sensitized group (Table 2, Fig. 1). Looking at the overall graft survival and including patient death as graft loss, a similar difference was obtained (Fig. 2), although without statistical significance.

When looking at graft outcome in the sensitized patients, the only significant negative factor was donor age below 55 years. Cold ischemia time above 20 h and DR antigen mismatch tended to have an influence on graft survival but was not significant. Recipients over 65 years, gender, PRA > 50 %, and total antigen mismatch did not significantly affect the outcome. We have calculated overall graft survival in our patients, excluding donors over 55 years, kidneys with longer cold ischemia time than 20 h, and two-antigen DR mismatch.

The overall graft survival between sensitized and non-sensitized groups was then almost equivalent (Table 3). Neither the rejection frequency nor the percentage of patients free from rejection or frequency of early rejections varied between sensitized and non-sensitized groups. Also, creatinine levels at 1 year were fully comparable, but at the 4-year follow-up the sensitized group had significantly better values.

In the sensitized group, grafts with no onset (i. e., never functioning) were strikingly more frequent, this difference also accounted for an increase in early loss of graft. Delayed graft function was also more apparent in the sensitized population. Analysis of grafts which never functioned among the sensitized patients showed that all but one were totally DR antigen mismatched. The cold ischemia time tended to be longer and donors tended to be older in the no-onset group, although not significantly. An interesting finding was that the no-on-

Table 3 Comparison of overall graft survival (%) when excluding patients with negative factors for graft outcome

	Non-sensitized, 1 year	Sensitized, 1 year	Non-sensitized, 4 years	Sensitized, 4 years
Total	82.0	70.1	65.9	54.2
Excluding no-onset	84.1	76.5	67.6	59.1
Excluding donors over 55 years	85.2	79.3	71.1	61.7
Excluding cold ischemia time over 20 h	84.2	75.0	66.0	59.5
Excluding two-DR antigen mismatch	80.0	78.5	66.6	64.8
Excluding donors over 55 years, cold ischemia time over 20 h, two-DR antigen mismatch	84.3	81.2	72.7	72.4

Table 4 Sensitized patients grouped on the basis of functioning or no-onset (primary non-function) grafts

	Functioning graft	No onset	
n	77	7	
Age (years)	44.1 ± 12.9	46.5 ± 11.9	NS
Retransplant	70.1 %	57.1 %	NS
Donor age (years)	42.9 ± 17.1	56.8 ± 11.8	< 0.05
Cold ischemia time (min)	1100 ± 284	1332 ± 420	0.05
Patients with peak PRA above 50 %	33.8 %	28.6 %	NS
Kidneys received via exchange program	28.6 %	42.9 %	NS
Peak PRA (T-cell, %)	59.2 ± 22.2	56.0 ± 24.7	NS
Latest PRA (T-cell, %)	27.0 ± 24.0	41.7 ± 32.5	NS
Change in PRA peak, latest (% PTA)	− 32.2 ± 24.7	− 14.3 ± 12.9	0.06
Mismatch HLA-A, -B, -DR	4.2 ± 1.2	4.1 ± 1.9	NS
Mismatch HLA-DR	1.3 ± 0.7	1.7 ± 0.8	NS

Table 5 Comparison of overall graft survival (%) for different risk groups

	One year	Four years
All ($n = 402$)	79.5	63.4
Sensitized ($n = 84$)	70.1	54.2
Diabetic ($n = 96$)	79.1	55.1
Systemic lupus erythematosus, rheumatoid arthritis ($n = 18$)	54.3	43.5
Recipient over 65 years ($n = 31$)	77.4	48.7

set group, despite similar peak PRA% as the functioning graft group, displayed different PRA% in current serum (Table 4).

In a subgroup consisting of 20 patients treated with plasmapheresis pretransplantation, we found significantly higher peak PRA levels than in the rest of the sensitized group. Three grafts (15 %) never functioned and a total of five (25 %) was lost within 1 month. The delayed graft function rate was 35 %. This treatment did reveal an overall graft survival at 1 year of 65 % and at 4 years of 57 %.

Discussion

The question of denying a sensitized patient the opportunity of a kidney transplant is highly controversial. In the literature, most reports published show a trend or significance for a better graft survival in the non-sensitized population [2, 8, 14]. Our own results, with an overall 1-year graft survival of 70.1 % for sensitized compared to 82.0 % for non-sensitized recipients are not significantly lower. Although the numerical difference cannot be ignored, the figures are not dramatically lower than for other risk groups such as diabetic patients, rheumatoid disease sufferers and the elderly (Table 5). The difference noted at 1 year in comparison with other risk groups is often diminished at 4 years due to the higher mortality in the other groups. We conclude that our previous liberal policy of accepting sensitized patients on the waiting list for kidney transplantation, irrespective of the number of previous grafts, PAR levels or blood group, is justified. The aim should be, instead, to improve the result for this group of patients.

Many of the previous publications aim to justify a wider usage of exchange schemes to achieve a better HLA match. In our patients, no attempts at HLA

S53

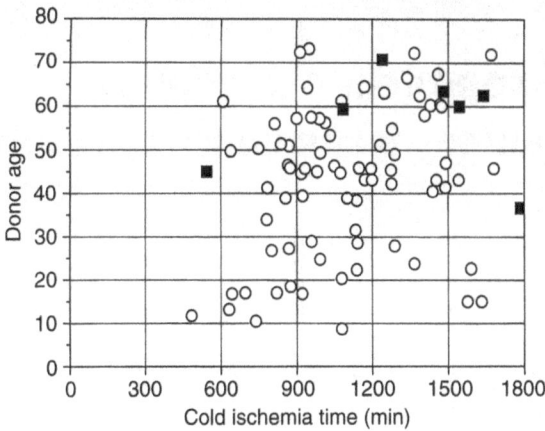

Fig. 3 Sensitized patients dependending on donor age and cold ischemia time. Grafts which never functioned are indicated by *solid boxes*, others *open circles*

matching were done (Table 1). Nevertheless, our results both for sensitized and non-sensitized groups are comparable to those of others, although the six-antigen-matched recipients reported by others show a better 1-year graft survival [12]. A policy aiming at very good matching has, however, the disadvantage of a long time on the waiting list [14] and long cold ischemia times also tend to have a negative influence on primary non-function (Fig. 3) as well as on graft survival. Therefore, a more extensive exchange program to improve HLA match does not appear to be of any advantage. One exception might be DR matching. Our results indicate that sensitized patients transplanted with two DR mismatches do worse, including a higher frequency of recipients undergoing primary non-function and lower graft survival. Thus, one way of further improving the trans-

plant results for HLA-sensitized patients would be to aim for a two-antigen DR match.

Primary non-function is one of the major problems in transplanting sensitized recipients [3]. The main cause for no-onset could be of immunological origin [4] and could therefore perhaps be prevented with better cross-matchtechniques in the future [11]. Although none of our cases showed positive B-cell cross-match or flow cytometric cross-match, we highly recommend the usage of these tests, as previous reports have shown a better graft survival [6, 13]. Another strategy for the prevention of the primary non-function, assuming the cause to be an antibody-mediated rejection, is to use an aggressive treatment with plasmapheresis and polyclonal antibodies, although we still need further evidence before recommending such a combative regime. Graft survival among sensitized recipients is more affected by negative risk factors than the normal transplant population and donors over 55 years of age present an even greater risk and, if possible, should be avoided.

In summary, this retrospective review of our experience employing a liberal policy of accepting sensitized patients for kidney transplantation, has encouraged us to continue this liberal approach. The graft survival is about 10 % lower for the sensitized cohort, which we feel is acceptable. To maintain and improve these results, the use of sensitive cross-match techniques such as flow cytometric cross-match, is highly recommended. Other factors, such as avoiding kidneys from elderly donors in this group and aiming at DR-matching kidneys, might further improve the results. Furthermore, new immunosuppressant drugs could hopefully be beneficial for this patient group and make it even more justified to freely accept HLA-sensitized patients.

References

1. Alarabi AA, Wikström B, Backman U, et al (1993) Pretransplantation immunoadsorption therapy in patients immunized with human lymphocyte antigen. Artif Organs 17: 702–707
2. Charpentier B, Hiesse C, Faycal K, et al (1992) How to deal with the hyperimmunized potential recipients. Kidney Int Suppl 38: 176–181
3. Gjertson DW (1993) Center-dependent transplantation factors. Clin Transplant: 445–468
4. Iwaki Y, Terasaki PI (1987) Primary nonfunction in human cadaver kidney transplantation: evidence for hidden hyperacute rejection. Clin Transpl 1: 125–131
5. Madsen M, Adsmussen P, Brekke I, et al (1994) Scandiatransplant year book (in press)
6. Mahoney R (1990) The flow cytometric crossmatch and early renal transplant loss. Transplantation 3: 527–535
7. Norman DJ (1991) Outcome of renal transplantation at Oregon Health Sciences University. Clin Transplant: 153–157
8. Ogura K (1992) Sensitization. Clin Transplant: 357–369
9. Opelz G (1986) Clin Transplant Newslett: June
10. Rankin GW, Wang XM, Terasaki PI (1990) Sensitization to kidney transplants. Clin Transplant: 417–424
11. Smit JA, Stark JH, Margolius, et al (1991) The relevance of more sensitive ancillary crossmatch techniques in predicting early cadaver renal graft outcome. Transpl Int 4: 77–81
12. Terasaki PI, Park MS, Takemoto S, et al (1989) Overview and epitope matching. Clin Transplant: 499–516
13. Wahlberg J, Bengtsson M, Bergström C, et al (1991) Impact of flow cytometric cross matching on the outcome of cadaveric kidney transplantation. Transpl Proc 26: 1752–1753
14. Washburn WK, Shaffer D, Conway P, et al (1959) A single-center experience with six-antigen matched kidney transplants. Arch Surg 130: 277–282
15. Zhou YC, Cecka JM (1991) Sensitization and renal transplantation. Clin Transplant: 313–323

Transpl Int (1996) 9 [Suppl 1]: S 54–S 57
© Springer-Verlag 1996

Marinus A. van den Dorpel
Hosam Ghanem
Jacqueline Rischen-Vos
Arie J. Man in 't Veld
Hans Jansen
Willem Weimar

Low-density lipoprotein oxidation is increased in kidney transplant recipients

M. A. van den Dorpel (✉)
Department of Internal Medicine I,
University Hospital Rotterdam-Dijkzigt,
Dr. Molewaterplein 40,
NL-3015 GD Rotterdam, The Netherlands
Tel. +31 10 463 34 51; Fax +31 10 436 63 72

M. A. van den Dorpel · H. Ghanem ·
J. Rischen-Vos · A. J. Man in 't Veld ·
H. Jansen · W. Weimar
Departments of Internal Medicine I and
III, University Hospital Rotterdam and
Department of Biochemistry, Erasmus
University Rotterdam, Rotterdam,
The Netherlands

Abstract Oxidative modification of low-density lipoproteins (LDL) plays an important role in the pathogenesis of atherosclerosis. In addition, there is evidence that chronic vascular allograft rejection may be mediated by oxidised LDL. Plasma lipoprotein concentrations and parameters of LDL oxidation were determined in 19 kidney transplant recipients and 19 healthy controls. Plasma triglycerides and total cholesterol was significantly higher in patients than in the controls. The mean LDL diameter was smaller in patients than in the controls (23.6 ± 0.71 nm vs 27.78 ± 1.16 nm, $P < 0.002$). Furthermore, the lag time of copper-induced in vitro LDL oxidation was shorter in patients than in the controls (101 ± 23 min vs 148 ± 81 min, $P = 0.02$). The titre and concentration of both IgG and IgM autoantibodies against malondialdehyde-modified LDL (MDA-LDL) were higher in the patients. We conclude that there is in vitro and in vivo evidence of increased LDL oxidation in renal transplant recipients. This might facilitate the progression of atherosclerosis and enhance the process of chronic vascular rejection.

Key words Kidney transplantation · Low-density lipoproteins · Atherosclerosis · Chronic vascular rejection

Introduction

The morbidity and mortality due to atherosclerotic cardiovascular disease is high in renal transplant recipients [1, 2]. Besides increased plasma lipoprotein concentrations, alterations in the composition and susceptibility to oxidation of lipoproteins may also play a role in atherosclerosis in kidney transplantation patients [2, 3]. Oxidative modification of low-density lipoproteins (LDL) probably precedes the uptake of LDL by macrophages and accelerates the accumulation of cholesterol in the arterial wall [4, 5]. In addition, oxidised LDL is highly immunogenic and elicits an inflammatory response which often accompanies atherosclerosis and closely resembles chronic vascular rejection [5–7].

The susceptibility of LDL to oxidation can be determined in vitro. A parameter for the susceptibility of LDL to oxidation is the time that elapses before lipid peroxidation products become detectable (lag time) after addition of the oxidant copper chloride [8]. The plasma concentration of autoantibodies against epitopes of oxidised LDL may also reflect in vivo LDL oxidation and appears to be correlated with the progression of atherosclerosis [9, 10].

The lipoproteins in the LDL density range are heterogeneous in size but can be separated by gel electrophoresis. If the LDL fraction contains mainly large LDL, this is designated as the LDL subclass pattern "A". The presence of mainly small LDL is indicated as the LDL subclass pattern "B" [11, 12]. The pattern B is associated with a high plasma triglyceride and a low HDL cholesterol concentration and is, partly, determined by genetic factors [11]. Subjects with the LDL subclass pattern B have an increased risk of coronary heart disease [13]. Small LDL is more prone to oxidative modification than larger LDL [14]. Therefore, the

Table 1 Patient characteristics (*Tx* transplantation, *CsA* cyclosporine A)

	Patients	Controls	P value
Male/female	13/6	13/6	NS
Age (years)	42.2 ± 12.3	47.3 ± 9.1	NS
Body mass index (kg/m^2)	24.9 ± 3.5	25.6 ± 3.1	NS
Time after Tx (months)	24 ± 5	–	–
CsA dose (mg/kg per day)	5.5 ± 1.7	–	–
Prednisone dose (mg/day)	9.6 ± 2.1	–	–
Serum creatinine (µmol/l)	154 ± 44	76 ± 9	0.05
Systolic pressure (mm Hg)	149 ± 20	139 ± 16	0.05
Diastolic pressure (mm Hg)	97 ± 14	83 ± 13	0.05

Table 2 Plasma lipid profile (mmol/l; mean ± SD)

Lipid	Patients	Controls	P value
Total cholesterol	5.91 ± 0.95	5.33 ± 0.50	0.017
Total triglyceride	2.40 ± 0.99	1.43 ± 0.65	0.001
LDL-cholesterol	3.73 ± 0.70	3.44 ± 0.44	0.13
HDL-cholesterol	1.09 ± 0.39	1.21 ± 0.23	0.28

LDL subclass pattern, the susceptibility of LDL to oxidation in vitro and the level of autoantibodies to epitopes of oxidised LDL seem to be indicators of in vivo LDL oxidation. In this study, we determined the LDL subclass pattern, the susceptibility of LDL to oxidation and the level of autoantibodies against oxidised LDL in the plasma of renal transplant recipients and matched controls.

Patients and methods

We studied 19 non-diabetic kidney transplant recipients with stable renal function and 19 matched healthy controls. At the time of blood sampling, none of the patients showed any signs of cardiovascular disease except hypertension. None of the control subjects had overt atherosclerosis or used antihypertensive drugs. Table 1 shows demographic data of patients and controls.

LDL for oxidation experiments were isolated by density gradient ultracentrifugation as described previously [15]. The plasma LDL cholesterol concentration was calculated using the Friedewald formula [16]. The LDL oxidation experiments were carried out as described by Esterbauer and our group [8, 15]. Oxidation was initiated by the addition of copper chloride solution (final concentration 1.66 µM). LDL oxidation was followed by monitoring the change in absorbance at 234 nm every 2 min for 16 h. The lag time was defined as the interval between initiation of the reaction and the intercept of the tangent to the slope of the absorbance curve with the time scale axis expressed in minutes.

The LDL subclass patterns were identified by electrophoresis on 2–16 % PAGE gels, as described by Austin et al. [13]. Concentrations of autoantibodies against malondialdehyde-modified LDL (MDA-LDL) were determined by ELISA as described previously [15]. Plasma cholesterol and triglycerides (Boehringer Mannheim, Mannheim, Germany) and creatinine (Sigma Diagnostics, St. Louis, USA) were determined using commercially avai-

lable test kits. Creatinine clearance was estimated from the plasma creatinine concentration by the Cockcroft-Gault formula. Data are presented as means ± SD. Statistical analysis was performed using Student's *T*-test or ANOVA followed by Bonferoni where appropriate. Correlations between variables were calculated using the Pearson correlation test. The level of significance was set at $P < 0.05$.

Results

Patient characteristics are shown in Table 1. Plasma triglyceride and cholesterol levels were significantly higher in renal transplant recipients than in controls (Table 2). LDL cholesterol tended to be higher in patients than in the controls. The mean size of the most prominent LDL fraction was significantly less in patients than in the controls (Table 3). The size of the LDL was inversely correlated with the plasma triglyceride ($r = -0.66$, $P < 0.001$) and weakly positively with HDL cholesterol ($r = 0.34$, $P < 0.05$). The LDL subclass pattern B was more frequently found in patients than in the controls (Table 3). The LDL subclass pattern A (mean particle diameter 25.09 ± 0.92 nm) was more frequently found in the control subjects. In kidney recipients, LDL was more susceptible to oxidation as reflected by a shorter lag time. In subjects with an LDL subclass pattern B, the lag phase was significantly shorter than in subjects with an LDL subclass pattern A (Table 3). In patients and controls with the same subclass pattern, the lag time tended to be shorter in the patients but the differences were not statistically significant (Table 3). Plasma concentrations of autoantibodies against MDA-LDL were significantly higher in renal transplant patients than in controls (Table 3). LDL subclass pattern B was associated with a higher IgM antibody concentration (pattern B vs. A 48.3 ± 17.6 mg/ml vs 26.2 ± 10.0 mg/ml ($P < 0.001$). Pattern A and pattern B subjects did not differ in IgG autoantibodies. There was no correlation between LDL cholesterol and any of the antibody parameters nor between the plasma cyclosporine A content and any of the determined variables (not shown).

Discussion

Kidney transplantation is associated with an increased occurrence of atherosclerotic cardiovascular disease. Several factors are associated with atherosclerosis, hypercholesterolemia being one of them [3, 4]. Oxidation of LDL is considered to be a major event in the development of atherosclerosis [4, 5]. We found that parameters of in vitro (lag phase of LDL oxidation) and in vivo (autoantibodies against MDA-LDL) LDL oxidation, consistently indicate the LDL oxidation is increased in these patients. This finding may be an additional cause

Table 3 Parameters of LDL oxidation

	Patients	Number	Controls	Number	P value
Lag time (min)	101 ± 23	–	148 ± 81	–	–
LDL size (nm)	23.65 ± 0.73	–	24.78 ± 1.16	–	< 0.05
Subclass pattern					
Lag time pattern A	122 ± 30	6	169 ± 80	13	–
Lag time pattern B	92 ± 11[a]	13	102 ± 21	6[b]	–
Anti-oxLDL Ab					
IgM (mg/l)	49.4 ± 15.9	–	24.4 ± 8.7	–	< 0.0001
IgG (mg/l)	5.6 ± 3.8	–	3.2 ± 1.9	–	< 0.02

[a] $P < 0.05$ lag time patients, pattern A vs B
[b] $P = 0.0502$, patients vs controls. Fisher's exact test

of the accelerated atherosclerosis in renal transplant patients. Increased lipid peroxidation has also been reported in cyclosporine-treated heart transplant recipients [17]. Apanay et al. found that high plasma cyclosporine levels were correlated with increased susceptibility to LDL oxidation in kidney transplant recipients [18].

Oxidative modification of lipoproteins has been suggested as a mediator of both acute and chronic vascular rejection [19]. Histologically, graft vascular disease closely resembles accelerated atherosclerosis. Oxidised LDL may act as a chemoattractant, trigger T lymphocyte activation and proliferation, and induce the expression of class II MHC antigens and cell adhesion molecules [20, 21]. There is also evidence that oxidised LDL leads to endothelial damage, enhanced platelet-derived growth factor expression and subsequently vascular smooth muscle cell proliferation [5, 11]. These features point towards a pathogenetic role of oxidised LDL in

chronic transplant rejection [11]. Supposing that increased LDL oxidation contributes to atherosclerosis, and possibly chronic rejection, in the transplant patients, a lowering of plasma triglycerides (leading to a shift of the LDL subclass pattern and subsequently less LDL oxidation) or administration of antioxidants may attenuate atherosclerosis and chronic rejection in renal transplant patients.

In conclusion, our results show that, in renal transplant recipients, there is increased incidence of the LDL subclass pattern B and an increased susceptibility to oxidative modification. Probably, LDL oxidation in vivo is also increased in the transplant patients as indicated by increased values of autoantibodies against MDA-LDL. These factors may play a role in the accelerated atherogenesis and graft vascular disease occurring after renal transplantation.

References

1. Braun WE (1990) Long-term complications of renal transplantation. Kidney Int 37: 1363–1378
2. Kasiske BL (1988) Risk factors for accelerated atherosclerosis in renal transplant recipients. Am J Med 84: 985–992
3. Moore R, Thomas D, Morgan E, Wheeler D, Griffin P, Salaman J, Rees A (1993) Abnormal lipid and lipoprotein profiles following renal transplantation. Transplant Proc 25: 1060–1061
4. Steinberg D, Parthasarathy S, Carew TE, Khoo JC, Witztum JL (1989) Beyond cholesterol: modifications of LDL that increase its atherogenicity. N Engl J Med 320: 916–924
5. Witztum JL, Steinberg D (1991) Role of oxidized low-density lipoproteins in atherogenesis. J Clin Invest 88: 1785–1792
6. Regnstrom J, Nilsson J, Tornvall P, Landou C, Hamsten A (1992) Susceptibility to low-density lipoprotein oxidation and coronary atherosclerosis in man. Lancet 339: 1183–1186
7. Appel G (1991) Lipid abnormalities in renal disease. Kidney Int 39: 169–183
8. Esterbauer H, Striegl G, Puhl H, Rotheneder M (1989) Continuous monitoring of in vitro oxidation of human LDL. Free Radic Res 6: 67–75
9. Palinski W, Ylä-Herttuala S, Rosenfeld ME, Butler SW, Socher SA, Parthasarathy S, Curtiss LK, Witztum JL (1990) Antisera and monoclonal antibodies specific for epitopes generated during oxidative modification of low density lipoprotein. Arteriosclerosis 10: 325–335
10. Jansen H, Ghanem H, Kuypers HSAM, Birkenhäger JC (1995) Autoantibodies against malondialdehyde-modified LDL are enhanced in subjects with an LDL subclass B pattern. Atherosclerosis 115: 255–262
11. Krauss RM, Burke DJ (1982) Identification of multiple subclasses of plasma low density lipoproteins in normal humans. J Lipid Res 23: 97–104
12. Rubenstein B, Steiner G (1976) Fractionation of human low density lipoprotein by column chromatography. Can J Biochem 22: 1023–1028
13. Austin MA, Breslow JL, Hennekens CH, Buring JE, Willett WC, Krauss RM (1988) Low density lipoprotein subclass patterns and the risk of myocardial infarction. J Am Med Assoc 260: 1917–1921
14. Chait A, Brazg RL, Tribble DL, Krauss RM (1993) Susceptibility of small, dense, low-density lipoproteins to oxidative modification in subjects with the atherogenic lipoprotein phenotype pattern B. Am J Med 94: 350–356
15. Ghanem H, van den Dorpel MA, Weimar W, Man in 't Veld AJ, El-kannishy MH, Jansen H (1996) Increased low density lipoprotein oxidation in stable kidney transplant recipients. Kidney Int (in press)

16. Friedewald WT, Levy RI, Fredrickson DS (1972) Estimation of low-density lipoprotein cholesterol in plasma, without use of the preparative ultracentrifuge. Clin Chem 18: 499–502
17. Chancerelle Y, de Lorgeril M, Viret R, Ciron B, Dureau G, Renaud S, Kergonou J-F (1991) Increased lipid peroxidation in cyclosporine-treated heart transplant recipients. Am J Cardiol 68: 813–816
18. Apanay DC, Neylan JF, Ragab MS, Sgoutas DS (1994) Cyclosporin increases the oxidizability of low-density lipoproteins in renal transplant recipients. Transplantation 58: 663–669
19. Taylor JE, Scott N, Hill A, Bridges A, Henderson IS, Stewart WK, Belch JJF (1993) Oxygen free radicals and platelet and granulocyte aggregability in renal transplant patients. Transplantation 55: 500–504
20. Hancock WH, Whitley DW, Tullius SG (1993) Transplantation 56: 643–649
21. Frostegard J, Wu R, Giscombe R, et al (1992) Induction of T-cell activation by oxidised low-density lipoprotein. Arterioscle Thromb 12: 461–467

Transpl Int (1996) 9 [Suppl 1]: S58–S62
© Springer-Verlag 1996

Thomas F. Müller
Christine M. Neumann
Christoph Greb
Michael Kraus
Harald Lange

The anaphylatoxin C5a, a new parameter in the diagnosis of renal allograft rejection

T. F. Müller · C. M. Neumann · C. Greb ·
Harald Lange (✉)
Department of Nephrology/Centre of
Internal Medicine,
Philipps-University of Marburg,
Baldinger Strasse 1,
D-35033 Marburg a. d. Lahn, Germany
Tel. 06421282709; Fax 0642121763

M. Kraus
Research Laboratories, Behringwerke AG,
Marburg, Germany

Abstract In the underlying study the diagnostic value of the anaphylatoxin C5a was evaluated in kidney transplantation. In 49 transplant patients the following parameters were measured daily for a mean period of 25.1 days: plasma C5a [P-C5a], urine C5a [U-C5a], serum amyloid A [SAA], serum neopterin [S-NEOP] and urine neopterin [U-NEOP]. Sensitivity, specificity and day of first significant parameter increase (exceeding a cut-off level of > 50 %) were evaluated retrospectively during 30 periods of rejection and 30 periods of stable graft function. U-C5a was the parameter with the highest sensitivity (84 %) and specificity (84 %), increasing in the mean 1.3 days before clinical diagnosis of rejection. Sensitivity and specificity of the other markers was lower: SAA 77 % and 77 %, U-NEOP 68 % and 65 %, S-NEOP 45 % and 77 %, and P-C5a 45 % and 48 %, respectively. During four instances of cytomegalovirus disease extremely high U-NEOP ($\geqslant$ = 1520 ± 518 μmol/mol creatinine) and slightly increased P-C5a levels ($\geqslant$ = 1.5 ± 1.4 ng/ml) occurred. Elevated urinary excretion of C5a seems to be a reliable and early marker of renal allograft rejection. In combination with SAA and U-NEOP, the daily assessment of U-C5a differentiates between viral infection and allograft rejection.

Key words Complement products · Anaphylatoxin C5a · Allograft rejection · Serum Amyloid A · Neopterin

Introduction

Parameters facilitating the differential diagnosis of a deterioration in graft function are needed [18]. The complement system is a very potent immune regulator [2, 17]. In the past, studies on complement activation in the field of organ transplantation were mainly focused on hyperacute rejections, especially after xenografting [20]. Early attempts to diagnose rejection episodes in human renal allografts by monitoring circulating, whole complement components failed [5]. Diagnostic approaches were primarily limited to the morphological analysis of complement deposits in tissues of grafted organs [1, 6, 8, 9]. Quite recently, complement products such as plasma C3d (28 Solling), C3a and the terminal complement complex TCC [12], and urine samples of C4d and TCC [3] were determined. Analysing these complement levels, which were not measured daily, no clear-cut correlation with the onset of acute rejection episodes was obtained.

In the following study, levels of the complement products C5a were measured in plasma (P) and urine (U) samples on a daily basis in patients following kidney transplantation. C5a is small molecule (MW: 11 kD) and a potent anaphylatoxin whose role has not yet been investigated in graft rejection [7, 14]. The diagnostic performance of P-C5a and U-C5a was compared with serum (S) and urine neopterin (S-NEOP and U-NEOP) and serum amyloid A (SAA). NEOP is a marker of the cellular immune response and elevated levels are primarily seen during rejection episodes and viral infections [10, 15, 19]. SAA is a protein of the acute phase response and peaks are found during acute allograft rejections [16, 19].

Patients and methods

Forty-nine consecutive patients (17 female, 32 male) received a cadaveric kidney transplant between April 1990 and March 1992 at the Philipps University of Marburg. Their mean age was 51.1 years. The total period of observation on the ward was 1229 days, with a mean of 25.1 days per patient.

Immunosuppressive protocol

As basic immunosuppressive therapy, prednisolone started with 80 mg on day 1 and was tapered to 20 mg on day 4 after transplantation. Ciclosporine (Sandoz) was started intravenously with 5 mg/kg body weight on day 1, continued orally at 10 mg/kg body weight and was adapted to blood levels of 200 to 250 ng per ml. The whole blood levels of Ciclosporine were determined by ELISA based on monoclonal antibodies. In primary non-functioning grafts, polyclonal rabbit anti T cell antibodies ATG (Fresenius) were given, Ciclosporine was reinstituted after recovery of graft function. Acute rejection episodes were treated by steroid pulses and in steroid-resistant rejections the monoclonal antibody OKT3 (Orthoclone, Cilag) was used.

Rejection episodes

Acute rejection episodes were diagnosed by a declining creatinine clearance when other non-immunological causes of graft failure were ruled out. In addition, a positive response to the immunosuppressive antirejection therapy was obligatory. Facultatively, fine needle as well as core needle biopsies were performed to support the clinical diagnosis. To allow comparisons between patients, the first day of clinically manifest rejection and the start of antirejection therapy was labelled as day 0. Subsequently, the days before and after day 0 were labelled, starting with day − 3 (i.e. three days before day 0) and ending with day + 2 (i.e. two days after day 0).

Stable graft function

Periods of stable graft function were defined as time intervals of at least 6 days duration where complications such as rejection episodes, viral infections, acute tubular necrosis, surgical interventions and therapies with mono- or polyclonal antibodies were ruled out by clinical and laboratory findings. The first 3 postoperative days were never considered for evaluation.

Blood collection

Daily, morning blood samples of 10 ml were drawn into EDTA tubes (Sarstedt) to which 0.25 ml aprotinin (Trasylol, Bayer; 20000 KIE/ml) were added. The samples were immediately cooled and centrifuged at 3000 g for 10 min at 4°C. Supernatants were separated into 300 μl fractions, frozen immediately and stored at − 70°C.

Urine collection

Daily samples of spontaneously voided morning urine (between 6 and 7 a.m.) were taken into sterile containers (Sarstedt) and again immediately cooled. In the laboratory, these samples wee separated into 300 μl fractions, frozen immediately and stored at − 70°C. In cases of pyuria or haematuria the urine samples were centrifuged beforehand.

Measurement of the Parameters

Anaphylatoxin (C5a)

Concentrations of C5a in plasma and urine were measured by a new enzyme immunoassay (EIA, Enzygnost C5a, Behringwerke AG, Marburg, Germany). For adjustment with a reference curve, known concentrations of purified C5 and C5a (Behringwerke AG, Marburg, FRG) were used as standards. In the C5a EIA, an anti-C5a monoclonal antibody (mAb) (561) was used as capture antibody and a horseradish-peroxidase labelled anti-C5a mAb (557) for detection as described by Klos et al. [13]. The intra- (within run) and interassay (between runs) coefficients of variance were 5.3 % and 6.5 %, respectively. The P-C5a levels were expressed in ng/ml. The U-C5a values were both measured in ng/ml as well as related to the daily urine volume and expressed in ng/d.

Neopterin (NEOP)

S-NEOP and U-NEOP levels were measured by radioimmunoassay (RIAcid, Henning/Brahms, Berlin, FRG). U-NEOP was related to creatinine excretion and expressed as μmol/mol creatinine. S-NEOP was measured in nmol/l.

Serum amyloid A (SAA)

A rapid immunonephelometric assay was developed to measure SAA levels, as previously described [11]. Basis of the test are highly specific antibodies raised against purified SAA, the antigen-antibody complexes being measured by laser nephelometer (Behringwerke AG, Marburg, FRG). The concentrations are expressed as mg/dl.

Analysis of the parameters

All markers investigated were measured on a daily basis. Clinical data as well as parameter values were displayed graphically for retrospective analysis. The postoperative courses were analysed and 6-day periods of interest were defined (day − 3 to day + 2) for rejection episodes and stable graft function. Each rejection episode was matched with a corresponding 6-day period of stable graft function of another patient. For each pair, the time of occurrence in the postoperative course as well as the number of HLA mismatches was matched. During the defined periods of interest (rejection/stable function) the individual parameter behaviour was analysed according to the criteria of a diagnostic test [4]. Changes in P-C5a, U-C5a, S-NEOP, U-NEOP and SAA were assessed as true positive (TP), false positive (FP), true negative (TN) or false negative (FN). Each parameter could show one TP or FN (during each rejection) and one FP or TN behaviour (during each period of stable function), respectively. The cut-off level for TP/FP and TN/FN parameter behaviour was a parameter increase of greater than 100 % from the pervious day. Sensitivity was calculated as TP/(FN + TP) and specificity as TN/(FP + TN). The day of first TP parameter increase related to day 0, i. e. the day of clinical diagnosis and start of rejection therapy, was calculated. Using the SAS statistical analysing system a k-sample median test (Brown-Mood) was performed to analyse the median parameter values during periods of stable graft function, rejection and viral infection.

Results

Example of an acute rejection episode and reactivated cytomegalovirus (CMV) infection

Figure 1 gives an example of an acute, steroid-resistant, reversible rejection episode, which was clinically diagnosed on postoperative day 28. The deterioration in graft function is shown by the increasing creatinine levels and accompanied by TP peaks, i. e. increases exceeding the 50 % cut-off level, of the parameters SAA, P-C5a and U-C5a. The U-NEOP levels are FN, a peak occurring on day 31 is due to the cytokine release induced by the OKT3 therapy. On day 45, CMV DNA was detected by PCR testing. Together with clinical symptoms a CMV disease could be verified. The viral infection is reflected in the increasing U-NEOP levels, exceeding levels of 1000 μmol/mol creatinine. In addition, a marked P-C5a peak is shown, quickly returning to baseline levels.

Median parameter values during periods of stable graft function, acute rejection and viral infection

Following the retrospective analysis of the parameter curves in the 49 patients, 30 acute, reversible rejection episodes were diagnosed. In 4 patients severe, clinically manifest CMV diseases occurred. These CMV infections were monitored for a total period of 53 days. Figure 2 shows the median values of the parameters SAA, U-C5a and U-NEOP obtained from the 6-day periods during the 30 rejections ($n = 180$), the 30 corresponding periods of stable graft function ($n = 180$) and 53 measurements during the four CMV infections. It is shown that the U-C5a median levels are significantly elevated during the rejection episodes in comparison to the stable graft function and infection periods. On the other hand, the viral infections are associated with significant elevations of the U-NEOP median values. The SAA median values did not discriminate significantly between the three clinical settings. The same applies for the parameters S-NEOP and P-C5as, the values are not shown.

Diagnostic qualities of the rejection parameters

Figure 3 summarises the diagnostic test qualities of the five markers by analysing the parameter behaviour dur-

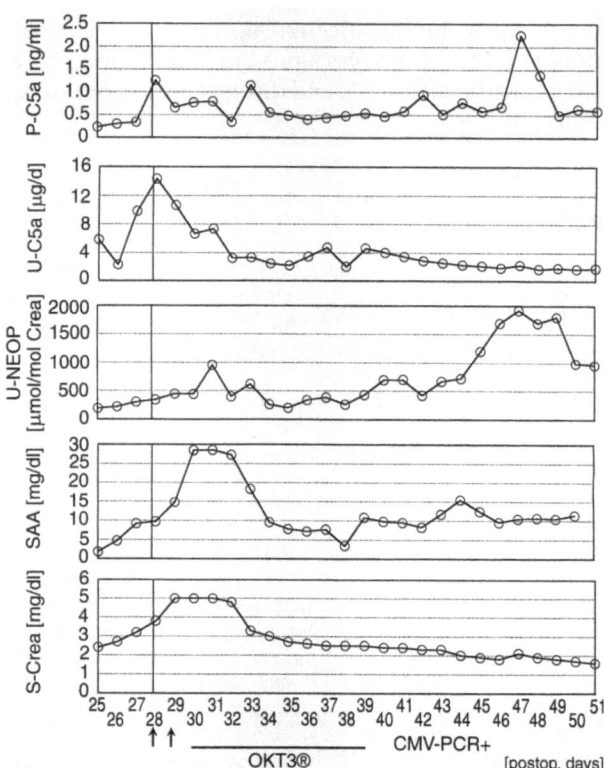

Fig. 1 Example of an acute rejection episode and reactivated cytomegalovirus (CMV) infection. Postoperative (day 25 to day 51) plasma C5a *(P-C5a)*, urine C5a *(U-C5a)*, urine neopterin *(U-NEOP)*, serum amyloid A *(SAA)* and serum creatinine *(S-Crea)* levels are shown in a patient with an acute, steroid-resistant rejection episode (↑ steroid pulse therapy on day 28 and day 29, OKT3® therapy from day 30 to day 39) and a reactivated CMV infection, diagnosed by a positive CMV-PCR on day 45

ing the 30 acute rejection episodes and 30 periods of stable graft function. U-C5a is the parameter with the highest sensitivity and specificity (84 %, respectively), followed by SAA with 77 % sensitivity and specificity. The diagnostic accuracy of U-NEOP, S-NEOP and P-C5a do not reach that level. In addition it is shown, that U-C5a is also the earliest predictor of an impending allograft rejection, increasing significantly in the mean 1.3 days before the clinical diagnosis of rejection is made. U-NEOP and SAA peaks occurred in the mean 0.5 days before the day of clinical diagnosis and start of antirejection therapy. Both, P-C5a and S-NEOP respond later in the rejection process.

Discussion

Recent studies suggest the major role of complement activation in allograft rejection. Substantial deposits of various complement components were found in renal allograft tissues during rejection processes [6, 8, 9]. Donor-specific, local complement synthesis could be dem-

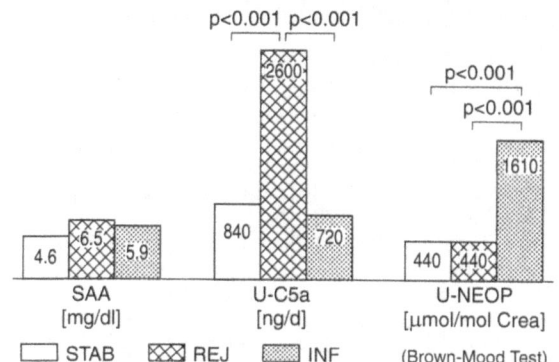

Fig. 2 Median parameter values during periods of stable graft function, acute rejection and viral infection. The median values of each parameter obtained from daily measurements during 30 periods of *acute rejection* (n = 180), 30 corresponding periods of stable graft function (n = 180) and 4 periods of clinically manifest CMV infection (n = 53) are given. The significance probability across the three different clinical situations is indicated

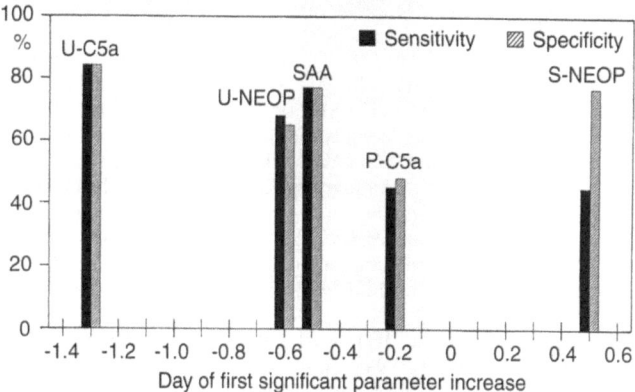

Fig. 3 Diagnostic qualities of the rejection parameters. Sensitivity, specificity and day of first significant increase (i.e. increase of > 50 % from level of the previous day) of the parameters obtained during 30 periods of acute allograft rejection and 30 corresponding periods of stable graft function are shown

onstrated in kidney transplantation [1, 2, 21]. Despite this strong morphological evidence, conflicting results are provided by several studies concerning the diagnostic value of circulating complement levels and split products. Once or twice weekly C3a, C3d, C1rsC1INH, C3b(Bb)P and sC5b-9 were measured. A clear-cut relationship to renal allograft rejections could not be established [12, 22]. In one study sC4d and sC5b-9 were measured in a few selected urine samples. Increased sC4d levels were found in steroid-resistant rejections and a further evaluation by longitudinal monitoring was suggested [3].

Therefore, daily measurements of the chemoattractant C5a were performed in plasma as well as urine samples of 49 renal transplant patients in the immediate postoperative course. The diagnostic value of P-C5a and U-C5a was compared with markers of the immune response in organ transplantation. SAA is a parameter of the acute phase reaction [16, 19]. S-NEOP and U-NEOP are markers of the cellular immune response [10, 15]. Analysing 30 periods of rejection and stable graft function, U-C5a was the parameter with the highest diagnostic accuracy in the detection of rejection episodes. In addition, it was the earliest predictor of an impending rejection. As a rejection marker, U-C5a was superior to SAA and U-NEOP. The circulating P-C5a levels showed a low sensitivity and specificity, and increases were seen predominantly during CMV infections. Viral infections were best detected by increases in the U-NEOP levels. There was no correlation between plasma and urine C5a levels.

These findings support the relevance of the complement system as an immune regulator [2]. The disproportionately high U-C5a levels in relation to the P-C5a levels favour the concept of the local immune synthesis in the allograft and agree with the intrarenal distribution of complement products, mainly located in the tubules [1, 21]. Therefore, the urine compartment is probably a better window than the blood compartment to look at complement activation associated with an immune response targeted against the renal allograft. This might, on the contrary, explain the increased P-C5a levels during systemic CMV diseases, which were not reflected by changes in the U-C5a excretion. Concerning the kinetics of the complement cascade and the quick turnover of complement components, short intervals between the determinations seem to be essential [23]. Probably the lack of diagnostic value in the detection of rejection episodes described for different complement products is partly due to the long intervals between the determinations.

In conclusion, U-C5a seems to be a reliable and early rejection parameter in kidney transplantation. In combination with SAA and U-NEOP, the daily monitoring of U-C5a facilitates the differential diagnosis between viral infection and acute rejection.

Acknowledgements We are indebted to the staff of the intensive care unit 12 for their excellent cooperation, especially in blood and urine collection.

References

1. Andrews PA, Finn JE, Lloyd CM, Zhou W, Mathieson PW, Sacks SH (1995) Expression and tissue localization of donor-specific complement C3 synthesized in human renal allografts. Eur J Immunol 25: 1087–1093
2. Andrews PA, Zhou W, Sacks SH (1995) Tissue synthesis of complement as an immune regulator. Mol Med Today 1: 202–207
3. Bechtel U, Scheuer R, Landgraf R, König A, Feucht HE (1995) Assessment of soluble adhesion molecules (sICAM-1, sVCAM-1, sELAM-1) and complement cleavage products (sC4d, sC5b-9) in urine. Clinical monitoring of renal recipients. Transplantation 58: 905–911
4. Büttner J (1977) Evaluation of the diagnostic value of clinical chemical tests. J Clin Chem Clin Biochem 15: 1–12
5. Carpenter CB (1974) Abnormalities of the complement system in clinical transplantation situations. Transplant Proc 6: 83–87
6. Cosyns JP, Kazatchkine MD, Bhakdi S, et al (1986) Immunohistochemical analysis of C3 cleavage fragments, factor H, and the C5b-9 terminal complex of complement in de novo membranous glomerulonephritis occurring in patients with renal transplant. Clin Nephrol 26: 203–208
7. Couser WG, Baker PJ, Adler S (1985) Complement and the direct mediation of immune glomerular injury. A new perspective. Kidney Int 28: 879–890
8. Feucht HE, Felber E, Gokel MJ, et al (1991) Vascular deposition of complement-split products in kidney allografts with cell-mediated rejection. Clin Exp Immunol 86: 464–470
9. Feucht HE, Schneeberger J, Hillebrand G, et al (1993) Capillary deposition of C4d complement fragment and early graft loss. Kidney Int 43: 1333–1338
10. Fuchs D, Hausen A, Reibnegger G, Werner ER, Dierich MP, Wachter H (1988) Neopterin as a marker for activated cell-mediated immunity. Imunology Today 9 (5): 150–155
11. Hocke G, Ebel H, Bittner K, Müller T, Kaffarnik H, Steinmetz A (1989) A rapid laser immunonephelometric assay for serum amyloid a (SAA) and its applictation to the diagnosis of kidney allograft rejection. Klin Wochenschr 67: 447–451
12. Kirschfink M, Wienert T, Rother K, Pomer S (1992) Complement activation in renal allograft recipients. Transpl Proc 24: 2556–2557
13. Klos A, Ihrig V, Messner M, Grabbe J, Bitter-Suermann D (1988) Detection of native human complement components C3 and C5 and their primary activation peptides C3a and C5a (anaphylatoxic peptides) by ELISAs with monoclonal antibodies. J Immunol Meth 111: 241–252
14. Kraus M (1995) Methodische Mitteilung. Komplementsystem. Diagn Lab 45: 79–84
15. Margreiter R, Fuchs D, Hausen A, Huber C, Reibnegger G, Spielberger M, Wachter H (1983) Neopterin as a new biochemical marker for diagnosis of allograft rejection. Experience based upon evaluation of 100 consecutive cases. Transplantation 36: 650–653
16. Maury CPJ, Teppo AM (1984) Comparative study of serum amyloid-related protein SAA, C-reactive protein and β2-microglobulin as markers of renal allograft rejection. Clin Nephrol 22 (6): 284–292
17. Mollnes TE, Lachmann PJ (1988) Regulation of complement. Scand J Immunol 27: 127–142
18. Müller MM, Andert SE, Winter PM, Holzinger CH (1990) Laboratory diagnostics in organ transplantation. Lab Med 14: 51–62
19. Müller T, Schindler S, Sprenger H, et al (1992) Prospective analysis of 10 different parameters of acute renal allograft rejection. Trans Proc 24: 2731–2734
20. Platt JL, Bach FH (1991) The barrier to xenotransplantation. Transplantation 52: 937–947
21. Seelen MAJ, Brooimans RA, van der Woude FJ, van Es LA, Daha MR (1993) IFN-γ mediates stimulation of complement C4 biosynthesis in human proximal tubular epithelial cells. Kidney Int 44: 50–57
22. Son WJ van, Bij W van der, Tegzess AM, et al (1989) Complement activation during an active cytomegalovirus infection after renal transplantation: Due to circulating immune complexes or alternative pathway activation? Clin Immunol Immunopathol 50: 109–121
23. Webster RO, Larsen GL, Henson PM (1982) In vivo clearance and tissue distribution of C5a and C5a des arginine complement fragments in rabbits. J Clin Invest 70: 1177–1183

Transpl Int (1996) 9 [Suppl 1]: S63–S67
© Springer-Verlag 1996

J. Kaden
B. Schütze
G. May

A critical analysis of soluble interleukin-2 receptor levels in kidney allograft recipients

J. Kaden (✉)
Friedrichshain Hospital,
Department of Laboratory Medicine,
Landsberger Allee 49, D-10249 Berlin,
Germany

B. Schütze
DPC Biermann GmbH, Hohe Strasse 2–4,
D-61231 Bad Nauheim, Germany

G. May
Kidney Transplant Centre,
Friedrichshain Hospital,
Landsberger Allee 49, D-10249 Berlin,
Germany

Abstract Soluble interleukin-2 receptor (sIL-2R) was measured by the Cellfree Kit (T Cell sciences) in 103 pretransplant and 1590 posttransplant samples from 103 patients with cadaveric kidney allografts. The mean values (± SD) detected in pretransplant sera were significantly higher (1932 ± 1389 U/ml) than in 72 healthy adults (267 ± 139 U/ml), but after transplantation they continuously fell towards normal levels within the first 3 postoperative weeks. Recipients with acute rejection episodes showed higher sIL-2R levels (1762 ± 904 U/ml) than those with stable transplants at discharge (937 ± 398 U/ml). Highest values were detected during antirejection therapy with antithymocyte globulin (4996 ± 2166 U/ml) or OKT3 (5905 ± 3910). Increases were also observed during bacterial and viral infections and even, in some cases, without any apparent cause. Because of this lack of specificity, elevated sIL-2R levels should be interpreted cautiously. Nevertheless, sIL-2R level can be useful for monitoring kidney allograft recipients. Increases point to a cellular immune activation process and can predict rejections or infections.

Key words Interleukin-2 receptor · Interleukin-6 · Kidney transplantation · Rejection

Introduction

Allograft rejection is one of the immune responses in which cytokines are considered to play an important role. The stimulation of T cells by foreign antigens results in cellular activation leading to de novo synthesis of interleukin (IL)-2 as well as expression of IL-2 receptor (IL-2R). Helper T cells (Th1 subset) appear to be the major source of IL-2. Membrane-bound IL-2R can be released in a soluble form (sIL-2R) and detected in vivo. This sIL-2R corresponds to a truncated extracellular part of the α chain of IL-2R. It is widely accepted that an elevated serum sIL-2R level reflects the degree of T cell activation. In the field of clinical kidney transplantation, a lot of effort has been made to improve monitoring of graft rejection by the determination of sIL-2R in serum [4, 6, 8, 19, 22, 23, 25–28] and urine [2, 5, 15]. Although most authors described elevated sIL-2R levels in connection with but hardly prior to rejection episodes [4, 6, 8, 19, 22, 23, 25, 27, 28], there were also reports of elevated sIL-2R levels in the immediate postoperative phase [28], during virus infections [4, 8, 19, 22, 27] or treatment with antilymphocytic antibodies [4, 8], and also without any apparent cause [22]. Therefore, in this study we investigated the pattern of IL-2R serum levels in 103 patients submitted for renal transplantation in order to clarify the usefulness of serial sIL-2R determinations and compared these results with the serum level of the proinflammatory cytokine IL-6 as an early indicator of inflammatory tissue injury.

Material and methods

Patients and protocol

One hundred and three patients (mean age 45 ± 11 years; females 32, males 71), who underwent cadaveric renal transplant (first, 93; second/third, 10) between July 1992 and August 1993 at the Kidney Transplant Centre Berlin-Friedrichshain were studied. The immunosuppressive regimen was identical for all recipients. It consisted of oral cyclosporine with the dose adjusted to maintain whole blood levels from 200 to 250 ng/ml, azathioprine (1 mg/kg per day) and methylprednisolone (MP) starting with 40 mg/day. In addition, all but one recipient received the Friedrichshain variant of ATG induction therapy, details are already published [13, 14]. Briefly, this induction consisted of an intraoperative high-dose single ATG or ALG bolus (ATG (Fresenius) 9 mg/kg [$n = 69$], lymphoglobulin (Merieux) 30 mg/kg [$n = 16$], ATGAM (Upjohn) 45 mg/kg [$n = 8$], pressimmun (Behringwerke AG) 60 mg/kg [$n = 10$]). In order to avoid a cytokine-release syndrome, 500 mg MP were given about 1 h pre-ATG/ALG. Rejection episodes were diagnosed by standard clinical and pathological criteria (including a progressive elevation of serum creatinine and urea nitrogen, accompanied by oliguria, albuminuria, IgG-uria, increase of graft size [sonography] and lymphocytic infiltrate [fine needle aspiration biopsy]) and treated with MP for 5 days at 5 mg/kg body weight. Attemps to reverse biopsy-proven MP-resistant rejections by ATG, using a dose-by-T cell-protocol (aspired values: 50–150 T cells/µl), were tried. The number of T cells were determined by flow cytometry (FACScan, Becton Dickinson, Heidelberg, Germany). OKT3 (CILAG, 10 days, 2.5 mg) was given as rescue therapy or primarily in cases of humoral/vascular rejections.

Detection of sIL-2R and IL-6

Soluble IL-2R levels were determined by means of the Cellfree IL-2R Kit (T cell Sciences, Cambridge, Mass., USA) and IL-6 by the Quantikine IL-6 Immunoassay (R & D Systems, Minneapolis, Mass., USA) according to the instructions of the manufacturers. In Germany, both immunoassays are distributed by DPC Biermann GmbH, Bad Nauheim. Serum for IL-2R and IL-6 assays were taken before transplantation and three times a week thereafter (always between 7.00 and 8.00 a.m.) up to discharge and stored at $-20\,°C$. Altogether 103 pretransplant sera and 1590 posttransplant sera were examined and the results compared with those obtained from 72 healthy adults.

Results

The range of sIL-2R levels in the serum of 72 normal individuals is between 17–737 U/ml, with a mean value of 267 U/ml. The upper normal limit $\geqslant +3$ SD) is 683 U/ml. IL-6 is not detectable in healthy subjects. The mean values ($\pm$ SD) of sIL-2R detected in pretransplant sera (i.e. sera from patients on chronic dialysis) were 1932 ± 1389 U/ml (Table 1). These values were significantly higher than in healthy adults (267 ± 139 U/ml, $P < 0.001$). The immediately posttransplant elevated sIL-2R serum levels (2109 ± 1212 U/ml) continuously fell towards normal levels within the first 3 weeks after

Table 1 Serum IL-2R levels in kidney transplant recipients (*CMV* cytomegalovirus, *sIL-2R* soluble interleukin-2 receptor)

Sample	Number	sIL-2R [U/ml]
Healthy adults	72	267 ± 139
Pretransplant (dialysis)	103	1932 ± 1389
Posttransplant (day 1–3)	93	2109 ± 1212
Stable transplant at discharge (event-free courses)	34	937 ± 398
Rejection		
Methylprednisolone (MP)-sensitive		
Pre-MP	16	1469 ± 911
During MP	16	1762 ± 904
MP-resistant		
Pre-ATG	6	3644 ± 2033
During ATG	6	4996 ± 2166
Humoral/vascular or MP-resistant		
Pre-OKT3	8	2111 ± 1867
During OKT3	8	5905 ± 3910
Infections		
CMV disease (mild) at the time of leukocytopenia	6	1081 ± 600
Bacterial infections (serious)	8	2593 ± 1764

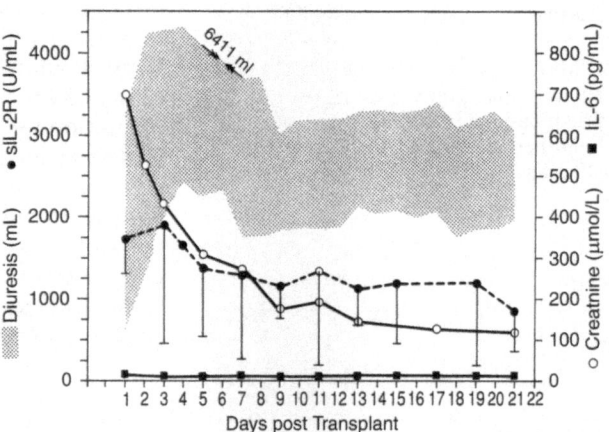

Fig. 1 Course of sIL-2R (mean $\pm$ SD) and IL-6 serum levels (mean $\pm$ SD) compared with serum creatinine (mean values) and diuresis ($\pm$ SD, *hatched area*) in 26 renal graft recipients with immediate early graft function, no rejection episodes and no infections in the early posttransplant period up to discharge from transplant centre

transplantation. Samples from patients with stable renal function (Fig. 1) after event-free courses showed values hardly above normal at discharge (937 ± 398 U/min), but significantly decreased as compared to pretransplant levels ($P < 0.01$). Recipients with acute cellular rejections episodes (Fig. 2) had significantly ($P < 0.01$) higher sIL-2R levels than stable patients (1762 ± 904 U/ml). In comparison to MP-sensitive rejections, in both MP-resistant and humoral/vascular rejections the sIL-

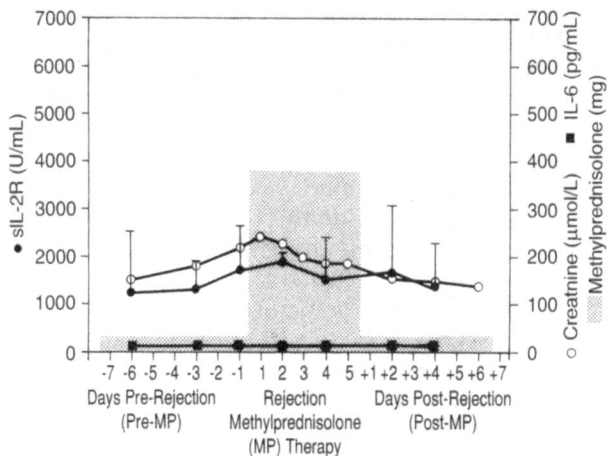

Fig. 2 Course of sIL-2R (mean ± SD) and IL-6 (mean ± SD) serum levels compared with serum creatinine (mean values) in 16 renal graft recipients with methylprednisolone(MP)-sensitive rejections. The treatment consisted of 5 mg MP/kg body weight for 5 consecutive days (MP dose = mean value)

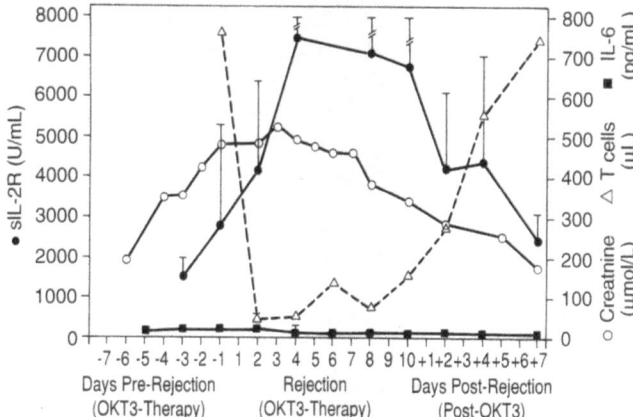

Fig. 3 Course of sIL-2R (mean ± SD) and IL-6 (mean ± SD) serum levels compared with serum creatinine (mean values) and T cell count (mean values of absolute numbers of CD3 positive cells) in eight renal graft recipients with methyl-prednisolone-resistant or humoral/vascular rejections during successful OKT3 therapy (2.5 mg/day for 10 consecutive days)

2R levels were significantly higher before antirejection therapy had begun (Table 1). Shortly after treatment with poly- or monoclonal anti-T cell antibodies (ATG or OKT3) sIL-2R levels further increased. The highest values were seen during OKT3 therapy (Fig. 3). In patients with mild cytomegalovirus (CMV) disease the sIL-2R levels were only slightly elevated at the time of leukocytopenia (1081 ± 600 U/ml). In contrast, serious bacterial infections (pneumonia, sepsis) were associated with marked but very different elevations of sIL-2R levels (2593 ± 1764).

With regard to the interpretation of elevated sIL-2R levels, the 103 sIL-2R serum peaks were grouped according to the clinical events and compared with the distribution of IL-6 peaks (Table 2). The data show that after transplantation two events are especially associated with sIL-2R serum level elevations, the immediate postoperative period (43/103 peaks, 41.7%) and rejection episodes (37/103 peaks, 35.9%). Because infectious diseases and even event-free phases could also be connected with increased sIL-2R levels, these data do not support the hypothesis that the sIL-2R level can be used to predict rejection. In comparison to sIL-2R, the IL-6 peaks showed a different distribution. Beside rejections and surgical trauma, 27% of IL-6 peaks are associ-

ated with infections, but also, in apparently uncomplicated courses, IL-6 can be detected at very low levels.

Discussion

In healthy individuals the sIL-2R mean value was determined to be 267 U/ml and, using the same kit, Pizzola [21] described mean values of approximately 250 U/ml. These values are likely to reflect the lymphocyte activation normally occurring upon physiological stimuli. The upper normal sIL-2R limit is 683 U/ml ($\geq$ + 3 SD). Only 2 out of 72 sIL-2R concentrations of the healthy control population were above this limit (734 and 729 U/ml). In contrast, only 2 out of 103 patients on chronic dialysis showed sIL-2R concentrations below this limit. This is in agreement with the findings of other investigators [4, 22, 27]. The reason for the sIL-2R elevation in chronic uraemia is not known. Köhler et al. [16] discussed a monocytic defect with an insufficient co-stimulatory signal transduction to T cells leading to a reduced IL-2 secretion with compensatory increase of IL-2R expression. This deficient production of IL-2 may partly explain the reduced response of uraemic lymphocytes in vitro [18]. In spite of the elevated sIL-

Table 2 Distribution of sIL-2R and IL-6 serum peaks in 103 kidney allograft recipients		sIL-2R peaks[a]			IL-6 peaks		
		n	%	$\geq$ ± s (U/ml)	n	%	$\geq$ ± s (pg/ml)
[a] Peak means the highest concentration in the posttransplant course independent of the height of the absolute value	Posttransplant (day 1–3)	43	41.7	2649 ± 1967	27	26.2	49 ± 70
	Rejection	37	35.9	4914 ± 3372	26	25.2	32 ± 20
	Infection	7	6.8	3397 ± 1800	28	27.1	37 ± 45
	Event-free phase	16	15.5	2193 ± 1623	22	21.4	10 ± 6

2R level, only 14.3 % of our patients showed pretransplant more than 8 % IL-2R$^+$ CD3$^+$ cells (mean ± 1 SD = 5.3 ± 3.7 %). Raskova et al. [24] described even a reduced expression of IL-2R in the plasma membrane of PHA-stimulated lymphocytes. Another explanation for the immune defect in chronic renal failure could be the binding of IL-2 by sIL-2R competing in this way with the membrane-bound IL-2R on T cells. In vitro experiments performed by Chopra et al. [3] support this hypothesis.

Soon after transplant there was a further, but not significant increase, of sIL-2R as compared to the pretransplant level. This fact seems to be related, to some extent, to the intraoperative high-dose ATG bolus; comparable results were found after heart transplantation [11]. Postoperatively, elevated sIL-2R serum levels were also described in patients undergoing major operations and discussed as non-specific response to the trauma of surgery [1, 17]. The elevation of sIL-2R which then interferes with IL-2-dependent immunity could play a role in postoperative immune deficiency [17]. The pre- and postoperatively elevated sIL-2R serum levels continuously fell towards normal levels within the first 3 weeks after transplantation. Samples from patients with stable renal function after event-free courses showed values hardly above normal at discharge (937 ± 398 U/ml). Patients with normal sIL-2R levels at discharge (≤ 683 U/ml, $n = 18$) had significantly less (3/18 vs 34/75, $P < 0.05$) need for rehospitalisation within the first year after grafting than patients ($n = 75$) with sIL-2R levels > 683 U/ml. There were no instances of rehospitalisation for rejection treatment in patients discharged with normal sIL-2R levels. In heart transplant recipients, a mean level < 1000 U/ml predicted long-term survival with a 76 % sensitivity, 79 % specificity and 88 % negative predictive value [29].

Patients with acute rejections had significantly higher sIL-2R levels than healthy individuals and stable patients. Rejections occurring early after transplantation will be difficult to detect because the background level is so high. In comparison to MP-sensitive rejections, the sIL-2R levels in MP-resistant or humoral/vascular rejections were clearly higher before antirejection therapy had begun. Shortly after treatment with poly- or monoclonal anti-T cell antibodies sIL-2R levels further increased. The highest values were seen after OKT3 therapy, therefore, reflecting the response to antirejection therapy. In agreement with Colvin et al. [4], our data also make no claim that the sIL-2R levels can be used to predict rejection. Comparable results were reported after heart [11, 12] and lung [9] transplantation. Nevertheless at the time of rejection most investigators observed elevated sIL-2R levels. Because infectious diseases in transplant recipients are also associated with elevated sIL-2R levels [4, 7, 8, 10, 19, 20, 22, 27], distinguishing between rejection and infection on the basis of sIL-2R serum level is not possible without knowledge of other clinical or laboratory parameters. Perkins et al. [20] recommend the exclusion of CMV and the confirmation of rejections by biopsy when sIL-2R levels increase. In our experience the simultaneous determination of IL-6 can be useful for distinguishing bacterial and viral infection. With regard to the interpretation of elevated sIL-2R levels, we should keep in mind that 16 out of 103 sIL-2R peaks (2193 ± 1623 U/ml) were not associated with clinical or otherwise detectable events. In these patients, the simultaneously determined IL-6 levels were not or only slightly elevated (10 ± 6 pg/ml) indicating no systemic inflammatory process. We conclude from our results that elevations of sIL-2R are not specific for allograft rejection, since increase of sIL-2R serum levels were also observed during bacterial and viral infections, after treatment with mono- and polyclonal antilymphocytic antibodies and even without any apparent cause. Because of this lack of specificity, elevated sIL-2R levels must be assessed carefully. Nevertheless sIL-2R level can be useful for monitoring kidney allograft recipients. Increases point to a cellular immune activation process and can predict rejections or infections.

References

1. Barton DPJ, Blanchard DK, Michelini-Norris B, Roberts WS, Hoffman MS, Fiorica JV, Nicosia SV, Cavanagh D, Djeu JY (1993) Serum soluble interleukin-2 receptor α levels in patients with gynecologic cancers: Early effect of surgery. Amer J Reprod Immunol 30: 202–206

2. Bock GH, Neu L, Long C, Patterson LT, Korb S, Gelpi J, Nelson DL (1994) An assessment of serum and urine soluble interleukin-2 receptor concentrations during renal transplant rejection. Am J Kidney Dis 23: 421–426

3. Chopra RK, Powers DC, Kendig NE, Adler WH, Nagel JE (1989) Soluble interleukin 2 receptors released from mitogen stimulated human peripheral blood lymphocytes bind interleukin 2 and inhibit IL2 dependent cell proliferation. Immunol Invest 18: 961–973

4. Colvin RB, Fuller TC, MacKeen L, Kung PC, Ip SH, Cosimi AB (1987) Plasma interleukin 2 receptor levels in renal allograft recipients. Clin Immunol Immunopathol 43: 273–276

5. Colvin RB, Preffer FI, Fuller TC, Brown MC, Ip SH, Kung PC, Cosini AB (1989) A critical analysis of serum and urine interleukin-2 receptor assays in renal allograft recipients. Transplantation 48: 800–804

6. Forsythe JLR, Shenton BK, Parrott NR, Taylor RMR, Proud G (1989) Plasma interleukin 2 receptor levels in renal allograft dysfunction. Transplantation 48: 155–157

7. Fraunberger P, Pfeiffer M, Haller M, Hoffmann RM, Zwiebel FM, Überfuhr P, Jauch KW, Nagel D, Walli AK, Seidel D (1995) Cytokine and cytokine-receptor profiles after liver and heart transplantation. Transplant Proc 27: 2023–2027

8. Hacini J, Berthoux F, Berthoux P, Vindimian M, Lambert C, Laurent B, Alamartine E, Guérin C (1992) Monitoring of serum cytokines in renal transplantation: respective value of neopterin (N), soluble interleukin 2 receptor (sIL-2R), and tumor necrosis factor alpha (TNFα) in the different clinical situation. In: Touraine JL, Traeger J, Bétuel H, Dubernard JM, Revillard JP, Dupuy C (eds) Transplantation and clinical immunology XXIV. Elsevier Science Publishers, Amsterdam London New York, pp 165–169

9. Humbert M, Emilie D, Cerrina J, Simonneau G, Rain B, Fattal S, Le Roy Ladurie F, Dartevelle P, Duroux P, Galanaud P (1991) Soluble interleukin 2 receptor and neopterin serum levels after lung/heart – lung transplantations – absence of predictive value for late allograft rejection. Transplantation 52: 1092–1094

10. Ippoliti G (1995) Behavior of serum cytokine levels and peripheral lymphocyte subsets after H-LTx. Transplant Proc 27: 2021–2022

11. Ippoliti G, Vinante F, Rovati B, Di Franco L, Martinelli L, Goggi C, Viganó M, Pizzolo G (1990) Serum levels of soluble interleukin-2 receptor (sIL-2R) fail to correlate with the occurrence and degree of rejection in heart transplant patients. Clin Transplant 4: 1–4

12. Jutte NHPM, Hesse CJ, Balk AHMM, Mochtar B, Weimar W (1990) Sequential measurements of soluble interleukin 2 receptor levels in plasma of heart transplant recipients. Transplantation 50: 328–330

13. Kaden J, May G, Schönemann C, Müller P, Groth J, Seeger W, Seibt F, Henkert M, Lippert J (1992) Effect of ATG prophylaxis in sensitized and non-sensitized kidney graft recipients. Transplant Int 5 [1]: 75–78

14. Kaden J, May G, Müller P, Groth J, Strobelt V, Eger E, Wohlfahrt L (1995) Intraoperative high-dose anti-T-lymphocyte globulin bolus in addition to triple-drug therapy improves kidney graft survival. Transplant Proc 27: 1060–1061

15. Kaden J, Willsch C, Spehr V, Kaden K, Strobelt V, May G (1995) Nachweis und diagnostische Wertigkeit von IL-8 im Harn von Nierentransplantatempfängern. Transplant Med 7: 114–122

16. Köhler H, Girndt M, Dumann H, Klingel R (1993) Immundefekt bei Niereninsuffizienz. II. Mechanismen des „urämischen" Immundefekts. Dtsch Med Wochenschr 118: 790–795

17. Lahat N, Shtiller R, Zlotnick AY, Merin G (1993) Early IL-2/sIL-2R surge following surgery leads to temporary immune refractoriness. Clin Exp Immunol 92: 482–486

18. Langhoff E, Ladefoged J, Odum N (1986) Effect of interleukin-2 and methylprednisolone on in vitro transformation of uremic lymphocytes. Int Arch Allergy Appl Immunol 81: 5–11

19. Malcus C, Pouteil-Noble C, Touraine F, Raffaele P, Touraine JL (1990) Plasma soluble interleukin-2 receptor (IL-2Rs) level and activation markers in blood in the follow-up of renal allograft patients. Transplant Proc 22: 1865–1866

20. Perkins JD, Munn SR, Barr D, Ferguson DC, Carpenter HA (1990) Evidence that the soluble interleukin 2 receptor level may determine the optimal time for cystoscopically directed biopsy in pancreatico-duodenal allograft recipients. Transplantation 49: 363–366

21. Pizzolo G (1988) The soluble interleukin-2 receptor as a new biological marker in diseases. Immunol Clin 7: 13–21

22. Plaza JJ, Blum G, Ortiz A, Hernando L, Feijoo E, Sanz J, Garcia R, Egido J, Ortiz F (1992) Usefulness of serum interleukin 2 receptor levels in renal allograft recipients. Transplant Proc 24: 63–64

23. Pollak R, Fabrega AJ, Vasquez E, Sanchez J, Mulero CB, Williams RH (1995) Measurement of serum-soluble interleukin 2 receptor levels following renal transplantation. Transplantation 59: 926–927

24. Raskova J, Ghobrial I, Shea SM, Ebert EC, Eisinger RP, Raska K (1986) T cells in patients undergoing chronic hemodialysis: Mitogenic response suppressor activity and interleukin-2 production and receptor generation. Diagn Immunol 4: 209–216

25. Schroeder TJ, Helling T, McKenna RM, Rush D, Jeffrey JR, Brewer B, Martin LA, Traylor D, Fisher RA, First MR, Muth KL (1992) A multicenter study to evaluate a novel assay for quantification of soluble interleukin 2 receptor in renal transplant recipients. Transplantation 53: 34–40

26. Simpson MA, Madras PN, Cornaby AJ, Etienne T, Dempsey RA, Clowes GHA, Monaco AP (1989) Sequential determinations of urinary cytology and plasma and urinary lymphokines in the management of renal allograft recipients. Transplantation 47: 218–223

27. Stockenhuber F, Steininger R, Apperl A, Muehlbacher F, Patek E, Sautner T, Sertl K, Graninger W, Hauser AC, Balcke P (1990) Soluble interleukin-2 receptor: A novel parameter of renal graft rejection. Transplant Proc 22: 165–166

28. Tice DG, Heintz S, Scruggs B, Hubbell C, Szmalc FS (1993) Immune monitoring: Does the reality fulfill the promise? Transplant Proc 25: 2654

29. Young JB, Lloyd KS, Windsor NT, Cocanougher B, Weilbaecher DG, Kleiman NS, Smart FW, Nelson DL, Lawrence EC (1991) Elevated soluble interleukin-2 receptor levels early after heart transplantation and long-term survival and development of coronary arteriopathy. J Heart Lung Transplant 10: 243–250

Transpl Int (1996) 9 [Suppl 1]: S68–S72
© Springer-Verlag 1996

KIDNEY

E. Sárváry
P. Borka
B. Sulyok
A. Péter
Z. Vass
G. Rákóczy
L. Selmeci
L. Takács
J. Járay
F. Perner

Diagnostic value of urinary enzyme determination in renal transplantation

E. Sárváry (✉) · P. Borka · B. Sulyok ·
A. Péter · Z. Vass · J. Járay · F. Perner
Transplantation and Surgical Clinic,
Semmelweis Medical University,
23–25 Baross street,
H-1082 Budapest, Hungary

G. Rákóczy
First Department of Pediatrics,
Semmelweis Medical University,
Budapest, Hungary

L. Selmeci
Cardiovascular Surgical Clinic,
Semmelweis Medical University,
Budapest, Hungary

L. Takács
Department of Biomedical Sciences,
Thousand Oaks, USA

Abstract The measurement of enzyme activity in urine provides a sensitive assessment for renal tubular cell damage. The present study was undertaken to evaluate the clinical value of the determination of tubular brush-border-associated enzymes, alkaline phosphatase (AP), gamma-glutamyl transferase (GGT), leucine aminopeptidase (LAP), and dipeptidyl peptidase IV (DPP), of patients with normal graft function (NOR, $n = 20$), with acute tubular necrosis (ATN, $n = 11$), with an acute rejection episode (*ARE*, $n = 17$) after transplantation, and of healthy persons ($n = 20$). The second urine of the morning was collected daily during the patients' stay in hospital. The enzyme activities were measured at 25 °C and were expressed as U/mmol creatinine. The enzymuria in NOR is higher than in healthy controls, but is still in the normal range. By 5 days after transplantation the initial increased excretion declines as the graft function improves. Elevated enzymuria (DPP 0.69 ± 0.56, AP 3.06 ± 3.24, GGT 4.16 ± 4.13, and LAP 1.39 ± 1.27) was observed during the rejection episodes. Two days before clinical diagnosis of rejection, the release of DPP-IV and GGT increases to double, and the AP and LAP increases to 3 times the value on the fourth day before rejection. Successful treatment of rejection coincided with a quick return by the third day of the rejection period to the previous enzyme distribution. In ATN no decrease of enzymuria occurs and the excretion is much higher than in ARE. Our method with the every day monitoring of kidney graft function offers the possibility for the early diagnosis of acute rejection.

Key words Enzymuria · Dipeptidyl aminopeptidase IV · Alkaline phosphatase · Gamma-glutamyl transferase · Leucine aminopeptidase

Introduction

Nowadays renal transplantation provides a well-established treatment for patients with end-stage renal disease. On the basis of present evidence many immunological, inflammatory, and enzymatic abnormalities are noted after transplantation. Detection of these problems can be used for diagnostic and therapeutic purposes [1, 3, 4, 7]. Kidney transplants are frequently followed by rejection (35–40 %). The clinical signs can be only detected when relatively large deterioration had happened in the renal tissue [1, 2, 4, 6]. In the past decade, the evaluation of urinary enzymes has played a key role in the non-invasive diagnosis of rejection. Diagnostic significance of urinary enzymes increased due to adoption of the new, nephrotoxic immunsuppressive therapy, because the clinical signs of rejection became less characteristic and so the diagnosis become more difficult.

Deterioration of graft function can be caused by acute rejection episode(s) (ARE), acute tubular necro-

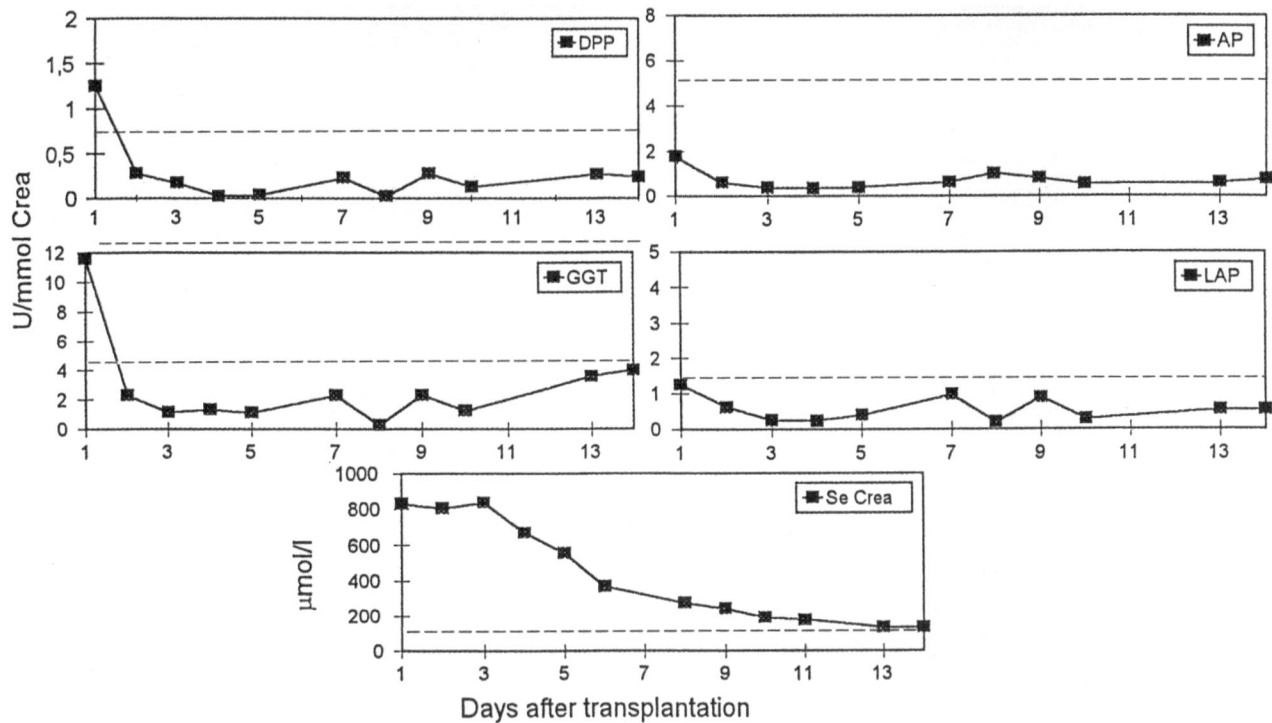

Fig. 1 Excretion patterns of brush border enzymes and serum creatinine concentration in an allograft recipient with normal graft function (y-*axis* shows the enzyme activities in U/mmol creatinine, *horizontal dotted lines* mark the upper reference limits of normal range)

sis (ATN), the cyclosporin (CyA)-induced nephrotoxicity, and surgical complications. It is difficult to make a prompt differential diagnosis because the symptoms are very similar in some cases. Our study was undertaken:

1. To find those enzymes which have a diagnostic and predictive value for rejection in the posttransplant period of renal transplant patients
2. To determine the dynamic changes of the different enzyme concentrations in the different complications (ARE, ATN) leading to deterioration of the graft function
3. To apply our results to the selection of the proper treatment and to monitor and promptly predict the usefulness of therapy (e.g. steroid "shot")
4. To create the enzyme diagnostic laboratory background for the clinicans to help them to discriminate between the different complications before the clinical symptoms occur, without expensive and dangerous invasive investigations.

The application of enzyme diagnostic methods in everyday practice would be beneficial from the point of view of the patients, because it can improve the chance of longer graft survival and this leads to a significant drop in the hospital costs.

Patients and methods

Healthy controls

The reference population (controls) consisted of 20 healthy persons (female = 11, male 9, age = 24–43 years) chosen from the staff and medical students of our clinic. They had no cardiac, liver, or renal disease, diabetes, or hypertension, and had normal blood cell counts, normal urine analysis, and normal findings in serum urea and creatinine. They were not on any medication for a week before the time of sampling. The female volunteers were neither pregnant nor menstruating at the time of sample collection.

Renal transplant patients

Samples from 54 renal transplant patients were collected and evaluated. Patients were on our standard immunsuppressive protocol of cyclosporin A (CyA) and IV methylprednisolone. After admission the patients were classified into three groups according to the diagnosis of the clinicians:
1. Patients ($n = 17$) with ARE were described as having fever (mostly in the mornings), rising serum creatinine, diminished daily urine volume, graft tenderness and enlargement, and increased resistance index. When there was a strong clinical suspicion of rejection antirejection therapy was started.
2. Patients ($n = 11$) with ATN were characterized by high serum creatinine, greatly diminished daily urine volume or no urine at all. These patients required dialysis following transplantation without any sign of other types of kidney diseases.
3. The uncomplicated group (NOR) of transplanted patients ($n = 20$) were classified as having an immediate onset of renal function and a spontaneous decrease in serum creatinine level immediately after transplantation.

Six investigated patients (OTHER) could not be classified into any group mentioned above. "Shot" therapy was applied for these

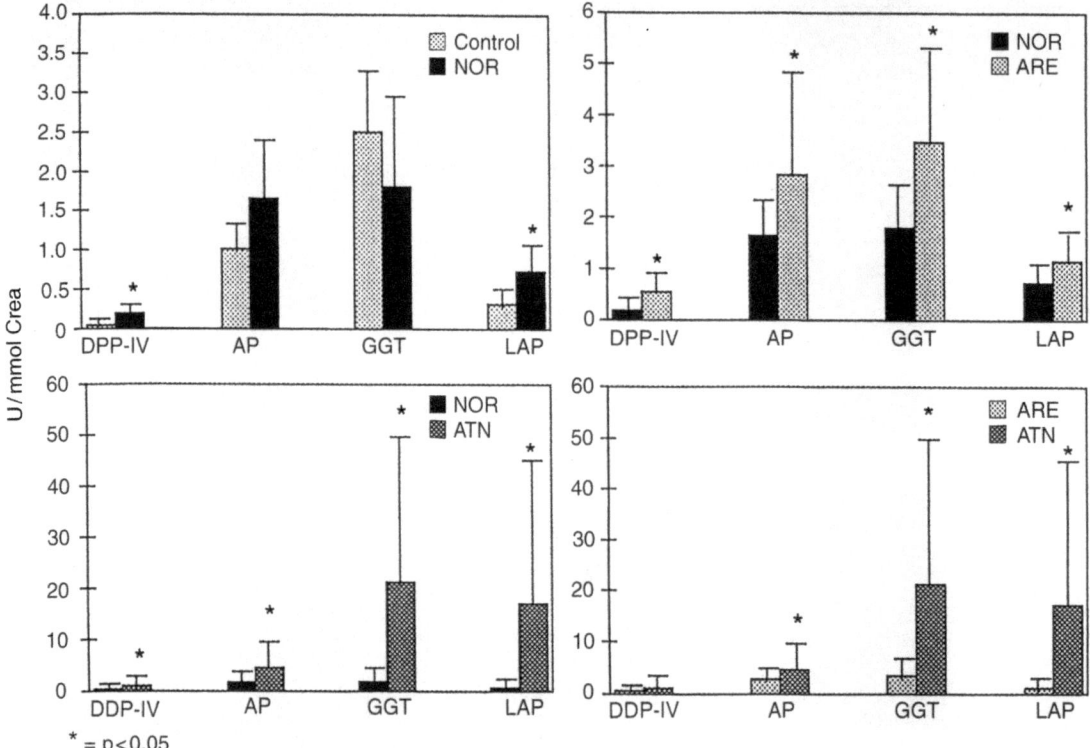

* = p<0.05

Fig. 2 The average enzyme activities are compared in the different groups; control vs patients with normal graft function (NOR), NOR vs patients with acute rejection episode (ARE), NOR vs patients with acute tubular necrosis (ATN), ARE vs ATN. (y-*axis* represents the enzyme activities in U/mmol creatinine, $P < 0.05$)

Table 1 Average enzymuria (U/mmol creatinine) of all investigated groups (*NOR* patients having immediate onset renal function posttransplantation, *ARE* patients having acute rejection episodes, *ATN* patients having acute tubular necrosis, *DPP-IV* dipeptidyl peptidase IV, *AP* alkaline phosphatase, *GGT* gamma-glutamyl transferase, *LAP* leucine aminopeptidase)

	DPP-IV	AP	GGT	LAP
Control	0.053	1.008	2.504	0.313
NOR	0.186	1.645	1.803	0.728
ARE	0.551	2.837	3.472	1.158
ATN	1.063	4.497	21.246	17.101
ARE/NOR (%)	352	178	222	185
ATN/NOR (%)	572	273	1180	2349
ATN/ARE (%)	162	159	612	148

patients, however, they had other problems but the symptoms were similar to rejection. They had no acute rejection episode diagnosed by clinicians retrospectively [5].

Collection of samples

The second midstream urines of the morning (2 ml) were collected from both control subjects and patients during the patients' stay in the hospital (2–3 weeks). The samples were centrifuged (2000 × g

for 15 min), the creatinine concentration measured (Jaffe method-VP Super System, single channel, ABBOT Laboratories Diagnostic Division Texas, USA) and the supernatants were stored at 4 °C until the day of measurement.

Determination of enzyme activities

The determination of enzyme activities were measured kinetically on an ELISA reader (Anthos Reader 2001, Anthos Labtec Instrument) 405 nm, 25 °C, by monitoring the increase of absorbance due to the release of chromogenic (the 4-nitroanilin/or at the ALP: 4-nitrophenol) substrates. The activities were expressed as U/l. In order to account for variations due to urine concentration without collecting 24-hour specimens, urinary enzyme/creatinine ratios were calculated and expressed as U/mmol creatinine. This method compensates for varying rates of urinary flow. The reference intervals of these enzymes at 25 °C are: DPP-IV 0.13–1.08, AP 0.03–0.32, GGT: 0.8–4.01, and LAP: 0.1–0.61.

The onset of rejection was indicated by the first day of "shot" therapy. The 4-day period before and the 4–6 days following rejection were investigated Students' *T*-probe was applied for statistical analysis and the differences were significance if $P < 0.05$.

Results

The investigated enzymes have controversial diagnostic value in the 4–5 postoperative days, although they can indicate the ability of the graft to regenerate (Fig. 1). In the NOR group the significant enzymuria in the early postoperative period decreases to within the normal range by the fifth day (Fig. 1). The enzymuria, except

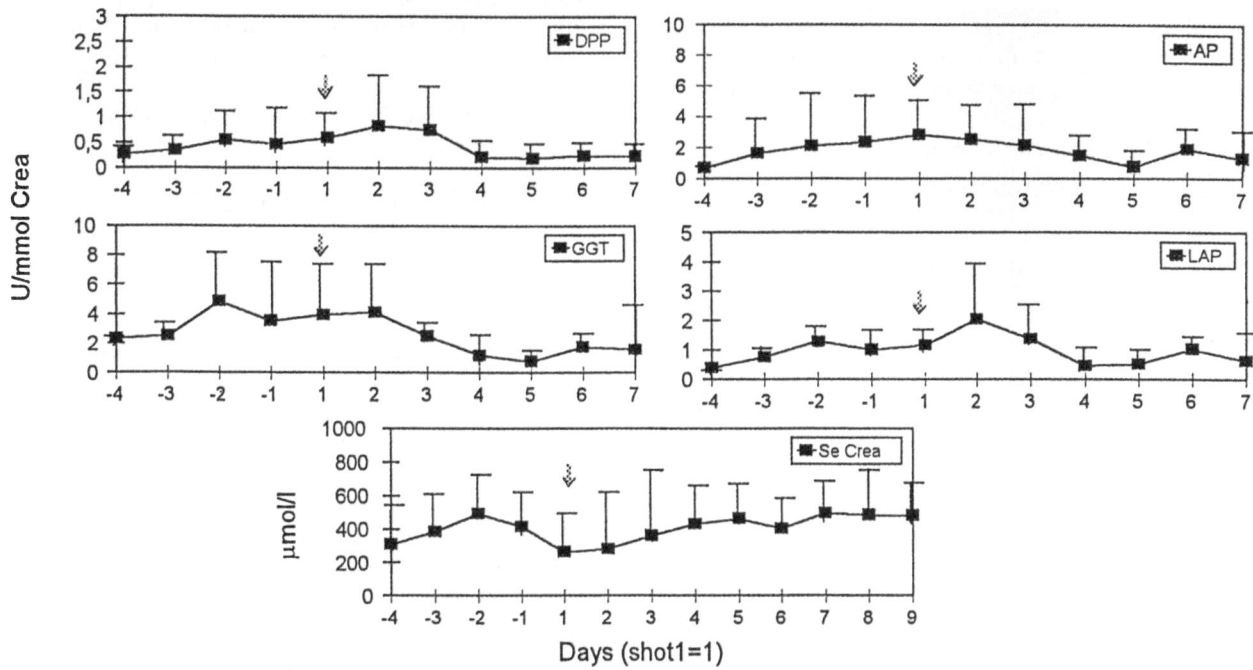

Fig. 3 Excretion patterns of brush border enzymes and serum creatinine concentration in patients with ARE before, during, and after "shot" therapy. (y-*axis* shows the enzyme activities in U/mmol creatinine, ↓ indicates the onset of rejection)

Table 2 Enzyme activities of ARE patients ($n = 17$) before during and after rejection episode. (Data are given as a % of the level 4 days before onset of rejection episode). "Shot" therapy was begun an day 1

Napok	DPP-IV (%)	AP (%)	GGT (%)	LAP (%)
– 4	100	100	100	100
– 3	126	239	107	190
– 2	208	306	206	324
– 1	172	343	151	251
1	221	408	168	292
2	308	364	174	514
3	282	310	107	345
4	77	213	50	112
5	72	111	33	131
6	91	272	75	257
7	89	186	67	155

for GGT, is slightly elevated when compared with the healthy controls (Fig. 2, Table 1). In the ATN group the prompt enzymuria does not decrease, it can even rise further (Fig. 2, Table 1). The measured and calculated enzymuria is several times higher than in the NOR ARE groups (Fig. 2, Table 1). In the ARE group, the immediate postoperative elevated enzymuria decreases similarly to the NOR group, then it starts to rise as a consequence of acute rejection. The enzymuria pre-

cedes the occurrance of clinical symptoms of acute rejection by 1–3 days (Figs. 2, 3, Table 1, 2). Two days before clinical diagnosis of rejection, the release of DPP-IV and GGT increases to double, and the AP and LAP increases to 3 times the value on the 4th day before rejection (Fig. 3, Table 2). The highest level of these enzymes was observed on the second day of the rejection period (Fig. 3, Table 2). On the third day of the rejection period the enzymuria decreases significantly showing the beneficial effect of "shot" therapy (Table 2). The enzyme activities of other group (OTHER) were under the reference limit before and during "shot" therapy.

Discussion

We evaluated the urinary enzyme activities to find those enzymes which have a diagnostic and predictive value for acute rejection in the early posttransplant period of renal transplant patients. Nowadays, applied immunsuppression therapy requires a new approach in the measurement of tubular brush border enzymes in the urine. The determination of urinary enzymes offers a good possibility for the diagnosis of different pathological alterations of renal grafts. Acute rejection episodes in kidney transplant patients with conventional immunsuppression therapy (azathioprine + prednisolone) were often predicted by an increasing enzymuria of certain brush border enzymes. The CyA therapy was followed by a more effective immunsuppression but also a higher degree of nephrotoxicity. Since then the clinical and laboratory diagnosis of acute rejection periods proved to be more difficult because as the frequency of acute rejection episodes decreased significantly, the clinical signs became less characteristic, and the nephrotoxicity meant a "noisy" background for the urinary enzyme "signals".

Acute rejection episodes are the most frequent postoperative complication of kidney transplantation so the early diagnosis and treatment is very important. The regular monitoring of these investigated urinary enzyme activities throughout the posttransplant period would be valuable in indicating graft function and in predicting effectiveness of the rejection treatment. Their simplicity, sensitivity, and non-invasive nature make the assay of urinary enzymes a powerful addition to the clinician's diagnostic armoury.

Acknowledgements The authors thank Mrs. Marta Lakatos for her excellent technical assistance.

References

1. Corbett R, Gardner GJ, Kind PRN, Thompson AE, Price R (1983) Comparison of urinary N-acetyl-beta-D-gucosaminidase and urinary fibrin degradation products for diagnosis of rejection after renal transplantation. Clin Chim Acta 128: 141–150
2. Dance N, Prince PG, Cattel WR, Landsell J, Richards B (1970) The excretion of N-acetyl-beta-D-gucosaminidase and galactosidase by patients with renal disease. Clin Chim Acta 27: 87–92
3. Dyck RF, Cardella CJ, Sacks MA (1979) Urinary lysosomal enzyme excretion after renal allotransplantation. Clin Chim Acta 91: 111–116
4. Horpacsy G, Zinsmeyer J, Schroder K, Mebel M (1977) Value of determining urinary enzymes after human kidney transplantation. Early warning of rejection or not? Clin Chem 23: 770–771
5. Jung K, Pergande M, Schreiber G, Schroder K (1983) Stability of enzymes in urine at 37 °C. Clin Chim Acta 131: 185–191
6. Whiting PH, Nicholls AJ, Catto GRD, Edward N, Engeset J (1980) Patterns of N-acetyl-beta-D-glucosaminidase excretion after renal transplantation. Clin Chim Acta 108: 1–7
7. Whiting PH, Peterson J, Power DA, Stewart RDM, Catto GRD, Edward N (1983) Diagnostic value of urinary N-acetyl-beta-D-glucosaminidase its isoenzymes and the fractional excretion of sodium following renal transplantation. Clin Chim Acta 130: 369–376

Transpl Int (1996) 9 [Suppl 1]: S 73–S 75
© Springer-Verlag 1996

J. Fangmann
K. Oldhafer
G. Offner
R. Pichlmayr

Retroperitoneal placement of living related adult renal grafts in children less than 5 years of age – a feasible technique?

J. Fangmann (✉) · K. Oldhafer ·
R. Pichlmayr
Klinik für Abdominal- und
Transplantationschirurgie,
Medizinische Hochschule Hannover,
Konstanty-Gutschow-Strasse 8,
D-30623 Hannover, Germany

G. Offner
Abteilung II für Kinderheilkunde,
Medizinische Hochschule Hannover,
D-30623 Hannover, Germany

Abstract The extraperitoneal approach was used for transplantation of adult renal grafts in eight children under 5 years, three of them weighing less than 10 kg. Usually, children of this size are approached transperitoneally. The modified procedure included partial mobilization of the right liver to provide enough space for retroperitoneal graft placement and positioning of the vascular anastomoses, invariably to the aorta and caval vein. With this regimen, no significant space problems were encountered in recipients as small as 9 kg, and particularly, neither arterial nor venous complications occurred. Currently, at a mean follow-up of 2.4 years, all patients are alive with well-functioning grafts. Thus, the extraperitoneal approach represents a feasible and successful procedure in the pediatric living related renal transplantation setting for recipients under 10 kg of weight.

Key words Kidney transplantation · Living donors · Children

Introduction

Living related pediatric renal transplantation is technically characterized by an extreme disparity in size of adult grafts and small recipients. Whereas in recipient children weighing more than 20 kg [10] the transplant procedure essentially is the same as for adults using the extraperitoneal approach, in small children and infants below this weight limit, a priori assumptions of space problems have led to the predominant practice of intraabdominal placement of the grafts [2, 8, 9]. Since the transperitoneal approach is associated with considerable disadvantages and thus is not considered to represent the optimal placement of the graft, we have modified the technique of the adult-type extraperitoneal approach. This paper describes the results by using this modified procedure in pediatric living related renal transplantations for small recipient children less than 5 years of age.

Patients and methods

Patients

The series between April 1991 and September 1995 presented here included seven boys and one girl less than 5 years of age transplanted with adult grafts from living related donors, in two cases from the mother and in six cases from the father. Except for one case, exclusively right donor kidneys were used. The mean age of the recipients was 3.0 ± 1.0 years (range 1.4–4.8 years); five of them were younger than 3 years. The mean weight of the entire series was 11.4 ± 2.0 kg (range 9.3–15.3 kg), three children weighing less than 10 kg. Seven children had been on dialysis prior to transplantation, and one boy, 17 months old, received a preemptive transplantation.

Surgical technique

In all recipients we employed a modified technique of the adult-type procedure. Surgery was carried out via an extraperitoneal approach from the right iliac fossa up to the retrohepatic space.

A standard oblique incision in the right lower quadrant of the abdomen from just above the symphysis pubis has been employed, which was extended cephalad to the costal margin to increase exposure for the disproportionately sized adult renal grafts. The external oblique aponeurosis and the muscle layer were divided in line with the skin incision, including the transversal fascia, without injuring the peritoneum. The peritoneum then was reflected off the psoas muscle medially, thus exposing the distal aorta and vena cava inferior including the iliac vessels in the retroperitoneal space. Depending on the size mismatch between the donor kidney and the recipient, the right retrohepatic area had to be mobilized as well and the peritoneum was retracted off. This maneuver created a large enough space to place an adult donor kidney retroperitoneally even in very small recipients weighing less than 10 kg. In addition, positioning of the graft may be facilitated by native nephrectomy, as indicated in the presence of chronically infected kidneys, uncontrolled nephrotic syndrome or extremely large polycystic diseased kidneys. Renal grafts placed in this manner will occupy the entire space between the bladder and the right retrohepatic area.

All grafts, irrespective of the side (left or right kidney), were invariably placed into the right iliac fossa, thus achieving an easy access to the inferior caval vein for venous anastomosis. This is especially important in the presence of a short renal vein, which would not allow an anastomosis to be performed from the left iliac fossa.

The venous anastomosis is always performed first in an end-to-side fashion, invariably to the distal caval vein. Venotomy is performed by a linear incision of the approximate size of the renal vein diameter; additionally, a small elliptical patch of the anterior venous wall may be excised. It is of great importance to shorten the renal vein as much as possible since the abdominal closure may exert considerable compression on the anastomoses, leading to impairment of the venous drainage as well as kinking, which may occur if the renal vein is too long. For the venous anastomosis, 6/0-monofilament running prolene suture was used. The renal artery, without an aortic patch, was anastomosed end-to-side, invariably to the distal aorta between the bifurcation and the branching of the mesenteric artery, anteriorly passing the caval vein. For the anastomosis, 6/0- or 7/0-running prolene suture was used. In the case of multiple arteries, we preferred separate anastomoses, with the superior artery anastomosed to the aorta and the inferior renal artery to the common iliac artery.

Urinary tract continuity was restored by means of an extravesical ureteroneocystostomy, as originated by Gregoir, using 6/0-polydioxanone suture.

Results

Of the eight renal grafts, seven functioned immediately after reperfusion was reinstituted. One graft showed a delayed onset of function for approximately 24 h, but the patient did not require hemodialysis. The pocket which was created in the iliac fossa cephalad up to the retrohepatic area after reflection of the peritoneum was large enough for all the adult grafts in the recipients as small as 9.3 kg. In all but one case, abdominal closure could be done directly without significant tension or any impairment of the arterial supply or venous drainage. In that single case, a boy of 2.8 years and 11 kg, an interposition of a vicryl mesh was needed for closure. Within 2 weeks, however, a secondary approximation of the skin could be accomplished.

No vascular complications were encountered, specifically no arterial or venous thrombosis occurred either in the early postoperative course or during the entire follow-up period. The patients have been followed for 1–4.5 years with a mean follow-up of 2.4 years. One-year graft survival was 100 %. Currently, all patients are alive with well-functioning grafts.

The only surgical complication we encountered in this series was one urinary leakage noted on day 5 postoperatively due to distal ureteral necrosis. The patient had to undergo ureteral reimplantation.

Discussion

Kidney transplantation in small children less than 5 years of age has been reported to be associated with a considerable number of surgical complications, often leading to technical failure and subsequent overall poor results [1, 2, 4–6]. In this context, the two main technical considerations are placement of the graft and positioning of the vascular anastomoses. Primarily depending on the size discrepancy between adult grafts and recipients, two surgical approaches are proposed, namely the intraperitoneal and the adult-type extraperitoneal procedures. Because of anticipated space problems using adult renal grafts, recipients weighing less than 20 kg have been recommended to be best approached transperitoneally with the kidney placed intraabdominally behind the right colon, as first described by Starzl et al. [10]. Recently, there have been reports [2, 7] showing transplantation of adult grafts via the extraperitoneal approach into children under 15 kg.

The results of the series of patients presented here demonstrate that the extraperitoneal approach represents a technically feasible, safe, and successful procedure for transplanting adult grafts into small children less than 5 years of age. It is of particular importance that this also holds true for children as small as 9 kg. However, the actual recipient weight limit for retroperitoneal graft placement remains to be determined.

Besides the extraperitoneal approach, the most critical factor that contributed to the success in our series is the positioning of the vascular anastomoses exclusively to the distal aorta and inferior caval vein. These vessels in small children are of approximately the same size as those of adult type renal vessels, and they therefore ensure adequate perfusion of the graft as well as sufficient venous drainage. Thus, a thrombosis of the graft, which has been reported to be a significant risk factor in pediatric renal transplantation [3], is prevented. Consequently, we have not encountered any immediate or late vascular complications in our entire series. In addition, an aggressive fluid replacement intraoperatively immediately before the release of the vascular clamps is important in order to avoid underperfusion of the graft, leading to non-technical thrombosis. Adult renal grafts sequester a significant percentage of the pediatric circulation blood volume.

Furthermore, the extraperitoneal graft placement offers major advantages compared to the transperitoneal approach, namely no intraabdominal adhesions, no small bowel obstructions or ileus, and thus a quicker mobilization of the patients. Possible bleedings and urinary leakage are restricted extraperitoneally, graft biopsy for monitoring is easy, and continuation of peritoneal dialysis is possible in cases of delayed graft function.

In conclusion, we therefore recommend the extraperitoneal approach with vascular anastomoses to aorta and caval vein in the pediatric living related transplantation setting as the standard technique. With this regimen we have realized 100 % 1-year graft and patient survival. However, small children assigned for transplantation remain a fragile group of patients who require great commitment and close cooperation of physicians and surgeons.

Acknowledgements We are indebted to Dr. S. Tager, currently at the Surgical Department of the Medizinische Hochschule Hannover, for critical reading of the manuscript.

References

1. Arbus GS, Hardy BE, Balfe JW, Churchill BM, Steele BT, Baumal R, Curtis RN (1983) Cadaveric renal transplants in children under 6 years of age. Kidney Int Suppl 15, 24: S111
2. Fine RN, Ettenger R (1994) Renal transplantation in children. In: Morris PJ (ed) Kidney transplantation: principles and practice, 4th edn. W.B. Saunders, Philadelphia, pp 412–459
3. Harmon WE, Stablein D, Alexander SR, Tejani A (1991) Graft thrombosis in pediatric renal transplant recipients. Transplantation 51: 406
4. Hodson EM, Najarian JS, Kjellstrand CM, Simmons RL, Mauer SM (1978) Renal transplantation in children aged 1 to 5 years. Pediatrics 61: 458
5. McEnery PT, Stablein DM, Arbus G, Tejani A (1992) Renal transplantation in children. N Engl J Med 326: 1727
6. Moel DI, Butt KM (1981) Renal transplantation in children less than 2 years of age. J Pediatr 99: 535
7. Rosenthal JT, Ettenger RB, Ehrlich RM, Fine RN (1990) Technical factors contributing to successful kidney transplantation in small children. J Urol 144: 116
8. Sheldon CA, Najarian JS, Mauer SM (1985) Pediatric renal transplantation. Surg Clin North Am 65: 1589
9. Simmons RL, Najarian JS (1984) Kidney transplantation. In: Egdahl RH (ed) Comprehensive manuals of surgical specialties. Springer, Berlin Heidelberg New York
10. Starzl TE, Marchioro TL, Morgan WW, Waddell WR (1964) A technique for use of adult renal homograft in children. Surg Gynecol Obstet 119: 106

Transpl Int (1996) 9 [Suppl 1]: S 76–S 80
© Springer-Verlag 1996

J. H. C. Daemen
R. J. de Wit
M. W. G. A. Bronkhorst
M. L. Marcar
M. Yin
E. Heineman
G. Kootstra

Short-term outcome of kidney transplants from non-heart-beating donors after preservation by machine perfusion

J. H. C. Daemen · R. J. de Wit ·
M. W. G. A. Bronkhorst · M. L. Marcar ·
M. Yin · E. Heineman · G. Kootstra (✉)
Department of Surgery, University
Hospital Maastricht, P. O. Box 5800,
NL-6202 AZ Maastricht,
The Netherlands
Tel. +31 43 3 87 59 23; Fax +31 43 3 87 54 73

Abstract In this study, the short-term outcome of renal transplants from non-heart-beating donors (NHBD) preserved by machine perfusion (MP) is evaluated and compared to preservation by cold storage (CS). Twenty-two NHBD kidneys were procured during 1993 and 1994 after in situ perfusion with histidine-tryptophan ketoglutarate and preserved by continuous perfusion using University of Wisconsin organ preservation solution for MP as a perfusate. Between 1980 and 1992, 57 NHBD kidneys were procured and preserved by CS. Donors in the MP group sustained increased first warm ischemia times (WIT1) ($P < 0.1$) and recipients in the MP group suffered longer anastomosis time, worse HLA-DR mismatch, and more initial use of cyclosporin as immunosuppressant; all these factors are known to be deleterious to short-term outcome. Despite these unfavorable conditions, delayed function (DF) rate was decreased in the MP group, although not significantly. However, when considering only kidneys with WIT1 $\geq$ 45 min, short-term outcome was significantly better in the MP group ($P < 0.05$). We conclude that MP is superior for the preservation of NHBD kidneys, especially after prolonged warm ischemia.

Key words Non-heart-beating donors · Kidney transplantation · Short-term outcome · Machine perfusion · Delayed graft function

Introduction

In the search for ways to reduce the organ shortage, non-heart-beating donors (NHBD) are recognized as a valuable source of organs for transplantation. After irreversible cardiac arrest and the subsequent diagnosis of death, organs can be procured and used for transplantation, especially kidneys since they are known to tolerate ischemia well [1]. The University Hospital Maastricht, has had an NHBD program for over a decade and procures and transplants kidneys from NHBD [2]. Analysis of the transplantation outcome with these renal grafts showed a high incidence of delayed function (DF) due to acute tubular necrosis (ATN) when compared to grafts from heart-beating donors (HBD) [3]. From experimental data, it is known that preservation of ischemically damaged kidneys by machine perfusion (MP) is superior to simple cold storage (CS) [4, 5]. In order to reduce the DF rate of kidney grafts from NHBD we recently implemented MP as the preferred method of preservation. In this study, the results of 22 renal grafts from NHBD preserved by MP were evaluated and retrospectively compared with grafts from NHBD preserved by CS.

Materials and methods

Patients dying after irreversible circulatory arrest in the emergency room or ICU, were considered potential NHBD when meeting the following criteria: circulatory arrest no longer than 30 min excluding the time of effective resuscitation and a total resuscitation

Table 1 Donor and recipient data. Results are given as mean ± SEM or numbers (%) (*CS* cold storage preservation, *MP* machine perfusion preservation, *WIT1* first warm ischemia time, *CIT* cold ischemia time, *CyA* cyclosporin A)

	CS	MP	P value
Period	1980–1992	1993–1994	
Cases	57	22	
Donor data			
Age (years)	40.7 ± 2.3	45.8 ± 3.7	0.21
Creatinine (μmol/l)	101.6 ± 4.9	111.6 ± 9.4	0.35
WIT1 (min)	33.1 ± 2.9	52.0 ± 7.9	0.10
Recipient data			
Age (years)	44.9 ± 1.7	49.0 ± 3.1	0.19
CIT (h)	31.5 ± 1.1	30.2 ± 1.2	0.5
Anastomosis time (min)	36.2 ± 2.0	40.7 ± 3.4	0.05
Graft number	1.2 ± 0.1	1.1 ± 0.1	0.8
HLA-DR mismatch	0.3 ± 0.1	0.6 ± 0.1	0.03
CyA immunosuppression	35 (38 %)	18 (82 %)	0.05

Table 2 Short-term outcome up to 3 months posttransplantation. Results are given as mean ± SEM or numbers (%) (*DF* delayed function, *mo* months)

	CS	MP	P value
Cases	57	22	
Immediate function	15 (26 %)	8 (36 %)	
Delayed function	34 (60 %)	11 (50 %)	0.67
Primary non-function	8 (14 %)	3 (14 %)	
Urine output (ml/1st 24 h)	836.9 ± 154.1	1465.2 ± 540.2	0.66
Duration of DF (days)	17.2 ± 1.7	18.9 ± 2.8	0.63
Number of dialyses	6.0 ± 0.8	5.5 ± 1.2	0.84
Creatinine 1 mo (μmol/l)	338.5 ± 46.1	324.5 ± 69.4	0.58
Creatinine 3 mo (μmol/l)	194.2 ± 13.8	264.8 ± 44.8	0.39

time not longer than 2 h. The upper age limit was considered to be 65 years and the potential donors were not known to suffer from kidney disease, uncontrolled hypertension, or metastasizing malignancies. Patients with signs of sepsis or intravenous drug abuse were excluded. All donors became available either after an unsuccessful attempt at cardiopulmonary resuscitation (so called NHBD cat II) or sustained final cardiac arrest after withdrawal of ventilatory support (NHBD cat III) [6]. After consent, an in situ perfusion procedure using a double-balloon-triple-lumen cooling catheter (Porgès AJ 6516), according to a technique described before, was performed [7]. Afterwards, the kidneys were procured in the operating room. The organs were preserved by either CS, using Euro-Collins (EC), histidine-tryptophan ketoglutarate (HTK), or University of Wisconsin (UW) CS solutions, or by MP in a Gambro-PF3B perfusion machine using UW machine preservation solution as a perfusate [8]. The in situ flush out was performed using the respective CS solution or HTK in all MP cases. During MP, flow characteristics and enzyme loss were recorded to evaluate the viability of the kidney. Because of these parameters, among others, kidneys were discarded and not used [9]. Kidneys transplanted within the Eurotransplant area were included and data were collected by approaching the transplant centers.

Short-term posttransplant function was classified as: (a) immediate function (IF), i.e., immediate life-sustaining renal function

without posttransplant dialysis, (b) DF, i.e., renal function that ultimately was life-sustaining but required one or more dialysis sessions, and (c) primary non-function (PNF), i.e., renal function failed and the patient was never without dialysis. Renal function was recorded as serum creatinine at 1 and 3 months after transplantation; DF was quantified by urine output during the first 24 h posttransplant, the duration of DF (number of days), and the number of dialysis sessions required.

Because WIT1 tended to be longer in the MP group, the results of transplantation with kidneys with prolonged warm ischemia, i.e., WIT1 of 45 min or more, were analyzed separately. The results are given as mean ± SEM. Statistical analysis employed the chi-squared test with Yates' correction or Fisher's exact test, the Mann-Whitney U-test, and the Kruskal-Wallis one-way ANOVA test for differences between the groups, as appropriate. A P value of less than 0.05 was considered significant.

Results

Between July 1993 and December 1994, 22 kidneys were recovered from 14 NHBD, preserved by MP, and subsequently transplanted. In the control group, 57 kidneys from NHBD were transplanted after preservation by CS in the period 1980–1992. Causes of death showed more brain trauma in the CS group while more patients died after myocardial infarction in the MP group ($P = 0.001$). Data concerning donor and recipient factors are summarized in Table 1. Donor age was $40.7 ± 2.3$ years in the CS group and $45.8 ± 3.7$ years in the MP group ($P = 0.21$); last serum creatinine level of the donors was $101.6 ± 4.9$ and $111.6 ± 9.4$ μmol/l, respectively ($P = 0.35$). Kidneys in the CS group sustained a first warm ischemia time (WIT1), the time elapsing between cardiac arrest and the start of in situ cooling, of $33.1 ± 2.9$ min vs $52.0 ± 7.9$ min in the MP group ($P = 0.10$). Forty-two (74 %) organs were cold stored in EC, 14 (24 %) in HTK, and 1 (2 %) in UW; in the MP group, one pair of kidneys was initially flushed with EC.

Mean cold ischemia time (CIT) was $31.5 ± 1.1$ h for cold-stored grafts and $30.2 ± 1.2$ h for machine perfused grafts ($P = 0.50$). Recipient data in either group were comparable for age, sex, number of the graft, and peak level of panel-reactive antibodies. In the MP group, the mean HLA-DR mismatch was $0.6 ± 0.1$ vs $0.3 ± 0.1$ in the CS group ($P = 0.03$). Mean anastomosis time was shorter in the CS group ($36.2 ± 2.0$ min vs $40.7 ± 3.4$ min, $P = 0.05$).

Short-term posttransplant outcome is summarized in Table 2. Results were comparable for both groups, reflected by a similar immediate posttransplant urine output and equal duration of DF, number of dialysis sessions, and kidney function at 1 and 3 months.

In the separate analysis (concerning prolonged ischemia time defined as WIT1 of 45 min or more), 17 kidneys (30 %) in the CS group sustained prolonged warm ischemia (WIT1 $59.7 ± 4.3$ min) vs 10 kidneys (45 %) in the MP group (WIT1 $89.0 ± 6.2$ min,

Table 3 Donor and recipient data for kidneys with WIT1 of 45 min or more. Results are given as mean ± SEM or numbers (%)

	CS	MP	P value
Period	1980–1992	1993–1994	
Cases	17	10	
Donor data			
Age (years)	42.4 ± 3.9	52.6 ± 5.2	0.08
Creatinine (μmol/l)	114.6 ± 8.6	121.4 ± 5.4	0.44
WIT1 (min)	59.7 ± 4.3	89.0 ± 6.2	0.002
Recipient data			
Age	44.8 ± 3.8	51.7 ± 4.2	0.27
CIT (h)	30.8 ± 2.2	29.6 ± 1.9	0.56
Anastomosis time (min)	29.9 ± 2.3	47.5 ± 4.1	0.001
Graft number	1.3 ± 0.2	1.2 ± 0.1	1.0
HLA-DR mismatch	0.3 ± 0.1	0.5 ± 0.2	0.22
CyA immunosuppression	13 (76%)	8 (80%)	0.83

Table 4 Short-term outcome of kidneys with WIT1 of 45 min or more. Results are given as mean ± SEM or numbers (%)

	CS	MP	P value
Cases	17	10	
Immediate function	4 (23%)	5 (50%)	
Delayed function	13 (76%)	3 (30%)	0.02
Primary non-function	0 (0%)	2 (20%)	
Urine output (ml/1st 24 h)	959.5 ± 323.5	1734.8 ± 998.0	0.7
Duration of DF (days)	17.2 ± 2.4	12.7 ± 1.8	0.42
Number of dialyses	4.8 ± 0.9	5.3 ± 1.3	0.93
Creatinine 1 mo (μmol/l)	408.6 ± 76.9	197.3 ± 26.3	0.05
Creatinine 3 mo (μmol/l)	197.4 ± 23.0	163.3 ± 14.9	0.5

$P = 0.002$). Results are depicted in Table 3. All donor data were comparable; for recipient data again the anastomosis time was different (CS group 29.9 ± 2.3 min vs MP group 47.5 ± 4.1 min, $P = 0.001$).

In Table 4, the posttransplant outcome of kidney transplants with prolonged warm ischemia is summarized. It is shown that this outcome was better in the MP group when compared to the CS group ($P = 0.02$), reflected by a lower serum creatinine level at 1 month ($P = 0.05$); serum creatinine at 3 months showed statistically no significant difference ($P = 0.5$). The length of DF and the number of dialyses required were the same.

Discussion

Although kidneys from NHBD have been used ever since the first transplantation, ways have to be found to ameliorate the ischemic damage through optimal methods of preservation and minimization of reperfusion injury, in order to develop this valuable source of transplantable organs. Studies on the transplantation results with kidneys from NHBD show DF rates as high as 60–

75%, almost twice as high as for grafts from HBD [3, 10–15]. This delayed onset of renal function is unfavorable as DF masks the signs of early acute rejection, complicates the postoperative treatment, and the reinstitution of dialysis has a negative impact on the patient's psyche. Consequently, hospital stay will be prolonged and costs increased [16, 17]. The effect of DF on graft survival is controversial; some believe DF is associated with reduced graft survival, while others suggest that DF only in combination with acute rejection is responsible for a worse transplant outcome [18–23]. In spite of doubled DF rates, long-term graft and patient outcome did not differ between recipients of NHBD and HBD kidneys [3].

To reduce DF rates we introduced MP in 1993 as the method of preservation for NHBD kidneys using the UW preservation solution for MP as a perfusate. Nowadays, CS is accepted as the method of choice for the preservation of renal grafts; the advantages of preservation by continuous cold perfusion are most pronounced for prolonged preservation times and for kidneys from marginal donors with ischemic damage [4, 24]. Recent experimental work at our laboratories showed that preservation of ischemically damaged kidneys by MP was superior to preservation by CS. MP counteracts the intrarenal vascular resistance induced by ischemia, providing better reperfusion and delivering oxygen and nutrients to and removing waste products from the organ during preservation. This resulted in better survival of the animals and better preservation of the microcirculatory integrity [5, 25]. The superiority of MP has been confirmed in clinical transplantation on several occasions [26–29] and, recently, impressive results were reported with NHBD after preservation by MP. Kidneys were from NHBD cat III only and sustained considerably less ischemia than our series and showed merely 19–22% DF rate [30, 31]. In the present analysis, the DF rate in the MP group was 50% compared to 60% in the CS group.

Apart from donor type (cadaver vs living donor, and NHBD vs HBD) and the preservation mode, several other factors have been identified as risk factors for ATN and DF. Retransplantation, warm ischemia time, type of preservation solution, preservation time, and number of HLA-DR mismatches have all been supposed to worsen early posttransplant function [3, 16, 17, 23, 32, 33]. In this analysis several of these factors were studied and some appeared to be statistically significant different between the study group and historical controls. For the machine-perfused kidneys, the anastomosis time was longer as well as the WIT1; the evident worse match on HLA-DR antigens in the MP group further deteriorates the early posttransplant function of these grafts. The results of the comparison between the CS and MP groups, therefore, may be biased to the detriment of the MP group concerning transplant outcome. However, although considered to be more profoundly damaged than the NHBD kidneys in the CS group, the grafted kidneys preserved by MP showed equal short-term outcome when compared to grafts preserved by CS. In a previous analysis, we showed that the elevation of serum creatinine at 1 month posttransplant when compared to HBD, was transient and was neutralized at 3 months, not affecting long-term graft outcome [3].

In the last few years, increased efforts have been made to identify potential NHBD and it was noticed that in our program more NHBD cat II were accepted after long resuscitation efforts. This fact is reflected by the increased number of donors dying after myocardial infarction and unsuccessful resuscitation; at present about half in the MP group (period 1993–1994) against one-third in the CS group (period 1980–1992). The more recently effectuated donors may, therefore, have suffered essentially more ischemic damage while all kidneys procured were preserved by MP. Kidneys in the historical control group on the contrary, may be less damaged while all were preserved by CS. The separate analysis of NHBD grafts with WIT1 longer than 45 min, indeed showed that almost half of the kidneys in the MP group suffered prolonged WIT1 and that even within this subgroup WIT1 evidently was increased (89.0 ± 6.2 and 59.7 ± 4.3 min for MP and CS group, respectively; $P = 0.002$). In the prolonged ischemia group, the other donor and recipient data were more comparable in the CS and MP groups, thus minimizing their influence. Although in the subgroup kidneys preserved by MP still sustained more warm ischemic damage than their CS counterparts, the short-term results were significantly improved by MP. This improvement was reflected by a better serum creatinine level at 1 month. The number of days before kidney function was life sustaining, as well as the number of dialyses needed, did not differ among the groups, implying that MP did not effect the severity of DF once it had occurred. Using cyclosporin (CyA) in the immediate posttransplant period is known to prolong the duration of DF [17]. The length of DF is important since prolonged DF was observed to be detrimental to graft survival in NHBD kidney transplants [34]. In the MP group, more patients received CyA (82 % vs 63 %, $P = 0.05$) and this may oppose the positive action of perfusion preservation. The use of ATG as induction immunosuppression and the delayed introduction of CyA until acceptable kidney function is established, could decrease the duration of DF [33].

A very simple and effective way to reduce the ischemic damage to the organs in NHBD is to reduce the WIT1. Since in an opting-in legislation consent is needed to start in situ cooling, WIT1 sometimes is very long while the gap between diagnosis of death and starting the donation procedure is bridged by cardiac massage and artificial ventilation. A presumed-consent law, or at least legal consent to start in situ cooling if the relatives cannot be approached immediately, will reduce ischemic damage considerably and, thus, improve transplant results.

NHBD kidneys and their recipients need special attention with regard to preservation and postoperative treatment. High DF rates are of major concern and must be reduced to improve graft prognosis. The CS group in this analysis suffered less severe ischemic attacks than the MP group. Nevertheless, short-term outcome was at least equal in both groups; for kidneys that sustained prolonged ischemia, however, MP was superior despite more unfavorable donor conditions. To verify these results and study the impact of MP on long-term outcome, a retrospective study with matched controls, along with a prospective study, is currently in process. We conclude that continuous cold perfusion is superior to simple cold storage as the preservation mode for NHBD kidneys, especially after prolonged warm ischemic periods.

Acknowledgements The authors would like to thank the Eurotransplant Foundation and the collaborating Transplant Centers for their cooperation.

References

1. Maessen JG (1988) The stunned kidney: postischemic renal failure and adenine nucleotide homeostasis. In: Maessen JG (ed) Evaluation of ischemic injury in donor kidneys: an experimental study. Wibro dissertatiedrukkerij, Roermond, pp 81–88

2. Daemen JHC, Kootstra G, Wijnen RMH, Yin M, Heineman E (1995) Nonheart-beating donors: the Maastricht experience. In: Terasaki PI, Cecka JM (eds) Clinical transplants 1994. UCLA Tissue Typing Laboratory, Los Angeles, pp 303–316

3. Wijnen RMH, Booster MH, Stubenitsky BM, De Boer J, Heineman E, Kootstra G (1995) Outcome of transplantation of non-heart-beating donor kidneys. Lancet 345: 1067–1070

4. Johnson RWG, Anderson M, Morley AR, Taylor RMR, Swinney J (1972) Transplantation 13: 174–179

5. Booster MH, Wijnen RMH, Yin M, Tiebosch ATM, Heineman E, Maessen JG, Buurman WA, Kurvers HAJM, Stubenitsky BM, Bonke H, Kootstra G (1993) Enhanced resistance to the effects of normothermic ischemia in kidneys using pulsatile machine perfusion. Transplant Proc 25: 3006–3011

6. Kootstra G, Daemen JHC, Oomen APA (1995) Categories of non-heart-beating donors. Transplant Proc 27: 2893–2894

7. Heineman E, Daemen JHC, Kootstra G (1995) Non-heart-beating donors: methods and techniques. Transplant Proc 27: 2895–2897

8. Hoffman RM, Stratta RJ, D'Alessandro AM, Sollinger HW, Kalayoglu M, Pirsch JD, Southard JH, Belzer FO (1989) Combined cold storage-perfusion preservation with a new synthetic perfusate. Transplantation 47: 32–37

9. Daemen JHC, Heineman E, Kootstra G (1995) Viability assessment of non-heart-beating donor kidneys during machine preservation. Transplant Proc 27: 2906–2908

10. Casavilla A, Ramirez C, Shapiro R, Nghiem D, Miracle K, Bronsther O, Randhawa P, Broznick B, Fung JJ, Starzl TE (1995) Experience with liver and kidney allografts from non-heart-beating donors. Transplantation 59: 197–203

11. Schlumpf R, Candinas D, Zollinger A, Keusch G, Retsch M, Decurtins M, Largiader F (1992) Kidney procurement from non-heartbeating donors: transplantation results. Transplant Int 5: S424–428

12. Valero R, Manalich M, Cabrer C, Salvador L, Garcia-Fages LC (1993) Organ procurement from non-heart-beating donors by total body cooling. Transplant Proc 25: 3091–3092

13. Castalao AM, Griñó JM, González C, Franco E, GilVernet S, Andrés E, Serón D, Torras J, Moreso F, Alsina J (1993) Update of our experience in long-term renal function of kidneys transplanted from non-heart-beating cadaver donors. Transplant Proc 25: 1513–1515

14. Varty K, Veitch PS, Morgan JDT, Kehinde EO, Donnelly PK, Bel PRF (1994) Kidney retrieval from asystolic donors: a valuable and viable resource of additional organs. Br Med J 308: 575

15. Vromen MAM, Leunissen KML, Persijn GG, Kootstra G (1988) Short- and long-term results with adult non-heart-beating donor kidneys. Transplant Proc 20: 743–745

16. Troppmann C, Gillingham KJ, Benedetti E, Stephen Almond P, Gruessner RWG, Najarian JS, Matas AJ (1995) Delayed graft function, acute rejection, and outcome after cadaver renal transplantation. Transplantation 59: 962–968

17. Canafax DM, Torres A, Fryd DS, Heil JE, Strand MH, Ascher NL, Payne WD, Sutherland DER, Simmons RL, Najarian JS (1986) The effects of delayed function on recipients of cadaver renal allografts. Transplantation 41: 177–181

18. Barry JM, Shively N, Hubert B, Hefty T, Norman DJ, Bennett WM (1988) Significance of delayed graft function in cyclosporine-treated recipients of cadaver kidney transplants. Transplantation 45: 346–348

19. Venkateswara Rao K, Andersen RC (1985) Delayed graft function has no detrimental effect on short-term or long-term outcome of cadaveric renal transplantation. Transplant Proc 17: 2818–2820

20. Bauma WD, Tang IYS, Maddux MS, Veremis SA, Pollak R, Mozes MF (1989) Delayed graft function following cadaver renal transplantation in the cyclosporine era: analysis of acute rejection and graft survival. Transplant Proc 21: 1276–1277

21. Howard RJ, Pfaff WW, Brunson ME, Scornik JC, Ramos EL, Peterson JC, Fennell RS, Croker BP (1994) Increased incidence of rejection in patients with delayed graft function. Clin Trnasplant 8: 527–531

22. Carpenter BJ, Rosenthal JT, Taylor RJ, Hakala TR (1985) The impact of acute tubular necrosis on graft outcome in patients receiving cyclosporine. Transplant Proc 17: 1282–1283

23. Ploeg RJ, Van Bockel JH, Langendijk PTH, Groenewegen M, Van der Woude FJ, Persijn GG, Thorogood J, Hermans J (1992) Effect of preservation solution on results of cadaveric kidney transplantation. Lancet 340: 129–137

24. McAnulty JF, Ploeg RJ, Southard JH, Belzer FO (1989) Successful five-day perfusion preservation of the canine kidney. Transplantation 47: 37–41

25. Booster MH, Yin M, Stubenitsky BM, Kemerink GJ, Van Kroonenburgh MJPG, Heidendal GAK, Halders SGEA, Heineman E, Buurman WA, Wijnen RMH, Tiebosch ATM, Bonke H, Kootstra G (1993) Beneficial effect of machine perfusion on the preservation of renal microcirculatory integrity in ischemically damaged kidneys. Transplant Proc 25: 3012–3016

26. Barber WH, Deierhoi MH, Phillips MG, Diethelm AG (1988) Preservation by pulsatile perfusion improves early renal allograft function. Transplant Proc 20: 865–868

27. Light JA, Kowalski AE, Gage F, Callender CO, Sasaki TM (1995) Immediate function and cost comparison between ice storage and pulsatile preservation in kidney recipients at one hospital. Transplant Proc 27: 2962–2964

28. Matsuno N, Sakurai E, Tamaki I, Uchiyama M, Kozaki K, Kozaki M (1994) The effect of machine perfusion preservation versus cold storage on the function of kidneys from non-heart-beating donors. Transplantation 57: 293–294

29. Kozaki M, Matsuno N, Tamaki T, Tanaka M, Kono K, Ito H, Uchiyama M, Tamaki I, Sakurai E (1991) Procurement of kidney grafts from non-heart-beating donors. Transplant Proc 23: 2575–2578

30. Orloff MS, Reed AI, Erturk E, Kruk RA, Paprocki SA, Cimbalo SC, Cerilli GJ (1994) Nonheartbeating cadaveric organ donation. Ann Surg 220: 578–585

31. D'Alessandro AM, Hoffmann RM, Knechtle SJ, Sollinger HW, Kalayoglu M, Pirsch JD, Belzer FO (1995) Controlled non-heart-beating renal donation in the cyclosporine era. Abstract, Third International Congress of the Society for Organ Sharing, Paris, France, 17–19 July

32. Halloran P, Aprile M, Farewell V, for the Ontario Renal Transplant Research Group (1988) Factors influencing early renal function in cadaver kidney transplants. Transplantation 45: 122–127

33. Zhou YC, Cecka JM (1994) Effect of HLA matching on renal transplant survival. In: Terasaki PI, Cecka JM (eds) Clinical transplants 1993, UCLA Tissue Typing Laboratory, Los Angeles, pp 499–510

34. Yokoyama I, Uchida K, Kobayashi T, Tominaga Y, Orihara A, Takagi H (1994) Effect of prolonged delayed graft function on long-term graft outcome in cadaveric kidney transplantation. Clin Transplant 8: 101–106

Transpl Int (1996) 9 [Suppl 1]: S 81–S 83
© Springer-Verlag 1996

M. J. Pacholczyk
B. Łągiewska
M. Szostek
A. Chmura
M. Morzycka-Michalik
D. Rowińska-Stryjecka
J. Wałaszewski
W. Rowiński

Transplantation of kidneys harvested from non-heart-beating donors: early and long-term results

M. J. Pacholczyk (✉) · B. Łągiewska ·
M. Szostek · A. Chmura · J. Wałaszewski ·
W. Rowiński
Department of General and
Transplantation Surgery, Warsaw Medical
School, Nowogrodzka 59, 02-006 Warsaw,
Poland
Fax 48 (02) 6 28 00 88

M. Morzycka-Michalik · D. Rowińska-
Skryjecka
Institute of Transplantology, Warsaw
Medical School, Nowogrodzka 59, 02-006
Warsaw, Poland

Abstract The purpose of this retrospective study was to evaluate results of non-heart-beating donor (NHBD) kidney transplantation. Between Jan 1986 and Dec 1994, 80 out of 582 cadaveric kidneys were harvested from NHBD (31.9 min ± 24 after cardiac arrest). The results in the NHBD group (76 recipients) were compared with those obtained after transplantation of kidneys harvested from heart-beating donors (HBD) with respect to early graft function, and the graft and recipient's survival. Both groups were matched for sex, age, PRA level, number of HLA mismatches, and cold ischemia time. Triple immunosuppression therapy was used in both groups. Acute tubular necrosis (ATN) was observed significantly more frequently in the NHBD group (50 of 76 recipients vs 33 of 100 in the HBD group). The striking finding of this study was that the occurrence of primary non-function was the same in both groups and that the main cause of it was acute rejection. The 1-year patient and graft survival rates were 98.7 % and 81.6 % for the NHBD group and 99 % and 90 % for the HBD group, respectively. There was also no statistical difference in the serum creatinine concentration in both groups. We concluded that despite an increased incidence of ATN in the NHBD kidney recipients, the long-term results are good and comparable with those in the HBD group.

Key words Non-heart-beating donors · Kidney transplantation

Introduction

For many years and for a variety of reasons kidneys have quite often been procured in our center from non-heart-beating donors (NHBD). The purpose of this retrospective study was to evaluate early and long-term results of kidney transplantation in recipients of kidneys retrieved from NHBD.

Materials and methods

Between January 1986 and December 1994, 582 cadaveric kidney transplants were performed in our department. During this period 84 kidneys were procured from NHBD and transplanted. Seventy-six recipients were incorporated into our study (NHBD group). In 8 cases, an HLR machine was used in the donor after cardiac arrest so those previously reported cases were excluded [3]. For comparison, we selected a group of 100 recipients (heart-beating donor HBD] group) matched with the NHBD group according to sex (female/male ratio), age, HLA mismatches (HLA-MM), and maximum panel-reactive antibody (PRA) level.

Donors

NHBD group

This group consisted of 38 donors (female/male: 13/25) aged 35.5 ± 16.4 years. All donors in this group were treated in various hospitals in the Warsaw area. The causes of death were as follows: 27 donors died from head injury, 8 from spontaneous cerebrovascular bleeding, 2 from anoxia (drowning and hanging), and 1 from drug poisoning; in all donors in this group brain-stem death was diagnosed. They were hemodynamically unstable (group C by UNOS) and required high doses of dopamine, exceeding 20 μg/kg

Table 1 Recipients' demographics. Relevant recipient data are shown as mean ± standard deviation (*NHBI*) non-heart-beating donor, *HB* heart-beating donor)

	NHBD	HBD
Number of recipients	76	100
Sex f/m	33/43	45/55
Age (years)	40.12 ± 10.94	39.06 ± 11.04
HLA mismatches A, B	2.15 ± 0.9	2.06 ± 0.8
DR	1.08 ± 0.55	1.1 ± 0.42
PRA maximum (%)	16.3 ± 20.9	20.6 ± 30.4
Anastomosis time (min)	34.8 ± 11.8	30.5 ± 8.07

per min. In all these cases cardiac arrest occurred before the transplant team arrived. Cardiac massage, mechanical ventilation, and heparin infusion were continued in all NHBD before in situ perfusion was started.

Euro-Collins (EC) or Ringer solution was used for in situ perfusion. The kidneys were removed en bloc with the abdominal aorta and vena cava and flushed again on the back table with EC in 58 cases or University of Wisconsin organ preservation (UW) solution in 18 cases. The warm ischemia time between cardiac arrest and in situ perfusion was from 10 to 120 min (mean 31 ± 24 min). The cold storage time ranged from 9 to 42 h (mean 25.6 ± 8.9 h).

HBD group

Incorporated in this group were 50 donors (female/male: 12/38) aged 31.3 ± 11.7 years; 30 had died from head injuries, 19 from a cerebrovascular accident, and 1 from an intracranial isolated tumor. All donors in this group were classified into group A and B (by UNOS) and the mean dose of dopamine was 10.8 ± 10 µg/kg per min. A standard procurement technique was used, including in situ perfusion (EC or Ringer), en bloc nephrectomy, and back table flushing with EC (68) or UW (32). The cold ischemia time ranged from 7 to 48 h (average 27.5 ± 7 h).

Recipients

Table 1 shows a summary and comparison of all relevant recipient data in the two groups. None of these data showed a statistically significant difference between the two examined groups of recipients. In both recipient groups, standard triple immunosuppressive protocol was used. Preoperatively all recipients received azathioprine, 3 mg/kg p. o. and methylprednisolone 500 mg i. v. on induction. Postoperatively azathioprine was given once a day (3 mg/kg) and the dose was modified according to the WBCC. Methylprednisolone was given 6 and 12 h after kidney reperfusion to a total dose of 1 g on the day of transplantation, followed by 0.5 g on day 2, 0.250 g on day 3, and an oral dose of prednisolone, 0.5 mg/kg, was gradually reduced during the first month. The first dose of cyclosporine A was administered 18 h after reperfusion at a daily dose of 6 mg/kg body weight.

Statistical analysis

Data are reported as the mean ± SD. Data were compared using the unpaired Student's *t*-test and chi-squared analysis.

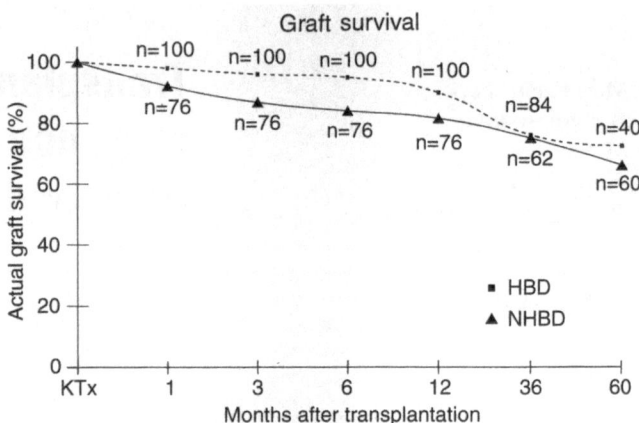

Fig. 1 Renal graft survival rates according to donors source: kidneys from heart-beating donors (*HBD*) vs non-heart-beating donors (*NHBD*) (*n* represents the total number of patients in the groups at each follow-up point, for whom survival rate was calculated)

Results

In the early postoperative period, 50 of 76 recipients (65.8 %) in the NHBD group and 33 of 100 recipients of the HBD group needed dialysis support. The mean time of hemodialysis (in days) was 16.8 ± 9.2 in the NHBD and 15.5 ± 8.4 in the HBD groups. The number of hemodialyses in the group of recipients who developed acute tubular necrosis (ATN) was 7.35 ± 3.2 and 7.05 ± 5.4 in the NHBD and HBD groups, respectively. Immediate graft function was observed in 23 recipients in the NHBD group (30.2 %) and in 64 recipients in the HBD group (64 %). There were three cases of primary nonfunction in the NHBD group (3.9 %) and three cases in the HBD group. The major cause of primary non-function in both groups (NHBD-2, HBD-2) was acute rejection following ATN (established by biopsy). In one case (NHBD), microscopy showed advanced graft necrosis. Renal artery thrombosis was found to be the direct cause of graft failure in one case in the HBD group.

In the early postoperative period (3 months), episodes of acute rejection confirmed by needle biopsy were observed in 50 of the 76 (65.8 %) recipients in the NHBD group and in 46 of the 100 recipients in the HBD group. The mean dose of steroids used for the treatment of acute rejection during the first 3 months was 5.4 ± 3.5 g in the NHBD group vs 4.0 ± 2.2 g in the HBD group.

The 1-year patient survival rate was 98.7 % for the NHBD group and 99 % for the HBD group. The 1-year graft survival rate was 81.6 % for the NHBD group and 90 % for the HBD group. The actual graft and patient survival rates at 3 and 5 years are shown in Figs. 1, 2. The courses of serum creatinine levels in the early and late postoperative periods for both groups are shown in Fig. 3.

During 5 years of observation, four patients died with a functioning graft in the NHBD group; one died at

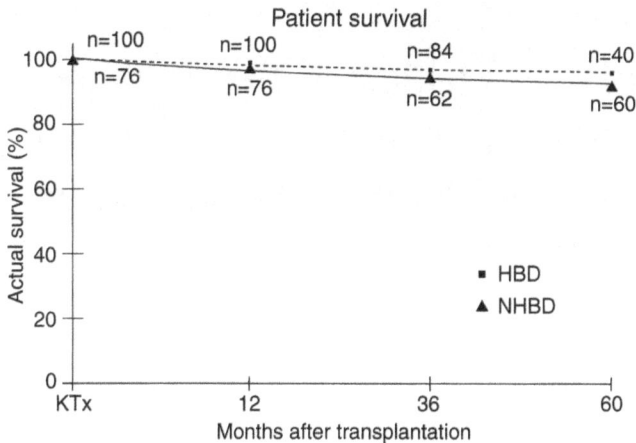

Fig. 2 Actual patient survival rates in *HBD* group vs *NHBD* (*n* represents the total number of patients in the groups at each follow-up point, for whom survival rate was calculated)

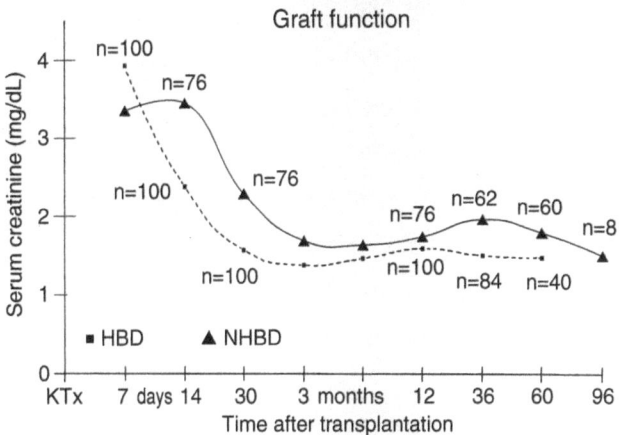

Fig. 3 Serum creatinine levels in the early (only for recipients who were not on dialysis at that time) and late postoperative periods (7, 14, and 30 days, 3, 6, 12, 36, 60 and 96 months after transplantation) in *NHBD* vs *HBD* groups

2 months from cytomegalovirus infection, and the other three died at 3 years from myocardial infarction (2) and pneumonia (1). In the HBD group, four recipients died; one died at 4 months from acute fulminant hepatitis (HCV), two patients died with functioning grafts at 2 years, one from a ruptured abdominal aortic aneurysm and one from myocardial infarction, and one died at home 3 years after transplantation from pneumonia.

Discussion

The purpose of this retrospective study was to compare the results of kidney transplantation in two groups of recipients: those who received kidneys from NHBD and those who received kidneys from HBD. Apart from the fact that delayed graft function was observed more frequently in the NHBD group ($P < 0.0003$), long-term follow-up showed that after 1, 3, and 5 years graft and patient survival were comparable with those in the HBD group [2, 4].

The important finding of our analysis was that the primary non-function rate in the NHBD group was no higher than that in the HBD group. The main cause of permanent graft failure in both groups was a combination of two factors, ischemia and acute rejection. In the first 3 months after transplantation, the episodes of acute rejection were observed more frequently in the NHBD group ($P < 0.03$). The cumulative dose (mean) of steroids used in NHBD recipients during this period was higher ($P < 0.03$) than in HBD recipients. Despite the increased occurrence of acute rejection in the NHBD group, long-term results were very good.

Therefore, we conclude that organ procurement from non-heart-beating donors should be performed and could be one of the ways of reducing the waiting list for renal transplantation [1, 4]. In all patients who have been diagnosed brain-stem dead, mechanical ventilation and cardiac massage should be continued in each case of sudden cardiac arrest, until surgical teams arrive.

Acknowledgements The paper was supported by the Committee for Scientific Research grants: E/7, E/18 and the Warsaw Medical School Grant: P-13.

References

1. Rowiński W, Wałaszewski J, Łągiewska B, Pacholczyk M (1993) Use of kidneys from marginal and non-heart-beating donors: warm ischemia per se is not the most detrimental factor. Transplant Proc 25 (1): 1511–1512
2. Schlumpf R, Kandinas D, Zollinger A, Keusch G, Retsch M, Decurtins M, Largiader F (1992) Kidney procurement from non-heartbeating donors: transplantation results. Transplant Int 5 (1): 424–428
3. Szostek M, Danielewicz R, Łągiewska B, Pacholczyk M, Rybicki Z, Michalak G, Adaynański L, Wałaszewski J, Rowiński W (1995) Successful transplantation of kidneys harvested from cadaver donor at 71 to 259 minutes following cardiac arrest. Transplant Proc 27 (5): 2902–2903
4. Wynen RMH, Booster M, Speatgens C, Yin M, Van Hooff JP, de Boer J, Kootstra G (1993) Long-term follow-up of transplanted non-heart-beating donor kidneys: preliminary results of a retrospective study. Transplant Proc 25 (1): 1522–1523

Transpl Int (1996) 9 [Suppl 1]: S 84–S 85
© Springer-Verlag 1996

KIDNEY

M. Szostek
M. Pacholczyk
B. Łągiewska
R. Danielewicz
J. Wałaszwski
W. Rowiński

Effective surface cooling of the kidney during vascular anastomosis decreases the risk of delayed kidney function after transplantation

M. Szostek (✉) · M. Pacholczyk ·
B. Łągiewska · R. Danielewicz ·
J. Wałaszwski · W. Rowiński
Warsaw Medical School, Department of
General and Transplantation Surgery,
Nowogrodzka 59, 02-006 Warsaw, Poland

Abstract The aim of the prospective study was to assess the exact kidney temperature and the effect of surface cooling of the kidney during the time of vascular anastomosis. Twenty-two renal graft recipients were incorporated into our study. We used an electronic temperature measurer provided with a needle-shaped probe pierced into the body of the kidney. The temperature was recorded every 5 min. The mean temperature of the kidney at the beginning of anastomosis (T_0) was $8.87 \pm 3.97\,°C$ and $17.95 \pm 5.1\,°C$ at the end (T_{end}). The striking finding of this study was that the mean T_{end} delayed kidney function-negative in [ATN(−)] recipients was significantly lower than in the ATN(+) group; respectively, $14.86 \pm 3.6\,°C$ and $19.71 \pm 5.07\,°C$. Therefore, we have divided all recipients according to T_{end} ($< 15\,°C$ and $> 15\,°C$) in an attempt to assess the direct influence of kidney temperature on early graft function. In nine cases, a temperature below $15\,°C$ was recorded and in 13 cases it exceeded $15\,°C$ at the end of anastomosis. The mean cold ischemia time and anastomosis time were not different in these recipients. Delayed graft function occurred in 14 recipients; in 3 of 9 (33.3 %) recipients from group $T_{end} < 15\,°C$; and in 11 of 13 (85 %) from group $T_{end} > 15\,°C$. One case of primary non-function was observed ($T_{end} > 15\,°C$). This study documents the value of effective cooling of the kidney during the time of vascular anastomosis. Since in most clinical reports the significance of the second warm ischemia was assessed only by the duration of the anastomosis, without measurement of the actual organ temperature, this may explain the different findings in our studies.

Key words Kidneys transplantation · Cooling technique

Introduction

Delayed kidney function after cadaveric kidney transplantation still remains an important problem complicating postoperative patients' management. Among the many factors which may contribute to the development of ischemic kidney damage, the most important can be attributed to profound metabolic, hormonal, and most of all, hemodynamic changes appearing during the preagonal period and to the warm ischemia [1, 3, 4]. This is especially true in countries where, despite legal regula-tions concerning brain death and exact definitions of its criteria, organ procurement takes place at a time when hemodynamic changes are quite advanced. Duration of cold storage (over 36 h) also contributes to ischemic organ damage [2]. The exact role of so-called second warm ischemia has been unclear. It has been often stated that if the duration of the vascular anastomosis procedure exceeds 40–45 min this may become an additional contributory factor to the development of ATN [4]. However, in a number of clinical studies, statistical analyses have not shown the significance of the second warm ischemia

(WIT2). The purpose of this clinical study was to assess the exact kidney temperature during the vascular anastomosis and to evaluate whether it has any influence on the development of delayed kidney function (ATN).

Patients and methods

Cadaver kidneys were harvested from 14 donors (female:male ratio 2:12) of mean age 33.1 ± 11.6 years. Hypotension (blood pressure < 80 mmHg) was observed in 7 of 14. The mean dose of dopamine administered to the donor in the last hour was 11.1 ± 7.6 µg/kg per min. During the last hour, urine output > 50 ml was observed in 10 of 14 donors. The mean serum creatinine concentration at the time of harvesting was 1.74 ± 0.84 mg/dl. The kidneys were retrieved en bloc, with the standard in situ perfusion (EC/Ringer) and backtable UW/EC (10/12) flushing. The mean time of cold preservation was 31.6 ± 6.9 h.

Cooling technique

During vascular anastomosis, all kidneys were placed inside the holding net, facilitating intraoperative maneuvers, with attached infusions set. Cold drip infusion (4 °C normal saline solution) was applied on the kidney surface during anastomosis. The time of vascular anastomosis lasted from 23 min to 65 min (mean 33.6 ± 9.2 min).

Temperature measurement

The kidney temperature was measured using an electronic measurer provided with a needle-shaped probe pierced (1-cm-deep) into the kidney cortex. The temperature was recorded every 5 min starting at the beginning of vascular anastomosis (kidney "out of ice", T_0) till the end of the anastomosis (end temperature, T_{end}).

The kidneys were transplanted to 22 recipients of mean age 38.5 ± 9.5 years. Six kidneys were transplanted out of our center. The maximum plasma renin activity (PRA) level (mean) in the reviewed group of recipients was 28.4 ± 29.3 %. Mean human leukocyte antigen (HLA) mismatches were 3.32 ± 0.95.

Results

The mean T_0 was 8.87 ± 3.97 °C. At the end of anastomosis, the T_{end} of the kidney was 18.95 ± 5.1 °C (range from 7.7 °C to 30 °C). The 1-min-temperature rise calculated for the whole group was 0.28 ± 0.14 °C. In 8 of the 22 kidney recipients (36.4 %), the graft functioned well immediately after transplantation. Delayed graft function was observed in 13 patients (59 %). One patient

treated with dialysis for ATN developed acute rejection resistant to steroids and lost the graft 56 days after transplantation.

The T_0 of the kidney in the ATN(–) and ATN(+) recipients was similar, 7.74 ± 4.11 °C and 9.52 ± 3.88 °C, respectively (not significant). The T_{end} in the ATN(–) patients was 14.86 ± 3.6 °C and was significantly ($P < 0.03$) lower than in ATN(+) recipients (19.71 ± 5.07 °C). The 1-min-temperature rises in the ATN(+) group was 0.29 ± 0.12 °C and 0.26 ± 0.19 °C in the ATN(–) group.

Since the mean kidney T_{end} in ATN(–) recipients was 14.9 °C, an analysis of the results was performed in the two groups divided according to $T_{end} < 15$ °C or > 15 °C. In nine cases, T_{end} was lower than 15 °C whereas in the remaining 13 cases it was above 15 °C.

The presence of hypotension in the donor, the mean dose of administered dopamine, the cold ischemia time, and the anastomosis time were no different in the two groups. Delayed graft function was observed in 3 of 9 recipients from the $T_{end} < 15$ °C group and 11 of 13 from the $T_{end} > 15$ °C group ($P < 0.03$).

Discussion

As shown in our studies, the kidney temperature at the beginning of anastomosis (T_0) ranged from 7.74 °C [ATN(–)] to 9.52 °C [ATN(+)]. The mean temperature of the organ at the end (T_{end}) of anastomosis was 14.9 °C, being statistically different in ATN(–) and ATN(+) kidneys (14.86 °C versus 19.71 °C, $P < 0.03$).

The analysis of various factors which may have been responsible for the development of ATN during the postoperative period showed that this complication occurred significantly less often in recipients of kidneys with $T_{end} < 15$ °C than in those with $T_{end} > 15$ °C. This documents the value of effective cooling of the kidney during the time of vascular anastomosis. Since in most clinical reports the significance of the second warm ischemia was assessed only by the duration of the anastomosis without measurement of the actual temperature of the organ, this may explain the different findings in our studies [3, 4].

Acknowledgements This work was supported by the Committee for Scientific Research grants numbers E/7 and E/18 and Warsaw Medical School grant number P-13.

References

1. Booster MH, Winjen RMH, Ming Y, Vroemen JPAM, Kootstra G (1993) In situ perfusion of kidneys from non-heart-beating donors. The Maastricht protocol. Transplant Proc 25: 1503–1504

2. Cicciarelli J, Iwaki Y, Mendez R, Asai P, Bogaard T, Khetan U, Mendez RG (1993) Effects of cold ischemia time on cadaver renal allografts. Transplant Proc 25: 1543–1546

3. Rowiński W, Wałaszweski J, Łągiewska B, Pacholczyk M (1993) Use of kidneys from marginal and non-heart-beating donors. Transplant Proc 25: 1511–1512

4. Wałaszewski J (1992) Multivariety analysis of the factors responsible for function of the kidney in early posttransplant period. Warsaw Medical School, Poland

Transpl Int (1996) 9 [Suppl 1]: S 86–S 89
© Springer-Verlag 1996

G. Nordén
I. Blohmé
G. Nyberg

Kidney transplantation to patients with congenital malformations of the distal urinary tract

G. Nordén (✉) · I. Blohmé · G. Nyberg
Transplant Unit,
Sahlgrenska University Hospital,
S-41345 Göteborg, Sweden
Fax + 4631-820557

Abstract Fourteen of 1000 consecutive kidney transplant patients had congenital malformations affecting the bladder or urethra: six had congenital valvulus of the urethra, two congenital sclerosis of the bladder outlet, and six a neurogenic bladder. Pretransplant surgey had been performed in all patients: reimplantation of ureter ($n = 11$), resection of congenital valvulus ($n = 7$), and nephrectomy ($n = 6$). Four patients had an intestinal bladder. Age was 0–17 (median 1) years at diagnosis. Follow-up time was 3–10 (median 5) years. Special transplant surgery techniques were required in five patients. Patient survival after 2 years was 100 % and graft survival 93 %. No graft was lost due to outflow obstruction, infection or other causes related to the underlying disorder. Late technical problems were seen in two patients. Urinary tract infections were reported in 13 patients before transplantation and in eight after. Results of transplantation were excellent. Infections and surgical problems had a minor impact on outcome.

Key words Kidney transplantation · Congenital malformation · Distal urinary tract

Introduction

Almost irrespective of the original disease, kidney transplantation is the superior treatment for patients with end-stage renal disease. However, the various renal diseases may influence the transplant procedure and outcome in different ways. In patients with distal urinary tract malformations, problems such as abnormal anatomy, bladder dysfunction, and urinary tract infection (UTI) might cause complications and thus have an impact on the outcome of transplantation. This report presents our experience of kidney transplantation in patients with congenital malformations affecting the distal urinary tract.

Patients and methods

We have reevaluated the underlying disease in 1000 consecutive patients who received 1095 kidney transplants in Göteborg between 1985 and 1993 [10]. This was done by retrieval of data from the patients' records in the Transplant Unit and the Renal Unit and/or Pediatric Units where they were first investigated. In this population, 14 patients had well-defined distal urinary tract malformations: congenital valvulus of the urethra, sclerosis of the bladder outlet, and neurogenic bladder. In the neurogenic bladder group, two patients had myelomeningocele, two spina bifida, one megaloureters with neurogenic bladder, and one patient had a neurogenic bladder with concomitant absence of perineal reflex and reduced sphincter tone in combination with moderate mental retardation. Hydronephrosis had been found in eight of the patients. Patients with hydronephrosis without defined malformation in the distal urinary tract are not included in this study. Demographic data are shown in Table 1.

The patients were 14–44 (median 25) years of age at the time of transplantation. Twelve transplants were first transplants and two, retransplants. Kidneys from living related donors were used in six recipients of primary transplants. Two patients had preemptive transplantations. All patients were supervised for UTI after the

Table 1 Demographic data for kidney transplanted patients with congenital malformations of the distal urinary tract ($n = 14$) separated according to type of malformation

Diagnosis	Number of patients	Male: female ratio	Diagnosis [age years, median (range)]	Start of renal replacement therapy [age years, median (range)]
Congenital valvulus of the urethra	6	6/0	1 (0–17)	22 (12–44)
Congenital sclerosis of the bladder outlet	2	2/0	2 (2–2)	25 (22–28)
Neurogenic bladder	6	4/2	3 (0–7)	30 (14–36)

Table 2 Pretransplant operations on the urinary tract in kidney transplanted patients with congenital malformations of the distal urinary tract ($n = 14$)

Type of operation	Number
Kidney	
Nephro- and/or ureterectomy, uni/bilateral	6
Ureter	
Cutaneous ureterostomy	3
Disconnection of cutaneous ureterostomies	1
Bladder	
Reimplantation of ureter(s)	12
Construction of intestinal bladder	
Bricker	2
Kock	2
Disconnection of Bricker bladder	1
Implantation of Scott's sphincter	1
Plastic operation of the bladder	1
Extirpation of bladder diverticle	1
Bladder neck incision/resection	4
Urethra	
Urethral valvulus operation	7
Exstirpation of urethral diverticle	1
Total	42

transplantation with a urine culture test at every out-patient control. Treatment was according to bacterial resistance patterns for short periods or with low-dose long-term prophylaxis.

Routinely, the ureter was anastomosed to the urinary bladder using an extravesical ureteroneocystotomy, as described by Röhl and Ziegler [12]. The immunosuppressive protocol was a combination of cyclosporine, prednisolone, and azathioprine [10]. Follow-up was until September 1995, which gives 3–10 (median 5) years of observation time.

Contemporary non-diabetic controls, two per patient, were picked from the consecutive file of patients, one by moving forwards, one backwards. Controls were matched for age ± 5 years, sex, kidney source (cadaveric donor or living donor), and transplant number.

Results

Pretransplant operations

Surgical intervention, aimed at correcting the congenital deformity or problem, had been performed before transplantation in all 14 patients on a total of 42 occasions: reimplantation of ureters, resection of congenital valves or bladder neck, construction of an intestinal bladder, and nephrectomy. These procedures are specified in Table 2. Operations were distributed in the whole pretransplant life-span with some procedures in infancy, others just prior to transplantation.

Special procedures at the transplantation

At the time of transplantation, three patients had ileal conduits: one a Bricker bladder, two a Kock's pouch with continent nipple. A fourth patient had previously had a Bricker bladder but at the time of transplantation this had been disconnected and the patient practised triple voiding and manual, suprapubical pressure.

As a consequence of the original disease, special procedures were required during the transplant operation in five patients (Table 3). A cutaneous ureterostomy was performed in one patient and ureteroileoanastomosis in the three patients with ileal conduits. The patient who had previously had a Bricker bladder used a suprapubical catheter to the bladder in the first postoperative period.

Bladder function

There was no immediate change of bladder status or capacity following kidney transplantation. Micturition was satisfactory in seven patients but seven had bladder dysfunction. Four of these had urinary diversion, namely the two patients with a Kock's pouch, the one with a Bricker conduit, and the one with a cutaneous ureterostomy before and after transplantation. Two patients applied triple voiding and/or external pressure. One patient with incontinence had used napkins and initially continued with them.

During the continued follow-up, the patient with napkins, 5 years after transplantation, received, to his own satisfaction, a suprapubical catheter. Another female patient with a neurogenic bladder and native voiding before transplantation started clean intermittent catheterization 3 years after transplantation.

Two patients had late technical problems necessitating additional surgery. Due to signs of outlet obstruction, one patient had a revision of a ureterostomy and one a transposition of ureter in an intestinal bladder and simultaneous augmentation of the bladder.

Table 3 Special surgical procedures during the transplant operation in kidney transplanted patients with congenital malformations

Type of operative procedure	Number	Reason for procedure
Ureteroileoanastomosis	2	Kock's bladder
	1	Bricker bladder
Cutaneous ureterostomy	1	Bladder incontinence
Suprapubic catheter	1	Neurovesical dysfunction

Outcome of transplantation

All patients were alive at the end of the study period. In the control group, one patient was dead due to malignant lymphoma and sepsis.

Graft survival at 2 years was 93 % in the patient group and 82 % in the control group (not significant). During the whole study period, five patients lost their grafts, two due to chronic vascular rejection and three due to chronic glomerulopathy, all confirmed by transplant biopsies. The underlying disease in four of these cases was congenital urethral valve disease. No graft was lost due to outflow obstruction, UTI or other causes related to the underlying disorder. Four of five patients have undergone retransplantation. These grafts function, as at September 1995, which means that 13/14 patients have functioning kidney transplants.

In the control patient group, nine grafts were lost during the study period: one acute rejection and arterial thrombosis, four chronic rejection, three recurrence of the original disease. One graft was never biopsied. Four of nine patients had a retransplant performed, and three patients are on the transplant waiting list.

UTI

In the pretransplant period, 13 patients had urinary infections: ten had a history of acute pyelonephritis or urosepsis and three had recurrent distal urinary infections with symptoms. Six patients were reported with previous vesico-ureteral reflux uremia (VUR). All of them had had acute pyelonephritis.

In the posttransplant period, 3–10 (median 5) years, eight patients have had infection problems. Six patients had prophylactic treatment with antibiotics, permanently or intermittently. Two patients had acute pyelonephritis and in one of them nephrectomy of the native kidneys was performed.

Discussion

Patients with distal urinary tract malformations constitute 1.4 % of our kidney transplanted population [10]. Only two of the patients reported in this paper was pediatric in the sense that they received transplants before the age of 18 years. Although congenital malformation of the distal urinary tract is "a childhood disease", our patients are adult at the time of kidney transplantation. This indicates that good medical treatment and surgical therapy had delayed and reduced the need for dialysis and kidney transplantation.

For comparison of incidences of congenital malformation of the distal urinary tract in different renal replacement therapy populations, the National Registries from United States of America, Canada, Japan, and Europe [5] are no help because they do not classify the patients into subgroups, only into groups headed, for example, chronic pyelonephritis or interstitial nephritis. In the registry from the North American Pediatric Renal Transplant Cooperative Study, where 2037 children (< 17 years) received kidney transplants from 1987 to 1992, 17 % had "obstructive uropathy" [9]. In the United States Renal Data System, 4.7 % of the patients had "congenital obstructive uropathy" as the cause of pediatric (< 20 years of age) end-stage renal disease (ESRD) [13]. These figures are also difficult to compare with ours due to ambiguities of definition.

There was no mortality in the patient group. This is probably related to their young age. Graft survival at 2 years was satisfactory and not different from the controls but superior to overall results of 75.6 % for the 1095 transplantations performed in the same period. The good graft survival is probably also an effect of youth. No graft loss was related to underlying disease. All retransplantations turned out successfully. A small series also reporting excellent results of kidney transplantations to patients with problems in the lower urinary tract has previously been published [3, 4, 6, 8].

In accordance with our results, Reinberg et al. [11] found that, in children who received kidney transplants because of posterior urethral valve uremia, failed grafts showed rejection, not obstructive lesions, when analyzed histologically. He also found a 5-year graft survival rate in these children comparable to that for children with VUR. Kalicinski et al. [7] found the same graft survival for transplanted children with "urologic" and "nonurologic" ESRD.

All patients had a history of repeated surgery from infancy to the day of transplantation. Correcting operations were performed with the hope of abolishing mechanical obstruction, preventing further VUR, and putting an end to recurrent infectious foci. Today, the trend is towards less surgey but early and intensive treatment of infections and hypertension [1, 2]. Due to the original disease and related problems, all patients were urologically extensively evaluated and treated before transplantation. This might be the reason why UTIs caused less problems after transplantation than before and no transplant-threatening infections were recorded.

A characteristic of this population is the bladder emptying problems, which are the cause of disease and uremia, the reason for several operations before transplantation, and an Achilles heel after transplantation. Our patients with Kock's bladder are regularly seen by urologist. Patients with native bladders are checked for the presence of residual urine volumes and the strategy for voiding is changed as indicated. In our patients, the bladder capacity was unchanged after transplantation,

but in the long-term one patient was able to start clean intermittent catheterization and a second received a suprapubical catheter.

Today's young patients with congenital malformations of the distal urinary tract will develop ESRD later in life, thanks to a greater awareness of the problem among pediatricians, physicians and surgeons, but also better and more effective treatment, especially handling of infections. In the case of ESRD there should be no hesitation about kidney transplantation because results are gratifying and, despite the previous history, the actual condition of these patients is of minor importance for the outcome.

References

1. Allen TD ed. (1992) International workshop on reflux and pyelonephritis. J Urol 148: 1639–1760
2. Birmingham reflux study group (1992) Prospective trial of operative versus non-operative treatment of severe vesico-ureteric reflux in children: five years' observation. Br Med J 295: 237–241
3. Bryant JE, Joseph DB, Kohaut C, Diethelm G (1991) Renal transplantation in children with posterior urethral valves. J Urol 146: 1585–1587
4. Cairns HS, Leaker B, Woodhouse CRJ, Rudge CJ, Neild GH (1991) Renal transplantation into abnormal urinary tract. Lancet 338: 1376–1379
5. D'Amico G, Striker GE (1995) Proceeding from the symposium on Renal replacement therapy throughout the world: the registries. Am J Kidney Dis 25: 113–118
6. Griffin PJA, Stephenson TP, Brough S, Salaman RJ (1994) Transplanting patients with abnormal urinary tracts. Transpl Int 7: 288–291
7. Kalicinski P, Kaminski A, Prokurat A, Smirska E, Szymkiewicz Cz, Kaminski W (1992) Kidney transplantation in children with end-stage renal disease caused by urologic abnormalities. Transplant Proc 24: 2760–2761
8. Kashi SH, Wynne KS, Sadek SA, Lodge JPA (1994) An evaluation of vesical urodynamics before renal transplantation and its effect on renal allograft function and survival. Transplantation 57: 1455–1457
9. McEnery PT, Alexander SR, Sullivan K, Tejani A (1992) Renal transplantation in children and adolescents: the 1992 Annual Report of the North American Pediatric Renal Transplant Cooperative Study. Pediatr Nephrol 7: 711–710
10. Nyberg G, Olausson M, Svalander C, Nordén G (1995) Original renal disease in a kidney transplant population. Scand J Urol Nephrol 29: 393–397
11. Reinberg Y, Gonzalez R, Fryd D, Mauer SM, Najarian JS (1988) The outcome of renal transplantation in children with posterior urethral valves. J Urol 140: 1491–1493
12. Röhl W, Ziegler M (1969) Die Ureteroneocystostomie bei der Nierentransplantation. Urologe A 8: 116–119
13. United States Renal Data System 1994 annual data report (1994) Am J Kidney Dis 24 (suppl 2): 112–127

Liver

Transpl Int (1996) 9 [Suppl 1]: S 93–S 96
© Springer-Verlag 1996

LIVER

M. Anthuber
S. Farkas
M. Rihl
M. D. Menger
F. W. Schildberg
K.-W. Jauch
K. Messmer

Impact of enalapril on microvascular perfusion and leukocyte adherence in a model of rat liver transplantation assessed by in vivo microscopy

M. Anthuber (✉) · F. W. Schildberg ·
K.-W. Jauch
Department of Surgery,
Klinikum Grosshadern,
Ludwig-Maximilians-University Munich,
Marchioninistr. 15, D-81377 Munich,
Germany

S. Farkas · M. Rihl · K. Messmer
Institute for Surgical Research,
Klinikum Grosshadern,
Ludwig-Maximilians-University Munich,
D-81377 Munich, Germany

M. D. Menger
Institute for Clinical-Experimental
Surgery, University of the Saarland,
D-66421 Homburg/Saar, Germany

Abstract ACE inhibitors have been proven to be effective in the reduction of ischemia/reperfusion damage after myocardial ischemia. In an attempt to investigate this effect in a model of syngeneic liver transplantation in the rat, we compared a control group with an ACE inhibitor treatment group, in which enalapril was given i. v. before and during reperfusion. By means of in vivo microscopy, sinusoidal perfusion rate, permanent leukocyte sticking in sinusoids and postsinusoidal venules, and leukocyte rolling in postsinusoidal venules were assessed. Liver function was evaluated by measuring bile output. The sinusoidal perfusion rate was significantly improved by enalapril treatment. Leukocyte sticking in both sinusoids and postsinusoidal venules was found to be remarkably reduced in enalapril-treated animals; the fraction of rolling leukocytes remained unchanged. Bile output was increased in enalapril-treated animals. These results demonstrated, in a model of rat liver transplantation, that ACE inhibition by enalapril is effective in reducing hepatic ischemia/reperfusion damage as assessed by the leukocyte-endothelium interaction using in vivo microscopy and postreperfusion bile production.

Key words Liver transplantation · Ischemia/reperfusion damage · Leukocyte-endothelium interaction · ACE inhibition

Introduction

After more than 20 years of clinical experience, liver transplantation is an established treatment modality for end-stage liver disease, with overall 3-year survival rates of almost 70 % [1, 2]. Selection of suitable recipients and selection of donors with satisfactory liver function are crucial elements for a successful outcome. However, primary graft dysfunction develops in up to 22 %, initiating a cascade of severe postoperative complications with considerable impact on mortality rates [1–3]. The pathophysiological bases for graft dysfunction are damages from cold ischemia, warm ischemia, and reperfusion.

Angiotensin-converting enzyme (ACE) inhibitors have been proven to be effective in reducing ischemia/reperfusion injury in experimental models of warm myocardial ischemia, and this is attributed not only to their

vasodilating effects, but also to the oxygen free radical scavenging properties of thiol-containing (SH-group) substances, for example captopril [4–6]. Vasodilation is mediated by inhibition of kininase II, leading to both a reduced production of vasoconstricting angiotensin II and an increase in bradykinin concentration [7]. Bradykinin by itself is the most potent endogenous stimulator of endothelial prostacyclin synthesis, which in turn enhances vasodilation [8, 9]. Furthermore prostacyclin has powerful antiaggregatory effects and, most importantly, possesses some, as yet not clearly understood, cytoprotective properties. In different models on ischemic, viral, and toxic liver damages, treatment with prostacyclin has resulted in amelioration of the insult to the liver [8–13]. On that basis and in an attempt to transfer the favorable effects of ACE inhibitors in myocardial ischemia to hepatic ischemia, we investigated in

Table 1 Body weight, liver wet weight, anhepatic period, and cold ischemic time in control (LTx) and enalapril-treated (LTx/Ena) groups. Results are given as mean (SEM)

Group	LTx	LTx/Ena
Body weight (g)	225.7 (6.9)	211.6 (3.0)
Liver wet weight (g)	7.2 (0.2)	7.6 (0.2)
Anhepatic period (min)	19.0 (0.3)	18.8 (0.7)
Cold ischemic time (h)	24.3 (0.0)	24.0 (0.2)

a model of syngeneic rat liver transplantation whether ACE inhibition by enalapril is effective in the amelioration of hepatic ischemia/reperfusion injury.

Material and methods

All experiments were performed with permission of the government authorities and in accordance with the German legislation on laboratory animal experiments.

Surgical technique

Syngeneic, male Lewis rats (donors: 150–200 g body weight; recipients: 190–250 g) underwent orthotopic liver transplantation according to the cuff technique described by Kamada and Calne [14]. In contrast to the original technique, the grafts were rearterialized as reported by Steffen with the modification described by Post, to allow for simultaneous arterial and portal-venous reperfusion [15, 16]. The total ischemic time was 24 h. Grafts were preserved by retrograde aortal flush with University of Wisconsin (UW) solution and stored in UW at a constant temperature of 4 °C. Prior to reperfusion the high-potassium UW solution was removed from the liver by flushing with Ringer's lactate solution at room temperature via the portal route.

A control group of untreated animals (LTx; $n = 10$), which received 0.9 % sodium chloride by an i.v. line in the internal jugular vein during reperfusion, was compared to a study group (LTx/Ena; $n = 8$) in which the animals were treated with enalapril (Xanef, Merck, Sharp & Dome, Munich, Germany) at a dosage of 0.1 mg/kg per hour i.v., starting 5 min before reperfusion and continuing until the end of the experiment. The mean arterial pressure was continuously monitored by an indwelling catheter in the left carotid artery.

In vivo microscopy (IVM)

For assessment of microvascular liver perfusion and the leukocyte-endothelium interaction, IVM was used according to the technique reported by Menger and coworkers [17]. In brief, 30 min after reperfusion and under the precondition of a stable mean arterial pressure of 50 mmHg, the left liver lobe was exteriorized and almost immobilized on a specially designed stage. To avoid major fluid loss and drying, the abdominal cavity was covered with a saran wrap. Sodium fluorescein (2.0 µmol/kg) and rhodamin 6G (0.1 µg/kg) were injected i.v. for fluorescent staining of hepatocytes and leukocytes, respectively. The following IVM parameters were assessed in ten randomly selected acinar areas and postsinusoidal venules, each:

1. Sinusoidal perfusion rate: percentage of perfused sinusoids of all sinusoids of a defined acinar area
2. Permanent leukocyte adherence ("sticker") in sinusoids and postsinusoidal venules: number of stickers per liver lobule, number of stickers per square millimeter of venular endothelial surface sticking for more than 20 s
3. Temporary leukocyte adherence ("roller") in postsinusoidal venules: percentage of rollers of the total number of moving leukocytes observed during the observation period of 20 s

Bile flow

To assess the bile production of the reperfused graft, as an indicator of reestablished liver function, a drain was fixed in the bile duct. The amount of bile draining over a period of 60 min was weighed, and, to allow for comparison between individual animals and groups, was related to 100 g of liver wet weight.

Statistics

Statistical differences between groups were calculated using Student's t-test for parametric data and the Mann-Whitney U-test for nonparametric data. Differences were considered significant at $P \leq 0.05$.

Results

In regard to body weight, liver wet weight, anhepatic period, and total ischemic time, there were no significant differences between the study groups (Table 1). Microvascular perfusion was significantly improved in enalapril-treated animals. The sinusoidal perfusion rate almost reached levels of sham-operated animals, which is 98–100 %. In addition, the number of sticking leukocytes was remarkably reduced in both sinusoids and postsinusoidal venules, indicative of a lesser degree of ischemia/reperfusion injury (Figs. 1 and 2). The fraction of rolling leukocytes in the postsinusoidal venules, however, remained unchanged despite enalapril treatment [LTx vs. LTx/Ena: 10.0 (2.1) % vs. 7.2 (1.4) %, mean (SEM)]. Bile flow, as an indicator of restored, energy-dependent liver function, was increased; however, the observed difference failed to reach a significant level [1.13 (0.3) vs. 0.43 (0.1); $P = 0.06$].

Discussion

In the technical proceeding of cadaveric liver transplantation, the inevitable periods of hypothermic anoxia and partial normothermic hypoxia, lack of hepatotrophic substrates, and toxic insult of oxygen free radicals result in organ damage known as ischemia/reperfusion injury, which may, in up to 22 %, clinically present as graft dysor nonfunction. Introduction of the UW solution by Belzer marked a considerable progress in liver preserva-

S95

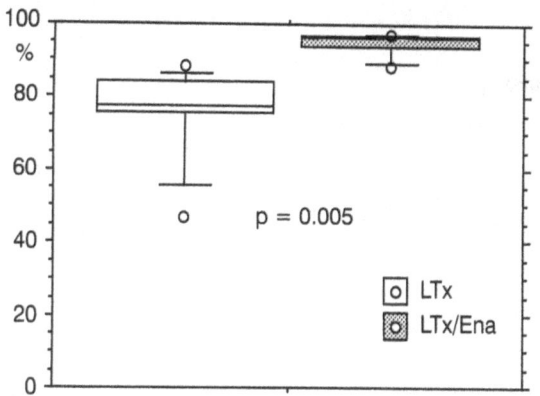

Fig.1 Sinusoidal perfusion (box plot: horizontal bars depict 10th, 25th, 50th, 75th and 90th percentile, circles show outliers)

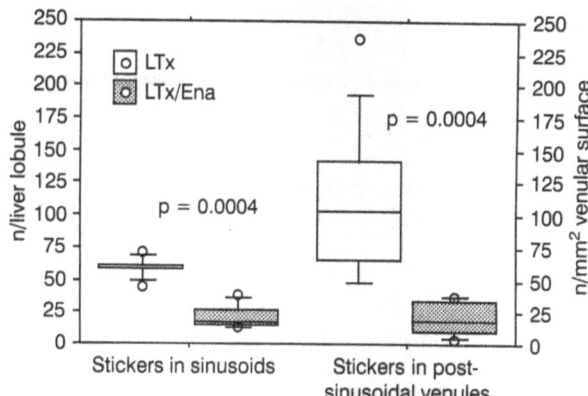

Fig.2 Leukocyte adherence in sinusoids and postsinusoidal venules (box plot: horizontal bars depict 10th, 25th, 50th, 75th and 90th percentile, circles show outliers)

tion; however, there still seems to be a lack of an optimal preservation concept [18]. To the best of current understanding of optimal organ preservation, the goal is not only to preserve the primary graft viability by simply flushing the liver with an appropriate ice-cold solution, but also, and probably more importantly, to undertake therapeutic interventions during the more harmful periods of warm ischemia, removal of the high-potassium UW solution and reperfusion.

Former studies have clearly demonstrated, that, by not only changing the solution for flushout of the UW solution prior to graft reperfusion, but also by treatment of the recipient with scavengers or calcium channel blockers, improvements in graft function and structural integrity can be accomplished [19–22]. In different models of temporary coronary blood flow occlusion, ischemia/reperfusion damage has been effectively reduced by different types of ACE inhibitors. For thiol-containing drugs, such as captopril, the effects are attributed to their ability to inactivate reactive oxygen species [23, 24]. The common property of all ACE inhibitors is, however, their vasodilative action, which is based on both an inhibition of angiotensin II production and reduced bradykinin metabolism. Vasodilation and the bradykinin-induced endothelial synthesis of antiaggregatory and cytoprotective prostacyclin may explain the observed beneficial effects.

In terms of microvascular perfusion, we showed by means of IVM that enalapril treatment starting before reperfusion and continuing for 2 h improves nutritive liver perfusion remarkably, almost reaching values of nontransplanted livers. The leukocyte-endothelium interaction was significantly reduced in different areas of the microvascular liver network, indicating amelioration of ischemia/reperfusion damage. Because enalapril does not contain a thiol group in its molecule, scavenging actions cannot explain the effects. Presumably, an impact on the angiotensin, bradykinin, and prostacyclin

metabolism is the underlying mechanism. As is known from earlier liver studies, the cytoprotective and platelet-inhibiting effect of prostacyclin may be of particular importance. Furthermore, prostaglandins of the E and I group are able to inhibit the activation of polymorphnuclear granulocytes, which in our model may explain the marked reduction in the leukocyte-endothelium interaction [25].

The findings of the IVM were in accordance with the result of the functional liver evaluation. Bile flow is known as a precise indicator of energy-dependent liver functions, and improvement may reflect better restoration of hepatic energy charge [26, 27]. Enalapril treatment was able to increase bile flow after reperfusion. The reason why the difference did not reach the level of significance may be related to the considerable variance in a group of only eight individuals and a collection period that was too short to demonstrate clearly the improvement.

Our study proved for the first time that the ACE inhibitor enalapril is able to reduce ischemia/reperfusion injury in a model of rat liver transplantation. The beneficial effects of enalapril observed in experiments on warm myocardial ischemia seem to be transferable to a model of rat liver transplantation, which includes a combination of cold and warm ischemia followed by reperfusion. However, these preliminary results need further confirmation. In particular, it has to be investigated in future studies whether the improvements can be attributed to changes in angiotensin, bradykinin, and prostacyclin metabolism, or whether enalapril, and possibly other substances of the ACE inhibitor group, possess some as yet unknown action of their own on ischemia/reperfusion injury.

References

1. Bismuth H, Azoulay D, Dennison A (1993) Recent developments in liver transplantation. Transplant Proc 25: 2191–2194
2. Neuhaus P, Blumhardt G, Bechstein WO, Keck H (1992) Progress in the field of liver transplantation in the last 10 years. Langenbecks Arch Chir Suppl Kongressbd 317: 209–216
3. Ploeg RJ, D'Alessandro AM, Knechtle SJ, Stegall MD, Pirsch JD, Hoffmann RM, et al (1993) Risk factors for primary dysfunction after lifer transplantation – a multivariate analysis. Transplantation 55: 807–813
4. de Graeff P, de Langen C, van Gilst W, Bel K, Scholtens E, Kingma J, et al (1988) Protective effects of captopril against ischemia/reperfusion-induced ventricular arrhythmias in vitro and in vivo. Am J Med 84: 67–74
5. Przyklenk K, Kloner R (1993) "Cardioprotection" by ACE-inhibitors in acute myocardial ischemia and infarction? Basic Res Cardiol 88 [Suppl 1]: 139–154
6. Scholkens BA, Linz W (1990) Cardioprotective effects of ACE inhibitors: experimental proof and clinical perspectives. Clin Physiol Biochem 8: 33–43
7. Schroer K (1992) Role of prostaglandins in the cardiovascular effects of bradykinin and angiotensin-converting enzyme inhibitors. J Cardiovasc Pharmacol 20 [Suppl 9]: 68
8. de Nucci G, Warner T, Vane JR (1988) Effect of captopril on the bradykinin-induced release of prostacyclin from guinea-pig lungs and bovine aortic endothelial cells. Br J Pharmacol 95: 783–788
9. Chen X, Pi X, Li D, Li Y, Deng H (1989) Prostacyclin-mediated cardioprotection of captopril and ramiprilate against lipidperoxidation in the rat. Prog Clin Biol Res 301: 167–173
10. Abecassis M, Falk JA, Makowka L, Dindzans VJ, Falk RE, Levy GA (1987) 16,16 Dimethyl prostaglandin E2 prevents the development of fulminant hepatitis and blocks the induction of monocyte/macrophage procoagulant activity after murine hepatitis virus strain 3 infection. J Clin Invest 80: 881–889
11. Alp M, Hickman R (1987) The effect of prostaglandins, branched-chain amino acids and other drugs on the outcome of experimental acute porcine hepatic failure. J Hepatol 4: 99–107
12. Araki H, Lefer AM (1980) Cytoprotective actions of prostacyclin during hypoxia in the isolated perfused cat liver. Am J Physiol 238: 176–181
13. Alvarez LA, de Hemptinne B, Hoebeke Y, Lambotte L (1987) Prostaglandin E2 increases the tolerance of the rat liver to warm ischemia in absence of splanchnic congestion. Transplant Proc 19: 4105–4109
14. Kamada N, Calne RY (1979) Orthotopic liver transplantation in the rat. Technique using cuff for portal vein anastomosis and biliary drainage. Transplantation 28: 47–56
15. Steffen R, Ferguson DM, Krom RA (1989) A new method for orthotopic rat liver transplantation with arterial cuff anastomosis to the recipient common hepatic artery. Transplantation 48: 166–168
16. Post S, Menger MD, Rentsch M, Gonzalez AP, Herfarth C, Messmer K (1992) The impact of arterialization on hepatic microcirculation and leukocyte accumulation after liver transplantation in the rat. Transplantation 54: 789–794
17. Menger MD, Marzi I, Messmer K (1991) In vivo fluorescence microscopy for quantitative analysis of the hepatic microcirculation in hamsters and rats. Eur Surg Res 23: 158–169
18. Belzer FO, D'Alessandro AM, Hoffmann RM, Knechtle SJ, Reed A, Pirsch JD, et al (1992) The use of UW solution in clinical transplantation. A 4-year experience. Ann Surg 215: 579–583
19. Gao WS, Takei Y, Marzi I, Lindert KA, Caldwell KJ, Currin RT, et al (1991) Carolina rinse solution – a new strategy to increase survival time after orthotopic liver transplantation in the rat. Transplantation 52: 417–424
20. Lemmens HP, Schoen MR, Blumhardt G, Filler D, Brandau O, Meissler M, et al (1993) Influence of SOD, catalase, and epoprostenol on 24-hour liver preservation in pigs. Transplant Proc 25: 2549–2553
21. Liang D, Thurman RG (1992) Protective effects of the calcium antagonists diltiazem and TA3090 against hepatic injury due to hypoxia. Biochem Pharmacol 44: 2207–2211
22. Post S, Rentsch M, Palma P, Gonzalez AP, Otto G, Menger MD (1992) Effect of Carolina rinse solution on Kupffer cell activation after reperfusion in rat liver transplantation. Transplant Proc 24: 2703
23. Chopra M, Scott N, McMurray J, McLay J, Bridges A, Smith WE, et al (1989) Captopril: a free radical scavenger. Br J Clin Pharmacol 27: 396–399
24. Chopra M, McMurray J, Stewart J, Dargie HJ, Smith WE (1990) Free radical scavenging: a potentially beneficial action of thiol-containing angiotensin converting enzyme inhibitors. Biochem Soc Trans 18: 1184–1185
25. Fantone JC, Kinnes DA (1983) Prostaglandin E1 and prostaglandin 12 modulation of superoxide production by human neutrophils. Biochem Biophys Res Commun 113: 506–512
26. Bowers BA, Branum GD, Rotolo FS, Watters CR, Meyers WC (1987) Bile flow – an index of ischemic injury. J Surg Res 42: 565–569
27. Sumimoto K, Inagaki K, Yamada K, Kawasaki T, Dohi K (1988) Reliable indices for the determination of viability of grafted liver immediately after orthotopic transplantation. Bile flow rate and cellular adenosine triphosphate level. Transplantation 46: 506–509

Transpl Int (1996) 9 [Suppl 1]: S97–S99
© Springer-Verlag 1996

LIVER

D. Seehofer
H. Baatz
J. Thiery
C. Hammer

Quantitative analysis of the microcirculation of xenogeneic haemoperfused rat livers by intravital microscopy

D. Seehofer · H. Baatz · C. Hammer (✉)
Institute for Surgical Research,
Marchioninistr. 15, D-81366 Munich,
Germany

J. Thiery
Institute for Clinical Chemistry,
University of Munich, Germany

Abstract Livers from male Sprague-Dawley rats were perfused with heparinised, unmodified isogeneic rat blood ($n = 6$) or xenogeneic human blood. The microcirculation of these livers, as the primary manifestation of hyperacute xenogeneic rejection, was directly observed and quantified by using fluorescence videomicroscopy. Bile flow and enzyme release of the isogeneic perfused livers were in the physiological range, whereas bile flow was significantly reduced and enzyme release increased during xenogeneic perfusion. In contrast to an almost physi-ological acinar (90.4 %) and sinusoidal (93.6 %) perfusion rate in the isogeneic group, a rapid breakdown of microcirculation with an acinar perfusion index of 47.5 % and a sinusoidal perfusion rate of 67.1 % were found in the xenogeneic group. This direct quantification of microcirculatory parameters is a step forward towards sensitive and early characterisation of the severity of the xenogeneic rejection of the liver.

Key words Xenograft · Microcirculation · Liver · Isolated perfusion · Rat

Introduction

Like most other immunological disease mechanisms, xenograft rejection is thought to manifest primarily at the level of the microcirculatory unit [1]. Despite extensive histological studies [2, 3] of hyperacute xenogeneic rejection (HXR), little is known about microhaemodynamic alterations during HXR. The purpose of this study was the direct observation and quantification, using intravital microscopy (IVM), of the microcirculation of rat livers perfused by human blood. This technique permits the dynamic investigation of the hepatic microcirculation in vital organs after staining the blood with different fluorescent dyes.

Materials and methods

Rat liver perfusion

Male Sprague-Dawley rats (250–300 g) were anaesthetised by intraperitoneal injection of pentobarbital sodium (60 mg/kg). After midline abdominal and subcostal incisions, the livers were prepared in situ to avoid relevant trauma or ischaemia. Livers were perfused using a modified technique of Miller et al. [4]. Briefly, the hepatic artery was ligated, and the common bile duct and portal vein were cannulated. Immediately after cannulation of the portal vein, the livers were flushed with 30 ml of cold lactated Ringer's solution and the rats were killed by exsanguination. The perfusion circuit was closed by cannulating the suprahepatic inferior caval vein and ligating the infrahepatic part of the inferior caval vein. After a total cold ischaemic time of less than 4 min, the livers were reperfused for 45 min at a constant flow rate of 1.15 ± 0.1 ml/min per gram of liver. The perfusate consisted of 35 ml heparinised (10 IU/ml) fresh isogeneic rat blood or xenogeneic human blood diluted to a haematocrit of 30 ± 2 % with hydroxyethyl-starch. The temperature, pH and portal pressure were monitored continuously during the course of the perfusion.

Four different groups were established: two perfusion groups (isogeneic or xenogeneic perfusion of a rat liver, $n = 6$) and two

Table 1 Microcirculatory parameters (mean ± SEM) during isogeneic and xenogeneic in situ perfusion of rat livers, assessed by intravital fluorescence microscopy

	Isogeneic perfusion (rat)	Xenogeneic perfusion (human)
Index of acinar perfusion (45 min)	90.4 ± 1.0 %	47.5 ± 2.1 %*
Sinusoidal perfusion		
Periportal	92.2 ± 1.0 %	59.0 ± 0.3 %*
Midzonal	92.1 ± 0.8 %	66.1 ± 0.3 %*
Pericentral	96.6 ± 0.7 %	76.1 ± 0.3 %*
Mean	93.6 ± 0.3 %	67.1 ± 0.3 %*
Adherent WBC in perfused sinusoids [n/lobule]		
Periportal	21.0 ± 1.2	9.3 ± 1.3
Midzonal	25.1 ± 1.0	7.3 ± 1.9
Pericentral	11.8 ± 1.1	3.8 ± 0.9
Mean	57.9 ± 1.5	20.4 ± 3.5
Sinusoidal diameter of perfused sinusoids (mean of the three liver zones)		
0–15 min	6.1 ± 0.1	6.7 ± 0.1*
15–45 min	6.5 ± 0.1	8.3 ± 0.3*
30–45 min	6.5 ± 0.1	9.2 ± 0.2*
Postsinusoidal venules		
WBC velocity [µm/sec]	1196 ± 75	890 ± 128*
Adherent WBC [n/mm²]	122 ± 27	55 ± 13*

* $P < 0.01$ (Mann-Whitney U-test)

control groups (perfusion of an anhepatic circuit with human blood or rat blood, $n = 5$). Blood samples were drawn at given time points for blood counts, biochemical analysis (GOT, LDH) and determination of titres of preformed natural antibodies by haemagglutination. As an indicator of liver function, bile was collected in intervals of 15 min.

Intravital microscopy

For IVM the right liver lobe was exteriorised on a specially designed mechanical stage and covered with a saran wrap to prevent drying of the tissue. The perfusate was stained with fluorescein sodium and rhodamine 6G. The microvessels of the liver were investigated directly using a microscope with epi-illumination and different filter blocks, a CCD video camera and a SVHS video recording unit. During perfusion eight to ten liver fields, postsinusoidal venules and portal venules were observed at a × 800 magnification (on the monitor) and videod. At the end of the perfusion, 30–50 acini were videod at a lower magnification (× 400). Quantification of the hepatic microcirculation was performed off line by frame-to-frame analysis of the videotapes as described elsewhere [5].

Results

During isogeneic in situ perfusion of rat livers, portal pressure remained in the physiological range, whereas perfusion with human blood resulted in a significantly increased portal pressure within the first minutes. The maximum pressure was reached in this group after 15 min, thereafter portal pressure decreased slowly to

values comparable to the isogeneic group. Bile flow as a gross indicator of liver function was severley depressed in the xenogeneic group but not in the isogeneic one. Biochemical analysis of the perfusate revealed no significant changes or unphysiological values in the isogeneic perfusion group, except for a marked rise in LDH due to haemolysis that was also present in the isogeneic control group. GOT and LDH showed no major changes in the xenogeneic control group, indicating a less expressed haemolysis of human blood compared to rat blood. In contrast, GOT and LDH increased significantly in the xenogeneic perfusion group, indicating severe parenchymal cell injury in the liver. A reduction in preformed natural antibodies (PNAB) to almost zero was found in the xenogeneic perfusion group, but not in the xenogeneic control group.

Isogeneic perfusion resulted in a slight reduction in white blood cell (WBC) counts after 45 min and in no reduction in platelet (PLT) counts compared to the control group. In contrast, most of the human WBC and PLT accumulated in the liver within the first 5 min – predominantly portal and periportal as observed by IVM – resulting in a rapid reduction in WBC and PLT counts in the perfusate. In situ perfusion of rat livers with isogeneic blood showed a homogenous perfusion of the liver and an almost physiological WBC behaviour, whereas in the xenogeneic group, 24 % of acini were not perfused and most of the remaining ones were irregularly perfused as reflected by a low index of acinar perfusion. The observed microcirculatory parameters can be seen in Table 1.

Discussion

In situ rat liver perfusion with isogeneic rat blood showed an almost intact microcirculation with a sinusoidal and acinar perfusion rate of over 90 %. The small reduction in the perfusion rate – which in normal livers in vivo is nearly 100 % – is considered to be due to the lack of hepatic arterial perfusion [6] or the formation of microemboli in extracorporeal perfusion systems [7], a fact that was confirmed by IVM. In postsinusoidal venules, WBC flow behaviour and WBC adherence were similar to the values of in vivo observations, indicating – together with normal bile flow and enzyme levels – no relevant ischaemic damage [5] of the liver. In contrast, xenogeneic perfusion resulted in a breakdown of the microcirculation within minutes. Comparable values for perfusion deficits are reached in allograft rejection in the rat only after 4–6 days [8]. The observed dilatation of sinusoids, which was expressed less in the first 15 min after reperfusion but was markedly so after 30 min, was in agreement with histological findings [Pascher et al., submitted for publication] of hyperaemic areas in xenografts.

The predominantly portal and periportal accumulation of WBC during HXR and its speed and extent was probably mediated by early complement activation [9, 10] enhancing thrombocyte aggregation [11], together with subsequent adhesion of WBC. This is in agreement with the binding of PNAB and the activation of complement predominantly in afferent vessels [2, 3; Pascher et al., submitted for publication]. Because no gold standard exists for evaluation of hepatic function [12], direct observation of the microcirculation and, in particular, determination of the sinusoidal and acinar perfusion rate is a step forward towards sensitive and early characterisation of the severity of rejection in xenogeneic models.

References

1. Menger MD, Lehr HA (1993) Scope and perspectives of intravital microscopy – bridge over from in vitro to in vivo. Immunol Today 14: 519–522
2. Collins BH, Chari RS, Magee JC, et al (1995) Immunpathology of porcine livers perfused with blood of humans with fulminant hepatic failure. Transplant Proc 27: 280–281
3. Makowka L, Wu GD, Hoffman A, et al (1994) Immunohistopathologic lesions associated with the rejection of a pig-to-human liver xenograft. Transplant Proc 26: 1074–1075
4. Miller LL, Bly CG, Watson ML, et al (1951) The dominant role of the liver in plasma protein synthesis. J Exp Med 94: 431–453
5. Post S, Palma P, Rentsch R, et al (1993) Hepatic reperfusion injury following cold ischemia in the rat: potentials of quantitative analysis by in vivo fluorescence microscopy. Prog Appl Microcirc 19: 152–166
6. Post S, Menger MD, Rentsch M, et al (1992) The impact of arterialization on hepatic microcirculation and leukocyte accumulation after liver transplantation in the rat. Transplantation 54: 789–794
7. Forty J, White DGJ, Wallwork J (1993) A technique for perfusion of an isolated working heart to investigate hyperacute discordant xenograft rejection. J Thorac Cardiovasc Surg 106: 307–316
8. Kawano K, Bowers JL, Kruskal JB, et al (1995) In vivo microscopic assessment of hepatic microcirculation during liver allograft rejection in the rat. Transplantation 59: 1241–1248
9. Vercellotti GM, Platt JL, Bach FH, et al (1991) Neutrophil adhesion to xenogeneic endothelium via iC3b. J Immunol 146: 730–734
10. Baldwin WM, Pruitt SK, Brauer RB, et al (1995) Complement in organ transplantation. Transplantation 59: 797–808
11. Robson SC, Kopp C, Lesnikoski B (1994) Platelets and xenograft rejection. Xeno 2: 38–46
12. Gores GJ, Kost LJ, LaRusso NF (1986) The isolated perfused rat liver: conceptual and practical considerations. Hepatology 6: 511–517

Transpl Int (1996) 9 [Suppl 1]: S100–S104
© Springer-Verlag 1996

LIVER

Beneficial effects of prostaglandin E_1 on hemodynamic changes during liver transplantation in pigs

M. Oishi
N. Tanaka
K. Orita

M. Oishi (✉) · N. Tanaka · K. Orita
First department of surgery, Okayama
University Medical School,
2-5-1 Shikata-cho, Okayama 700,
Japan

Abstract The vasodilative action of prostaglandin E_1 (PGE_1) on the systemic and pulmonary circulation was investigated in swine models of orthotopic liver transplantation. In the PGE_1-treated group ($n = 8$), PGE_1 (0.05 μg/kg per minute) was intravenously infused from the onset of the anhepatic stage to 30 min after revascularization. During the anhepatic stage, PGE_1 decreased systemic vascular resistance without a corresponding hypotension, so cardiac output was maintained at a higher level. In the control group ($n = 8$), pulmonary vascular resistance increased to 3 times the anhepatic value during reperfusion, accompanied by a decline in cardiac output with a 28 % decrease in blood pressure. In the PGE_1-treated group, on the other hand, pulmonary vascular resistance was maintained within the normal range without any associated decrease in cardiac output. The blood pressure decreased slightly by 12 %. In conclusion, in this model, PGE_1 increased cardiac output without hypotension during the anhepatic stage and also prevented postreperfusion pulmonary hypertension and the subsequent systemic hypotension.

Key words Liver transplantation · Pulmonary hypertension · Postreperfusion syndrome

Introduction

Prostaglandin E_1 (PGE_1) has been widely used in clinical liver transplantation because of its cytoprotective effect [1]. Recently, PGE_1 has been shown to protect the liver graft from antibody-mediated rejection [2]. On the other hand, PGE_1 has several actions on the circulatory system, including a direct vasodilator action on the peripheral vascular bed, a reflex increase in cardiac output due to the decrease in peripheral vascular resistance, and a direct positive inotropic action on the myocardium [3]. However, there have been only a limited number of studies of the effects of PGE_1 on vascular dynamics in liver transplantation [4]. Therefore, it would be interesting to examine how PGE_1 as a vasodilator affects the markedly changing and complicated hemodynamics in liver transplantation.

During the anhepatic stage of the operation, decreased venous return leads to a compensatory elevation in systemic vascular resistance in spite of the use of the venovenous bypass [5, 6]. In addition, the venovenous bypass itself causes an increase in systemic vascular resistance due to a non-physiological venous return. PGE_1 may suppress systemic vasoconstriction and maintain stable systemic hemodynamics.

In liver transplantation in pigs, marked pulmonary hypertension appears immediately after graft reperfusion [7, 8], with impaired hemodynamics after reperfusion. When PGE_1 is administered intravenously, it is almost completely metabolized in the lung during the first pass [9], exerting a vasodilative action predominantly on the pulmonary blood vessels and decreasing right ventricular afterload. Therefore, PGE_1 may suppress pulmonary hypertension in pigs undergoing liver transplantation. The species is generally recognized to be susceptible to pulmonary hypertension and lung edema. The pig accordingly appears to be a suitable animal for the study of pulmonary vasomotion [10]. The purpose of this study was to investigate the vasodilative action of PGE_1 during liver transplantation, particularly its effects on the hemodynamics during the anhepatic stage and on postreperfusion pulmonary hypertension.

Materials and methods

Animals

Thirty-two large white pigs weighing 20–25 kg were used to perform 16 orthotopic liver transplantations.

Anesthesia

Following premedication with 300 mg ketamine and 250 mg thiopental, each pig was orally intubated and ventilated to maintain the arterial Pco_2 at 30–40 mm Hg. Anesthesia was maintained with a mixture of nitrous oxide-oxygen (1:1) and halothane (0.5 %). Ringer's solution was infused intravenously through the right jugular vein at 20–25 ml/kg per hour and 400–800 ml whole blood was given to the recipient, depending on the amount of blood loss.

Donor and recipient operation

Liver transplantation was performed orthotopically as described previously [11]. The donor liver was perfused with 1500 ml of UW solution at 4 °C and also preserved with 500 ml of UW solution at 4 °C for 2 h. In the recipient, following laparotomy using a midline incision, the left iliac vein, portal vein, and left external jugular vein were prepared for placement of the venovenous bypass. During the anhepatic stage, the venovenous bypass was used at flow rates ranging from 600 to 1200 ml/min to prevent congestion in the gut and lower extremities. Before placement of the venous bypass, the pig received a bolus injection of 2000 IU heparin. The order of anastomoses was as follows: suprahepatic vena cava (4-0 polypropylene suture); portal vein using the growth factor procedure (6-0 polypropylene suture); aortic conduit after reperfusion of the liver (end-to-side with 6-0 polypropylene suture); infrahepatic vena cava (4-0 polypropylene suture). The liver was flushed with 300 ml of cold Ringer's solution prior to the portal vein anatomosis. The portal vein was anatomosed without removing the portal cannula for the venous bypass until the suturing of the last two or three stitches to keep the portal occlusion time as brief as possible (maximal period of portal occlusion, 1 min). All recipient operations were performed without technical problems, and the recipient pigs recovered uneventfully from the surgical procedure.

Experimental design

The recipients were divided into group A ($n = 8$), which received no further treatment, and group B ($n = 8$), which received PGE_1 (0.05 µg/kg per minute; Ono Pharmaceutical Ltd) intravenously from the onset of the anhepatic phase to 30 min after revascularization.

Monitoring

Electrocardiography was used to monitor heart rate (HR) and to detect arrhythmia. Mean arterial pressure (MAP) was measured using a catheter placed in the right external carotid artery. A 5-Fr Swan-Ganz catheter was inserted via the right external jugular vein to monitor mean pulmonary artery pressure (MPAP), central venous pressure (CVP), pulmonary capillary wedge pressure (PCWP), cardiac output (CO), systemic vascular resistance (SVR), and pulmonary vascular resistance (PVR). CO was measured by the thermodilution technique. As described in a previous report [5], the above hemodynamic profiles were measured at the following six sequential time points during surgery: 5 min before the onset of the anhepatic stage (II-5), 5 min after the onset of the anhepatic stage (II + 5); 5 min before the start of reperfusion (III − 5); 3, 30, and 60 min after the start of reperfusion (III + 3, III + 30, III + 60). Before and after reperfusion, blood samples were obtained via the arterial line for analysis of blood gases and also for measurement of serum electrolytes.

Statistical analysis

Values are expressed as the mean value or mean ± standard deviation (SD). The significance of differences between mean values were determined using Student's unpaired t-test. A P value of less than 0.05 was considered significant.

Results

Systemic and pulmonary hemodynamic variables and other factors affecting the hemodynamics are presented in Figs. 1–3 and Table 1. At the start of the venovenous bypass (II + 5) in group A, the reduced venous return caused an immediate decrease in CVP (34 %) and CO (27 %) and a compensatory increase in SVR (32 %) and PVR (35 %). Because of these compensatory responses, the MAP and MPAP were well maintained. The flow rate in the venovenous bypass was sufficient to maintain venous return (Table 1). At the end of the bypass (III − 5), the CVP was returned to almost its preanhepatic value with the infusion of fluid and blood, but adequate CO was not maintained despite the adequate preload. SVR and PVR showed a tendency to increase. Reperfusion of the liver graft in the control group caused a slight increase in CVP (5 %) and a marked increase in PVR (threefold) and MPAP (54 %). As a result of the increase in right ventricular afterload, the CO and MAP decreased by 30 % and 27.9 %, respectively (CO from 1.52 ± 0.28 to 1.07 ± 0.45 l/min, MAP from 101.4 ± 13.6 to 73.2 ± 19.4 mm Hg). During the anhepatic and reperfusion stage, the PCWP showed changes similar to those of the CVP (data not shown). No changes were observed in HR and cardiac rhythm.

In the PGE_1-treated pigs, hemodynamic changes similar to those in the control pigs were seen for the first 5 min of the anhepatic stage (II + 5). However, at the end of this stage (III − 5), the increases in SVR and PVR were suppressed and the CO was maintained at a

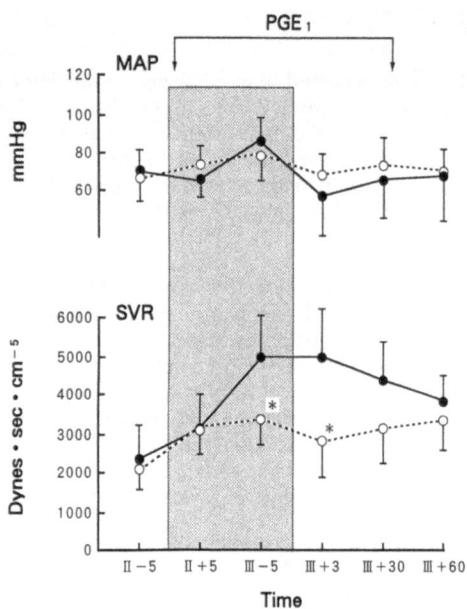

Fig. 1 Mean arterial pressure (MAP) and systemic vascular resistance (SVR) values (mean ± SD) measured in eight control (●) and eight PGE₁-treated pigs (○) at six sequential time points. The *shaded area* indicates the anhepatic period. * $P < 0.05$ compared with the control group

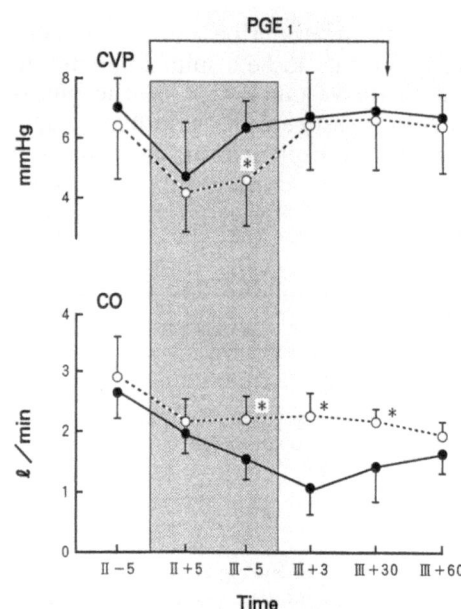

Fig. 3 Central venous pressure (CVP) and cardiac output (CO) values (mean ± SD) measured in eight control (●) and eight PGE₁-treated pigs (○) at six sequential time points. The *shaded area* indicates the anhepatic period. * $P < 0.05$ compared with the control group

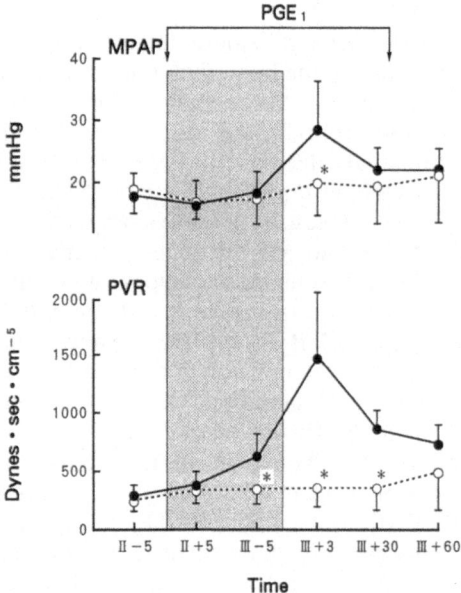

Fig. 2 Mean pulmonary arterial pressure (MPAP) and pulmonary vascular resistance (PVR) values (mean ± SD) measured in eight control (●) and eight PGE₁-treated pigs (○) at six sequential time points. The *shaded area* indicates the anhepatic period. * $P < 0.05$ compared with the control group

higher level than that in group A (1.52 ± 0.28 vs 2.17 ± 0.44 l/min, $P < 0.05$). As a result, hypotension did not occur in spite of the infusion of PGE₁. In addition, a high CO was obtained with a lower CVP compared with that in group A. There was no difference between the two groups in the extra volume administered during the anhepatic stage or in the flow rate of the venovenous bypass. At 3 min after the start of the reperfusion stage (III + 3), no changes in PVR or MPAP were observed, in contrast to group A. Consequently, CO was well maintained, showing a change from 2.17 ± 0.44 to 2.22 ± 0.52 l/min. Because PVR was low and consequently CO was high, the MAP showed only a slight change (from 95.3 ± 13.9 to 84.2 ± 13.1 mm Hg). A significant difference in the MAP between the two groups was not demonstrated at III + 3, but the percentage decrease in MAP, accompanied by revascularization, was significantly less in group B ($12.0 \pm 7.5\%$, $P < 0.05$) compared with that in group A ($27.9 \pm 16.2\%$). There was no difference between the groups in the degree of increase in blood potassium concentration, decrease in base excess, or drop in temperature. In the PGE₁-treated group, persistent wheezing or requirement for further blood transfusion was not observed.

Discussion

It has been reported that PGE₁ is effective in the treatment of primary nonfunction [1], humoral rejection,

Table 1 Summary of systemic variables in the two groups. Date are presented as mean ± SD. Group A is the control group and group B, the PGE$_1$-treated group

	A	B
Anhepatic time (min)	57 ± 7.8	54 ± 10.8
Bypass flow rate (ml/min)	0.78 ± 0.20	0.78 ± 0.14
Blood transfusion (ml)	550 ± 193	480 ± 160
Fluid infusion during anhepatic stage (ml)	420 ± 122	440 ± 108
Changes after reperfusion in:		
Potassium (mEq/l)	0.23 ± 1.29	0.33 ± 0.37
Base excess (mmol/l)	− 1.80 ± 1.38	− 1.53 ± 1.07
Temperature (°C)	− 1.26 ± 0.51	− 0.92 ± 0.25

and nephrotoxicity of FK506 following liver transplantation [2]. PGE$_1$ also has adverse effects, such as an inhibitory effect on platelet aggregation, hypotension, and severe diarrhea. In particular, hypotension limits the use of PGE$_1$ [1, 2]. In our study, the administration of PGE$_1$ (0.05 µg/kg per minute) during liver transplantation in pigs resulted in no decrease in MAP and did not result in a hemorrhagic diathesis.

Some previous clinical assessments [5, 6] have suggested that venous return is decreased in the anhepatic stage in spite of use of the venovenous bypass, which can lead to a decrease in CO and cause a compensatory elevation in SVR. Venovenous bypass is not totally effective in maintaining venous return. Another reason for the elevation in SVR is that the venovenous bypass itself leads to an increase in SVR due to a nonphysiological venous return. In our control group, the CVP and MAP returned to the preanhepatic values at the end of bypass, but the SVR showed a tendency to increase. This pattern indicated that the main reason for the increased SVR at the end of bypass is the nonphysiological venous return rather than a decreased venous return. We had anticipated that the administration of PGE$_1$, under such conditions as increased SVR, would be result in cardiovascular instability. Contrary to this expectation, stable hemodynamics were maintained without a decrease in MAP after the administration of PGE$_1$. This stable state may be sustained by the increased CO as a consequence of the vasodilator action of PGE$_1$. In addition, PGE$_1$ may exert a direct positive inotropic action on the myocardium during the anhepatic stage. From these results, we suggest that PGE$_1$ may have a cardiovascular support action during the anhepatic stage under venovenous bypass.

In the present study, reperfusion in liver transplantation in pigs was found to be associated with the onset of marked pulmonary hypertension causing systemic hypotension [7, 8]. PVR increased to about triple the level before reperfusion in the control group, CO was decreased by this phenomenon, and blood pressure decreased by 28 % compared to the level before reperfu-

sion. None of these pigs, however, showed bradyarrhythmia or rapid decreases in SVR. These results suggested that an elevation in PVR during reperfusion is the primary cause of systemic hypotension during reperfusion.

Post et al. [12] have reported that prostaglandin I$_2$ (PGI$_2$), prostaglandin E$_2$ (PGE$_2$), and thromboxane A$_2$ (TXA$_2$) are released from the transplanted liver during reperfusion following cold storage. PGI$_2$ and PGE$_2$ have a vasodilative action, whereas TXA$_2$ has a vasoconstrictive action. Therefore, the predominant vasomotor action depends on the ratio between PGI$_2$ and TXA$_2$. On the other hand, macrophages in pulmonary capillaries have been shown to metabolize arachidonic acid [13]. These intravascular macrophages appear to regulate the pressure in the pulmonary microcirculation by adjustment of the ratio between PGI$_2$ and TXA$_2$. There are interspecies differences in the size and number of the macrophages, which are larger in pigs than in other species [14, 15]. Since the sensitivity to TXA$_2$ is believed to be higher in the lungs of pigs than in humans, the postreperfusion pulmonary hypertension in pigs is thought to be caused by TXA$_2$ released from the transplanted liver during reperfusion.

Pettiet et al. [7] have reported that administration of a cyclooxygenase inhibitor, indomethacin, inhibits the synthesis of TXA$_2$ in the reperfused liver and suppresses pulmonary hypertension, as well as the postreperfusion syndrome. PGE$_1$ prevented pulmonary hypertension in this experiment, probably because PGE$_1$ efficiently antagonized the vasoconstrictive action of TXA$_2$. As a result, PGE$_1$ alleviated right ventricular afterload and subsequently prevented the decrease in CO in the postreperfusion stage. Although Blankensteijn [4] has reported deleterious effects of PGE$_1$ on the hemodynamics during liver transplantation, their experiment differed from ours in that the doses used in their experiment were smaller and the administration of PGE$_1$ was discontinued immediately before reperfusion.

Postreperfusion pulmonary hypertension is specific to pigs and is not found in humans. However, a similar phenomenon has caused trouble in some clinical settings. Pulmonary hypertension is not uncommon in end-stage liver disease [16]. In these patients, sudden occurrence of pulmonary hypertension during the operation is fatal [17]. In order to avoid mortality in these patients, administration of PGE$_1$ must be considered.

In summary, in this study in pigs a continuous infusion of PGE$_1$ increased CO without any adverse effect on the hemodynamics during the anhepatic stage and it also prevented pulmonary hypertension during reperfusion. Hence, we suggest that the administration of PGE$_1$ should be considered in clinical liver transplantation.

References

1. Greig PD, Woolf GM, Sinclair SB, et al (1989) Treatment of primary liver graft non-function with prostaglandin E_1. Transplantation 48: 453
2. Takaya S, Iwaki Y, Starzl TE (1992) Liver transplantation in positive cytotoxic crossmatch cases using FK506, high dose steroids, and prostaglandins E_1. Transplantation 54: 927
3. Nakao J, McCurdy IR (1967) Cardiovascular effects of prostaglandin E_1. J Pharmacol Exp Ther 156: 538
4. Blankensteijn JD, Schlejen PM, Groenland THN, Terpstra OT (1992) The effects of long-term graft preservation and prostaglandin E_1 on intraoperative hemodynamic changes in liver transplantation. Transplantation 54: 423
5. Rettke S, Janossy TA, Chantigian RC, et al (1989) Hemodynamic and metabolic changes in hepatic transplantation. Mayo Clin Proc 64: 232
6. Shaw BW, Martin DJ, Marquez JM, et al (1984) Venous bypass in clinical liver transplantation. Ann Surg 200: 524
7. Pittet J-F, Morel DR, Mentha G, Le Coultre C, Suter PM, Rohner A (1991) Protective effect of indomethacin in the development of the postreperfusion syndrome during liver transplantation. Transplant Proc 23: 2290
8. Miichi N (1989) Hemodynamic effects of anesthetic agents and bypass flow during orthotopic liver transplantation (in Japanese). Nippon Geka Gakkai Zasshi 90: 1907
9. Ferreira SH, Vane JR (1967) Prostaglandins, their disappearance from and release into the circulation. Nature 216: 868
10. Attinger EO, Cahill JM (1960) Cardiopulmonary mechanics in anesthetized pigs and dogs. Am J Physiol 198: 346
11. Sakagami K, Toda K, Nakai H, et al (1987) Improved techniques for orthotopic liver transplantation: a preliminary study. Hiroshima J Med Sci 36: 211
12. Post S, Goerig M, Otto G, et al (1990) Prostanoid release in experimental liver transplantation. Transplantation 49: 490
13. Bertram TA, Overby LH, Danilowicz R, Eling TE, Brody AR (1988) Pulmonary intravascular macrophages metabolize arachidonic acid in vitro. Am Rev Respir Dis 138: 936
14. Winkler GC, Cheville NF (1985) Monocytic origin and postnatal mitosis of intravascular macrophages in the porcine lung. J Leukocyte Biol 38: 471
15. Crocker SH, Lowery BD, Eddy DO. Wismar BL, Buesching WJ, Obenauf RN (1981) Pulmonary clearance of blood-borne bacteria. Surg Gynecol Obstet 153: 845
16. McDonnell PJ, Toye PA, Hutchins GM (1983) Primary pulmonary hypertension and cirrhosis: are they related? Am Rev Respir Dis 127: 437
17. De Wolfe AM, Scott VL, Gasior T, Kang Y (1993) Pulmonary hypertension and liver transplantation. Anesthesiology 78: 213

Transpl Int (1996) 9 [Suppl 1]: S 105–S 108
© Springer-Verlag 1996

LIVER

Tetsushi Kitagawa
Yonson Ku
Nobuya Kusunoki
Masahiro Tominaga
Ichiro Maeda
Takumi Fukumoto
Takeshi Iwasaki
Yoshikazu Kuroda
Yoichi Saitoh

Pharmacokinetics of intravenous adriamycin for anhepatic chemotherapy during liver transplantation

T. Kitagawa · Y. Ku (✉) · N. Kusunoki ·
M. Tominaga · I. Maeda · T. Fukumoto ·
T. Iwasaki · Y. Kuroda · Y. Saitoh
First Department of Surgery, Kobe
University School of Medicine, 7-5-2
Kusunoki-cho, Chuo-ku, Kobe 650, Japan

Abstract Frequent recurrence of hepatocellular carcinoma after liver transplantation indicates the necessity to eliminate patients with advanced disease and combine transplantation with some form of perioperative adjuvant chemotherapy. This study was undertaken to elucidate adriamycin pharmacokinetics for anhepatic chemotherapy during liver transplantation. Beagles of both sexes were allocated into two groups, controls ($n = 4$) and anhepatic animals with total hepatectomy under venovenous bypass ($n = 5$). In both groups, adriamycin was administered in 1 min at a dose of 1 mg/kg through the left antecubital vein and peripheral blood was obtained at intervals for up to 2 h to determine the plasma adriamycin levels. The animals were then sacrificed to determine tissue adriamycin levels in the liver, kidney, heart, lung, and skeletal muscle. Plasma adriamycin levels in anhepatic animals were significantly higher than those in controls at all measured time points after 10 min, resulting in a 50 % reduction of the mean total body clearance of adriamycin compared with controls ($P < 0.01$). However, there was no statistically significant difference in adriamycin levels between the two groups for all measured tissues except for the liver. Despite the complete lack of hepatic function, anhepatic animals showed only a 50 % reduction in total body clearance of adriamycin compared with normal controls, probably due to compensatory excretion from other organs such as the kidney. These results suggest that systemic chemotherapy with the standard dose of adriamycin may be tolerable during the anhepatic period of liver transplantation with enhanced tumoricidal effects on micrometastases.

Key words Anhepatic chemotherapy · Liver transplantation · Adriamycin pharmacokinetics · Malignant liver tumor

Introduction

Surgical removal is the only chance for cure in patients with hepatocellular carcinoma. Unfortunately, candidates for hepatectomy are limited to only 10–30 % of the patients at the time of diagnosis, either by virtue of the extent of the tumor or by the lack of hepatic functional reserve [1, 2]. Furthermore, even when resectable, recurrence rates after hepatectomy are unacceptably high [3, 4].

Orthotopic liver transplantation had been advocated as the ultimate treatment for the potential cure of the disease. Despite early enthusiasm, however, it became evident that recurrence either in the transplanted liver or in extrahepatic sites developed in the majority of patients [5, 6]. In response to dismal outcomes, several transplant centers have recently conducted pre-, intra-, and postoperative adjuvant chemotherapies to improve prognosis after liver transplantation [7–9]. As a logical extension to intraoperative systemic chemotherapy

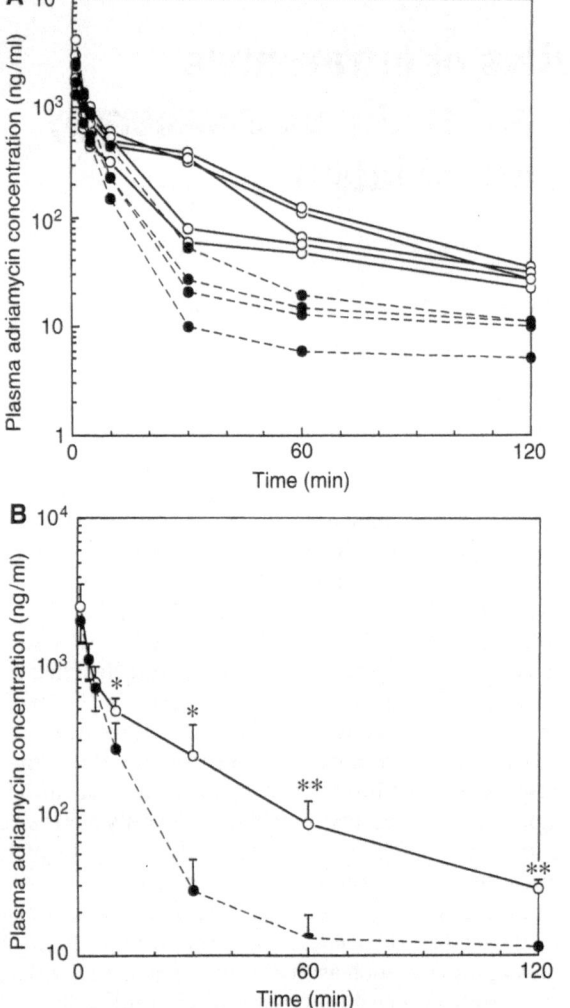

Fig. 1 A, B A semilogarithmic plot of the time course of plasma adriamycin concentrations. **A** Individual dog. **B** Mean ± SD in each group. (● Control dogs, ○ anhepatic dogs; * $P < 0.05$, ** $P < 0.01$ vs controls)

with orthotopic liver transplantation, anhepatic chemotherapy seems to emerge to give a tumoricidal impact on micrometastases that have spread beyond the liver. However, to our knowledge, anhepatic chemotherapy has not been described previously and its safety is still uncertain. We herein investigated the pharmacokinetics of adriamycin when administered during the anhepatic period of liver transplantation.

Materials and methods

Beagles of both sexes weighing 7.0–8.1 kg were used for this study. The animals were fasted overnight and anesthetized using pentobarbital, 25 mg/kg i.v., and pancuronium bromide, 0.1 mg/kg i.v., as an induction dose. After endotracheal intubation, animals were mechanically ventilated during the experiment. An arterial line

was placed into the left carotid artery for blood pressure and heart rate monitoring. Lactate-Ringer's solution (10 ml/kg body weight per h) was administered intravenously during the procedure. A midline laparotomy was simply performed in group 1, controls ($n = 4$). On the other hand, in group 2 anhepatic animals ($n = 5$), the liver was mobilized and isolated by dividing all of its peritoneal attachments. Subsequently a pump-driven venovenous bypass from the inferior vena cava and the portal vein to the left jugular vein was constructed, as described previously [10]. Under venovenous bypass, the supra- and infrahepatic inferior vena cava and the portal vein were clamped and the liver was removed.

In both groups, a 1-min bolus injection of adriamycin, 1 mg/kg was performed through the left antecubital vein. Blood samples were obtained from the carotid artery (for monitoring systemic drug levels) just before and 1, 3, 5, 10, 30, 60, 90, and 120 min after drug infusion. The animals were then sacrificed to determine tissue adriamycin levels in the liver (only for group 1), kidney, heart, lung, and skeletal muscle. Plasma adriamycin levels were determined by high-performance liquid chromatography (HPLC) using the method described previously [11]. In brief, aliquots of plasma were placed on mini-columns (Nucleosil 5C 18; Chemo Company, Japan). After washing, the drug was eluted and the eluent was dried under vacuo. Samples were then redissolved in mobile phase before injection into the HPLC. A routine internal standard of adriamycin was used to account for assay variability. Tissue adriamycin levels were analyzed by homogenizing the tissue and then performing a chloroform-methanol centrifugation extraction of adriamycin from the homogenate. The phase containing the extracted adriamycin was washed and eluted, and the eluent was dried under nitrogen. Samples were then redissolved in HPLC mobile phase and adriamycin levels were measured by routine HPLC. The area under the time concentration curve was calculated by the trapezium method.

Student's two-tailed t-test was used for statistical analysis of the results. Differences were considered significant at the 5 % level.

Results

No significant differences were found in mean arterial pressure and heart rate between the two groups throughout the experiment. The semilogarithmic plots of the plasma concentration-time data for adriamycin in both groups are illustrated in Fig. 1. The plasma levels reached peak values of 2.0 ± 0.6 (means ± SD) and 2.5 ± 1.1 µg/ml, respectively, in groups 1 and 2, 1 min after drug infusion. Thereafter, the levels in groups 1 and 2 promptly decreased to 0.7 ± 0.2 and 0.8 ± 0.2 at 5 min. During the initial 5 min, no significant difference was noted in plasma adriamycin levels between the two groups. Subsequently, group 2 animals had significantly higher plasma adriamycin levels at all measured time points from 10 to 120 min compared to group 1. As shown in Fig. 1 A, two distinctive phases were identified in each animal. During the distribution phase, the mean plasma half-lives were similar in both groups; the mean values were 3.2 ± 0.8 min and 2.4 ± 1.6 min, respectively, in groups 1 and 2. On the other hand, the mean elimination half-life of 62.7 ± 17.3 min in group 1 tended to be longer than that of 47.4 ± 19.8 min in group 2.

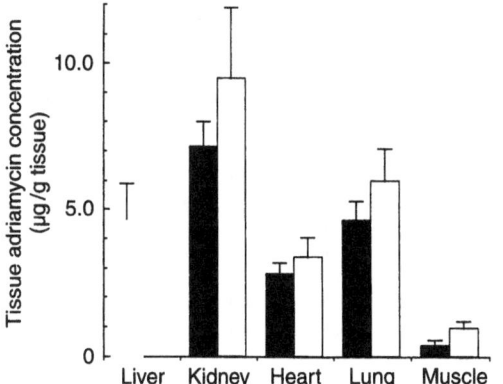

Fig. 2 Tissue adriamycin concentrations. (■ Control dogs, □ anhepatic dogs) Values are expressed as mean ± SD

The mean areas under the concentration-time curves were 12.4 ± 4.1 and 24.9 ± 8.0 µg/ml per min, respectively, in groups 1 and 2, showing a two-fold increase in group 2 compared with group 1 ($P < 0.01$). Conversely, the mean total body clearance of adriamycin showed a 50 % reduction in group 2 compared with group 1.

Figure 2 shows tissue adriamycin levels in five organs including the liver (only for group 1), kidney, heart, lung, and skeletal muscle. Tissue levels in the heart were 2.8 ± 0.4 and 3.4 ± 0.7 µg/g tissue, respectively, in groups 1 and 2, showing no statistically significant difference. Similarly, all other tissues, except for the liver, showed a higher drug level in group 2 than in group 1, although statistically this was not significant.

Discussion

Adriamycin has been widely used as a potent cytotoxic agent for the treatment of malignant liver tumors. Major dose-limiting toxicities of adriamycin include myelosuppression and delayed cardiac dysfunction, which become frequent when systemic plasma levels exceed 1.0 µg/ml [12] and a cumulative dose reaches around 500 mg/m^2 [13]. Previous studies demonstrated that the liver is the major organ rich in key enzymes responsible for adriamycin metabolism and that the drug is mainly excreted from the hepato-biliary system [14]. Thus, any

given dose may be more effective, but also more toxic, under the anhepatic condition. With these considerations in mind, we investigated adriamycin pharmacokinetics under the complete hepatectomized condition for safe and effective performance of anhepatic chemotherapy during liver transplantation.

Anhepatic chemotherapy has a theoretical advantage in that it could minimize drug exposure to the liver allograft. In the clinical setting, the liver allograft is subjected to a variety of insults such as ischemia during organ harvest, cold preservation, and subsequent reperfusion. Thus, it is unadvisable to administer a potentially hepatotoxic drug shortly after reperfusion. According to the plasma profile in this study, adriamycin levels reached a near steady-state by 60 min, even in anhepatic animals, and the values at 60 min were less than 3 % of the peak levels. Provided that the anhepatic period in orthotopic liver transplantation averages 60 min, it is reasonable to speculate that a bolus injection of adriamycin at the beginning of the anhepatic period would exhibit only a marginal toxic effect on the liver allograft.

As shown in Fig. 1, two distinctive phases consisting of the distribution and the elimination phases were identified in the concentration-time curve of anhepatic animals as well as normal controls. During the distribution phase, both groups showed similar plasma levels of adriamycin, reflecting a rapid tissue uptake of the drug in various organs during the first pass. As a result, there was no significant difference in the plasma half-life during this phase between the two groups. In contrast, during the elimination phase, plasma half-life tended to be shortened in anhepatic animals. It is most likely that higher plasma levels of adriamycin may enhance compensatory drug excretion through extrahepatic organs such as the kidney, although a definitive conclusion should wait further study investigating urinary drug excretion under anhepatic conditions.

In terms of total body clearance, anhepatic dogs exhibited only a 50 % reduction compared to that of normal controls. Furthermore, tissue adriamycin concentrations in five measured organs did not differ significantly between the two groups. These results indicate that the standard dose of adriamycin may be theoretically tolerable and enhance tumoricidal effects on extrahepatic micrometastases during the anhepatic period.

References

1. Okuda K, Otsuki T, Obata H (1985) Natural history of hepatocellular carcinoma and prognosis in relation to treatment. Study of 850 patients. Cancer 56: 918–928
2. The Liver Cancer Study Group of Japan (1987) Primary liver cancer in Japan. Sixth report. Cancer 60: 1400–1411
3. Belghiti J, Panis Y, Farges O, Benhamou JF, Fekete F (1991) Intrahepatic recurrence after resection of hepatocellular carcinoma complicating cirrhosis. Ann Surg 214: 114–117
4. Sasaki Y, Imaoka S, Fujita M (1987) Regional therapy in the management of intrahepatic recurrence after surgery for hepatoma. Ann Surg 206: 40–47
5. Iwatsuki S, Starzl TE, Seahan DG (1991) Hepatic resection versus transplantation for hepatocellular carcinoma. Ann Surg 214: 221–229

6. Olthoff KM, Millis JM, Rosove MH, Goldstein LI, Ramming KP, Busutill RW (1990) Is liver transplantation justified for the treatment of hepatic malignancies? Arch Surg 125: 1261–1268

7. Stone MJ, Klintmalm GB, Polter, Husberg BOS, Mennel RG, Ramsay MAE, Flemens EE, Goldstein RM (1993) Neoadjuvant chemotherapy and liver transplantation for hepatocellular carcinoma: results in 20 patients. Gastroenterology 104: 196–202

8. Carr BI, Starzl TE, Iwatsuki S, Van Thiel D (1991) Aggressive treatment for advanced hepatocellular carcinoma (HCC): high recurrence rates and prolonged survival. Hepatology 14: 103 A

9. Cherqui D, Piedbois P, Pierga J, Duvoux C, Vavasseur D (1994) Multimodal adjuvant treatment and liver transplantation for advanced hepatocellular carcinoma. Cancer 73: 2721–2726

10. Kam I, Lynch S, Todo S, Dewolf A, McSteen F, Jakab F, Ericzon BG (1986) Low flow venovenous bypass in small dogs and pediatric patients undergoing replacement of the liver. Surg Gynecol Obstet 163: 33–36

11. Robert J (1980) Extraction of anthracycline from biologic fluids for HPLC evaluation. J Liquid Chromatogr 3: 1561–1572

12. Legha SS, Benjamin RS, Mackay B (1982) Reduction of doxorubicin cardiotoxicity by prolonged continuous intravenous infusion. Ann Intern Med 96: 133–139

13. Benjamin RS, Wiernik PH, Bachur NR (1974) Adriamycin chemotherapy-efficacy, safety and pharmacologic basis of an intermittent single high-dose schedule. Cancer 33: 19–26

14. Loveless H, Arena E, Felsted RL (1978) Comparative mammalian metabolism of adriamycin and daunorubicin. Cancer Res 38: 593–598

Transpl Int (1996) 9 [Suppl 1]: S 109–S 111
© Springer-Verlag 1996

LIVER

G. Colella
G. F. Rondinara
L. De Carlis
C. V. Sansalone
A. O. Slim
P. Aseni
O. Rossetti
A. De Gasperi
E. Minola
R. Bottelli
L. S. Belli
G. Ideo
D. Forti

Liver transplantation for hepatocellular carcinoma: prognostic factors associated long-term survival

G. Colella (✉) · G. F. Rondinara ·
L. De Carlis · C. V. Sansalone · A. O. Slim ·
P. Aseni · O. Rossetti · A. De Gasperi ·
E. Minola · R. Bottelli · L. S. Belli · G. Ideo ·
D. Forti
Department of Abdominal
Organ Translation, Pizzamiglio II,
Ospedale Niguarda,
piazza Ospedale Maggiore, 3,
I-20162 Milano, Italy

Abstract Between December 1985 and February 1995, 260 orthotopic liver transplantations (OLTX) were performed on 238 patients at Niguarda Hospital. Sixty-three patients had hepatocellular carcinoma (HCC); in 13 of the patients HCC was incidental. All patients had negative lymph nodes. According to the Child classification, 13 patients were Child A, 30 Child B, and 18 Child C. According to the TNM classification, 11 patients were stage I, 22 stage II, 15 stage III, and 15 stage IVa. Pre-OLTX chemoembolization was performed on 25 patients. The perioperative mortality rate was 27 % (17 patients). Overall survival and disease-free actuarial survival rates at 1, 3, and 5 years were 94 %, 76 %, 76 %, and 83 %, 75 %, 75 %, respectively. Survival curves were compared for 16 different variables. No difference was observed for all parameters analyzed except tumor site, TNM stage, pre-OLTX AFP levels and vascular infiltration. These results seem to demonstrate that the OLTX for unresectable HCC can be considered in specifically selected cases as the treatment of choice. An adequate tumor staging is also necessary for a better patient selection in order to increase survival.

Key words Hepatocellular carcinoma · Liver transplantation

Introduction

In recent years, hepatocellular carcinoma (HCC) has been diagnosed and treated with increasing frequency by means of several options including alcoholization, transarterial chemoembolization, resective surgery, and orthotopic liver transplantation (OLTX) [1, 2, 4, 5, 7, 8]. Up to now, if extrahepatic tumor spread is excluded, a complete surgical excision is generally considered the treatment of choice for potentially resectable HCC [1, 2].

OLTX was considered a controversial indication for primary liver neoplasms because of high recurrence rate [3, 4, 6] but up to now a consistent number of OLTX are still performed for malignancies, principally for HCC in cirrhosis. Recently, a critical review of previous experience demonstrates a significant relationship between tumor stage and patient survival after OLTX for HCC in cirrhosis [2, 5, 7]. Furthermore, hepatic resection appears to achieve poor long-term survival, while OLTX has recently shown improving trends in results.

We report here a retrospective analysis of 10 years' experience in OLTX for HCC in cirrhosis in order to define indications for OLTX.

Besides TNM tumor staging, several variables were investigated and related to post-OLTX tumor survival in order better to define the selection and management of patients undergoing OLTX for HCC.

Patients and methods

Patients

Between December 1985 and June 1995, 260 OLTX were performed on 238 patients at the Department of General Surgery and Abdominal Organ Transplantation, Niguarda Hospital, Milan, Italy. Of these, 63 patients (53 male, 10 female, mean age 52 years,

Table 1 Characteristics of the series of patients

Age	Median (range)	52 years (22–61 years)
Sex	Male/female	53/10
HbsAg	Positive	19 (30%)
HCVAb	Positive	28 (44%)
AFP	20–400 ng/ml	19 (31%)
	> 400 ng/ml	12 (19%)
Cirrhosis stage	Child A	13 (21%)
	Child B	30 (49%)
	Child C	18 (30%)
Cirrhosis etiology	Viral	35 (57%)
	Alcoholic	12 (20%)
	Mixed	7 (11.5%)
	Unknown	7 (11.5%)

Table 2 Pathological characteristics

Size (diameter)	Median (range)	3 cm (1–15 cm)
Number	Solitary	35 (56%)
	Multiple	28 (44%)
Localization	Monolobar	48 (76%)
	Bilobar	15 (24%)
Capsule (51 patients evaluable)	Present/not infiltrated	14 (27%)
	Absent/infiltrated	37 (73%)
Vascular invasion (55 patients evaluable)	Macroscopic	2 (4%)
	Microscopic	13 (24%)
TNM stage	I	11 (17%)
	II	22 (35%)
	III	15 (24%)
	IVa	15 (24%)

Table 3 Orthotopic liver transplantations (OLTX) for hepatocellular carcinoma (HCC) in cirrhosis: prognostic factors for survival

		3 years survival	5 years survival	3 years tumor-free	P
TNM stage	I	100%	100%	100%	0.01
	II	93%	93%	93%	
	III	50%	–	56%	
	IVa	52%	–	58%	
Location	Monolateral	96%	96%	92%	< 0.01
	Bilateral	47%	47%	52%	
Vascular invasion	Absent	96%	96%	96%	0.02
	Micro	33%	–	38%	
	Macro	0%	0%	0%	
AFP level (ng/ml)	< 20	100%	100%	100%	< 0.001
	20–400	75%	–	91%	
	> 400	17%	17%	18%	

range 22–61 years) had an HCC at the time of OLTX (Table 1). In 13 patients, HCC was an incidental finding; HCC was discovered in a cirrhotic liver after OLTX for end-stage liver disease. Only 2 patients out of the 63 were not cirrhotics. No patient had either extrahepatic tumor spread or lymph node tumor invasion at pathological examination at the time of OLTX.

According to the Child classification, 13 patients were Child A, 30 Child B, and 18 Child C. Pathological characteristics

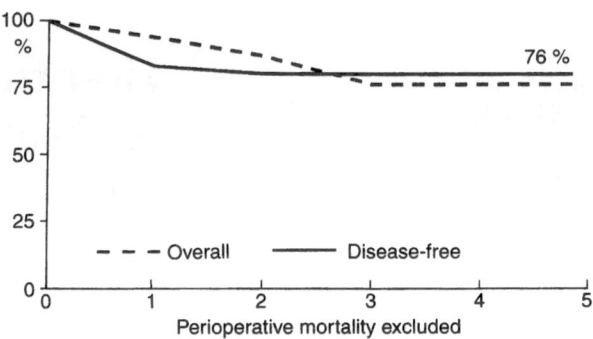

Fig. 1 Orthotopic liver transplantations for hepatocellular carcinoma in cirrhosis: actuarial survival

and tumor stage according to the TNM classification are reported in Table 2.

Pre-OLTX transarterial chemoembolization (TAE) was performed in 26 patients.

All patients underwent quadruple immunosuppression therapy in the early post-OLTX period and received cyclosporine (Cya) for chronic immunosuppression in the absence of clinical contraindication or severe rejection.

Statistical analysis

Perioperative mortality rate within 3 months was 27% (17 patients). Actuarial survival curves were calculated for the remaining 46 patients (median follow-up, 45 months) as cumulative survival rates by the Kaplan-Meier method and analyzed by the log-rank and Mantel-Haenszel tests.

Survival curves were compared for sex, age (< 50, > 50 years), tumor location (mono-, bilateral), diameter (< 3, > 3 cm), mono- or plurifocality, capsule status, pre-OLTX AFP level (< 20, 20–400, > 400 ng/ml), micro- or macro-vascular infiltration, incidental tumor, TNM stage, Child classification, pre-OLTX chemoembolization, additional immunosuppression for acute rejection, and etiology of cirrhosis.

Results

Overall survival and disease-free actuarial survival rates at 1, 3, and 5 years were 94%, 75%, 75%, and 83%, 76%, 76%, respectively (Fig. 1). Seven patients had tumor recurrence at 4, 5, 5, 7, 8, 9, and 15 months. Sites of recurrence (multiple in four cases) were liver (three patients), bone (three patients), lung (two patients), and brain (two patients); in three patients, recurrence was both hepatic and extrahepatic. All patients with tumor recurrence died within 34 months after OLTX, whereas all the patients alive are free of disease.

All the patient-related characteristics examined (age, sex, etiology of cirrhosis, Child stage) are not significantly related to tumor recurrence or patient survival.

Among the different tumor-related variables, tumor location (mono-, bilateral), TNM stage, pre-OLTX AFP levels, and vascular infiltration are significantly related to tumor recurrence and patient survival (Ta-

Table 4 OLTX for HCC in cirrhosis: prognostic factors for survival (*NS* not significant)

		3 years survival	5 years survival	3 years tumor-free	*P*
Capsule	Complete	100 %	100 %	100 %	NS
	Absent/ infiltrated	70 %	70 %	70 %	
Number of lesions	Single	90 %	90 %	87 %	NS
	Multiple	56 %	–	67 %	
Diagnosis	Incidental	100 %	100 %	100 %	NS
HCC	Pre-OLTX	67 %	67 %	73 %	
Diameter	< 3 cm	89 %	89 %	90 %	NS
	> 3 cm	60 %	60 %	66 %	

ble 3), while the number of lesions, capsule, diameter, and incidental HCC are not significantly related to tumor recurrence and patient survival (Table 4). All those patients (three) with a tumoral thrombus in a main portal vein branch suffered tumor recurrence within 1 year. Microvascular tumor invasion detected at pathological examination of whole liver specimens was associated with a 3-year disease-free survival rate of 38 %. On the contrary, 96 % of patients without micro- or macrovascular tumor invasion were disease-free after 3 years. Advanced HCC, considered as TNM stage T3–T4 or a bilateral tumor, had 3-year tumor-free survival rates of 56 % (T3), 58 % (T4), and 52 % (bilateral). In our series, no patients (32) with normal AFP levels suffered tumor recurrence after OLTX, while for six out of nine patients with AFP levels greater then 400 ng/ml recurrence was within 15 months, with a 3-year survival rate of 18 %. No patients with an incidental HCC or a completely encapsulated HCC suffered recurrence after OLTX. Patients with a solitary HCC or with HCC less than 3 cm diameter had 3-year tumor-free survival rates of 87 % and 90 % (73 % and 66 % for non-incidental and more than 3-cm diam-

eter HCC). No differences in patient survival and tumor-free survival were evident for treatment-related variables; in particular, pre-OLTX chemoembolization and immunosuppression do not seem to affect recurrence rate.

Discussion

Indication to OLTX for HCC in cirrhosis is generally considered because of the low resection rate of HCC due to tumor location or liver impairment. OLTX undoubtedly has the capacity to cure both HCC and cirrhosis. Some HCC patterns are correlated with tumor recurrence and patients' survival [2, 5, 7]. Our results confirm this observation.

The TNM stage, the vascular invasion, the pre-OLTX AFP levels, and bilateral HCC are prognostic factors for survival after OLTX. Some of these parameters, such as AFP levels, are easy to verify before OLTX and can be utilized as selection criteria for candidates. Other parameters, such as TNM staging, can be used to complete the selection. Others, such as the extent of microvascular invasion, cannot be defined at the time of OLTX, and cannot be used as selection criteria for candidates, but have a prognostic value in the indication for adjuvant therapy.

These results seem to demonstrate that OLTX for unresectable HCC can be considered the treatment of choice for specifically selected patients. Because of the low recurrence rate after OLTX, this indication can be extended to young patients with potentially resectable HCC in cirrhosis. These patients are, in fact, considered suitable candidates for OLTX in some transplantation centers.

In conclusion, unresectable HCC in cirrhosis can be considered as the treatment of choice for selected patients; indication to OLTX for patients with a resectable HCC is still to be defined.

References

1. Bismuth H, Morino M, Sherlock (1992) Primary treatment of hepatocellular carcinoma by arterial chemoembolization. Am J Surg 163: 387–394
2. Bismuth H, Chiche L, Adam R, Castaing D, Diamond T, Dennison A (1993) Surgical treatment of hepatocellular carcinoma in cirrhosis: liver resection or transplantation? Transplant Proc 25: 1066–1067
3. Calne RY (1982) Liver transplantation for liver cancer. World J Surg 6: 76–80
4. Iwatsuki S, Gordon RD, Shaw BW, Starzl TE (1985) Role of liver transplantation in cancer therapy. Ann Surg 202: 401–407
5. Iwatsuki S, Starzl TE, Shean DG, Yokoyama I, Demetris AJ, Todo S, Van Thiel DH, Carr B, Selby R, Madariaga J (1991) Hepatic resection versus transplantation for hepatocellular carcinoma. Ann Surg 214: 221–229
6. O'Grady LG, Polson RJ, Rolles K, Calne RY, Williams R (1988) Liver transplantation for malignant disease: results of 98 consecutive patients. Ann Surg 207: 373–379
7. Ringe B, Pichlmayr R, Wittekind C (1991) Experience in liver resection and transplantation in 198 patients. World J Surg 15: 270–285
8. The Liver Cancer Study Group of Japan: primary Liver Cancer in Japan (1990) Clinicopathological features and results of surgical treatment. Ann Surg 211: 277–287

Transpl Int (1996) 9 [Suppl 1]: S 112–S 114
© Springer-Verlag 1996

LIVER

Francesco Crafa
Jean Gugenheim
Angela Ruggiero
Stefano Pepe
Jean Mouiel

DNA flow cytometry in patients undergoing liver transplantation for hepatocellular carcinoma

F. Crafa · J. Gugenheim · J. Mouiel
Department of Liver Transplantation,
University of Sophia Antipolis,
Saint-Roch Hospital, Nice, France

A. Ruggiero · S. Pepe
Department of Oncology,
II University of Medicine and Surgery,
Naples, Italy

J. Gugenheim (✉)
Hôpital St Roch,
Service de Chirurgie Digestive,
Transplantation Hepatique et
Videochirurgie, 5 Rue Pierre Devoluy,
F-06006 Nice, Cedex 1, France

Abstract The purpose of the study was to analyse patterns of DNA content in hepatocellular carcinomas (HCC) submitted to orthotopic liver transplantation (OLT). Paraffin-embedded archival material from 15 patients (ten men, five women, mean age 51 ± 1.78 years) transplanted in St-Roch Hospital between 1988 and 1991 was available for laboratory evaluation by flow cytometry. Five out of 15 were incidental HCC. The analysis was performed by a FACSscan flow cytometer coupled to a Hewlett-Packard computer. The cellular DNA content was defined as diploid or aneuploid in the presence of a single (DNA index of 1) or two distinct (DNA index different from 1) G_0/G_1 peaks, respectively. All incidental HCC (five patients) were diploid, the tumour size was 1.2 ± 0.2 cm, the number of nodules was 1.4 ± 0.24 and the mortality rate was 40 %. No death in the incidental HCC group was related to neoplastic recurrence. In the remaining ten patients transplanted for HCC, we observed 50 % diploid tumours, the tumour size was 5.2 ± 1.55 cm and the number of nodules was 2.7 ± 0.56. In this group six patients died of neoplastic recurrence (two were diploid and four aneuploid). The diameter of the neoplasm in diploid patients who died of neoplastic recurrence was over 5 cm and the number of nodules was over three. Moreover, in aneuploid patients who died of neoplastic recurrence, the diameter of the neoplasm was less than 5 cm in three cases and the number of nodules was less than three in two patients. This study indicates that incidental HCC may be a less aggressive malignancy and may have a better prognosis. In this group, no patient recurred after OLT and all tumours were diploid. Aneuploidy, tumour size (> 5 cm) and number of lesions (> 3) are prognostic indicators for neoplastic recurrence in patients transplanted for hepatocellular carcinoma.

Key words Hepatocellular carcinoma · Incidental hepatocarcinoma · Orthotopic liver transplantation · Nuclear DNA content (ploidy)

Introduction

In order to design an effective therapy against a malignant tumour it is important to understand its biological behaviour. DNA flow cytometry (DNA-FCM) is an objective, quantitative technique which can measure both the degree of quantitative abnormalities of DNA content (ploidy) and the tumour proliferation rate, defined as the percentage of cells in S-phase [1]. Although many studies have investigated the relationship between DNA-FCM and the outcome of resected hepatocellular carcinoma (HCC) [2, 3], no report has been published on transplanted HCC. The purpose of this study was to analyse patterns of DNA content in HCC submitted to orthotopic liver transplantation (OLT) and to correlate ploidy status with patients' survival.

Patients and methods

Patients

Retrospective DNA-FCM was performed on paraffin-embedded HCC specimens from 15 patients transplanted in St-Roch Hospital between 1988 and 1991. Ten out of 15 patients were men and the mean age was 51.33 ± 1.78 years. Five out of 15 were incidental HCC (three men, two women, mean age 50 ± 4.76 years). According to the Child-Pugh classification, 60 % of these patients had a grade C disease and 40 % had a grade B involvement. We have described in detail our technique of OLT in hepatic malignancy [4]. All patients received triple therapy immunosuppression with azathioprine, cyclosporin A and methylprednisolone [5]. Long-term passive immunoprophylaxis was realised in HbsAg-positive patients.

Flow cytometry

Flow cytometry was performed on nuclear suspensions prepared from 50-μm sections of formalin-fixed, paraffin-embedded tissue of HCC. To determine the percentage of tumour cells in the tissue analysed, adjacent 4-μm-thick histological sections were removed before and after the 50-μm sections used for flow cytometry analysis. Briefly, the sections were dewaxed with xylene, rehydrated through 90, 80, 70 and 50 % ethanol, washed twice in deionised H$_2$O and minced in 2 ml of 0.5 % pepsin (Sigma Chemicals, St. Louis, Mo., USA) in 0.9 % NaCl (pH 1.5) at $37\,^{\circ}$C for 30 min. The samples were filtered through a 30-mm pore-size polyester filter and stained in propidium iodine solution [1] for 30 min at room temperature in the dark (all chemicals were from Sigma Chemicals). Before the analysis, the nuclear suspension were syringed 2–3 times through a 25 G needle to prevent nuclear clumps. A total of 40 000 events was analysed on a FACSscan flow cytometer (Becton-Dickinson, San José, Calif., USA) and data on DNA content were collected and stored as list mode files using the CELLFIT software (Becton-Dickinson), without background substraction. Before each DNA-FCM procedure, the FL2 channel was calibrated with normal paraffin-embedded liver tissue. The fluorescence intensity of the G_0/G_1 peak of the normal cell population was set on channel 200. Given the lack of a standard procedure to calculate the DNA index (IDNA) in DNA-FCM from paraffin-embedded tissue, the G_0/G_1 peak with the smallest DNA content was equated with the normal diploid cells in the samples. IDNA was calculated dividing the mode channel value of the aneuploid G_0/G_1 peak with the mode channel value of the euploid G_0/G_1 peak. DNA aneuploidy was documented only if there was clear evidence of a second > G_0/G_1 peak. Histograms were taken into consideration only if the median CV of the diploid G_0/G_1 peak was equal to or less than 7 %.

Statistical analysis

Results were expressed as means $\pm$ SEM.

Results

All incidental HCC (five patients) were diploid, the tumour size was 1.2 ± 0.2 cm and the number of nodules was 1.4 ± 0.24. In this group we observed two deaths related to septic complication (1 and 4 months after OLT), the remaining patients are alive and free of neoplastic disease (follow-up 73, 66, 65 months from OLT). In the remaining ten patients transplanted for HCC, we observed 50 % diploid tumours, the tumour size was 5.2 ± 1.55 cm and the number of nodules was 2.7 ± 0.56. In this group the mortality rate was 90 %. Six patients died of neoplastic recurrence at 6, 12, 12, 15, 22 and 42 months after OLT (two were diploid and four aneuploid). The diameter of the neoplasm in diploid patients who died from neoplastic recurrence was over 5 cm and the number of nodules was over three. In aneuploid patients who died from neoplastic recurrence, the diameter of the neoplasm was less than 5 cm in three cases and the number of nodules was less than three in two patients. The remaining deaths, in patients transplanted for HCC, were related to septic complications (two patients) and PNF (one patient). One patient (diploid) in the HCC group is still alive and free from neoplastic disease at the time of this report (follow-up 69 months)

Discussion

Although having a wide coefficient of variation and more cell debris, DNA-FCM using paraffin blocks has good correlation between DNA indices with flow cytometry using fresh tissue [6]. It has been reported that ploidy correlates significantly with survival rates in surgically resected HCC [2, 7, 8]. Moreover it has been shown that the DNA pattern also correlates with tumour size [7–9] and the pTNM index [8]. Nevertheless, no study has been published on DNA analysis in patients transplanted for HCC. OLT seems to be a logical treatment for HCC unaccompanied by extrahepatic disease and a growing body of evidence suggest that OLT could be the best treatment for small HCC in cirrhotic livers. Small incidental tumours found in the liver resected at OLT do not seem to recur after transplantation [10]. A recent study also suggests that patients with resectable tumours (< 3 cm) were the best candidates for OLT [11]. In our study, all incidental HCC were diploid and no recurrence of neoplastic disease was observed. Heterogeneity of the ploidy seems to reflect the biological behaviour of the tumour, usually characterised either by the existence of clones with different malignant potential or by the rapid emergence of drug resistance in the individual tumour [3]. We can speculate that the observed homogeneity of the ploidy status in association with the small size of the tumour in incidental HCC m℥ responsible for the absence of neoplastic recurrence ⅃as been reported that tumour size, portal venous i᛫ ⅂sion, intrahepatic metastasis, atypia of tumour cells, serum αFP levels, microscopic invasion into the tumour capsule and vascular invasion, clinical stage (pTNM) are related to recurrence [12–14]. In our study we observed six neoplastic recurrences in the HCC group and two of these occurred in diploid patients. Several possible explanations can be considered for recurrence in large diploid HCC. Ploidy status estimates the quantitative changes in chromosomes by measuring the DNA content. It is difficult to identify small genetic defects in the chromosomes or the presence of small chromosomes. Likewise, balanced translocation, chromosomal rearrangement without change in chromosomal value, point mutations or deletions are difficult to detect [3]. In conclusion, the prognosis of patients seemed to be influenced by ploidy status and also by the number of tumours and tumour size. The nuclear DNA content can be precisely and rapidly evaluated by flow cytometry, from preoperative specimens [2] or from surgically resected tissues. It is expected that aggressive adjuvant therapy [13] in cases with an aneuploid DNA pattern may improve the results of the current treatment of HCC.

References

1. Pepe S, Ruggiero A, De Laurentis M, et al (1995) DNA-flow cytometry (ploidy and S-phase fraction) as prognostic factors in a retrospective series of 515 primary breast cancers. Oncol Rep 2: 345–350
2. Cottier M, Jouffre C, Maubon I, et al (1994) Prospective flow cytometric DNA analysis of hepatocellular carcinoma specimens collected by ultrasound-guided fine needle aspiration. Cancer 74: 599–605
3. Ng I, Lai E, Ho J, et al (1994) Flow cytometric analysis of DNA ploidy in hepatocellular carcinoma. Anat Pathol 102: 80–86
4. Gugenheim J, Crafa F, Fabiani P, et al (1992) Transplantation hépatique pour carcinome hépatocellulaire: résultats à moyen terme. Presse Medicale 21: 1846–1848
5. Gugenheim J, Samuel D, Saliba F, et al (1987) Use of flexible triple drug immunosuppressive therapy in liver transplantation. Transplant Proc 19: 3805–3808
6. Hedeley DW (1989) Flow cytometry using paraffin-embedded tissue: five years on. Cytometry 10: 229–241
7. Fujimoto J, Okamoto E, Yamanaka N, et al (1991) Flow cytometric DNA analysis of hepatocellular carcinoma. Cancer 67: 939–944
8. Ishizu H (1989) Flow cytometric analysis of the nuclear DNA content of hepatocellular carcinoma. Jpn J Surg 19: 662–673
9. Ezaki T, Kanematsu T, Okamura T, et al (1988) DNA analysis of hepatocellular carcinoma and clinicopathologic implications. Cancer 61: 106–109
10. Belghitti J, Panis Y, Farges O, et al (1991) Intrahepatic recurrence after resection of hepatocellular carcinoma complicating cirrhosis. Ann Surg 214: 114–117
11. Bismuth H, Chiche L, Adam R, et al (1993) Liver resection versus transplantation for hepatocellular carcinoma in cirrhotic patients. Ann Surg 218: 145–151
12. Eisuke A, Takashi M, Takashi M, et al (1995) Risk factors for intrahepatic recurrence in human small hepatocellular carcinoma. Gastroenterology 108: 768–775
13. Cherqui D, Piedbois P, Pierga JY, et al (1994) Multimodal treatment and liver transplantation for advanced hepatocellular carcinoma. A pilot study. Cancer 73: 2721–2726
14. Iwatsuki S, Starzl TE, Sheahan DG, et al (1991) Hepatic resection versus transplantation for hepatocellular carcinoma. Ann Surg 214: 221–229

Transpl Int (1996) 9 [Suppl 1]: S 115–S 119
© Springer-Verlag 1996

LIVER

M. Knoop
W. O. Bechstein
H. Schrem
H. Lobeck
U. Hopf
P. Neuhaus

Clinical significance of recurrent primary biliary cirrhosis after liver transplantation

M. Knoop (✉) · W. O. Bechstein ·
H. Schrem · P. Neuhaus
Department of Surgery, Virchow Clinics,
Humboldt University of Berlin,
Augustenburger Platz 1, D-13353 Berlin,
Germany

H. Lobeck
Department of Pathology, Virchow Clinics,
Humboldt University of Berlin, Germany

U. Hopf
Department of Hepatology,
Virchow Clinics,
Humboldt University of Berlin, Germany

Abstract Primary biliary cirrhosis (PBC) represents a classic indication for orthotopic liver transplantation (OLT); as an autoimmune disease, however, the existence and incidence of recurrent PBC is a matter of significant controversy. Between September 1988 and September 1994 a total of 544 OLTs was performed at our institution. Forty-nine patients (40 female) with a median age of 50.5 years and previous surgery in 36.4 %, received a liver graft for PBC. The mean serum bilirubin level was 8.9 mg/dl (range 0.7–29.7). Immunosuppression was commenced as a cyclosporine A-based quadruple therapy or with FK 506 and prednisolone. Protocol liver biopsies were taken at defined intervals posttransplant. Two patients died due to *Legionella* pneumonia and hypoxic brain damage 2 and 8 weeks after OLT, resulting in an actuarial 5-year survival rate of 95 % with 47/49 patients being alive compared to 83.5 % of all other liver recipients. Evidence of recurrence of PBC, as defined by elevated cholestatic parameters and histological features of PBC, was found in four patients, another five patients showed only histological signs. Recurrence of PBC, which might compromise the long-term outcome after OLT, was suspected in 4/47 patients (8.5 %). This evidence of recurrent PBC is in conflict with findings of other groups that did not report recurrent PBC. OLT is still the optimal therapy for advanced PBC, with an excellent prognosis.

Key words Liver transplantation · Primary biliary cirrhosis

Introduction

Among end-stage liver diseases, primary biliary cirrhosis (PBC) represents one of the most common indications for orthotopic liver transplantation (OLT). PBC, which is characterized by a chronic, slowly progressive inflammatory destruction of small intrahepatic bile ducts, is considered as a classic indication for OLT, with 5-year survival rates of over 70 % [15]. The course of the disease is usually prolonged over an asymptomatic and symptomatic period leading to a sudden terminal deterioration of liver function that is usually not associated with significant impairment of other vital organs. Due to the inflammatory, autoimmune character of PBC, medical treatment consists of immunosuppressive and inflammatory drugs with, however, only marginal success [3, 10]. In contrast, ursodeoxycholic acid has been shown to decrease the severity of cholestasis [12, 14, 18, 19].

The indication for OLT in PBC is given in the case of rising serum bilirubin levels (> 8–10 mg/dl), recurrent esophageal hemorrhage, irretractable ascites, progressive hepatic osteodystrophy, pruritus, muscle dystrophy, vitamin depletion (A, D, E, K), hepatic encephalopathy or recurrent spontaneous bacterial peritonitis. Beyond these symptoms, PBC bears a significant risk of developing into hepatocellular carcinoma [16]. By follow-up of patients receiving conservative treatment, parame-

Table 1 Indications for orthotopic liver transplantation September 1988–September 1994, University Hospital Rudolf Virchow (*PBC* primary biliary cirrhosis, *PSC* primary sclerosing cholangitis)

Preoperative condition	Number of patients	Total
Postnecrotic cirrhosis		252
HbsAg positive	72	
HbsAg + delta positive	11	
NANB, Hepatitis C	89	
Alcoholic cirrhosis	80	
Fulminant liver failure		34
PBC		49
PSC		29
Others		180
Total		544

ters have been identified on which prognostic models are based that predict quite accurately the individual course of PBC [4, 5, 8, 20]. Taken the calculated life expectancy of an individual patient into account, choosing the appropriate time for OLT has become easier and safer. A common feature of the different prognostic models is the high significance of serum bilirubin as the most important single prognostic parameter.

While there is no doubt that advanced PBC is an excellent indication for OLT [2], considerable scientific dispute has gathered on the existence and recurrence of PBC in liver recipients. In this retrospective study we analyzed the peri- and postoperative course of patients with PBC after liver transplantation and possible recurrence of the underlying disease.

Patients and methods

Patients

Between September 1988 and September 1994 a total of 544 OLT was performed at the Department of Surgery, University Hospital Rudolf Virchow, Free University of Berlin. Forty-nine patients underwent primary OLT for PBC. The other indications for OLT are listed in Table 1.

Liver transplantation

All OLT were performed using standard surgical techniques. All grafts were preserved using University of Wisconsin solution. A veno-venous bypass was used during the anhepatic phase and all vascular anastomoses were completed before reperfusion of the graft. The bile duct anastomosis was accomplished as side-to-side choledocho-choledochostomy using a T-tube for 42 days.

Immunosuppressive therapy

Immunosuppression was given according to our conventional protocol with a cyclosporine A (CsA)-based quadruple induction therapy for the first 7 days and continuation as triple therapy thereafter, or with FK 506 and prednisolone as part of the European multicenter trial of FK 506. The quadruple protocol consisted of CsA, azathioprine, prednisolone, and of rabbit antithymocyte globulin (ATG).

Rejection therapy

Rejection was diagnosed by histopathological evidence, deteriorating liver function, and changes in the amount and composition of bile. Acute rejection was treated by i.v. bolus application of 500 mg methylprednisolone for 3 days and OKT3 mAb for steroid-resistant or severe recurrent rejection. Non-responders to rejection therapy were switched to FK 506 rescue therapy. If OKT3 and FK 506 rescue therapy failed, patients were candidates for retransplantation.

General medication

Before administration of i.v. CsA and ATG, patients received dimethindene (4 mg) and ranitidine (50 mg). Anti-infectious prophylaxis consisted of systemic antibiotic therapy for 2 days (4 × 1 g cefotaxim, 3 × 40–80 mg gernebcin, 2 × 500 mg metronidazol) and selective bowel decontamination (100 mg polymyxin B, 80 mg gernebcin, and 0.5 MU Nystatin 4 times/day) starting at least 5 days prior to transplantation, and given for at least 3 weeks posttransplant. The identical antibiotic combination was used as an oral paste 4 times/day. Microbial screening was performed routinely twice a week by testing body fluids (including bile) and orifices. Specific antibiotics were given according to sensitivity tests (predominantly vancomycin and imipenem due to positive selection of enterococci and gram-positive bacteria after selective bowel decontamination). Antiviral prophylaxis consisted of acyclovir against herpes for the first 6 postoperative weeks. All patients received 10 g of Ig 7S and anti- (CMV) hyperimmunoglobulin on postoperative days (PODs) 1 and 14, and daily medication of 500 mg ursodeoxycholic acid, vitamins, and minerals.

Histology

The histological criteria of recurrent PBC are delineated in Table 2.

Results

Patient characteristics

Patients with PBC had a median age of 50.5 years, females being predominant (77.5 %, 40/49) and previous operations, mainly cholecystectomy, had been performed in 36.4 %. The median serum bilirubin level was 8.9 mg/dl. All patients received AB0-compatible grafts. HLA antigen mismatches between donor and recipient were not analyzed.

Table 2 Histological criteria for recurrence of PBC; differential diagnosis of bile duct alterations

Criteria	PBC grade I/II	Chronic rejection	Chronic cholangitis
Number of bile ducts	⇒/⇑	⇓	⇑
Basal membranes	Destroyed	Intact	Intact
Epithelium	Altered	Altered	Altered
Lumen	Narrow	Narrow	Large
Cholestasis	Mild	Indifferent	Elevated

Survival

Kaplan-Meier estimates for 3-, 6-, 12-month and 1 to 5-year patient survival in the PBC group were 95.83 % for all intervals since two patients died 2 and 8 weeks posttransplant due to *Legionella* pneumonia and hypoxic brain damage after a prolonged course of intensive care with various complications. These two patients were excluded from this analysis. No other patient with PBC died during this 5-year period. One patient had to be retransplanted on POD 3 for initial non-function of the graft, resulting in a 5-year graft survival of 94 % (47/50) in the PBC group.

The 5-year survival rate of all other patients transplanted between September 1988 and September 1994 is 83.5 %.

Recurrent PBC

In 4/47 patients there were histological signs of recurrent PBC (8.5 %) that correlated with elevated aP and serum bilirubin (4–10 mg/dl). In five patients there were histological signs of recurrent PBC with, however, apparent normal liver function (10.6 %). PBC-specific epitheloid granulomas, however, were not found in both groups. A common feature in these nine patients was the finding of non-suppurative destructive cholangitis (19.1 %), which is typical for PBC stage II but is also seen in ischemic-type biliary lesions or in the early stage of chronic rejection. In eight patients, elevated cholestatic parameters were not accompanied by histological findings indicative of recurrent PBC. AMA titers have not been analyzed in these patients yet. One patient has developed cirrhosis, obviously due to recurrent PBC, but has not been retransplanted yet.

Discussion

Concerning the treatment of end-stage PBC by liver transplantation, three points are of great importance: prognostic models for conservative therapy of the disease to determine the individually optimal time for transplantation; disease-specific aspects and their rele-

vance for liver transplantation; and the prognosis after liver transplantation, with special emphasis on the recurrence of PBC.

Prognostic models

Prognostic models to predict the survival of conservatively treated, non-transplanted patients with PBC have been developed by long-term follow-up and identification of important parameters. Christensen et al. [5] and Dickson et al. (Mayo model) [8] described models which have bilirubin, age, and albumin as parameters in common. Markus et al. [15] compared the outcome of liver recipients with PBC to a group of patients with conservative treatment. By using the Mayo model they found from 3 months posttransplant onwards a higher survival probability in the transplant group and concluded that OLT is an efficacious treatment for advanced PBC. Bonsel et al. [4] compared the actuarial survival of 30 patients with PBC in Child-Pugh stages B and C after OLT to the calculated survival rate if these patients had been treated conservatively. The Christensen model, the Mayo model, and his own model (AZG, Akademisch Ziekenhuis Groningen) were used. During a follow-up period of 7 years, a growing advantage of OLT versus medical therapy emerged. The three models revealed remarkably consistent results. Since the models are based on data from just one time during the course of the disease, criticism was raised concerning the precision of prediction of survival. Christensen et al. [6] presented an improved model by incorporating follow-up data that changed their former model from a time-fixed to a time-dependent one, with a more accurate predictive capability.

The common feature of all statistical models is the significance of a raised serum bilirubin level. However, if patients receive ursodeoxycholic acid, bilirubin loses, to a certain extent, its predictive value and is replaced by the determination of hyaluronic acid and type III procollagen amino-terminal peptide [19]. Accordingly, prognostic models for the need for OLT should be adapted if patients receive ursodeoxycholic acid. A recent trial showed that long-term therapy with ursodeoxycholic acid slows the progression of PBC and reduces the need for OLT [19].

Disease-specific aspects

Disease-specific aspects of PBC that reduce the quality of life drastically are osteoporosis, with fracturing, and severe pruritus due to cholestasis. While the jaundice disappears soon after OLT if no complications arise, the duration of osteopenia after OLT and its reversibility has not been well investigated. A histomorphometric study of premenopausal women with PBC showed that bone formation at the remodeling site is reduced and that the overall level of bone remodeling and turnover is influenced by the degree of hepatic dysfunction [13]. The degree of hepatic osteodystrophy in female PBC patients and its reversibility by OLT was analyzed by measuring bone density pre- and posttransplant [9]. The density of spine bodies was reduced by 7 % compared to controls. Three months after OLT there was a further decline and a significant incidence of atraumatic fractures. One year after OLT the preoperative baseline was reached and after 2 years the initial level was surpassed by 5 %. The further decline in the early period after OLT is certainly caused by high doses of corticosteroids, which subsequently tapered off, and coincides with the consolidation of hepatic metabolism in the medium term after OLT.

Prognosis after liver transplantation

The excellent outcome of OLT for PBC in our study with a 5-year survival of 95.6 % is in accord with similar reports in the literature [15]. To assess the long-term effect of OLT for PBC, detection of recurrence of the underlying disease is of extreme importance. There is still controversy whether PBC which recurs after OLT can be attributed in part to non-standardized criteria for the diagnosis of recurrence. In OLT for PBC it is essential to differentiate between chronic allograft rejection and recurrence of PBC. PBC, chronic allograft rejection, and graft-versus-host disease share common histopathological features. Neuberger et al. [17] reported on three patients who had undergone OLT more than 3.5 years previously and had apparently developed a recurrence of PBC. This suggestion was based on histopathological findings such as reduction of small bile ducts and portal inflammation, a clinical course after OLT resembling PBC with mild jaundice, and detection of AMA. Demetris et al. [7], however, found in a large group of liver recipients with PBC a higher incidence of chronic rejection but no evidence of recurrent PBC, according to Neuberger's criteria. A recent study by Balan et al. [1] demonstrated histological evidence of recurrent PBC in approximately 10 % of the liver recipients for PBC but no evidence of progressive disease. In 19 PBC patients, followed-up for 11 years, no distinctive histological nor serological findings for recurrent PBC were detectable [11]. The role of posttransplant AMA titers and the PBC-specific subtypes, anti-PDH-E2 and anti-BCKD-E2, and their correlation to recurrence of PBC is still unclear.

Conflicting reports on the recurrence of PBC after liver transplantation may reflect differences in patient selection, medical management, and immunosuppressive therapy. Cyclosporine A, for example, may postpone the onset of recurrent PBC, as seen in precirrhotic patients. A much longer observation period may be necessary to definitely prove or rule out the existence of recurrent PBC.

References

1. Balan V, Batts KP, Porayko MK, et al (1993) Histological evidence for recurrence of primary biliary cirrhosis after liver transplantation. Hepatology 18: 1392–1398
2. Benhamou JP (1994) Indications for liver transplantation in primary biliary cirrhosis. Hepatology 20: 11S–13S
3. Beukers R, Schalm SW (1992) Immunosuppressive therapy for primary biliary cirrhosis. J Hepatol 14: 1–6
4. Bonsel GJ, IJ Klompmaker, Veer F van'T, et al (1990) Use of prognostic models for assessment of value of liver transplantation in primary biliary cirrhosis. Lancet 335: 493–497
5. Christensen E, Neuberger J, Crowe J, et al (1985) Beneficial effect of azathioprine and prediction of prognosis in primary biliary cirrhosis: final results of an international trial. Gastroenterology 89: 1084–1091
6. Christensen E, Altman DG, Neuberger J, et al (1993) Updating prognosis in primary biliary cirrhosis using a time-dependent Cox regression model. PBC1 and PBC2 trial groups. Gastroenterology 105: 1865–1876
7. Demetris AJ, Markus BH, Esquive C, et al (1988) Pathologic analysis of liver transplantation for primary biliary cirrhosis. Hepatology 8: 939–947
8. Dickson ER, Grambsch PM, Fleming TR, et al (1989) Prognosis in primary biliary cirrhosis: model for decision making. Hepatology 10: 1–7
9. Eastell R, Dickson ER, Hodgson SF, et al (1991) Rates of vertebral bone loss before and after liver transplantation in women with primary biliary cirrhosis. Hepatology 14: 296–300
10. Fennerty MB (1993) Primary sclerosing cholangitis and primary biliary cirrhosis. How effective is medical therapy? Postgrad Med 94: 81–88
11. Gouw ASH, Haagsma EB, Manns M, et al (1994) Is there recurrence of primary biliary cirrhosis after liver transplantation? A clinicopathologic study in long-term survivors. J Hepatol 20: 500–507
12. Heathcote EJ, Cauch-Dudek K, Walker V, et al (1994) The Canadian multicenter double-blind randomized controlled trial of ursodeoxycholic acid in primary biliary cirrhosis. Hepatology 19: 1149–1156
13. Hodgson SF, Dickson ER, Eastell R, et al (1993) Rates of cancelleous bone remodeling and turnover in osteopenia associated with primary biliary cirrhosis. Bone 14: 819–827
14. Lindor KD, Dickson ER, Baldus WP, et al (1994) Ursodeoxycholic acid in the treatment of primary biliary cirrhosis. Gastroenterology 106: 1284–1290
15. Markus BH, Dickson ER, Grambsch PM, et al (1989) Efficacy of liver transplantation in patients with primary biliary cirrhosis. N Engl J Med 320: 1709–1713

16. Melia WM, Johnson PJ, Neuberger J, et al (1984) Hepatocellular carcinoma in primary biliary cirrhosis: detection by alpha fetoprotein estimation. Gastroenterology 87: 660–663

17. Neuberger J, Portmann B, MacDougall BRD, et al (1982) Recurrence of primary biliary cirrhosis after liver transplantation. N Engl J Med 306: 1–4

18. Poupon RE, Balkau B, Eschwege E, et al, UDCA PBC Study Group (1991) A multicenter, controlled trial of ursodiol for the treatment of primary biliary cirrhosis. N Engl J Med 324: 1548–1554

19. Poupon RE, Balkau B, Guechot J, et al (1994) Predictive factors in ursodeoxycholic acid-treated patients with primary biliary cirrhosis: role of serum markers of connective tissue. Hepatology 19: 636–640

20. Rydning ?hrumpf E, Abdelnoor M, et al (19?? ?tors of prognostic importance ? ?nary biliary cirrhosis. Scand J ? enterol 25: 119–126

Transpl Int (1996) 9 [Suppl 1]: S 120–S 125
© Springer-Verlag 1996

LIVER

N. P. Mora
M. Jiménez
J. Buján
R. Arahuetes
F. Jurado
J. M. Bellón
M. L. Leret
F. J. Tendillo
J. L. Castillo-Olivares

Hepatic resuscitation after warm anoxia: one approach for increasing the donor pool for liver transplantation

N. P. Mora (✉)
Liver Transplant Unit, Clinica Puerta de Hierro, Reina Victoria 35, 7D, 28003 Madrid, Spain

N. P. Mora · M. Jiménez · F. J. Tendillo ·
J. L. Castillo-Olivares
Experimental Surgery Service, Clinica Puerta de Hierro, San Martin de Porres, 4, 28035 Madrid, Spain

J. Buján · F. Jurado · J. M. Bellón
Department of Morphological Sciences and Surgery, School of Medicine, University of Alcalá de Henares, Alcalá de Henares, Madrid, Spain

R. Arahuetes · M. L. Leret
Department of Animal Biology, Universidad Complutense de Madrid, Madrid, Spain

Abstract The deleterious effects of warm anoxia on the liver are seen to be irreversible if cooling and transplantation (LT) follow immediately after. The aim of our study is to demonstrate that livers subjected to anoxia may be suitable for LT if a period of resuscitation is interposed before the cooling process. Forty female Large White pigs were used. Preservation (Euro-Collins solution) and LT technique were the same in all 20 procedures. All donors underwent clamping of the porta hepatis at the end of harvesting dissection. In the so-called "resuscitated" groups (A_R and B_R), the clamp was released for a period of time before the liver was cooled. Then, all livers underwent 2 h of cold ischemia followed by LT. Ul-trastructural study showed better maintenance of mitochondria and sinusoidal cell integrity in resuscitated livers after LT. Liver synthesis of total adenine nucleotides, graft function and recipient survival were found to be better in the "resuscitated" groups. In conclusion, anoxic livers may be retrieved for LT if a resuscitation period (i. e. aerobic perfusion) is allowed prior to cold preservation. Longer periods of warm anoxia are needed to further support these preliminary results.

Key words Anoxia · Cardiac arrest · Liver transplantation · Resuscitation · Warm ischemia

Introduction

The progress of clinical liver transplantation (LT) over the last 15 years is unquestionable. The efficiency of immunosuppressive drugs, refinements in surgical technique, and the introduction of the University of Wisconsin organ preservation solution (UW) are among the responsible factors [1, 2, 9]. Nevertheless, the real access of liver patients to transplantation is seriously limited by the shortage of available donor organs. In fact, the demand for organ donors has increased in recent years while the supply has reached a plateau or decreased [6]. Previous authors have suggested the possibility of resuscitating livers after warm ischemic injury [7]. This would make it possible to use cardiac arrest donors as a new source of organs for LT.

The deleterious effects of warm anoxia on the liver are seen to be irreversible if cooling and transplantation follow immediately after. The aim of our study is to demonstrate that livers subjected to anoxia may be suitable for LT if a period of resuscitation is interposed before the cooling process. We also attempt to study in depth the effects of warm ischemia (WI) followed by cold ischemia and subsequent LT.

Methods

Technical aspects

Forty female Large White pigs (15–20 kg) were used in 20 orthotopic LT procedures. At the end of harvesting dissection, all donors underwent a period of hepatic WI (clamping of the porta

Table 1 Time employed in each phase of the preservation-transplantation process (*WI* warm ischemia, *R* resuscitation, *CT* cold ischemia time, *ST* vascular suture time, *TT* total ischemia time)

Group	Wi (min)	R (min)	CT (min)	ST (min)	TT (min)
A	5	0	98 ± 12	53 ± 5	151 ± 16
A_R	5	5	91 ± 5	50 ± 5	140 ± 6
B	10	0	88 ± 14	55 ± 3	143 ± 13
B_R	10	10	85 ± 11	52 ± 3	137 ± 10

Table 2 Tissue TAN and ATP levels in anoxic liver grafts (*WI* warm ischemia, *R* resuscitation, *TAN* total adenine nucleotides (µmol/mg of liver tissue), *ATP* adenosine triphosphate, *P* end of preservation, *T* transplanted liver)

Group	WI + R (min)	% Baseline TAN		% Baseline ATP	
		P	T	P	T
A	5 + 0	78 ± 25	76 ± 16	73 ± 41	51 ± 34
A_R	5 + 10	75 ± 18	110 ± 78[*1]	46 ± 19	86 ± 19[*4]
B	10 + 0	54 ± 13	66 ± 17	70 ± 17	73 ± 30
B_R	10 + 10	78 ± 6[*2]	92 ± 25[*3]	81 ± 36	81 ± 5

[*1] $P < 0.01$ vs A; [*2] $P < 0.01$ vs B; [*3] $P = 0.08$ vs B; [*4] $P = 0.09$ vs A

Table 3 Graft function and survival with anoxic donor livers (*WI* warm ischemia, *R* resuscitation, *AST* aspartate aminotransferase, *BIL* bilirubin output)

Group	WI + R (min)	AST (24 h)	BIL (24 h) (cc)	Six-day survival
A	5 + 0	1736 + 774	64 + 35	1/5
A_R	5 + 10	1026 + 332	114 + 54*	5/5**
B	10 + 0	[a]	20 + 44	0/5[a]
B_R	10 + 10	1321 + 752	104 + 36*	3/5

* $P < 0.05$ vs B; ** $P < 0.05$ vs A
[a] All but one animal died within 24 h after LT

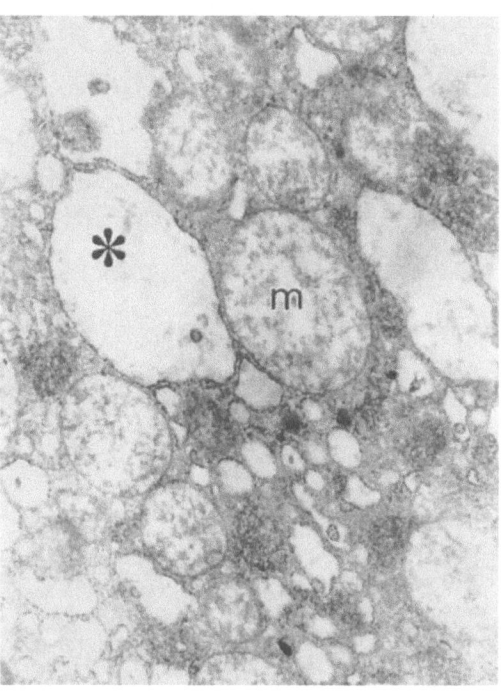

Fig. 1 Swollen mitochondria *(m)* and disorganized crests near dilated endothelial reticulum cisternae (*) can be seen in some hepatocytes subjected to 5 min of ischemia without resuscitation. TEM × 12000

hepatis) followed, or not, by a period of resuscitation (R) (clamp release) before liver cooling. All donor livers were flushed with Euro-Collins solution and stored at 4 °C before LT.

Spontaneous porto-jugular bypass was established before the anhepatic phase. Heparin was not used. Arterial reconstruction was done with an end-to-end anastomosis between the donor celiac trunk and the recipient hepatic artery. Surgical loops (2 × 1) were used for this purpose. No biliary reconstruction was performed. A silicon tube was introduced into the donor bile duct and exteriorized through the abdominal wall for measuring the 24-h biliary output after each LT.

Animal groups

The animals were divided into four different groups, A, A_R, B, and B_R, according to the WI period and the presence or absence of the R period (Table 1). Aside from this, there were no differences among groups with respect to cold ischemia time (CT), vascular suture time (ST) or total ischemia time (TT = CT + ST) (Table 1).

Graft assessment

Liver biopsies were taken from each graft as follows: at baseline (B), the end of harvesting dissection; at the end of preservation (P), just before graft reperfusion; and in the transplanted liver (T), 1 h after graft reperfusion.

Morphological and ultrastructural studies

The morphological and ultrastructural studies were done by transmission electron microscopy. The samples were fragmented into small sections, fixed in 3 % glutaraldehyde for 2 h and placed in Milloning buffer (pH 7.3). For the ultrastructural study, the samples were postfixed in 2 % osmium tetroxide, dehydrated in a grade series of acetones and embedded in Araldite for thin sectioning. Afterwards, their contrast was enhanced with lead citrate and they were examined under a Zeiss 109 transmission electron microscope.

HPLC assay

ATP, ADP, and AMP levels in liver tissue were determined in each liver biopsy by HPLC assay. Total adenine nucleotide (TAN) levels were calculated by summing ATP + ADP + AMP.

Additional determinations

Plasma aspartate aminotransferase (AST) levels were compared 24 h after LT. Biliary output was collected and recorded for the same period of time in each recipient.

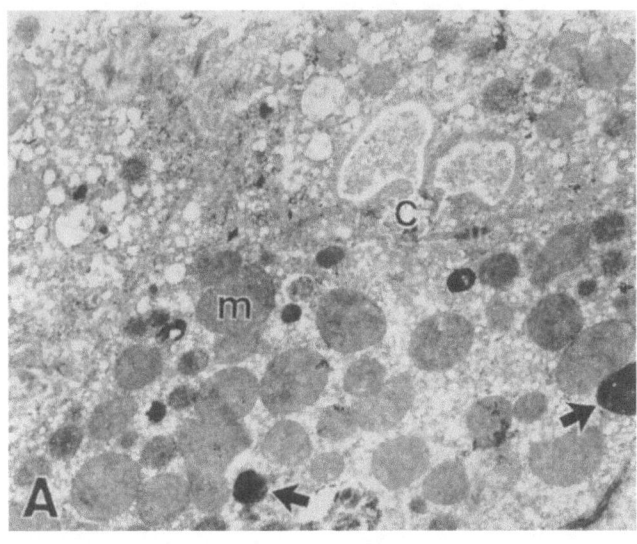

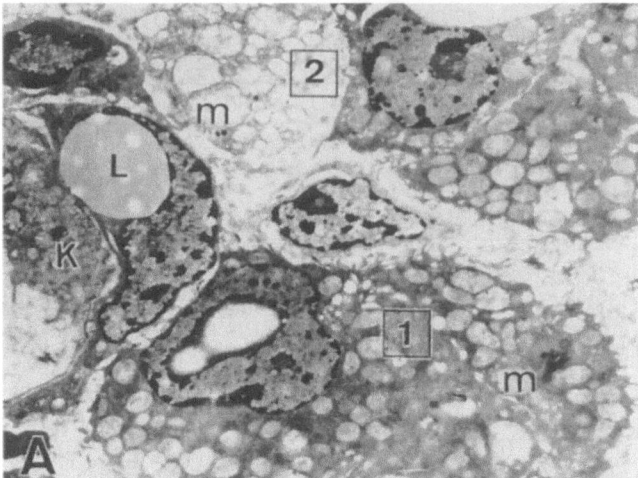

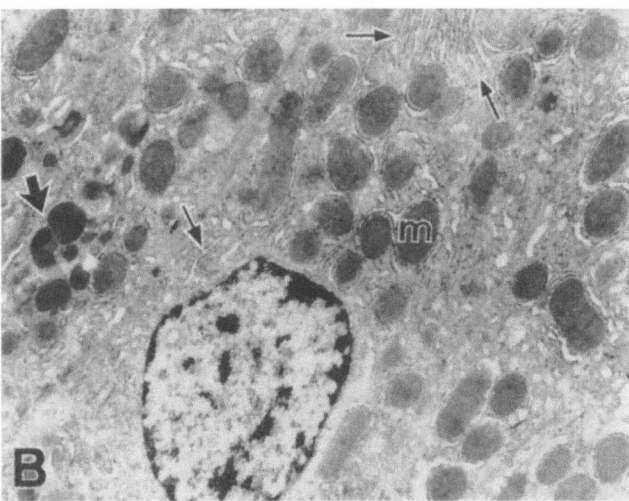

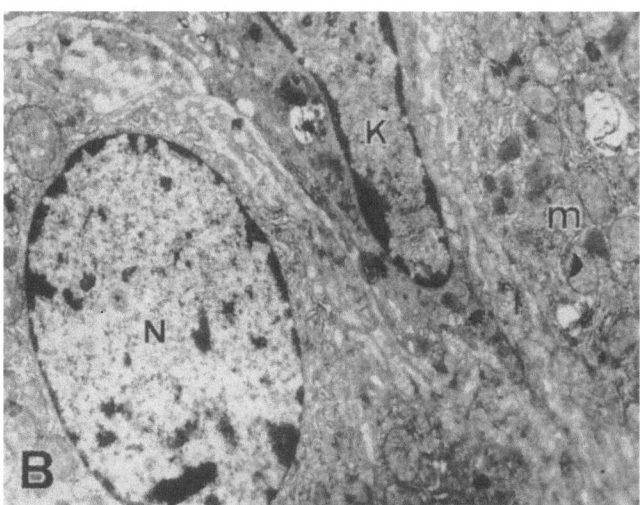

Fig. 2 A Group A(P). Microvesiculated hepatocytes, with swollen mitochondria and lysosomes. **B** Group A_R(P). Hepatocyte showing no noteworthy morphological changes after 5 min of resuscitation. (*m* mitochondria, *small arrows* rough endoplasmic reticulum, *large arrows* lysosomes, *C* hepatic canaliculi) TEM × 7000

Fig. 3 A Group A(T). Dark-colored hepatocytes *(1)* exhibiting condensed cytoplasm, little vesiculation and small, light-colored mitochondria *(m)*, next to a light-colored, vacuolated hepatocyte *(2)* with swollen, ruptured mitochondria. (*L* Fat-storing cell with a large lipid droplet, *K* Kupffer cell) TEM × 3000 **B** Group A_R(T). Hepatocytes with typical morphology and normal mitochondria *(m)* next to a Kupffer cell *(K)*. (*N* Hepatocyte nucleus) TEM × 7000

Statistical study

The statistical analysis consisted of Student's *t*-test for parametric data and the Mann-Whitney test for nonparametric data. Fisher's exact test was used to compare survival rates among the groups. A *P* value of less than 0.05 was considered to be significant.

Results

The HPLC findings and rate of survival are summarized in Tables 2, 3. The ultrastructural study revealed that livers subjected to 5 min of anoxia without resuscitation at the end of preservation, group A(P), showed varying degrees of ultrastructural change. Two types of cellular

lesion could be clearly distinguished. Some hepatocytes presented microvesiculation, dilatation of the smooth endoplasmic reticulum (SER) and swollen mitochondria (Fig. 1), having disorganized crests, different degrees of lysosome activation, and a light-colored nucleus with fragmented chromatin. Others presented a few peripheral vacuoles and several transversal cisternae in the SER, while the mitochondria and nucleus had undergone little change (Fig. 2 A). In both cases, the hepatocytes had a smooth sinusoidal pole, with no microvilli protruding toward Disse's space. The sinusoid endothelial cells presented a rounded nucleus, condensed mitochondria, a few vacuoles, and numerous micropinocy-

Fig. 4 A, B Group A(T).
A Vacuolated endothelial cells *(EC)*, Disse's space *(D)* with numerous microvesicles and light-colored hepatocytes with vesicles *(v)*, and swollen mitochondria *(m)*. **B** Activated Kupffer cell *(K)* next to an endothelial cell *(EC)* having an elongated nucleus. TEM × 7000

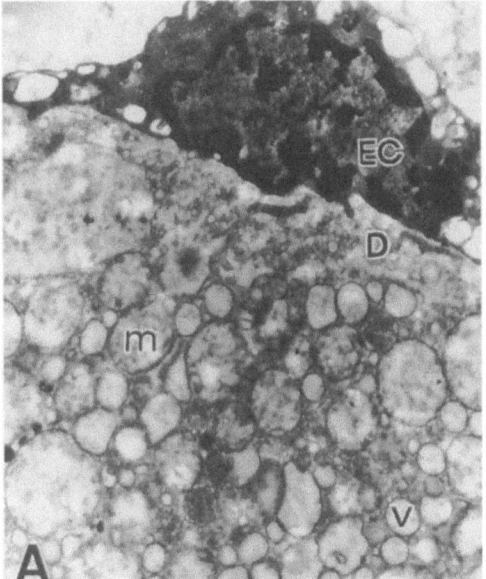
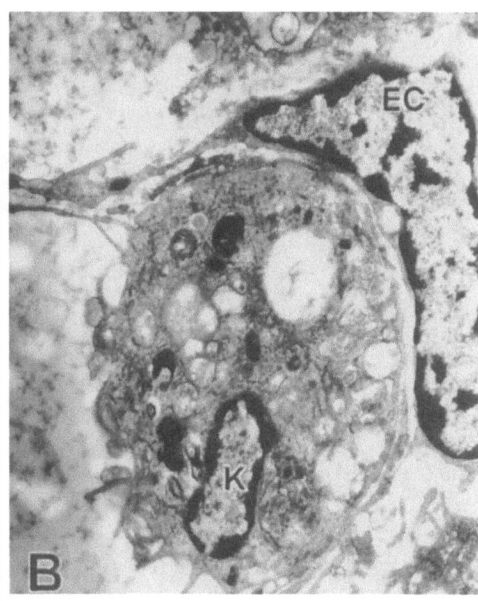

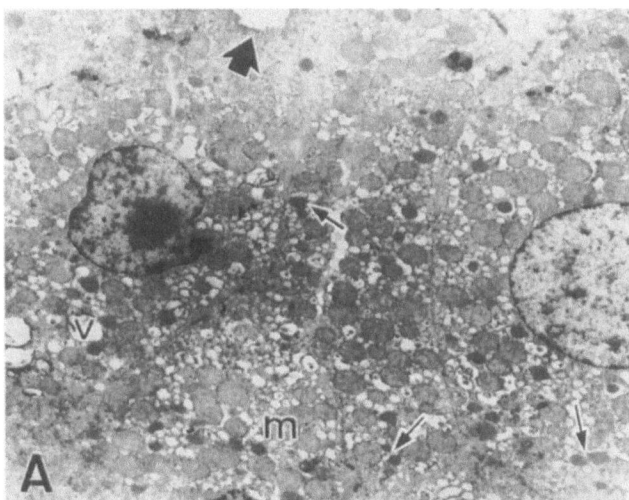
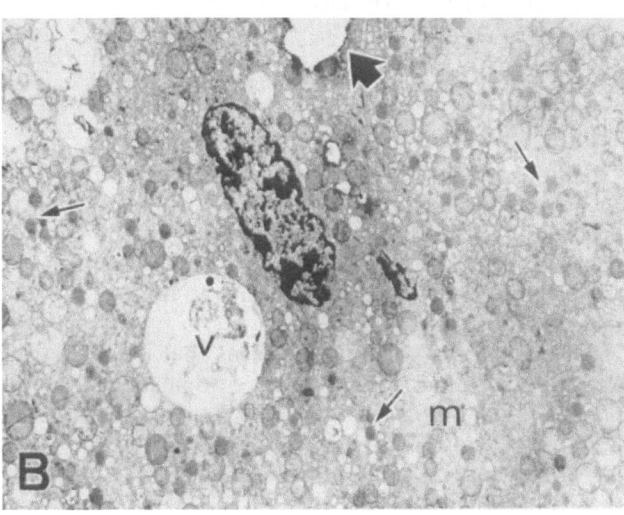

totic vesicles. However, when the liver was subjected to a short period of resuscitation (5 min) prior to cooling, group $A_R(P)$, the changes observed in the hepatocytes were less marked, consisting of mild inflammation with increased SER (Fig. 2 B).

One hour after transplantation and revascularization of the graft with no resuscitation, group A(T), the differences between the two types of hepatocytes described above had become more marked (Fig. 3 A). In those of the first type, the vesiculation of the cytoplasm and inflammation of the mitochondria were more generalized, and rupture of the inner mitochondrial structure was observed. The second type of hepatocyte tended to greater cytoplasmic condensation; SER activity had decreased, while the content of the vacuoles appeared to have been concentrated in one or two larger ones. The hepatocytes had contracted thus widening the intercellular spaces and canaliculi. Disse's space was dilated and fat-storing and endothelial cells with tiny vacuoles were observed (Fig. 4 A). At this stage, the Kupffer cells were seen to be highly active (Fig. 4 B). In grafts that had undergone resuscitation after transplantation, group $A_R(T)$, the hepatocytes presented nearly normal morphology (Fig. 3 B).

When the liver remained anoxic for 10 min without post-ischemic resuscitation, group B(P), the tissue exhibited greater changes (Fig. 5 A). The hepatic canaliculi were markedly dilated, with distension of the hepatocel-

◀ **Fig. 5 A** Group B(P). Dilated hepatic canaliculi *(large arrow)* and the hepatocellular border devoid of microvilli. The hepatocytes present vacuoles *(v)* of different sizes, swollen mitochondria *(m)* and a few lysosomes *(small arrow)*. TEM × 3000. **B** Group $B_R(P)$. Microvesiculated hepatocyte showing a large vacuole *(v)*

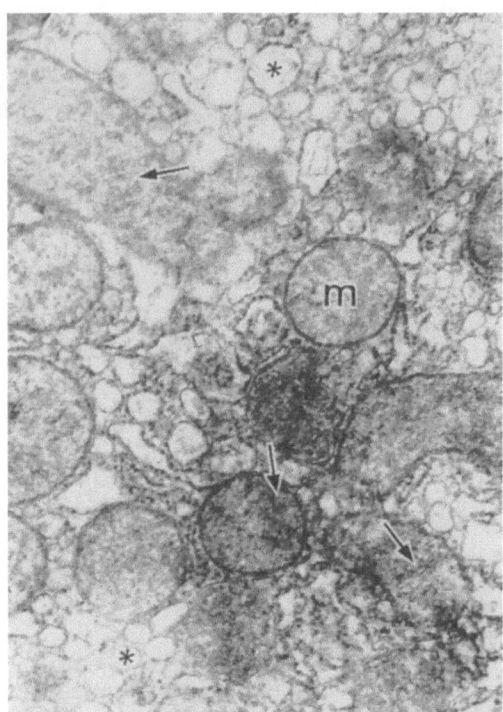

Fig. 6 Group B(P). Swollen mitochondria *(m)* with light-colored matrix and fragmented crests *(arrows),* next to numerous smooth endoplasmic reticulum transversal cisternae (*). TEM × 20000

lular microvilli and widened intercellular spaces. The hepatocytes presented a few vacuoles and numerous transversal cisternae in the SER, swollen, light-colored mitochondria (Fig. 6), and changes in the nucleus. When anoxia was followed by 10 min of resuscitation, group B_R(P), the hepatocytes showed areas of normal structure, as opposed to others in which the vacuolation and the SER dilatation persisted (Fig. 5 B). Following revascularization of the ischemic organ, group B(T) (Fig. 7 A), the hepatocytes retracted, the cytoplasm became denser, and the microvesiculation was diminished; however, the canaliculi and the intercellular spaces remained dilated, and the hepatocytes presented vacuolation and dilatation of the SER. When the organ had undergone 10 min of resuscitation, group B_R(T), the structural changes produced in the tissue by the lack of oxygenation had not been totally normalized. The canaliculi remained dilated, although the dilatation of the hepatocellular SER was less marked and the vacuoles had fused into one or more of greater size, arranged in the direction of the sinusoid (Fig. 7 B). The endothelium remained stable, although a few cells had become rounded.

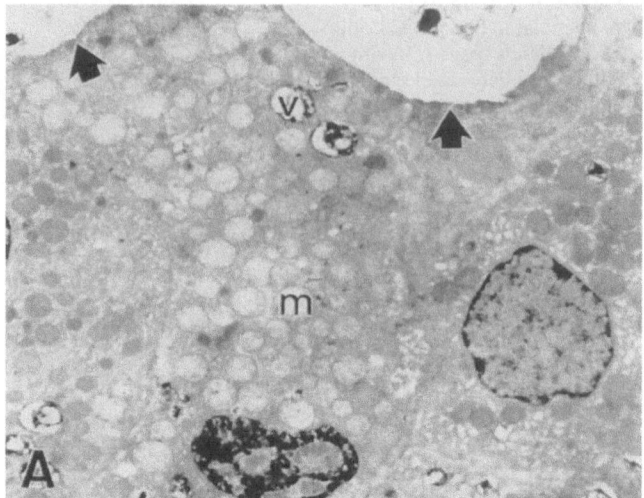

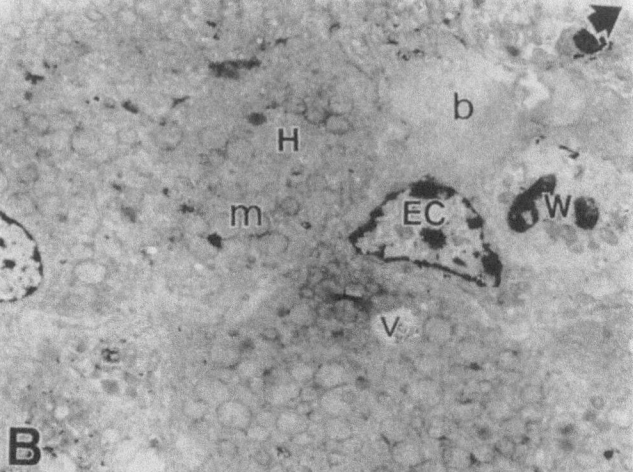

Fig. 7 A Group B(T). Following revascularization, the hepatocytes present few vacuoles arranged in the direction of the sinusoid and slightly swollen mitochondria *(m)*. Dilated hepatic canaliculi *(arrows)*. TEM × 3000. **B** Group B_R(T). Hepatocytes *(H)* next to a sinusoid surrounded by a normal endothelial cell *(EC)*; the lumen is occupied by a white cell *(W)* and a few bubbles *(b)*

Discussion

The number of organs available for liver grafting needs to be increased if transplantation is to be a realistic life-saving therapy for those patients with end-stage liver disease. Cardiac arrest donors and xenografts are the proposed new sources of organs to make this possible.

There exists a general consensus that if cold preservation follows immediately after cardiac arrest, the donor liver will not resume adequate function in the recipient. Meanwhile, there is widespread acceptance of the assertion that the liver can tolerate WI [4, 5], meaning that WI lesions may be reversible.

In a previous study, Schön et al. [7] have demonstrated the reversibility of WI by subjecting ischemic livers to machine perfusion. We have found no additional studies dealing with experimental LT after an insult of that kind. Shirakura et al. [8], working with dogs, also used a perfusion machine to resuscitate different organs retrieved from cardiac arrest donors prior to grafting. Nevertheless, the study does not report on LT.

We demonstrated that livers subjected to 5 min of anoxia could be fully recovered if a 5-min aerobic period was interposed before flushing and cold preservation. All A_R animals survived. Ultrastructural changes and tissue TAN levels were totally corrected soon after transplantation.

When the WI period was extended to 10 min, liver non-function occurring in the first 24 postoperative hours was common. Ten minutes of resuscitation (group B_R) was found to improve survival rates and biliary output, but the results cannot be considered optimal. In fact, TAN synthesis recovery did not reach statistical significance when compared to non-resuscitated livers (group B). The recovery of tissue TAN levels has been suggested as a viability prediction factor in LT [3]. Livers in both groups failed to fully resolve the ultrastructural lesions found at the end of preservation.

We conclude that 5 min of aerobic recovery is enough to resuscitate livers subjected to 5 min of WI. Livers that undergo 10 min of WI appear to require a longer period to achieve optimal graft function. Trials combining longer WI periods with longer periods of resuscitation should be performed to give consistency to these findings. We suggest that parallel results may be obtained with brief perfusion periods if an adequate machine is available.

Acknowledgements The authors wish to thank M. Messman for her editorial help. This work was supported by grant number 94/0392 from the Spanish Health Research Fund (F. I. S.).

References

1. First MR (1992) Transplantation in the nineties. Transplantation 53: 1–11
2. Groth CG, Ohlman S, Gannedahl G, Ericzon BG (1993) New immunosuppressive drugs in transplantation. Transplant Proc 25: 2681–2683
3. Hamamoto I, Takaya S, Todo S, Fujita S, Gulik M van, Nakamura K, Irish WD, Starzl TE (1993) Can adenine nucleotides predict primary nonfunction of the human liver graft? Transplant Proc 25: 3036–3037
4. Harris KA, Wallace AC, Wall WJ (1982) Tolerance of the liver to ischemia in the pig. J Surg Res 33: 524–530
5. Huguet C, Nordlinger B, Bloch P, Conard J (1978) Tolerance of the human liver to prolonged normothermic ischemia. Arch Surg 113: 1448
6. Lemasters JJ, Bunzendahl H, Thurman RG (1995) Reperfusion injury to donor livers stored for transplantation. Liver Transplant Surg 1: 124–138
7. Schön MR, Hunt CJ, Pegg DE, Wight DG (1993) The possibility of resuscitating livers after warm ischemic injury. Transplantation 56: 24–31
8. Shirakura R, Kamiike W, Matsumura A, Miyagawa S, Fukushima N, Hatanaka N, Chang JC, Shimizu S, Sueki H, Amemiya A, Matsumiya G, Izutani Y, Miyata M, Nakano S, Nakahara K, Shimazaki Y, Matsuda H (1993) Multiorgan procurement from non-heart-beating donors by use of Osaka University cocktail, Osaka rinse solution, and the portable cardiopulmonary bypass machine. Transplant Proc 25: 3093–3094
9. Southard JH, Belzer FO (1993) The University of Wisconsin organ preservation solution: components, comparisons, and modifications. Transplant Rev 7: 176–190

Transpl Int (1996) 9 [Suppl 1]: S126–S131
© Springer-Verlag 1996

LIVER

A. R. Mueller
K.-P. Platz
I. Wiehe
F. Monticelli
J. Lierath
M. Keitel
R. Streich
W.-O. Bechstein
P. Neuhaus

Cytokine pattern in patients with infections after liver transplantation

A. R. Mueller (✉) · K.-P. Platz · I. Wiehe ·
F. Monticelli · J. Lierath · W.-O. Bechstein ·
P. Neuhaus
Department of Surgery, Virchow Klinikum,
Humboldt University of Berlin,
Augustenburger Platz 1, D-13353 Berlin,
Germany
Tel. + 49-(0) 30-4 50-5 20 01;
Fax + 49-(0) 30-4 50-5 29 00

M. Keitel · R. Streich
Department of Anesthesiology, Virchow
Klinikum, Humboldt University of Berlin,
Berlin, Germany

Abstract Severe infections are the most frequent cause of death after liver transplantation. Determination of new parameters may increase the knowledge of pathophysiological mechanisms of infection. For this purpose, 81 patients with 85 liver transplants were monitored for various new parameters on a daily basis. Patients with severe infections ($n = 10$) were compared with patients with mild or asymptomatic cholangitis ($n = 11$) and with patients with an uneventful postoperative course ($n = 37$). One-year patient survival was 88.9 %; in five patients, death was related to serious infections. Mean neopterin, soluble tumor necrosis factor-RII (sTNF-RII), and hyaluronic acid levels were significantly elevated in patients with serious infections compared with the other two groups ($P \leq 0.01$). A further increase in sTNF-RII and neopterin levels was observed in patients with lethal infections ($P \leq 0.01$ versus surviving patients with serious infection). An increase in neopterin levels was observed prior to severe infection, and in six of ten patients, this increase occurred as early as during the reperfusion period. Soluble TNF-RII and hyaluronic acid levels also increased significantly prior to severe infection. Interleukin (IL)-6, soluble intercellular adhesion molecule-1 (sICAM-1), and sIL-2R increased in patients with serious infection and cholangitis to a similar extent. As part of an overwhelming immune response, a significant increase in IL-6, sIL-2R, and also IL-1β levels occurred during the late phase of lethal infection ($P \leq 0.01$ versus surviving patients with serious infection). Routine monitoring of these parameters may improve current diagnostic tools and possibly lead to earlier detection of patients at risk after liver transplantation.

Key words Liver transplantation · Infection · Cytokines · Neopterin · Hyaluronic acid

Introduction

Atypical, bacterial, and fungal infections are one of the most serious complications of immunocompromised patients, and are the most frequent cause of death after liver transplantation [1–3]. The aim of this study was to investigate various new parameters during and after transplantation in order to gain increased knowledge on the pathophysiological mechanism of infection. Most cytokines, adhesion molecules, and also neopterin are known to be rather non-specific and their levels increase with stimulation or alteration of the immune response caused by acute allograft rejection, graft-versus-host disease, viral infections, and bacterial sepsis, as well as tumor disease [4–7]. However, there may be significant differences in the pattern of these parameters for each disease. In the present study, we show that there are significant differences in cytokine patterns in patients with serious infections compared with the other two groups, and that some parameters may be indicative of serious infections as early as during reperfusion, while others may detect patients who subsequently died.

Materials and methods

Patients

Between August 1993 and July 1994, 81 patients receiving 85 orthotopic liver transplants were prospectively monitored for various new parameters. Indications for liver transplantation included 5 patients with acute liver failure due to fulminant hepatitis B (HBV) and hepatitis C (HCV) infections, or intoxication, 23 patients with HBV and HCV cirrhosis, 16 patients with alcoholic cirrhosis, 11 with primary biliary cirrhosis, 8 with cryptogenic cirrhosis, 4 patients with autoimmune cirrhosis, and 15 patients with various other indications. Six patients who were undergoing retransplantation were also included: 1 initial non-function (INF), 1 refractory acute rejection, 1 chronic rejection, and 1 early graft failure following recombinant tissue-type plasminogen activator (rt-PA) lysis therapy and disseminated intravascular coagulopathy (DIC) due to lung artery embolism; 2 patients entered the study at the time of retransplantation: 1 patients with chronic rejection and 1 with HBV recurrence. The study was approved by the ethics commitee of the Humboldt University of Berlin and informed consent was received from each patient prior to participation in the study.

Immunosuppression

Immunosuppression was commenced as quadruple therapy comprizing cyclosporine A (CsA), azathioprine, prednisolone, and ALG (anti-lymphocyte immunoglobulin, Merrieur, France; $n = 24$) or interleukin (IL)-2 receptor antagonist BT563 (Biotest, Dreieich, Germany; $n = 47$) for the first 7 or 12 postoperative days, respectively, and was continued as triple therapy thereafter [8]. Twelve patients received no induction therapy. Two patients undergoing retransplantation who had been previously converted to FK506 because of steroid-resistant and chronic rejection received FK506 (Prograf, Fujisawa, Osaka, Japan) in conjunction with prednisolone.

Management of rejection

Diagnosis of acute rejection was based on clinical (fever, change of color, and amount of bile production) and laboratory (aspartate transaminase, alanine transaminase, bilirubin, γGT, and alkaline phosphatase) findings and was confirmed by histological evaluation of graft biopsies. Patients received methylprednisolone for treatment of acute rejection at a dosage of 500 mg/day for 3 days and FK506 or the combination of FK506 and OKT3 monoclonal antibody (Cilag, Sulzbach, Germany) for steroid-resistant or severe recurrent rejection [9].

Management of infection

Cytomegalovirus (CMV) infection was diagnosed by routinely performed PCR techniques and treated with gancyclovir. If pneumonia was suspected following clinical examination or chest X-ray, di-agnostic bronchoscopy was performed to confirm diagnosis and allow appropriate antibiotic, antiviral, or antifungal treatment. Infections were defined as serious when more than two secondary organ failures, including acute renal failure (ARF), acute respiratory insufficiency (ARI), liver failure, DIC, sepsis or systemic inflammatory response syndrome (SIRS), requirement of cathecholamines, neurological disorders, or acute and chronic rejection, were present.

Clinical and experimental monitoring

Laboratory investigations and clinically adverse events were evaluated on a daily basis for the first month, and, subsequently, after 3, 6, 9, and 12 months. Experimental parameters were determined at the same time points, and additionally at predefined time points during transplantation and after reperfusion: 15 min, 2, 6, 12, 18, 24, 36, 48, and 72 h. Heparinized blood was immediately stored on ice and centrifuged at 4°C for 10 min within 30 min of retrieval. Plasma was stored at –70°C until measured. Commercially available immunoassays with 96-well microtiter plates were used: neopterin (ELItest Neopterin, B. R. A. H. M. S. Diagnostica, Berlin, Germany); IL-1β, IL-6, and IL-10 (Biozol, Eching, Germany); sIL-2R, soluble tumor necrosis factor (sTNF)-RII, and soluble intercellular adhesion molecule-1 (sICAM-1) (DPC Biermann, Bad Nauheim, Germany). Hyaluronic acid was determined by radioimmunoassay (Kabi Pharmacia, Uppsala Sweden). The normal ranges ($n = 45$) of various plasma levels for healthy subjects were: 6.2 ± 0.3 nmol/l for neopterin; 0.0 pg/ml for IL-1β; 28.8 ± 0.9 pg/ml for IL-6; 4.7 ± 0.3 pg/ml for IL-10; 380 ± 20.6 U/l for sIL-2R; 1450 ± 52.7 pg/ml for sTNF-RII; 129 ± 24.1 ng/ml for sICAM-1; and 19.4 ± 2.5 µg/l for hyaluronic acid.

Statistical analysis

Kaplan Meier estimates, Wilcoxon, chi-square tests and analysis of variance were used as indicated. Results were expressed as means ± standard error of the mean.

Results

Survival

Actuarial 1-month and 1-year patient and graft survival was 97.5 % (79/81) and 88.9 % (72/81) for patients, and 94.1 % (80/85) and 84.7 % (72/81) for grafts, respectively. During the first year after transplantation, nine patients died; in five patients death was related to serious infections, two patients died because of fulminant HBV recurrence, one patient because of fulminant HCV, and one because of tumor recurrence.

Postoperative complications

Twenty-eight patients (34.7 %) developed acute rejection during the first month after transplantation; in 14 cases rejection was steroid-resistant and required treatment with FK506 (8 patients) or a combination of

Table 1 Serious infections after liver transplantation. (*LTX* Liver transplantation, *HCV* hepatitis C virus, *CR* chronic rejection, *NANB* non-A, non-B, *INF* initial non-function, *KTx* kidney transplantation, *CMV* cytomegalovirus, *ARF* acute renal failure, *ARI* acute respiratory insufficiency, *DIC* disseminated intravascular coagulopathy, *GI* gastrointestinal, *SIRS* systemic inflammatory response syndrome)

Patient number	Indication for LTX	Infection	Organ failure	Survival
1	ALV, fulminant hepatitis A	Atypical pneumonia, *Aspergillus* infection	ARF, ARI, cathecholamines, liver failure, coma	No
2	(1) ALV, unknown; (2) liver failure: re-LTX	*Enterococcus* sepsis, *Aspergillus* sepsis	Lung artery embolism, DIC, ARI, ARF, cathecholamines, coma, Guillam-Barre syndrome	No
3	(1) HCV cirrhosis; (2) CR: re-LTX	*Pseudomonas* sepsis	CR, ARF, ARI, cathecholamines, coma, GI bleeding	No
4	ALV, fulminant NANB hepatitis	*Aspergillus* pneumonia, *Staphylococcus aureus* sepsis	Steroid-resistant rejection, ARF, ARI, coma, extrapontine myelinolysis	No
5	Klatskin tumor, LTX + Whipple procedure	Necrotizing pancreatitis, peritonitis, CMV pneumonia	Septic liver failure, ARF, ARI, coma, cathecholamines, anastomotic leak	No
6	Alcoholic cirrhosis	*Aspergillus* pneumonia, unknown sepsis	CR, ARF, ARI, SIRS, cathecholamines, coma	Yes
7	(1) Autoimmune cirrhosis; (2) INF: re-LTX	*Enterococcus* pneumonia/sepsis	ARI, ARF, coma, acute rejection	Yes
8	Cryptogenic cirrhosis	Atypical pneumonia	ARI, ARF, cathecholamines	Yes
9	Alcoholic cirrhosis	*Pneumocystis carinii* pneumonia	ARI, ARF, cathecholamines, acute rejection	Yes
10	Oxalosis, LTX + KTX	*Legionella* pneumonia	ARI, cathecholamines, ARF	Yes

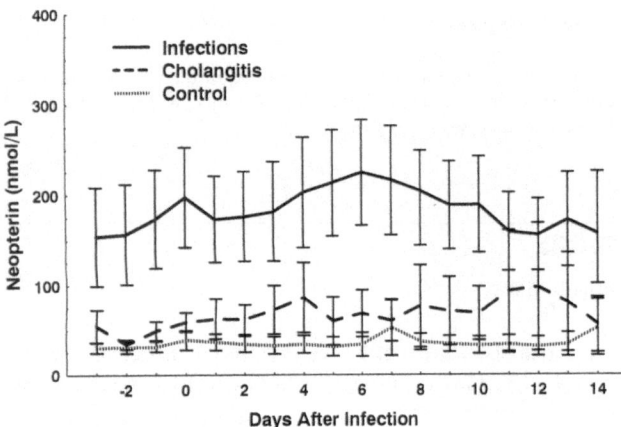

Fig. 1 Neopterin levels in patients with serious infection ($n = 10$), asymptomatic or mild cholangitis ($n = 11$), and an uneventful postoperative course ($n = 37$). $P \leq 0.01$ for serious infections versus cholangitis and uneventful postoperative course

FK506 and OKT3 (6 patients). Ten patients developed serious infections; five patients subsequently died (Table 1). Eleven patients with asymptomatic or mild cholangitis but no signs of concomitant acute allograft rejection were included in the control group together with the 37 patients with an uneventful postoperative course.

Neopterin

Mean neopterin levels were significantly increased in patients with serious infections (192 ± 48.2 nmol/l; $P \leq 0.01$) compared with patients with asymptomatic cholangitis (64.8 ± 27.1 nmol/l) and with patients with an uneventful postoperative course (43.1 ± 13.5 nmol/l) (Fig. 1). A further increase was observed in all five patients who subsequently died (245 ± 51.2 nmol/l versus 103 ± 50.8 nmol/l in surviving patients). In six of ten patients with serious infection, mean neopterin levels rose significantly during the early reperfusion period (149 ± 60.4 nmol/l versus 25.7 ± 6.9 nmol/l in patients with an uneventful postoperative course). There was no correlation, however, between neopterin levels and the extent of reperfusion injury.

Soluble TNF-RII

A significant increase in mean sTNF-RII occurred in patients with serious infections as early as 3 days prior to infection (25522 ± 6744 pg/ml; $P \leq 0.01$) compared with patients with cholangitis (14328 ± 3087 pg/ml) and with patients with an uneventful postoperative course (7352 ± 822 pg/ml) (Fig. 2). Higher mean sTNF-RII levels were observed during the first week of infection in

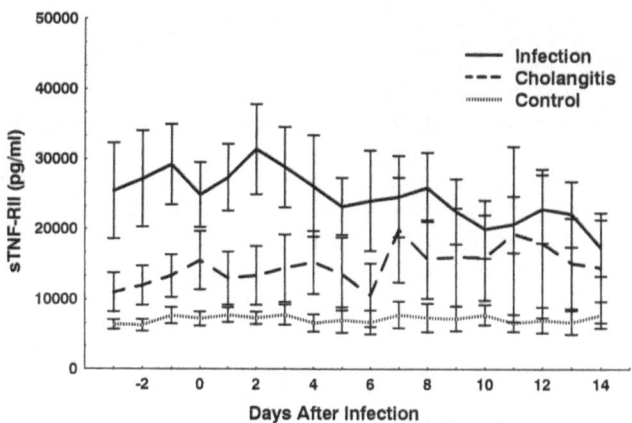

Fig.2 Soluble tumor necrosis factor-RII *(sTNF-RII)* levels in patients with serious infection ($n = 10$), asymptomatic or mild cholangitis ($n = 11$), and an uneventful postoperative course ($n = 37$). $P \leq 0.01$ for serious infections versus cholangitis and uneventful postoperative course

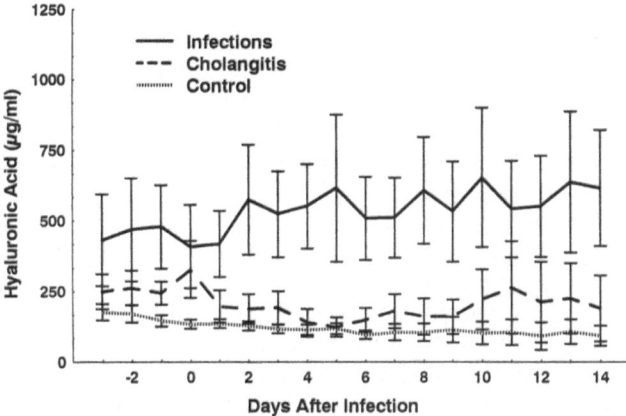

Fig.3 Hyaluronic acid levels in patients with serious infection ($n = 10$), asymptomatic or mild cholangitis ($n = 11$), and an uneventful postoperative course ($n = 37$). $P \leq 0.01$ for serious infections versus cholangitis and uneventful postoperative course

four of five patients who died (26929 ± 6455 versus 20217 ± 5832 pg/ml in surviving patients). Soluble TNF-RII was significantly increased in all transplanted patients compared with healthy subjects.

IL-1β, IL-6, IL-10, and sIL-2R

IL-1β was virtually absent in all but four of five patients experiencing lethal infections (31.8 ± 19.2 pg/ml versus 2.1 ± 0.1 pg/ml in surviving patients; $P \leq 0.01$). IL-1β levels increased during the second week of infection and persisted until death. IL-6 was increased in patients with serious infections and cholangitis (191 ± 47.9 pg/ml and 220 ± 76.4 pg/ml, respectively) to a similar extent as that in patients with an uneventful postoperative course (35.1 ± 16.2 pg/ml). During the second and third week of

infection, a progressive rise occurred in all five patients who died (384 ± 88.9 pg/ml versus 122 ± 31.3 pg/ml in surviving patients; $P \leq 0.01$). Mean levels of IL-10 were significantly elevated in patients with serious infections (114 ± 25.1 pg/ml; $P \leq 0.01$) compared with patients experiencing cholangitis (68.6 ± 24.8 pg/ml) and with an uneventful postoperative course (37.9 ± 9.7 pg/ml). A significant rise of IL-10 was observed during the entire infectious period in all five patients who died (152 ± 54.8 pg/ml versus 46.5 ± 12.9 pg/ml in surviving patients; $P \leq 0.01$). Soluble IL-2R was higher in patients with serious infections and cholangitis (3018 ± 698 U/l and 3829 ± 599 U/l, respectively) than in patients with an uneventful postoperative course (1460 ± 187 U/l). A further increase was observed in four of the five patients who died (3839 ± 897 U/l versus 2411 ± 743 U/l in surviving patients; $P \leq 0.01$).

Hyaluronic acid

Hyaluronic acid levels were significantly increased in all patients with serious infections (518 ± 94 µg/l; $P \leq 0.01$) compared with patients with cholangitis (227 ± 34 µg/l) and patients with an uneventful postoperative course (121 ± 26 µg/l) (Fig.3). Differences between surviving and non-surviving patients with severe infections were minor (P not significant).

Soluble ICAM-1

Mean sICAM-1 levels were predominantly increased in patients with asymptomatic or mild cholangitis (1123 ± 189 ng/ml versus 908 ± 198 ng/ml in patients with severe infections and 690 ± 78.3 ng/ml in patients with an uneventful postoperative course). Slightly higher mean sICAM-1 levels were observed in patients with lethal infection.

Discussion

Within recent years, liver transplantation has become a highly successful treatment for end-stage liver disease and irreversible acute liver failure [8–11]. New approaches may now concentrate on patients at risk. Since atypical, fungal, and bacterial infections are still the predominant cause of death, in the present prospective study we attempted to analyze whether determination of new parameters, i.e., cytokines, adhesion molecules, and neopterin may be of value in improving the currently established monitoring of serious infections after liver transplantation.

Neopterin, an intermediate of tetrahydrobiopterin synthesis, is predominantly produced by interferon

(IFN)-γ-activated macrophages [12]. Neopterin increased more than 3 days prior to severe infection. Thus, neopterin may be considered as an early indicator of infectious complications after liver transplantation. The highest neopterin levels were observed in patients with a lethal outcome, while recovering patients showed a decrease in neopterin with recovery of clinical status. Besides retransplantation and, possibly, chronic rejection, which also led to a rise in neopterin levels, neopterin was highly specific for infection, which is in accordance with observations by others [13].

A variety of studies have shown an increase of the pro-inflammatory cytokines, IL-1β and TNF-α, in non-transplanted patients with serious infection, sepsis, and SIRS. In some studies, these cytokines and the counter-regulatory cytokine IL-6, correlated with severity of disease and ultimate outcome of infection [14, 15]. As a reflection of the activation of the pro-inflammatory cytokines, sTNF-RII increased significantly prior to serious infection. A further rise was observed in non-surviving patients, indicating a positive correlation of sTNF-RII increase with the severity of infection. Soluble TNF-RII has been shown to correlate with TNF-α production [16]. Because of its longer half-life, determination of sTNF-RII may more reliably reflect TNF-α production than determination of the cytokine itself. IL-1β was not detected except in four of five patients who died. This conforms to observations by others where, in non-transplanted, critically ill patients, although there was no increase in TNF-α and IL-1β levels during the early course of severe infection, high levels of the respective cytokine receptors were observed [17]. Vast production of endogen sIL-1Ra (receptor antagonist) may cope well with the early IL-1β production and may prohibit detection of IL-1β in these patients [18].

IL-6, which is known to increase after stimulation and secretion of endotoxin, TNF-α, IL-1β, and interferons, is produced by various cell types including endothelial cells and macrophages [19]. Although IL-6 levels failed to correlate with severity of infection, since it also increased during asymptomatic cholangitis, there was a marked IL-6 production during the late course of infection in all five patients who died. Increased sICAM-1 levels seemed to be more closely associated with cholangitis, although this group contained no patients with severe cholangitis. This may be explained by a high expression of ICAM-1 on bile ducts, as has been shown in liver biopsies during infection [20].

An increase of the downregulatory TH$_2$ cytokine, IL-10, was most pronounced in patients with lethal infection. IL-10, which is produced by monocytes and CD4$^+$ T-cell subsets [21, 22], is thought to have strong anti-inflammatory activity, by suppressing macrophage activity, as well as the release of reactive oxygen intermediates (ROI) and of reactive nitrogen intermediates (NO) [23, 24]. Furthermore, IL-10 has been shown to downregulate the activity of pro-inflammatory cytokines including TNF-α, IL-1β, and IL-8 [22, 25].

Next to stimulation of inflammatory cytokines, we also observed an increase in immunostimulatory TH$_1$ cytokines as reflected by an increase in sIL-2R in most patients with lethal infections. IL-1 and TNF have been shown to stimulate T- and B-lymphocytes and may thereby augment the specific immune response and IL-2 production [26]. The therapeutic dilemma of severe infection with signs of overimmunosuppression of the immunocompromised host and the stimulation of the specific immune response by the activated cytokine network may make selective inhibition of cytokines or their receptors desirable in the future.

Hyaluronic acid (HA), a high molecular weight protein, is located in the loose connective tissue at the inside of plasma membranes. It plays an important role in organisation of the extracellular matrix, cell-cell interactions, and inflammation [27–29]. HA increases upon stimulation with IL-1 [29]. Increased HA levels may most likely result from increased production by inflammatory cells such as fibroblasts [27, 28]. However, in patients with impaired septic liver dysfunction, a decreased catabolism of HA may also be possible, since liver endothelial cells are the predominant site of uptake and degradation of HA [27].

Neopterin and sTNF-RII are eliminated by the kidneys and acute renal failure may result in elevation of circulating plasma levels [3, 30]. There was indeed a positive correlation of both parameters with BUN and serum creatinine. However, there was no increase in neopterin and sTNF-RII levels in patients with ARF related to CsA toxicity or other origins than infection, indicating that the predominant source of neopterin and sTNF-RII during infection was an increased production.

Although most of these parameters are not specific for infections, we found a distinct timing and pattern of the respective parameters during infection and other diseases, including rejection. Furthermore, the extent of increase in neopterin and sTNF-RII levels detected patients at risk for lethal outcome as early as prior to, or with the onset of severe infection. In conclusion, we think that determination of cytokines, neopterin, and hyaluronic acid after liver transplantation is of great value and may influence postoperative management with respect to intensified infectious screening and earlier therapeutic approaches in high risk patients.

References

1. Mora NP, Gonwa TA, Goldstein RM, et al (1992) Risk of postoperative infection after liver transplantation: a univariate and stepwise logistic regression analysis of risk factors in 150 consecutive patients. Clin Transplant 46: 443–449

2. Hadley S, Samore MH, Lewis WD, et al (1995) Major infectious complications after orthotopic liver transplantation and comparison of outcomes in patients receiving cyclosporine or FK506 as primary immunosuppression. Transplantation 59: 851–859

3. Paya CV, Wiesner RH, Hermans PE, et al (1993) Risk factors for cytomegalovirus and severe bacterial infections following liver transplantation: a prospective multivariate time-dependent analysis. J Hepatol 18: 185–192

4. Henderson DC, Sheldon J, Riches P, Hobbs JR (1991) Cytokine induction of neopterin production. Clin Exp Immunol 83: 479–482

5. Fuchs D, Hausen A, Reibnegger G, et al (1988) Neopterin as a marker for cell-mediated immunity: application in HIV infection. Immunol Today 9: 150–155

6. Függer R, Hamilton G, Steininger R, et al (1991) Intraoperative estimation of endotoxin, TNFα, and IL-6 in orthotopic liver transplantation and their relation to rejection and postoperative infection. Transplantation 52: 302–306

7. Gehr G, Braun T, Lesslauer W (1992) Cytokines, receptors, and inhibitors. Clin Invest Med 70: 64

8. Neuhaus P, Bechstein WO, Blumhardt G, et al (1993) Comparison of quadruple immunosuppression after liver transplantation with ATG or IL-2 receptor antibody. Transplantation 55: 1320–1327

9. Neuhaus P, Blumhardt G, Bechstein WO, et al (1995) Comparison of FK506- and cyclosporine A-based immunosuppression in primary orthotopic liver transplantation. A single center experience. Transplantation 59: 31–40

10. Starzl TE, Todo S, Fung J, et al (1989) FK506 for liver, kidney, and pancreas transplantation. Lancet II: 1000

11. European FK506 Multicentre Liver Study Group (1994) Randomized trial comparing tacrolimus (FK506) and cyclosporin in prevention of liver allograft rejection. Lancet 344: 423–428

12. Ziegler I (1985) Synthesis and interferon-γ controlled release of pteridines during activation of human peripheral blood mononuclear cells. Biochem Biophys Res Commun 132: 404–411

13. Tilg H, Vogel W, Alitzky WE, et al (1989) Neopterin excretion after liver transplantation and its value in differential diagnosis of complications. Transplantation 48: 594–599

14. Waage A, Halstensen A, Expevik T (1987) Association between tumor necrosis factor in serum and fatal outcome in patients with meningococcal disease. Lancet 1: 355

15. Dinarello CA (1993) Anti-interleukin-1 strategies in the treatment of septic shock syndrome. In: Baumgartner JD, Calandra T, Carlet J (eds) Mediators of sepsis from pathophysiology to therapeutic approaches. Medicin-Sciences Flammarion, Paris, France, pp 112–121

16. Spinas GA, Keller U, Brockhaus M (1992) Release of soluble receptors for tumor necrosis factor (TNF) in relation to circulating TNF during experimental endotoxinemia. J Clin Invest 90: 533–536

17. Rogy MA, Coyle SM, Oldenburg HSA, et al (1994) Persistently soluble tumor necrosis factor receptor and interleukin-1 receptor antagonist levels in critically ill patients. J Am Coll Surg 178: 132–138

18. Dinarello CA, Thompson RC (1991) Blocking IL-1: effects of IL-1 receptor antagonist in vitro and in vivo. Immunol Today 12: 404–410

19. Ray A, Tratter SB, Santhanam U, et al (1989) Regulation of expression of interleukin-6: molecular and clinical studies. Ann NY Acad Sci 557: 353–371

20. Steinhoff G, Behrend M, Schrader B, et al (1993) Expression patterns of leukocyte adhesion molecules on human liver endothelia. Lack of ELAM-1 and CD62 inducibility on sinusoidal endothelia and distinct distribution of VCAM-1, ICAM-1, ICAM-2, and LFA-3. Am J Pathol 142: 481–488

21. Yssel H, Waal Malefyt R de, Roncarlo MG, et al (1992) IL-10 is produced by subsets of human CD4$^+$ T cell clones and pheripheral blood T cells. J Immunol 149: 2378–2384

22. Donkier V, Flament V, Gerard C, et al (1994) Modulation of the release of cytokines and reduction of the shock syndrome induced by anti-CD3 monoclonal antibody in mice by interleukin 10. Transplantation 1436–1439

23. Bogdan C, Vododvotz Y, Nathan C (1991) Macrophage deactivation by interleukin 10. J Exp Med 174: 1549–1555

24. Cunha FQ, Moncada S, Liew FY (1992) Interleukin 10 (IL-10) inhibits the induction of nitric oxide synthase by interferon-γ in murine macrophages. Biochem Biophys Res Commun 182: 1155–1163

25. Waal Malefyt R de, Abrams J, Bennett B, et al (1991) Interleukin 10 (IL-10) inhibits cytokine synthesis by human monocytes: an autoregulatory role of IL-10 produced by monocytes. J Exp Med 174: 1209–1220

26. Oppenheim JJ, Ruscetti FW, Faltynek C (1991) Cytokines. In: Stites DP, Terr AI (eds) Basic human immunology. Appleton and Lange, Norwalk, Calif., pp 78–100

27. Laurent TC (1987) Biochemistry of hyaluronan. Acta Otolaryngol Suppl (Stockh) 442: 7–24

28. Laurent TC, Fraser JRE (1992) Hyaluronan. FASEBJ 6: 2397–2404

29. Hamura Y, Ito A, Okada Y, Mori Y (1989) Hyaluronic acid metabolism in inflamed mesenterium of guinea pig. Res Commun Mol Pathol Pharmacol 66: 311–327

30. Ward RA, Gordon L (1993) Soluble tumor necrosis factor receptors are increased in hemodialysis patients. ASAIOJ: M782–M786

Transpl Int (1996) 9 [Suppl 1]: S 132–S 134
© Springer-Verlag 1996

LIVER

Th. Gruenberger
S. Winkler
F. Garro
M. Barlan
W. Huber
E. Roth
R. Steininger
F. Muehlbacher

Prediction of graft dysfunction by analysis of liver biopsies after cold storage

S. Winkler · F. Garro · M. Barlan · W. Huber ·
E. Roth · R. Steininger · F. Muehlbacher
Department of Transplantation Surgery
University of Vienna, Austria

T. Gruenberger (✉)
Department of General Surgery,
University of Vienna,
Waehringer Guertel 18–20, A-1090 Vienna,
Austria

Abstract Failure of the hepatic allograft continues to be a serious life-threatening risk for the recipient. Because no effective method of extracorporeal support is available for these patients, early retransplantation is the only alternative that offers the potential for survival. The aim of this prospective analysis was to search for a predictor of primary non-function of hepatic allografts before reperfusion. From March to June 1993 we investigated 19 liver biopsies which were obtained during the preparation of the donor liver in the back table bath immediately before the implantation of the organ. All organs were preserved by UW solution. Biopsies were stored at −80 °C, the working-up process was started by dividing the biopsy into several portions for the determination of fat (petrol-ether extraction), water (weighing before thawing and after drying) and free amino acids (OPA-HPLC method). Graft function was categorized into three groups: (1) good function; (2) fair function; (3) primary non-function (PNF). In addition to known risk factors for delayed graft function such as a long stay of the donor in intensive care and a prolonged anhepatic period of the recipient, we were able to demonstrate that organs with malfunction had a higher fat and water content. Donor livers developing PNF showed a trend towards higher total and subdivided amino acids, which could be explained by the incapacity of the liver to utilize available substrates for gluconeogenesis.

Key words Liver transplantation ·
Liver biopsy · Primary non-function

Introduction

Although orthotopic liver transplantation has become an established therapy for patients with end-stage liver disease, several problems remain to be solved. Despite improvements in organ retrieval, preservation and controlled reperfusion, primary non-function still occurs in 2–20 % of the patients [5, 11]. Multiple factors are involved in graft dysfunction and some of them have been identified as predictors for delayed graft function [7, 9], but none of these so-called predictors is a potent indicator for the development of primary non-function. One important factor in the suitability of the liver graft seems to be the nutritional status of the donor [2, 3]. This factor should be considered because many donors have a period of hyponutrition before organ harvesting, correlating with the length of stay in an intensive care unit (ICU).

The aim of our prospective study was to address the period after cold storage immediately before organ replacement to determine whether the organ had sustained any grave injury.

Materials and methods

From March to June 1993 during a series of 19 consecutive orthotopic liver transplantations we obtained liver biopsies from the fourth segment. Biopsies were taken at the time of unwrapping the liver from the storage pack and were immediately stored at

-80°C. All organs were preserved with the University of Wisconsin (UW) solution after the standard procurement of organ retrieval and in situ liver perfusion with up to 5000 ml of UW solution during the donor operation. The working-up process was started by dividing the biopsies into several portions for the determination of fat, water, and free amino acids. Fat was measured by the method of petrol-ether extraction, water content was measured by weighing the liver piece before thawing and after drying, and the free amino acids were measured by the OPA-HPLC method. Results of the measurement of the free amino acids were divided into those for total amino acids, essential amino acids, aromatic amino acids, and branched-chain amino acids to observe any subgroup differences. The results of the preparation of the liver biopsies were compared with the postoperative function of the transplanted livers. Two further risk factors for delayed postoperative graft function were taken into consideration, the length of donor stay at the ICU before organ procurement and the length of the intraoperative anhepatic period during the liver transplantation. Postoperative graft function was categorized as described before [7] and divided into three groups: (1) good function (GOT under 1000 U/l, spontaneous PT higher than 50 %, bile production above 100 ml/day); (2) fair function (highest GOT above 1000 U/l, clotting factor support, bile production under 100 ml/day); and (3) primary non-function (death without retransplantation within 7 days because of complete liver failure.

Results

Distribution of the postoperative organ function showed 13 livers (68 %) having good function 4 livers (21 %) with fair function, and 2 livers (11 %) with primary non-function (PNF). Concerning the water content of the biopsies, we observed a mean of 313 g/100 g fat-free substance (FFS) with a standard deviation of ± 89 g/100 g FFS in the group of organs with good postoperative liver function. The biopsies of the livers showing fair postoperative graft function had a water content of 289 ± 37 g/100 g FFS. The liver biopsies of the two livers with postoperative non-function had a water content of 335 ± 8 g/100 g FFS. Examination of the fat content within the liver biopsies of the three groups showed the following results: biopsies of organs with good postoperative function had a fat content of 8.45 ± 4.2 g/100 g FFS, biopsies of organs with fair function, 7.25 ± 2.6 g/100 g FFS, and biopsies of organs which were complicated by postoperative non-function had a fat content of 19.55 ± 5.1 g/100 g FFS. Concentrations of amino acids in the liver grafts after cold storage showed the following results. Total amino acids allocated to the three groups: good function, 8.717 ± 2.162 mmol/100 g FFS; fair function, 8.021 ± 3.454 mmol/100 g FFS; PNF, 11.140 ± 0.211 mmol/100 g FFS. Essential amino acids (tyrosine, valine, methionine, tryptophan, isoleucine, phenylalanine, leucine, lysine), divided into the three groups: good function, 1.539 ± 0.555 mmol/100 g FFS; fair function, 1.357 ± 0.781 mmol/100 g FFS; PNF, 1.734 ± 0.305 mmol/100 g FFS. Aromatic amino acids (tyrosine, phenylalanine), distributed among the three

groups: good function, 0.095 ± 0.05 mmol/100 g FFS; fair function 0.13 ± 0.029 mmol/100 g FFS; PNF, 0.12 ± 0.016 mmol/100 g FFS. Branched-chain amino acids, divided into the three groups: good function, 0.301 ± 0.16 mmol/100 g FFS; fair function, 0.376 ± 0.071 mmol/100 g FFS; PNF, 0.419 ± 0.127 mmol/100 g FFS.

In addition to these results of the liver biopsies we found the following correlation to the ICU-stay of the donor and the intraoperative anhepatic period. Divided into the three groups, ICU-stay of the donor showed the following results: good function, 1.9 ± 1.3 days; fair function, 2.8 ± 2.1 days; PNF, 4.5 ± 0.7 days. Good working organs were transplanted with an anhepatic period of 84 ± 17 min, organs showing fair function with an anhepatic period of 90 ± 10 min, and the organs which were classified as having no postoperative function had an anhepatic period of 125 ± 43 min.

Discussion

The increasing demand of organs for liver transplantation has led to the utilization of older donors, of minimal steatotic livers, of livers from donors after a longer period of hypotension and of donors after a longer ICU-stay. Therefore the risk of development of a PNF of the transplanted organ remains high. Since preservation injury is not completely understood, we want to know if there is any predicting factor which could be identified by the examination of a biopsy taken after cold storage. High donor liver fat content has been reported to be associated with the development of PNF [1, 12], and our investigation confirmed this finding; as in other reported analyses we were able to identify a strong correlation between fat content of the liver and development of postoperative PNF. Although the differences were not statistically significant, there was a trend towards higher water content in the livers developing PNF. Cell injury and subsequent cell swelling may be an explanation for the development of PNF. Amino acid content in the liver has not been evaluated as a possible predictor for postoperative graft function so far. Other investigators have examined amino acids in the preservation fluid and found a strong correlation between the amount of amino acids and the development of graft dysfunction [4]. Another group has investigated the normalization of plasma amino acids immediately after liver transplantation and found that abnormalities of the amino acid content should be restored within 3 h after transplantation, in other cases, PNF should be strongly suspected [8]. Our own data showed a significantly higher amino acid content in the biopsies obtained from livers which developed postoperative PNF. As a possible explanation for these findings we could assume an incapacity of the liver to utilize available substrates for gluconeogenesis and anaerobic energy charge. The donor-related risk factor of length of ICU stay before organ retrieval could again be identified as an independent factor associated with the appearance of PNF if the donor stayed for longer than 4 days in the ICU [6, 7, 10]. Another results of our previous study, which was associated with a higher rate of PNF, the prolonged anhepatic period, was again clearly above the critical time of 90 min in the PNF group.

Although we were able to confirm previous studies and their findings of indicators for postoperative organ failure, we could not identify a new predictor of PNF by these analyses of liver biopsies obtained after cold storage of the organ.

References

1. Adam R, Reynes M, Johann M, et al (1991) Transplant Proc 23/1: 1538
2. Adam R, Astarcioglu I, Gigou M, et al (1992) Transplantation 54: 753
3. Boudjema K, Lindell SL, Southard JH, et al (1990) Transplantation 50/6: 943
4. Calmus Y, Cynober L, Dousset B, et al (1995) Gastroenterology 108: 1510
5. D'Alessandro AM, Kalayoglu M, Sollinger HW, et al (1990) Transplant Proc 22: 474
6. Greig PD, Woolf GD, Sinclair SB, et al (1990) Transplant Proc 22: 2072
7. Gruenberger T, Steininger R, Sautner T, et al (1994) Transplant Int 7/1: 672
8. Hisanaga M, Nakajimy Y, Segawa M, et al (1991) J Surg Res 50: 139
9. Ploeg RJ, D'Alesandro AM, Knechtle SJ, et al (1993) Transplantation 55: 807
10. Pruim J, Worden WF van, Knol E, et al (1989) Transplant Proc 21: 2383
11. Todo S, Nery J, Yanaga K, et al (1989) J Amer Med Assoc 261: 711
12. Todo S, Demetris AJ, Makawka L, et al (1989) Transplantation 47: 903

Transpl Int (1996) 9 [Suppl 1]: S135–S139
© Springer-Verlag 1996

LIVER

Th. Kraus
M. Schuller
F. Klee
M. Bredt
A. Mehrabi
G. Hartter
A. Mißbichler
G. Otto

Validation of endothelin (ET) immunoreactivity in human bile by HPLC. Comparison of biliary ET concentration in liver transplant recipients with values obtained during cholecystectomy

Th. W. Kraus (✉)
Chirurgische Universitätsklinik
Heidelberg, Im Neuenheimer Feld 110,
D-69120 Heidelberg, Germany

Th. Kraus · F. Klee · M. Bredt · A. Mehrabi ·
G. Otto
Surgery Department and Salem-Hospital,
University of Heidelberg, Germany

M. Schuller · G. Hartter
Institute for Occupational Medicine,
University of Vienna, Austria

A. Mißbichler
Biomedica GmbH, Vienna, Austria

Abstract High endothelin (ET) concentrations were recently detected in human bile after orthotopic liver transplantation (OLT). In the present study we compared biliary ET/big-ET levels measured by radioimmunoassay (RIA) in liver graft recipients ($n = 37$) with levels measured in non-transplant patients during cholecystectomy ($n = 38$) to clarify the influence of transplantation on the levels of biliary ET peptides. HPLC elution profiles of biliary ET were analyzed for characterization of ET peptide composition and validation of RIA analysis in bile extracts. Mean ET/big-ET levels in the common bile duct after OLT were significantly elevated (ET, 20.9 ± 15; big-ET, 39.2 ± 19 fmol/ml) compared to levels in non-transplant patients (ET, 5.7 ± 4.9; big-ET, 12 ± 8 fmol/ml).

Highest ET/big-ET levels were measured in the gall bladder during cholecystectomy (ET, 61.7 ± 41; big-ET, 75 ± 28 fmol/ml). ET and big-ET levels were correlated by linear regression. HPLC analysis reveals the presence of high levels of ET/big-ET in human bile. Biliary ET mostly represents ET-1. High biliary ET levels after OLT appear to be derived from active endothelial secretion and probably reflect hepatic endothelial stress after preservation/reperfusion. High biliary ET levels could be involved in the mediation of functional cholestatic syndromes after OLT.

Key words Endothelin/big-endothelin · bile · Liver transplantation · Cholestasis · Motility

Introduction

Endothelin-1 (ET) and its precursor big-endothelin (big-ET) are secreted by endothelial cells and have vascular, non-vascular, autocrine, and hormonal effects. Most striking is a strong contractile effect on smooth muscle cells and vasculature. Multiple unspecific stimuli such as ischemia, hypoxia, mechanical stress or inflammation have been shown to induce ET generation in endothelial cells of ubiquitous location [17, 23]. Hepatic ET secretion has been documented by autoradiographic studies, liver cell cultures, and perfusion experiments. The liver appears to be a major site for ET clearance from systemic circulation by receptor binding and cellu-

lar incorporation [1, 5]. Whether biliary excretion of ET peptides is a relevant ET clearance mechanism has not been fully investigated. The existence, source, and physiological relevance of ET peptides in human bile are still controversially discussed in the literature [10]. We have recently published the detection of comparably high concentrations of both ET and big-ET in human bile after orthotopic liver transplantation (OLT), which can be interpreted as a model of severe hepatic endothelial stress [15]. To clarify the influence of liver transplantation on the levels and composition of ET peptides in bile secretion, we have compared biliary ET/big-ET concentrations detected after OLT with levels measured in non-transplant patients. As ET measurement in bile extracts by radioimmunoassay (RIA) has not been validated in detail, a separation of ET peptides in bile by high-pressure liquid chromatography (HPLC) was performed, comparing elution profiles of bile extracts with purified ET/big-ET peptides.

Materials, patients and methods

Bile samples

Bile samples were collected from two distinct clinical groups (Table 1). Samples were obtained from 37 liver transplant recipients in the early postoperative course (days 1–5) after OLT (two samples per patient) and from 39 patients during elective cholecystectomy for treatment of symptomatic cholecystolithiasis. A total of 113 bile samples was analyzed. Samples in transplant recipients were obtained by sterile syringe aspiration from the bile drain, which was implanted during OLT for stenting of the side-to-side choledocho-choledochostomy. Attention was paid to collect fresh bile only. Bile samples were not taken from the reservoir bag. Samples from non-transplant patients were either obtained by direct puncture of the gall bladder or by aspiration of bile from the common bile duct via canulation of the cystic duct (Table 1).

Patient groups

Indications for OLT included alcoholic cirrhosis ($n = 8$), chronic hepatitis ($n = 12$), cholangio/hepatocellular carcinoma ($n = 7$), primary biliary cirrhosis ($n = 6$), and miscellaneous entities ($n = 4$). Mean patient age was 43 ± 13 years, overall female/male sex ratio was 1:2. UW solution was used for preservation. Mean cold ischemia time was 12 ± 3 h. Postoperative immunosuppression involved methylprednisolone (100 mg/day), azathioprine (2 mg/kg per day), cyclosporine A (blood levels 250–400 mg/dl by HPLC) and FK 506 (0.15 mg/kg i. v.). Indication for cholecystectomy was symptomatic cholecystolithiasis. Inflammation of the gall bladder was graded histologically by a pathologist. Patients were differentiated into the presence ($n = 18$) or absence ($n = 13$) of acute inflammation according to the degree of polynuclear cellular infiltration. Mean patient age was 53 ± 13 years: male/female ratio, 2:3. Patients with empyema were excluded.

ET/big-ET analysis

All bile samples were immediately frozen in sterile polystyrene tubes at $-40\,^{\circ}$C until analysis. ET/big-ET concentration was measured in duplicate in all samples and HPLC fractions by commercial RIA (Biomedica, Austria). Technical details of the RIAs have been published previously [8, 19]. Prior to RIA analysis, ET peptides were extracted from bile samples using preconditioned Sep-Pak-C18 extraction cartridges (Water Millipore) to avoid interference by other plasma components and to enrich the ET peptide component in the sample.

HPLC analysis

Pooled bile from five patients was separated by reversed-phase chromatography. For HPLC injection, dried bile extracts (Speedvac) were redissolved in 0.15 % BSA solution, separated on a Nucleosil 100 5 C18 column (150 × 4 mm; Forschungszentrum Sei-

Table 1 Mean concentrations $\pm$ SD (fmol/ml) of endothelin *(ET-1)* and big ET peptides in human bile in the different clinical groups investigated. All differences were statistically significant. (A versus B $P < 0.001$, A versus C $P < 0.006$, B versus C $P < 0.005$; Wilcoxon test)

Patient groups	Sample aspiration site	ET-1	big-ET
A Liver transplant ($n = 37$)	Common bile duct (bile drain aspiration)	20.9 ± 15	39.2 ± 19
B Cholecystectomy ($n = 8$)	Common bile duct (cystic duct canulation)	5.7 ± 4.9	12.1 ± 8
C Cholecystectomy ($n = 31$)	Gall bladder (direct puncture)	61.7 ± 41	75.4 ± 28

bersdorf, Austria), and fractions monitored at 1-min intervals with a UV/visible detector (absorption 214 nm). The concentration of ET/big-ET in separated bile extracts was analyzed in all HPLC fractions (volume 1 ml) and compared with elution profiles of purified ET/big-ET peptides. The retention time for ET-1 (fractions 1–38) was 15.5 min, for big-ET (fragments 22–38) was 25.8 min.

Statistical analysis

Data are presented as mean values $\pm$ SD. ET values in different groups were compared by the Wilcoxon signed rank test. Correlation between ET and big-ET was analyzed by linear regression. P values > 0.05 were considered statistically significant.

Results

ET and big-ET peptides were detected in all human bile samples investigated. Mean ET and big-ET levels measured in bile, drained from the common bile duct in the early postoperative course after OLT, were significantly higher compared to levels detected in the common bile duct during cholecystectomy in non-transplant patients. Highest ET/big-ET levels were measured in bile, directly aspirated from the gall bladder. Levels in the gall bladder markedly exceeded levels detected in the common bile duct in both groups. Mean levels of ET and big-ET detected in the different groups investigated are shown in Table 1.

Biliary big-ET concentration always exceeded synchronous biliary ET concentration. Synchronous biliary ET and big-ET levels were correlated by linear regression in all bile compartments and patient groups analyzed (transplant patients, $r = 0.79$, $P > 0.001$; non-transplant patients, bile duct values, $r = 0.6$, $P < 0.04$, common bile duct values, $r = 0.8$, $P < 0.0001$). ET levels in the gall bladder did not correlate with the grade of histological inflammation.

Chromatographic characterization of bile extracts by reversed-phase HPLC revealed identical elution profiles for biliary ET, synthetic human ET, and big-ET (fractions 23–27). Separation of bile extracts by HPLC and analysis of fractions by RIA thus reveals the exis-

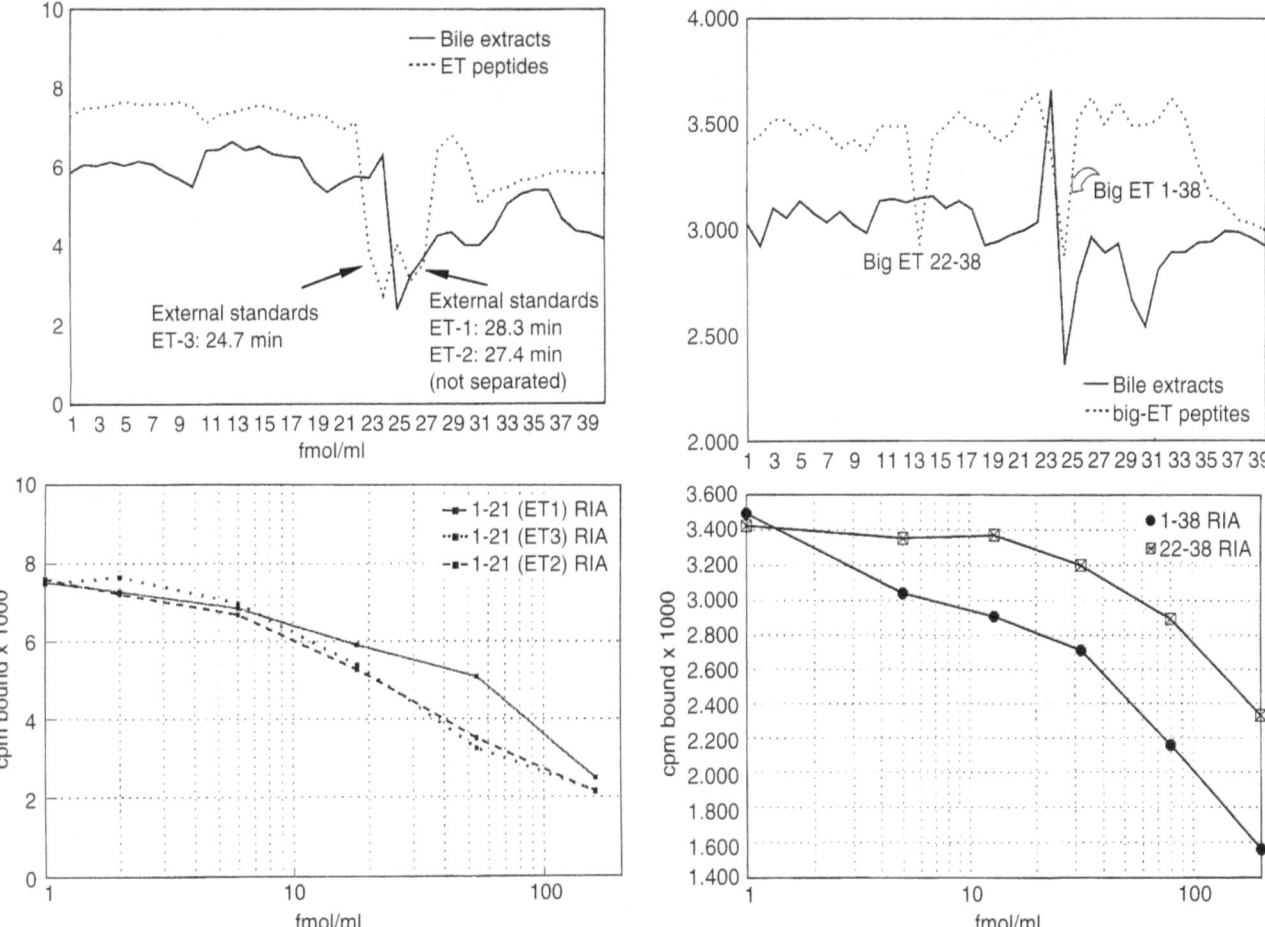

Fig. 1 Elution profiles of purified endothelin *(ET)* peptides *(dotted line)* and ET in bile extracts *(solid line)* after HPLC separation. *Below,* standard curves of bound radioactivity (percentage of total activity) of the radioimmunoassays *(RIAs)* used for ET analysis in HPLC fractions. Total ET immunoreactivity was 135 fmol/ml

Fig. 2 Elution profiles of purified big-ET *(dotted line)* and big-ET in bile extracts *(solid line)* after HPLC separation. *Below,* standard curves of bound radioactivity (percentage of total activity) of the RIAs used for big-ET/big-ET fragment analysis in HPLC fractions. Total big-ET immunoreactivity was 29 fmol/ml

tence of high amounts of ET and big-ET in human bile. Biliary ET mostly represents ET-1. No big-ET (fragment 22–38) could be detected in human bile. Additional elution signals were found in all assays in fractions 29–34, particularly in the big-ET RIA. Elution profiles of ET and big-ET peptides, including standard curves of the purified peptides are shown in Figs. 1 and 2.

Discussion

Only limited research has so far been focussed on the physiology and source of ET peptides in human bile. We know that cultured human epithelial cells of the gall bladder, intra- and extrahepatic bile ducts, and epithelial lining cells of hepatic cysts are able to synthesize and secrete ET [10]. These findings suggest that ET is locally produced in the biliary tract in vivo and secreted

into the bile duct system by a paracrine route. Whether hepatic ET clearance by biliary excretion is a relevant mechanism has not been fully investigated. As all isoforms of ET are potent contractile agonists for smooth muscle cells in a wide variety of tissues, including the gall bladder and bile ducts, biliary ET levels could possess a physiological role in the regulation of choledochal motility and gall bladder contraction [3, 9, 11, 12, 21]. No reference values for ET levels in bile from different clinical groups have been available so far. The specific influence of OLT on biliary ET/big-ET levels could therefore only be estimated. In the current study we have shown that mean ET concentrations in bile collected from the common bile duct during the early postoperative period after OLT significantly exceeded mean ET levels detected during cholecystectomy in nontransplant patients.

Increased biliary levels after OLT could either reflect endothelial stress of the liver graft after cold preservation and reperfusion [6, 7, 20] or just mirror elevated systemic postoperative ET levels and hepatic ET clearance functions. Systemic ET levels after OLT have been previosly investigated by various authors [13, 14, 16, 22]. Published levels in systemic circulation were far lower than biliary concentrations detected after OLT [15]. The fact that biliary ET levels in patients with symptomatic cholecystolithiasis also proved to be significantly lower, despite the regular presence of marked epithelial inflammation, suggests a dominant sinusoidal endothelial generation of biliary ET peptides within the liver graft. As a marked concentration gradient from gall bladder to the common bile duct was found, any future comparison of biliary ET levels in different groups should always refer to the exact source of the bile sample investigated. Pathological grading of histological gall bladder inflammation did not correlate with biliary ET levels. The remarkable quantity of ET peptides detected in the gall bladder can most probably be explained by a secondary concentration effect, caused by active epithelial water resorbtion. Biliary ET and big-ET levels were significantly correlated by linear regression in transplant and non-transplant patients, both in the common bile duct and gall bladder compartments. As big-ET is the precursor of ET, and in the case of local generation usually found in equimolar concentration [17, 23], this again points to the predominance of local hepatic ET generation. Cyclosporine could have modified biliary ET levels, as it is known to produce cholestasis and, furthermore, has been reported to increase ET levels. ET may thus potentiate the cholestatic action of cyclosporine [2, 4, 14, 18].

According to the HPLC elution profiles of ET peptides in bile extracts, ET peptides measured in human bile probably mostly represent ET-1. A clearcut differentiation between ET-1, -2 and -3 would have required the further separation of fractions 23–27, necessitating the analysis of a further extended bile volume. The additional signals in HPLC fractions 29–34 most probably represent ET propeptides or aggregates and not unidentified ET metabolites, as the peaks could also be detected in a big-ET ELISA system (our unpublished data). The HPLC elution profiles detected demonstrate the validity of the RIAs used for analysis of bile extracts.

Biliary ET secretion could be associated with, if not causative of, a large variety of functional cholestatic syndromes associated with various hepatic disorders or occasionally encountered in the postoperative course after OLT. Whether there is a diagnostic or even prognostic value of single or repetitive ET measurements in bile after OLT for estimation of the individual patient's course or for characterization of graft function and preservation damage, should now be investigated in more detail.

References

1. Anggard E, Galton S, Rae G (1989) The fate of radioiodinated endothelin-1 and endothelin-3 in the rat. J Cardiovasc Pharmacol 13: 31140–31143
2. Benigni A, Morigi M, Perico N (1992) The acute effect of FK506 and cyclosporine on endothelial cell function and renal vascular resistance. Transplantation 54: 775–780
3. Bluhm RE, Frazer MG, Vore M, Pinson CW, Badr KF (1993) Endothelins 1 and 3: potent cholestatic agents secreted and excreted by the liver that interact with cyclosporine. Hepatology 18: 961–968
4. Copeland KR, Yatscoff RW (1992) Comparison of the effects of cyclosporine and its metabolites on the release of prostacyclin and endothelin from mesangial cells. Transplantation 53: 640–645
5. Fukuroda T, Fujikawa T, Ozaki S, Ishikawa K, Yano M, Nishikibe M (1994) Clearance of circulating endothelin-1 by ETB receptors in rats. Biochem Biophys Res Commun 199: 1461–1465
6. Gianello P, Fishbein J, Besse T, Gustin T, Chatzopoulos C, Ketelslegers JM, Lambotte L, Squifflet JP (1994) Measurement of the vasoconstrictive substances endothelin, angiotensin II, and thromboxane B2 in cold storage solution can reveal previous renal ischemic insults. Transplant 7: 11–16
7. Goto M, Takei Y, Kawano S, Nagano K, Tsuji S, Masuda E, Nishimura Y, Okumura S, Kashiwagi T (1994) Endothelin-1 is involved in the pathogenesis of ischemia/reperfusion liver injury by hepatic microcirculatory disturbances. Hepatology 19: 675–681
8. Hartter E, Woloszczuk W (1989) Radioimmunoassay of endothelin. Lancet 22: 909
9. Housset C, Rockey DC, Bissell DM (1993) Endothelin receptors in rat liver: lipocytes as a contractile target for endothelin-1. Proc Natl Acad Sci USA 90: 9266–9270
10. Housset C, Carayon A, Housset B, Legendre C, Hannoun L, Poupon R (1993) Endothelin-1 secretion by human gallbladder epithelial cells in primary culture. Lab Invest 69: 750–755
11. Isales CM, Nathanson MH, Bruck R (1993) Endothelin-1 induces cholestasis which is mediated by an increase in portal pressure. Biochem Biophys Res Commun 191: 1244–1251
12. Kamimura Y, Sawada N, Aoki M, Mori M (1993) Endothelin-1 induces contraction of bile canaliculi in isolated rat hepatocytes. Biochem Biophys Res Commun 191: 817–822
13. Kraus T, Mehrabi A, Klar E, Mathias D, Arnold J, Otto G, Herfarth Ch (1992) Peri- and postoperative plasma kinetics of big endothelin and endothelin 1/2 after liver transplantation. Transplant Proc 24: 2569–2571
14. Kraus Th, Mehrabi A, Klar E, Arnold J, Sido B, Otto G, Herfarth Ch (1994) Intraoperative evaluation of big-endothelin plasma levels during liver transplantation in different vascular compartments. Transplant Int 7 (Suppl 1): 144–149

15. Kraus Th, Klee F, Mehrabi A, Bleyl J, Klar E, Otto G, Herfarth Ch (1995) Endothelin 1/2 and big-endothelin concentrations in bile samples during the early postoperative period after orthotopic liver transplantation. Transplant Proc 27: 1258–1260

16. Lerman A, Click RL, Narr BJ, Wiesner RH, Krom RA, Textor SC, Burnett J (1991) Elevation of plasma endothelin associated with systemic hypertension in humans following orthotopic liver transplantation. Transplantation 51: 646–650

17. Masaki T (1993) Endothelins: homeostatic and compensatory actions in the circulatory and endocrine system. Endocrine Rev 14: 256–268

18. Mouquet C, Benalia H, Carayon A, Bitker MO, Luciani J, Viars P (1994) Is the vasoconstrictive effect of cyclosporine mediated by endothelin in kidney transplantation? Transplant Proc 26: 277–278

19. Schuller M, Stetter R, Skrabal S, Missbichler A, Woloszczuk W, Hartter E (1991) Radioimmunoassay of immunoreactive C-terminal big-endothelin. Eur J Clin Chem Clin Biochem 29: 147–150

20. Stansby G, Fuller B, Jeremy J, Cheetham K, Rolles K (1993) Endothelin release – a facet of reperfusion injury in clinical liver transplantation? Transplantation 56: 239–240

21. Tanaka A, Katagiri K, Hoshino M, Hayakawa T, Takeuchi T (1994) Endothelin-1 stimulates bile acid secretion and vesicular transport in the isolated perfused rat liver. Am J Physiol 266: 1–12

22. Textor SC, Wilson DJ, Lerman A, Romero JC, Burnett J, Wiesner R, Dickson ER, Krom RA (1992) Renal hemodynamics, urinary eicosanoids, and endothelin after liver transplantation. Transplantation 54: 74–80

23. Yanagisawa M, Kurihara H, Kimura S, Tomobe Y, Kobayashi M, Mitsiu Y, Yazaki Y, Goto K, Masaki T (1988) A novel potent vasoconstrictor peptide produces by vascular endothelial cells. Nature 332: 411–414

Transpl Int (1996) 9 [Suppl 1]: S 140–S 143
© Springer-Verlag 1996

LIVER

E. Klar
T. Kraus
M. Bredt
B. Osswald
N. Senninger
C. Herfarth
G. Otto

First clinical realization of continuous monitoring of liver microcirculation after transplantation by thermodiffusion

E. Klar (✉) · T. Kraus · M. Bredt ·
B. Osswald · N. Senninger · C. Herfarth ·
G. Otto
Chirurgische Universitätsklinik, University
of Heidelberg, Im Neuenheimer Feld 110,
D-69115 Heidelberg, Germany,
Tel. +49 6221 566202; Fax +49 6221 411666

Abstract To date, no method is available for the continuous long-term monitoring of liver microcirculation in patients. Experimentally, thermodiffusion has been validated in the quantification of hepatic perfusion. In an attempt to investigate the practicability of thermodiffusion technology in patients after liver transplantation thermodiffusion probes were inserted into the graft in seven patients during liver transplantation. Continous monitoring started intraoperatively and was performed until day 7, when the probes were extracted transcutaneously. No probe-related complications (i.e., hemorrhage, infection) were observed. In four patients with normal graft function, liver perfusion recovered within 12 h from the intraoperative reduction to a range between 85 and 93 ml/100 g per min. In contrast, primary graft failure ($n = 1$) was characterized by a con-

stant decrease of hepatic perfusion (< 50 ml/100 g per min). In prolonged reperfusion injury ($n = 1$), a second peak of transaminases was paralled by an impairment of liver microcirculation. In one patient, R2 rejection on day 7 was preceded by a drop in hepatic perfusion 48 h earlier. Thus, thermodiffusion is a safe and reliable method for the continuous quantification of liver microcirculation after transplantation in patients. Measurements are reproducible for at least 7 days. Changes in hepatic perfusion during postoperative complications can be detected. The characteristics of microcirculatory disorders will have to be defined in a larger number of patients.

Key words Liver transplantation · Liver microcirculation · Thermodiffusion · Clinical monitoring · Liver graft function

Introduction

Hepatic microcirculation plays a pathophysiological key role during the early postoperative phase after liver transplantation [1]. The methods currently available for the assessment of liver perfusion preclude clinical application after abdominal closure. We have recently validated a newly developed thermodiffusion probe allowing for continuous monitoring of the hepatic microcirculation for at least 1 week postoperatively [2]. In the present study we tested the clinical practicability of the thermodiffusion method with regard to the assessment of liver perfusion after transplantation.

Patients and methods

The study was approved by the Ethics Committee of the Medical Faculty of Heidelberg and complied with the Declaration of Helsinki. Before surgery a written consent to implant the probes was obtained from each patient. One thermodiffusion probe was inserted into liver segment IV B of seven patients and exited transcutaneously during liver transplantation 60 min after arterial reperfusion. The mean age of the patients was 40 years ranging, from

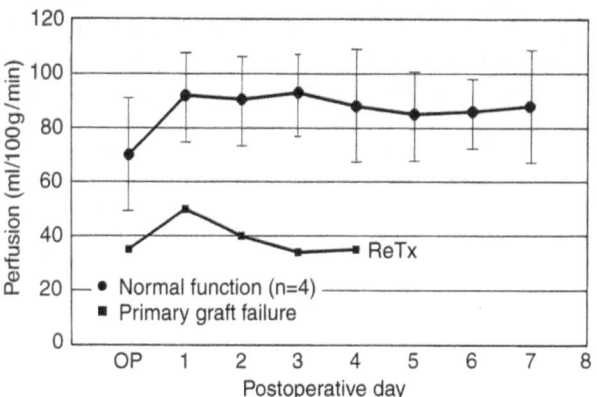

Fig. 1 Hepatic perfusion after liver transplantation. The upper curve represents four patients with normal graft function (*n* = 4). After an intraoperative reduction, liver perfusion increased within 12 h to a near-normal level, which was maintained during 7 days postoperatively. In contrast, primary graft failure was characterized by a primary reduction in liver perfusion without tendency to recover. (*Re Tx* Retransplantation)

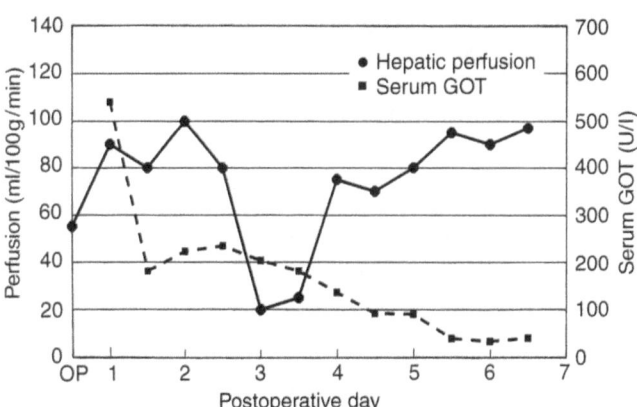

Fig. 2 Hepatic perfusion and serum GOT in a patient developing a second peak of serum transaminases after reperfusion. The increase of GOT is paralleled by a reduction in liver perfusion. Simultaneous normalization of both parameters following day 4 continued with an uneventful course thereafter

14 to 60 years. The underlying liver disease for transplantation was alcoholic cirrhosis (*n* = 3), cirrhosis due to autoimmune hepatitis (*n* = 1), acute liver failure of unknown etiology (*n* = 1), fulminant hepatitis B (*n* = 1), and fibrolamellar carcinoma (*n* = 1). Four patients had an uneventful postoperative course. In one patient, primary graft failure occurred, necessitating retransplantation on postoperative day 5. One patient developed early rejection on day 7, proven by biopsy. In one patient, a prolonged reperfusion injury was documented by a second peak of transaminases on day 2. The probe was extracted on postoperative day 7; a swab was taken for bacteriology.

The mechanism of thermodiffusion technology (Thermal Technologies, Cambridge, Mass.) as used in this study is the quantification of heating power required to maintain a temperature increment of 2 °C above the surrounding tissue. Thermal conductivity by local perfusion can be calculated from the difference of the effective thermal conductivity minus the intrinsic conductivity. The probe (diameter 0.9 mm) has a self-heated thermal transducer at the tip as well as a thermistor, 7 mm proximal. The intraparenchymal radius of measurement is dependent on the quality of perfusion: 2.7 mm at fast capillary flow, 4.5 mm under low flow conditions. Continuous monitoring of perfusion is based on one measurements. Perfusion data are displayed as mean values of 20-min sampling periods.

Results

Normal function (*n* = 4)

There was an increase in hepatic perfusion from 70 ± 20 ml/100 g per min to 92 ± 17 ml/100 g per min during a 12-h period after reperfusion. Liver perfusion was recorded within a stable range between 85 ± 17 ml/100 g per min and 93 ± 16 ml/100 g per min until the end of the observation period (Fig. 1).

Primary graft failure (*n* = 1)

Hepatic perfusion was primarily reduced without tendency to recover until retransplantation (34–50 ml/100 g per min (Fig. 1).

Prolonged reperfusion injury (*n* = 1)

After initial recovery of liver perfusion to 90 ml/100 g per min, a secondary reduction to 21 ml/100 g per min was recorded on day 3, in parallel with a second peak of transaminases. After normalization of transaminases and liver perfusion, the postoperative course was uneventful (Fig. 2).

Rejection (*n* = 1)

Intraoperatively, as well as during postoperative days 1–4, liver perfusion was comparable to the patient group with normal graft function. On day 5, a considerable reduction in perfusion from 80 to 35 ml/100 g per min was recorded. Due to a rise in transaminases on day 7, a liver biopsy was performed revealing R2 rejection (Fig. 3).

All patients

On day 7, extraction of the probe was performed without complications. Bacterial contamination of the probe could be excluded in all patients.

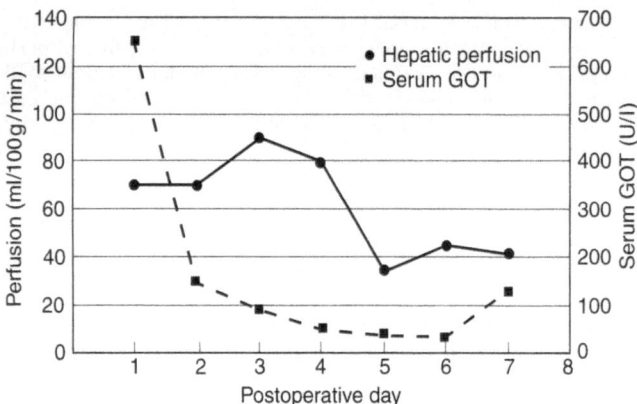

Fig. 3 Drastic reduction of liver perfusion on day 5 after transplantation. Increase of serum GOT on day 7. Liver biopsy revealed R2 rejection

Discussion

Thermodiffusion has been previously validated in pigs as a reliable method for the continuous monitoring of hepatic microcirculation following liver transplantation [2]. The measurements at baseline conditions as well as during intermittent occlusion of hepatic artery and/or portal vein were reproducible during the observation period of 7 days.

The main finding of the current study is that the clinical application of thermodiffusion is reliable and safe. No complications (e.g., hemorrhage) were observed during insertion or extraction of the probes. The measurements in the group of patients with normal graft function followed the characteristic pattern observed from experimental studies in pigs [2, 3]. Hepatic perfusion recovered from an initial reduction to stable values between 85 and 93 ml/100 g per min over subsequent days. Total liver blood flow in man, as measured by portal venous and hepatic arterial flow, has been reported to be 120 ml/100 g per min [4]. The difference in liver perfusion recorded here could well be explained by an increase of shunt perfusion via arterioportal-venous anastomoses visualized in the rat by scanning electron microscopy [5] and documented functionally in man [6]. By means of H2-clearance, shunt perfusion has been shown to increase to 38 % of total liver blood flow early after reperfusion in pigs [7].

A constant reduction of liver perfusion was recorded in primary graft failure from the first measurement intraoperatively until retransplantation on day 5. This finding is consistent with the angiographic picture encountered in primary graft failure, the "leafless-tree" phenomenon, i.e., failure to visualize peripheral arterial branches in the liver parenchyma as a result of an increase in intracapsular pressure with subsequent parenchymal necrosis [8]. One patient in our study developed a second peak of transaminases after an initial continuous decrease, which was ascribed to prolonged preservation injury. In parallel, a decrease in hepatic perfusion was recorded by thermodiffusion for 2 days, followed by normalization of both parameters. One patient developed early acute rejection, which was suspected by a rise in transaminases on postoperative day 7 and confirmed (R2) by biopsy. In fact, on day 5, a decrease of hepatic perfusion was noted.

Injury of hepatic sinusoidal endothelium is the primary effect of ischemia-reperfusion injury and has been documented by conventional and scanning electron microscopy [9–12]. So far, functional assessment of hepatic microcirculation has been performed mainly experimentally by means of intravital microscopy [13, 14], laser doppler flowmetry [15], and gas clearance techniques using [85]Kr [4, 16] or hydrogen [3]. Intravital microscopy is not applicable clinically; laser doppler flowmetry, [85]Kr, and hydrogen clearance can only be used intraoperatively. Other clearance techniques, such as the use of indocyanine green [4, 17], represent indirect methods measuring total liver blood flow but not perfusion and are restricted to single measurements. Intraparenchymal laser doppler flowmetry has the drawback of covering only a small surface range of the liver tissue (1–2 mm³), which may not be representative in the presence of redistribution phenomena, as documented after reperfusion [18]. In contrast, a larger tissue volume is integrated by thermodiffusion measurements ranging between 82 and 381 mm³ in a flow-dependent fashion. Recently, an extractable autofocus doppler flow probe has been described allowing continuous blood flow measurement of hepatic artery and portal vein after liver transplantation in man [19]. Possible risks of the method originate from the mechanical irritation of the blood vessels: induction of vasospasm or kinking, with subsequent thrombosis.

In summary, it could be demonstrated that thermodiffusion is clinically applicable to the continuous monitoring of liver perfusion after transplantation. In accordance with the experimental validation of the method, measurements are reproducible for at least 1 week postoperatively. Hemorrhage upon extraction or contamination of the probe has not been encountered so far. Changes of liver perfusion in connection with reperfusion injury, primary graft failure, or rejection can be detected. Characteristic patterns of capillary flow impairment have to be evaluated in a larger series of patients with complicated postoperative course. Thermodiffusion is a promising method to further define the pathophysiological role of hepatic microcirculation after liver transplantation in man.

References

1. Kim YI, Kai T, Kawano T, et al (1992) Predictive value of liver tissue flow in assessment of the viability of liver grafts after extended preservation in pigs. Transplant Int 5 (Suppl 1): S382–S387
2. Klar E, Kraus T, Bleyl J, et al (1995) Thermodiffusion as a novel method for continuous monitoring of hepatic microcirculation after liver transplantation. Transplant Proc 27: 2610–2612
3. Manner M, Schult W, Senninger N et al (1990) Evaluation of preservation damage after porcine liver transplantation by assessment of hepatic microcirculation. Transplantation 50: 940–943
4. Mathie RT, Nagorney DM, Blumgart LH (1989) Liver blood flow: physiology, measurement and clinical relevance. Anat Pathophysiol 98: 73–87
5. Yamamoto K, Sherman I, Phillips MJ, Fisher MM (1985) Three-dimensional observations of the hepatic arterial terminations in rat, hamster and human liver by scanning electron microscopy of microvascular casts. Hepatology 5: 452–456
6. Hoefs JC, Reynolds TB, Pare P, Sakimura I (1984) A new method for the measurement of intrahepatic shunts. J Lab Clin Med 103: 446–461
7. Manner M, Senninger N, Thies J, et al (1991) Intrahepatic shunt predicts graft function after liver transplantation in pigs. In: Engemann R, Hamelman H (eds) Experimental and clinical liver transplantation. Elsevier Science Publishers, Amsterdam, pp 83–86
8. Hermann A, Hoffmann V, Richter GM, et al (1995) The leafless tree sign: a specific angiographic finding after liver transplantation suggesting acute liver necrosis. Eur Radiol 5: S242–243
9. Caldwell-Kenkel JC, Currin RT, Tanaka Y, et al (1989) Reperfusion injury to endothelial cells following cold ischemic storage of rat livers. Hepatology 10: 292–299
10. Lim PS, Andrews FJ, Christophi C, O'Brien PE (1994) Microvascular changes in liver after ischemia-reperfusion injury. Protection with misoprostol. Dig Dis Sci 39: 1683–1690
11. Thurmann Rg, Marzi I, Seitz G, et al (1988) Hepatic reperfusion injury following orthotopic liver transplantation in the rat. Transplantation 46: 502–506
12. Jaeschke H, Farhood A (1991) Neutrophil and Kupffer cell induced oxidant stress and ischemia-reperfusion injury in rat liver. Am J Physiol 260: G355–G362
13. Marzi I, Takei Y, Knee J, et al (1990) Assessment of reperfusion injury by intravital fluorescence microscopy following liver transplantation in the rat. Transplant Proc 22: 2004–2005
14. Post S, Palma P, Rentsch M, et al (1993) Differential impact of Carolina rinse and University of Wisconsin solutions on microcirculation, leukocyte adhesion, Kupffer cell activity and biliary excretion after liver transplantation. Hepatology 18: 1490–1497
15. Wheatley AM, Zhao D (1993) Intraoperative assessment by laser doppler flowmetry of hepatic perfusion during orthotopic liver transplantation in the rat. Transplantation 56: 1315–1318
16. Leibermann DP, Mathie RT, Harper AM, Blumgart LH (1978) The hepatic arterial and portal venous circulations of the liver studied with a krypton-85 clearance technique. J Surg Res 25: 154–162
17. Altmayer P, Grundmann U, Ziehmer M, et al (1991) Cardiac output and liver blood flow in humans: effect of the volatile anesthetic halothane. Methods Find Exp Clin Pharmacol 13: 709–714
18. Sheperd AP, Riedel GL, Kiel JW, et al (1987) Evaluation of an infrared laser-Doppler blood flowmeter. Am J Physiol 252: G832–G839
19. Zurbrügg HR, De P, Bachmann S, et al (1994) Continous blood flow measurements after liver transplantation: first clinical experience. Transplant Proc 26: 2218–2226

Transpl Int (1996) 9 [Suppl 1]: S 144–S 150
© Springer-Verlag 1996

Two-year data from the European multicentre tacrolimus (FK 506) liver study

Roger Williams
Peter Neuhaus
Henri Bismuth
Paul McMaster
Rudolf Pichlmayr
Roy Calne
Gerd Otto
Carl Groth

R. Williams (✉)
Institute of Liver Studies, King's College
Hospital, London SE5 9PJ, UK
Fax +44 171 346 3167

P. Neuhaus
Virchow-Klinikum, Universitätsklinikum
der Humboldt-Universität, Berlin,
Germany

H. Bismuth
Centre Hepato-Biliaire, Hôpital Paul
Brousse, Villejuif, France

P. McMaster
The Liver and Hepatobiliary Unit, Queen
Elizabeth Hospital, Birmingham, UK

R. Pichlmayr
Klinik für Abdominal- und
Transplantationschirurgie, Medizinische
Hochschule, Hannover, Germany

R. Calne
Department of Surgery, Addenbrooke's
Hospital, Cambridge, UK

G. Otto
Chirurgische Klinik, Ruprecht-Karls-
Universität, Heidelberg, Germany

C. G. Groth
Department of Transplantation Surgery,
Huddinge Hospital, Stockholm, Sweden

Abstract To provide a more definitive assessment of the efficacy and safety of tacrolimus therapy in comparison with cyclosporin, the extended follow-up of the European multicentre study is reported. Two-year Kaplan-Meier estimates indicated significant reductions in acute (tacrolimus 45.4 %, cyclosporin 55.8 %; $P = 0.006$), refractory (1.2 % versus 6.4 %; $P = 0.003$) and chronic rejection (2.0 % versus 6.9 %; $P = 0.015$) despite significantly lower steroid usage in patients receiving tacrolimus therapy. Patient and graft survival rates (80.6 % versus 74.8 % and 74.5 % versus 70.0 %, respectively) were also superior, although these failed to reach statistical significance. Safety profiles were comparable for most major categories (including renal, neurological and glucose metabolic disorders) and in certain aspects were more favourable for tacrolimus. Hypertension (28.0 % versus 39.6 %, $P < 0.01$) and cytomegalovirus infection (14.8 % versus 22.3 %, $P < 0.01$), two events with important long-term clinical consequences, were reported signif-icantly less frequently. Hirsutism (0.0 % versus 8.7 %, $P < 0.01$) and gum hyperplasia (0.0 % versus 2.3 %, $P < 0.05$) were absent in patients receiving tacrolimus. Tacrolimus appears to provide effective and safe long-term immunosuppression.

Key words Tacrolimus · Cyclosporin · Comparative study · Primary liver transplantation · Immunosuppressive treatment failure

Introduction

Preliminary clinical studies conducted at the University of Pittsburgh demonstrated that tacrolimus (FK 506) was both safe and effective when administered as primary therapy to liver transplant recipients. Comparison with an historical cohort of cyclosporin-treated controls indicated that tacrolimus therapy was associated with significantly better patient and graft survival rates and a significant reduction in the incidence of rejection [16]. A prospective, controlled study was subsequently undertaken by the same group; patient and graft survival rates at 12 months were reported to be 93 % and 90 %, respectively, for patients receiving tacrolimus therapy compared with 81 % and 70 % for the cyclosporin control group [8].

Based on these encouraging results, two international, open-label, multicentre, randomised comparative studies were conducted (one in Europe and the second in the United States). Their objective was to compare the efficacy and safety of tacrolimus- and cyclosporin-based therapy in patients undergoing primary liver transplantation. Details of the results at both 6 months [2, 4, 5, 9, 11, 12, 17] and 1 year [1, 3, 6, 7, 10, 14, 15] have been published previously. This report presents the continued follow-up of the 529 patients evaluated in the European multicentre trial.

Methods

Patient eligibility

This study was conducted at eight centres in four European countries (France, Germany, Sweden and the United Kingdom). Male and female patients, 18–70 years of age, with end-stage liver disease requiring transplantation were eligible for entry. Patients were excluded if they had serological evidence of HIV, diagnoses of active neoplastic disease or primary liver cancer with evidence of metastases, arteritis or vasculitis, if they were undergoing multiple organ transplantation or had previously received a liver allograft. Women who were pregnant or who were using inadequate contraceptive measures were also excluded. Formal approval for the conduct of the study was obtained from the ethics committees of the participating centres prior to enrolment and informed consent was received from each patient. This study was performed in accordance with the Declaration of Helsinki.

Prior to transplantation, patients were equally and randomly assigned to treatment within centres. Patients were stratified for the presence of fulminant hepatic failure. Treatment consisted of either tacrolimus and low-dose steroids or the optimal, centre-specific cyclosporin-based regimen (cyclosporin, azathioprine, steroids ± ALG). Full details of the immunosuppressive regimens administered have been published previously [1, 6].

Evaluation of efficacy and safety: statistical analysis

The primary efficacy variables were the incidences of acute, refractory acute and chronic rejection, steroid usage, and patient and graft survival. Safety was assessed in terms of spontaneously reported adverse events and/or significant changes in laboratory parameters, irrespective of any causality in relation to the study medication.

The sample size (414 evaluable patients, 207 per treatment group) was calculated to detect a 10 % difference in survival rates at 12 months between tacrolimus- and cyclosporin-treated patients with a power of at least 80 % (log-rank test), assuming an 80 % 1-year survival rate for patients receiving conventional therapy. The time to the first biopsy-proven rejection, and patient and graft survival were summarised by Kaplan-Meier methodology; differences between the survival curves were analysed with the generalised Wilcoxon test. The incidences of rejection were compared with the Cochran-Mantel-Haenszel procedure, the Mann-Whitney U-test was used to compare cumulative steroid doses and Fisher's exact test was applied to test for any differences in adverse event incidence rates.

Results

Five hundred and forty-five patients (294 men, 251 women, aged 15–68 years) were enrolled into this study between September 1990 and February 1992. Sixteen of these patients (tacrolimus 5, cyclosporin 11) did not receive study medication and were excluded from the efficacy analysis. A further 5 patients were misrandomised (tacrolimus 3, cyclosporin 2); data from these patients were evaluated and were attributed to the treatment that they received. The population for analysis, therefore, constituted 529 patients, 264 of whom received treatment with tacrolimus and 265 with cyclosporin.

The mean age of the patients was similar for both treatment groups although the proportion of male and female patients differed ($P = 0.021$). The two treatment groups were well matched in terms of baseline characteristics (primary diagnoses, stage of hepatic encephalopathy, urgency of transplant, mean donor age, assessment of liver prior to reperfusion, total ischaemia time and preservation fluid utilised).

The median oral tacrolimus dose administered was progressively reduced throughout the course of the study (month 1: 0.152 mg/kg; months 2–3: 0.142 mg/kg; months 4–6: 0.116 mg/kg; months 7–12: 0.089 mg/kg; months 13–18: 0.073 mg/kg; months 19–24: 0.069 mg/kg). A similar decline in median oral cyclosporin doses was also noted changing from 8.01 mg/kg during month 1 to 3.47 mg/kg for the 19–24-month period.

Two hundred and nine patients (39.5 %) were withdrawn from the study during the 24-month treatment period [tacrolimus 98 (37.1 %), cyclosporin 111 (41.9 %)], 19 of whom were withdrawn between months 13 and 24 [tacrolimus 11 (4.2 %), cyclosporin 8 (3.0 %)]. The proportion of patients withdrawn as a result of experiencing adverse events was marginally higher in the tacrolimus treatment group than in patients receiving cyclosporin therapy [tacrolimus 82 (31.1 %), cyclosporin 67 (25.3 %)]. In contrast, the number of patients withdrawn as a result of 'intractable' rejection was significantly lower in the tacrolimus treatment group [tacrolimus 7 (2.7 %), cyclosporin 27 (10.2 %); $P < 0.001$].

Efficacy analysis

Rejection

Kaplan-Meier estimates of the primary efficacy endpoints at 24 months indicated that there were significant reductions in the incidences of acute (Fig. 1, $P = 0.006$), refractory acute ($P = 0.003$) and chronic rejection ($P = 0.015$) for patients receiving tacrolimus therapy.

A total of 285 acute rejection episodes were reported (tacrolimus 133, cyclosporin 152), 204 of which were ex-

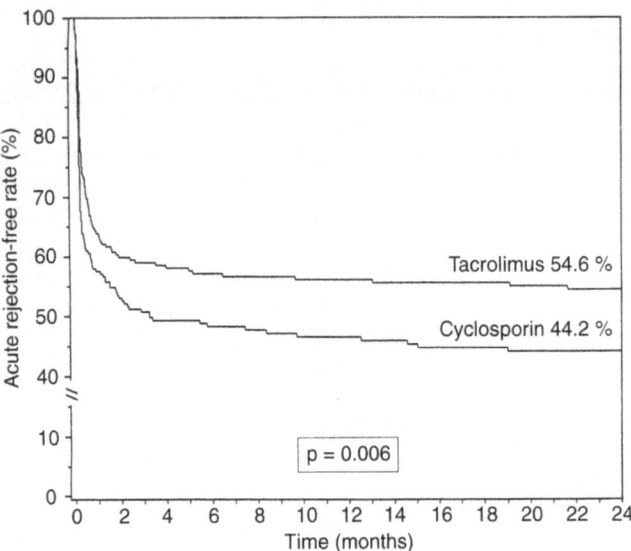

Fig. 1 Kaplan-Meier estimates of patients with acute rejection

Table 1 Immunosuppressive treatment failures

	Number of patients (%)		P value
	Tacrolimus	Cyclosporin	
Refractory acute rejection	3 (1.1)	16 (6.0)	0.005
Chronic rejection	4 (1.5)	14 (5.3)	0.032

Table 2 Steroid usage

Prednisone dose (mg per day)	Percentage of patients	
	Tacrolimus (n = 166)	Cyclosporin (n = 153)
0	48.2	22.9
> 0–≤ 2.5	6.6	14.4
> 2.5–≤ 5.0	24.1	30.7
> 5.0–≤ 7.5	4.8	8.5
> 7.5–≤ 10.0	11.4	14.4
> 10.0–≤ 12.5	2.4	3.3
> 12.5–≤ 15.0	1.8	3.3
> 15.0–≤ 20.0	0.0	2.6
> 20.0	0.6	0.0
Mean dose	3.35 ± 4.31	5.16 ± 4.42

treated patients. The severity of these acute rejection episodes, as assessed histologically, was also reduced in patients receiving tacrolimus therapy with fewer patients experiencing grades of moderate, moderate/severe and severe rejection.

Immunosuppressive treatment failures (Table 1)

Thirty cyclosporin-treated patients were classified as immunosuppressive treatment failures (i.e. with diagnoses of either refractory acute or chronic rejection), of whom 14 were converted to tacrolimus therapy, 2 continued to receive treatment with cyclosporin, 11 were retransplanted and 3 died. Of the 14 switched to tacrolimus therapy, 8 were alive with their original graft (including 4 who were converted with histologically-proven chronic rejection), 1 was retransplanted and 5 had died by the end of the 24-month follow-up period. Seven tacrolimus-treated patients were considered to be immunosuppressive treatment failures, 3 of whom were converted to cyclosporin therapy in an attempt to salvage their graft (1 patient died and 2 required retransplanting). Of the remaining 4, 1 patient died, 2 underwent retransplantation (both of whom were alive at the end of the follow-up period), and 1 continued to receive treatment with tacrolimus (again, this patient was alive at month 24).

Steroid usage

The cumulative steroid dose during the 24-month treatment period, administered either as prophylaxis or for the treatment of rejection, was significantly reduced in the tacrolimus treatment group. The median intravenous dose was 21.5 mg/kg for tacrolimus-treated patients and 28.0 mg/kg for patients receiving cyclosporin therapy ($P = 0.028$). Corresponding figures for oral usage were 71.0 mg/kg and 87.6 mg/kg, respectively ($P = 0.008$). Details of the maintenance steroid dose administered at month 24 and the number of patients remaining in the study in whom steroid therapy was successfully withdrawn are presented in Table 2.

Patient and graft survival

Patient death was self-explanatory whereas graft failure reflected the combined losses resulting from retransplantation and/or death. Kaplan-Meier estimates of 24-month patient and graft survival were approximately 5 % higher in patients receiving tacrolimus therapy but this difference failed to reach statistical significance (Fig. 2). One hundred and nineteen deaths were recorded during the 24-month follow-up period, but only

perienced during the first four weeks of treatment (tacrolimus 95, cyclosporin 109). A further 58 episodes (tacrolimus 27, cyclosporin 31) were reported before the end of month 6, 11 (tacrolimus 6, cyclosporin 5) between months 7 and 12, and 12 (tacrolimus 5, cyclosporin 7) between months 13 and 24. Of the 133 episodes of acute rejection experienced by patients receiving tacrolimus therapy, 105 (78.9 %) resolved following treatment with supplemental steroids alone compared with 108 of the 152 episodes (71.1 %) in cyclosporin-

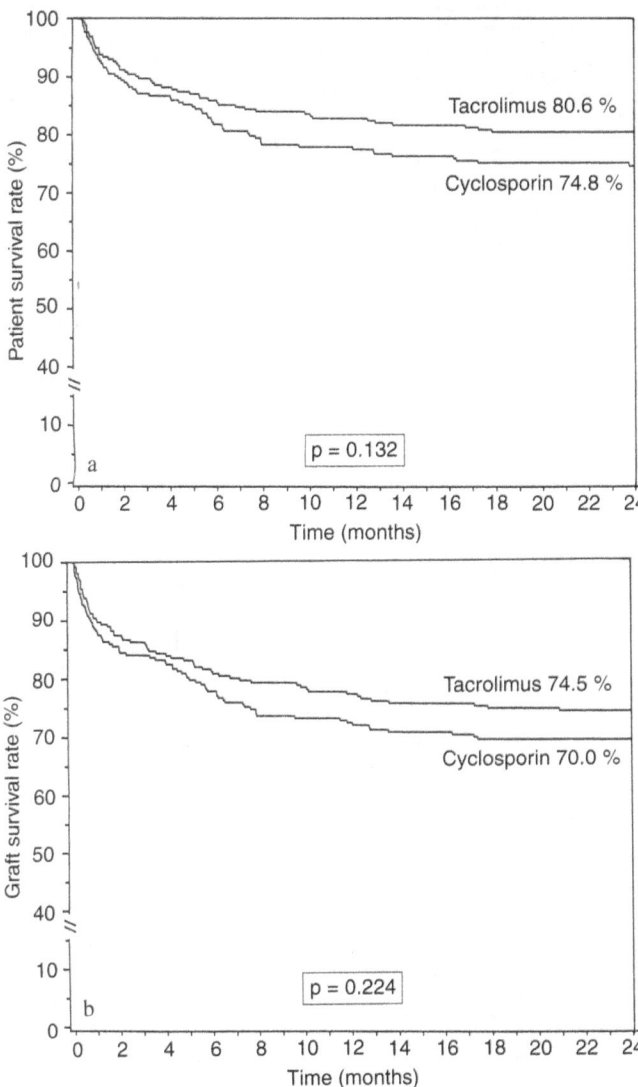

Fig. 2 a, b Kaplan-Meier estimates of **a** patient survival and **b** graft survival for the tacrolimus and cyclosporin treatment groups

Table 3 Causes of patient and graft loss

	Number of patients (%)	
	Tacrolimus ($n = 179$)	Cyclosporin ($n = 166$)
Causes of death		
Bronchopneumonia	0 (0.0)	1 (0.6)
Cardiovascular failure	1 (0.6)	0 (0.0)
Hepatic infarction	0 (0.0)	1 (0.6)
Hepatitis B recurrence	1 (0.6)	0 (0.0)
Hypoxic brain damage	0 (0.0)	1 (0.6)
Metastases – cholangiocarcinoma	0 (0.0)	1 (0.6)
Prolonged septicaemic breakdown	0 (0.0)	1 (0.6)
Recurrent hepatocellular carcinoma	1 (0.6)	3 (1.8)
Septic shock	1 (0.6)	0 (0.0)
Urosepsis	1 (0.6)	0 (0.0)
Causes of graft failure		
Death	4 (2.2)	6 (3.6)
Retransplantation		
Chronic rejection	0 (0.0)	2 (1.2)
Fulminant hepatitis	1 (0.6)	0 (0.0)
Ischaemic-type biliary lesion	1 (0.6)	0 (0.0)
Recurrence of Budd-chiari disease	1 (0.6)	0 (0.0)

13 of these were encountered between months 13 and 24. In total, 57 patients were retransplanted, 25 (9.5%) from the tacrolimus treatment group compared with 32 (12.1%) receiving cyclosporin therapy. Nine of the 25 tacrolimus-treated patients (36.0%) subsequently died compared with 19 of the 32 patients (59.4%) receiving cyclosporin. Causes of patient and graft loss during the second year of the study are listed in Table 3.

Safety analysis

Over the 24-month treatment period, 82 tacrolimus-treated patients (31.1%) experienced adverse events that led to withdrawal compared with 67 patients (25.3%) receiving cyclosporin therapy. The majority of these events occurred within the initial 6-month treatment period (with approximately 50% of these occurring within the first month). Subsequently, 19 patients (tacrolimus 10, cyclosporin 9) were withdrawn between months 7 and 12, and a further 14 (tacrolimus 6, cyclosporin 8) between months 13 and 24.

Adverse event occurrence rates listed below (Tables 4–6) are for those events assessed as being causally related to treatment. Events, for example, reported during month 2 that only subsequently resolved at month 14 would have been counted for the purposes of the analysis during months 2–6, 7–12 and 13–18, respectively.

In terms of the adverse events reported during the second year of this study, there was little difference between the two treatment groups in their incidence, type or nature. No significant differences were observed in the occurrence of abnormal renal function (a term incorporating the COSTART codes abnormal kidney function, and increased creatinine and blood urea concentrations), glucose metabolism disorders (hyperglycaemia and diabetes mellitus combined) and neurological complications (except tremor which was more prevalent in the tacrolimus treatment group between months 13 and 18) (Table 4). Hypertension, however, was experienced by significantly fewer patients receiving tacrolimus therapy both between months 13 and 18, and 19–24.

The incidences of infection and benign and malignant neoplasm were analysed over the 24-month treatment period (Tables 5, 6, respectively). Two of the main clinical categories of infection, namely cholangitis and

Table 4 Frequency of adverse events

Adverse event	Percentage of patients Months 13–18		P value	Percentage of patients Months 19–24		P value
	Tacrolimus (n = 179)	Cyclosporin (n = 166)		Tacrolimus (n = 168)	Cyclosporin (n = 153)	
Renal impairment						
Abnormal renal function	23.5	21.7		20.8	21.6	
Hypertension	19.0	31.9	0.006	18.5	28.8	0.035
Changes in glucose metabolism						
Hyperglycaemia/diabetes mellitus	16.8	11.4		16.1	9.4	
Neurological complications						
Headache	16.2	18.7		20.2	20.9	
Insomnia	5.6	6.6		5.4	1.3	
Paraesthesia	6.1	4.2		4.2	4.6	
Tremor	33.5	18.7	0.002	21.4	16.3	

Table 5 Frequency of infectious complications

Adverse event	Percentage of patients		P value
	Months 1–24		
	Tacrolimus (n = 264)	Cyclosporin (n = 265)	
Cholangitis	14.8	15.8	
Cytomegalovirus infection	14.8	22.3	0.033
Pneumonia	13.6	20.4	
Urinary tract infection	16.3	15.8	

Table 6 Frequency of benign and malignant neoplasm

Adverse event	Percentage of patients	
	Months 1–24	
	Tacrolimus (n = 264)	Cyclosporin (n = 265)
Breast neoplasm	0.4	0.0
Lymphoma-like reaction	0.8	0.4
Other neoplasms	2.3	3.4
Skin benign neoplasm	0.0	1.1

urinary tract infection, did not differ in incidence between the two treatment groups. Pneumonia was reported less frequently and the incidence of cytomegalovirus (CMV) infection was significantly reduced in patients receiving tacrolimus therapy (tacrolimus 14.8 %, cyclosporin 22.3 %; $P = 0.033$). Neoplasms had been diagnosed in 22 patients by month 24 (Table 6), 9 of whom received tacrolimus and 13 cyclosporin therapy.

Hirsutism (tacrolimus 0.0 %, cyclosporin 8.7 %; $P < 0.01$) and gum hyperplasia (tacrolimus 0.0 %, cyclosporin 2.3 %; $P < 0.05$) were both reported by significantly fewer patients receiving tacrolimus therapy.

Discussion

In contrast to the US multicentre study, severely decompensated cirrhotic patients with renal impairment, patients with primary carcinoma of the liver and severely ill patients with fulminant hepatic failure were included in this trial. This accounts for the somewhat lower overall patient and graft survival figures (1-year patient and graft survival rates for the US study were 88 % and 82 %, respectively, for the tacrolimus treatment group 88 % and 79 % for patients receiving cyclosporin therapy [15]). With the exception of children, the exclusion criteria used in the trial reported here were limited to

those patients in whom it would normally be considered inadvisable to perform primary liver transplantation. The study population was, therefore, representative of patients requiring transplantation in everyday clinical practice.

The primary determinant of treatment efficacy was the prevention of rejection. Tacrolimus therapy was associated with a significant reduction in the frequency of rejection (acute, refractory and chronic) despite significantly lower steroid usage. The decreased incidence in immunosuppressive treatment failure for patients receiving tacrolimus therapy is of considerable clinical benefit and was reflected by a reduced requirement for retransplantation.

The improvement in overall patient and graft survival for the tacrolimus treatment group failed to reach statistical significance, but this was, at least in part, related to the use of an intent-to-treat analysis [13]. Those patients converted from cyclosporin to tacrolimus therapy as a result of inadequate rejection control, and in whom grafts were subsequently 'salvaged', were nevertheless assigned to the cyclosporin arm for the final comparison.

One might have expected a higher incidence of infection to be associated with the greater immunosuppressive potency of tacrolimus therapy. This was not apparent; the main clinical categories of infection did not differ and there was a significant reduction in the incidence of CMV infection in tacrolimus-treated patients. This latter observation is an important finding in terms of reducing patient morbidity.

It is unclear whether the reduced incidence of hypertension observed in this study was the result of lower steroid usage or whether this represents an intrinsic benefit associated with tacrolimus therapy. In either eventuality, it is a significant advantage for patients receiving treatment with tacrolimus therapy over conventional cyclosporin-based immunosuppression. This advantage will be of particular benefit for the paediatric population but could have important long-term clinical consequences for all patients receiving tacrolimus therapy.

Insulin usage and the development of new-onset diabetes mellitus have in many cases been attributed to steroid therapy; however, the diabetogenic effects of both tacrolimus and cyclosporin have been documented previously. The extended follow-up of the present study would tend to indicate that there is no significant difference in the degree of diabetogenicity between the two immunosuppressive regimens administered during the course of this study.

The clinical significance of the reported neurological and nephrological events have been discussed previously [3, 7]: the conclusions drawn being that the type, incidence and severity of these events were comparable between the tacrolimus and cyclosporin treatment groups. Minor neurological symptoms (including tremor, headache, insomnia, and paraesthesia) were not considered to have significant clinical relevance and did not appear to interfere with daily activities whereas major complications were considered to be reversible. Acute renal failure appeared to be reversible with no long-term damage being observed.

Again on the positive side for tacrolimus, the absence of hirsutism and gum hypertrophy is very much welcomed by the patient.

It should be borne in mind that none of the eight participating centres had previous clinical experience of administering tacrolimus therapy when this trial was initiated. During the early part of the study, tacrolimus therapeutic drug monitoring proved to be somewhat problematic as the available technique (ELISA) was both time consuming and unreliable. With little or no blood level information available, dose modifications were implemented following signs of rejection or suspicion of drug-related toxicity. Early experience indicated that the doses recommended initially were inappropriately high and this led to a marked reduction in the dose of tacrolimus being administered. Only later was a rapid and locally available assay introduced to assist with therapeutic drug monitoring. In contrast, cyclosporin blood concentrations were used to determine, and subsequently adjust, the dose both during the early post-operative period and throughout the course of the study. If tacrolimus blood level monitoring had been available from the outset of this study then some of the problems encountered in the early postoperative period may have been prevented. In addition, as further clinical experience is gained with tacrolimus, it has to be expected that the overall risk-benefit ratio will improve.

In conclusion, the demonstrated superiority of tacrolimus therapy over the 2-year follow-up period in terms of significant reductions in the incidence of acute, refractory acute and chronic rejection, is translated into a shorter and less problematic convalescent period. The reduced requirement for corticosteroids is also of direct benefit to the patient. The safety profile associated with tacrolimus therapy, although similar to that for cyclosporin in major categories, is in certain respects more favourable provided that careful attention is paid to the doses administered on the basis of clinical and blood level assessments.

Acknowledgements This study was sponsored by Fujisawa Pharmaceutical Co. Ltd., Osaka, Japan.

References

1. Bismuth H for the European FK 506 multicenter liver study group (1995) Comparison of FK 506- and cyclosporine-based immunosuppression: FK 506 therapy significantly reduces the incidence of acute, steroid-resistant, refractory, and chronic rejection whilst possessing a comparable safety profile. Transplant Proc 27: 45–49

2. Bismuth H, Samuel D, Neuhaus P, McMaster P, Calne R, Pichlmayr R, Otto G, Williams R, Groth C (1994) Focus on intractable rejection: 6-month results of the European multicentre study of FK 506 and cyclosporin A. Transplant Int 7 [Suppl 1]: S3–S6

3. Christe W (1994) Neurological disorders in liver and kidney transplant recipients. Transplant Proc 26: 3175–3176

4. Devlin J, Williams R, Neuhaus P, McMaster P, Calne R, Pichlmayr R, Otto G, Bismuth H, Groth C (1994) Renal complications and development of hypertension in the European study of FK 506 and cyclosporin in primary liver transplant recipients. Transplant Int 7 [Suppl 1]: S22–S26

5. Ericzon B, Groth C, Bismuth H, Calne R, McMaster P, Neuhaus P, Otto G, Pichlmayr R, Williams R (1994) Glucose metabolism in liver transplant recipients treated with FK 506 or cyclosporin in the European multicentre study. Transplant Int 7 [Suppl 1]: S11–S14

6. European FK 506 multicentre liver study group (1994) Randomised trial comparing tacrolimus (FK 506) and cyclosporin in prevention of liver allograft rejection. Lancet 344: 423–428

7. Frei U, Wagner K (1994) Renal function in liver transplant patients receiving FK 506 or cyclosporin A immunosuppressive therapy. Transplant Proc 26: 3270–3271

8. Fung J, Abu-Elmagd K, Jain A, Gordon R, Tzakis A, Todo S, Takaya S, Alessiani M, Demetris A, Bronster O, Martin M, Mieles L, Selby R, Reyes J, Doyle H, Stieber A, Casavilla A, Starzl T (1991) A randomized trial of primary liver transplantation under immunosuppression with FK 506 vs cyclosporine. Transplant Proc 23: 2977–2983

9. McMaster P (1994) Patient and graft survival in the European multicentre liver study – FK 506 vs cyclosporin A. Transplant Int 7 [Suppl 1]: S32–S36

10. Neuhaus PJ (1994) Optimised first-line FK 506-based protocol in liver transplantation: experience from the University Hospital Rudolf Virchow, Berlin. Transplant Proc 26: 3264–3266

11. Neuhaus P, McMaster P, Calne R, Pichlmayr R, Otto G, Williams R, Bismuth H, Groth C (1994) Neurological complications in the European multicentre study of FK 506 and cyclosporin in primary liver transplantation. Transplant Int 7 [Suppl 1]: S27–S31

12. Otto G, Bleyl J, Neuhaus P, McMaster P, Calne R, Pichlmayr R, Williams R, Bismuth H, Groth C (1994) Corticosteroids and concomitant medication in the European multicentre study of FK 506 and cyclosporin in primary liver transplantation. Transplant Int 7 [Suppl 1]: S7–S10

13. Starzl TE, Donner A, Eliasziw M, Stitt L, Meier P, Fung JJ, McMichael JP, Todo S (1995) Randomized trialomania? The multicenter liver transplant trials. Lancet 346: 1346–1350

14. The European FK 506 multicentre liver study group (1994) Reduced incidence of acute, refractory acute, and chronic rejection after liver transplantation with FK 506-based immunosuppression. Transplant Proc 26: 3260–3263

15. The U.S. multicenter FK 506 liver study group (1994) A comparison of tacrolimus (FK 506) and cyclosporine for immunosuppression in liver transplantation. N Engl J Med 331: 1110–1115

16. Todo S, Fung JJ, Tzakis A, Demetris AJ, Jain A, Alessiani M, Takaya S, Day R, Gordon R, Starzl TE (1991) One hundred ten consecutive primary orthotopic liver transplants under FK 506 in adults. Transplant Proc 23: 1397–1402

17. Winkler M, Pichlmayr R, Neuhaus P, McMaster P, Calne R, Otto G, Williams R, Bismuth H, Groth C (1994) Optimal FK 506 dosage in patients under primary immunosuppression following liver transplantation. Transplant Int 7 [Suppl 1]: S58–S63

Transpl Int (1996) 9 [Suppl 1]: S 151–S 154
© Springer-Verlag 1996

Th. Gruenberger
Th. Windhager
M. Gnant
M. Mittlböck
R. Steininger
F. Herbst
F. Muehlbacher

Tumor recurrence after oLTX

Th. Gruenberger · Th. Windhager ·
M. Gnant · M. Mittlböck · R. Steininger ·
F. Herbst · F. Muehlbacher
Department of Transplantation Surgery,
University of Vienna, Austria

Th. Gruenberger (✉)
Department of General Surgery,
University of Vienna,
Waehringer Guertel 18–20,
A-1090 Vienna, Austria

Abstract Although early survival
following transplantation for primary hepatic cancer is excellent,
previously reported high recurrence
rates have generally discouraged liver replacement for this condition.
The aim of this retrospective analysis was to examine the influence of
risk factors on the development of
early tumor recurrence. Between
December 1982 and June 1995, 480
liver transplantations were performed at a single institution. Out of
these, 103 patients had unresectable
primary hepatic cancer (88 hepatocellular cancer; HCCA; 20 %) and
15 had cholangiocellular cancer
(CHCA; 4 %). The influence of the
following tumor-associated risk factors was assessed: tumor size, tumor
distribution within the liver, grading,
pseudocapsular formation, vascular
invasion, lymph node metastasis,
and cirrhotic alteration. The diagnosis of tumor recurrence was made
using various radiological imaging
techniques, reelavation of serum al-
phafetoprotein, or autopsy. For patient survival and disease-free period, data analysis was performed by
the method of Kaplan-Meier. The
Cox model was used for multivariate
analysis; a P-value of less than 0.05
was considered to be significant. The
mean age of the 103 patients was 54
years (range 15–63 a). There were 22
female and 81 male patients. The
follow-up period ranged between 4
and 108 months. Twenty-nine patients (50 %) died during the follow-
up period due to recurrence of disease. The survival rates of the 88 patients with HCCA were 57 %, 34 %,
and 26 % at 1, 3, and 5 years, respectively, after orthotopic liver
transplantation (oLTX; follow-up
36 month). Of the 15 pts with
CHCA the rates were 53 %, 33 %,
and 33 %, respectively, with a median follow-up of 60 months. The influence of the risk factors studied
showed a significantly longer disease-free period for the following
tumor characteristics: grading below
or equal 2 ($P = 0.009$) and absence
of vascular invasion ($P = 0.04$). Regarding a median survival rate of 2–
4 months for patients with unresectable malignant liver tumors, these
results confirmed the indication for
oLTX, especially if the patient does
not compete with someone on the
waiting list for benign liver disease.

Key words Liver transplantation ·
Primary hepatic cancer · Outcome

Introduction

Worldwide, primary hepatic carcinoma is a common malignant tumor with variable incidence. Compared to the natural course of the disease, it has been clearly demonstrated that surgical tumor removal offers the only chance for long-term cure [1]. Without surgical resection the tumor biology leads to survival times of a maximum of 6 months. Only 20–40 % of primary liver malignancies are resectable conventionally because of bilobular tumor spread at the time of diagnosis or underlying advanced liver cirrhosis. Orthotopic liver transplantation has been considered as the only therapeutic possibility to achieve acceptable survival times, but high recurrence rates have been reported and therefore have impaired the good early survival rates [2, 3]. Therefore, some centers have recommended that patients with unresectable primary cancers and advanced-stage tumors should not be candidates for liver transplantation [3]. Other studies have shown that the rate of tumor recurrence is influenced by tumor size, the number of tumors, histological type and differentiation, and the presence of vascular or lymph node involvement [1, 4–6]. A review of the recently puplished data suggests that there is again a trend in favour of liver transplantation at an early stage of the hepatic cancer, where resection has been the method of choice for a long time because of survival rates that are comparable to those for benign conditions requiring liver transplantation [7]. Another option for better long-term disease-free survival in advanced hepatocellular malignancies is multimodal treatment with neoadjuvant chemotherapy and subsequent liver transplantation, which has been reported with 3-year survival rates of over 60 % [8–10]. This therapeutic option seems to be the method of choice for the majority of the cancer patients transferred to transplant centers because the proportion of patients treatable by other surgical methods is infinitely small.

We report on a series of 103 orthotopic liver transplants of otherwise unresectable primary hepatic cancers that were transplanted at our unit throughout the last 14 years and a subgroup of patients who received neoadjuvant chemotherapy, consisting of doxorubicin, throughout the last year. The aim of this study was to evaluate tumor characteristics and determine their potential risk in regard to recurrence rates after complete removal of the tumor. Is the neoadjuvant chemotherapeutic treatment a possible way to destroy undetected micrometastases, allowing these patients to lead a long life without recurrence of their tumor?

Material and methods

From December 1982 to June 1995, 480 patients were treated by total hepatectomy and subsequent transplantation at the transplantation department of the University of Vienna. Of these 480 transplants, the indication for liver replacement in 103 patients was a primary malignant tumor of the liver that was not treatable by resection because of underlying cirrhosis or tumor spread. In 88 patients, the indication was primary hepatocellular carcinoma (HCCA) and in 15 patients, primary cholangiocellular carcinoma (CHCA).

The HCCA group consisted of 72 male and 16 female patients with a mean age of 54 years (14–67 a). The CHCA group included 9 male and 6 female patients with a mean age of 50 years (31–62 a). All patients had a preoperative diagnosis of solitary liver tumor without metastatic disease. Preoperative investigations included chest radiography, hepatic doppler ultrasonography, computerized tomography, bone scintigraphy, and echocardiography. Orthotopic liver transplantation was done in the standardized way without using veno-venous bypass. Immunosuppression consisted of induction therapy with antithymocyte globulin (ATG-Fresenius) followed by cyclosporin and prednisolone, using azathioprine as a third therapeutic agent only in case of histologically proven rejection. In the recent transplants starting in January 1995, we introduced a neoadjuvant chemotherapeutic approach consisting of up to five cycles of doxorubicin 15 mg/m² i. v. preoperatively, one intraoperative cycle of doxorubicin 15 mg/m² i. v. after induction of general anaesthesia and before manipulation of the liver and, again, doxorubicin therapy 15 mg/m² i. v. in the postoperative period when the recipient's condition had stabilized, normally starting 2 weeks after transplantation and thereafter every second week up to a total dosage of 300 mg/m².

We collected the following pathological variables to get information about their possible prognostic relevance: histological diagnosis of the primary tumor and the associated liver disease, grade of tumor differentiation, intrahepatic tumor size (maximum diameter in centimeters), number and location of the nodules, presence or absence of vascular invasion, tumor thrombosis of the portal vein, and lymph node involvement. Patients were routinely seen at our outpatient department monthly for the first 6 months after transplantation, thereafter every 3 months until the second year of follow-up, and then semi-annually. Blood samples were routinely controlled at every visit, liver ultrasonography and chest radiography were done half yearly, and computerized tomography and bone scintigraphy in case of suspected recurrence of the primary carcinoma.

Statistical analysis was calculated using the univariate model in the first step (chi-square test), entering variables found to be significant in the multivariate Cox regression model. Overall survival was summerized using the Kaplan-Meier method.

Results

Considering the 30-day mortality rate, we had 1 death (7 %) in the CHCA group and 13 deaths (14.8 %) in the HCCA group. Reasons for that were cardiac complications, sepsis, and nonfunction of the hepatic graft complicated by no available organ for retransplantation. The overall survival rates 1, 3, and 5 years after transplantation were 53 %, 33 %, and 33 %, respectively, in the CHCA group after a median follow-up of 60 months and 57 %, 34 %, and 26 %, respectively, in the HCCA group after a median follow-up of 36 months. The disease-free survival rates at the same times were 72%, 52%, and 39%, respectively, in the CHCA group and 85%, 56%, and 43%, respectively, in the HCCA group. Median survival times after transplantation were 18 months in the HCCA group and 14 months in the CHCA group. Death due to recurrence of disease was observed in 48% of the patients in the HCCA group and in 55% of the patients in the CHCA group.

Histological evaluation revealed multicentricity in 74% of the patients in the HCCA group and in 71% of the patients in the CHCA group. Overall survival was not statistically significantly better in either unifocal group. The median tumor diameter was 5 cm (0.5–27 cm) in the HCCA group and 11.5 cm (2–23 cm) in the CHCA group. As we had only a small number of patients in both treatment groups with a median tumor diameter below 5 cm, disease-free survival was not found to be statistically significantly better in these patients. An associated cirrhotic alteration of the liver was present in 78% of the HCCA group and in 7% in the CHCA group. No statistical benefit was observed in nonchirrhotic patients. A significantly better overall survival was observed in patients without vascular invasion. On histological examination, 66% of the tumors did not show vascular invasion and 34% of the tumors did show vascular invasion. After a median follow-up of 36 months, 81% of the patients without vascular invasion had no signs of recurrence compared to only 63% of the patients with vascular invasion of the tumor at histological examination ($P = 0.04$, Mantel-Cox).

The second histopathological variable that was found to be significant in the multivariate model was the grading of the tumor. Twenty-three percent of the patients in the HCCA group had a good differentiation (grade I) of the tumor, 55% had a moderate (grade II), and 22% had poor tumor differentiation (grade III). Comparing grades I and II tumors with grade III tumors revealed a significantly better disease-free survival in the more differentiated tumor group ($P = 0.009$). A 3-year disease-free survival of 82% in the grade I tumor patients compared to 68% in the grade II and 50% in the grade III tumor patients was observed.

An improved disease-free survival in the so-far very small group of patients entered into the neoadjuvant chemotherapeutic program was not observed because the follow-up was too short; nevertheless, we have not seen any recurrent tumor, and one of the explanted livers showed complete remission after preoperative doxorubicin therapy.

Discussion

Primary hepatic cancer remains difficult to treat. Early disease is diagnosed infrequently and survival after the onset of symptoms is extremly poor. Many treatment modalities have been applied, but without surgical ablation, chemoembolization, chemotherapy, and radiation remain palliative at best. The present study was a retrospective analysis of patient's outcome after liver transplantation for primary hepatic cancer at our unit throughout the last 14 years. The results demonstrated better overall survival compared to other treatment options for advanced liver malignancy. Nevertheless, we have to confess that recurrence is the crucial point for this disease. Median overall survival times of 18 months for our large number of stage III and IVa patients could be considered excellent results in comparison to those of other groups [11]. The data presented here showed that postoperative tumor recurrence rates correlate significantly with the differentiation of the hepatoma and the presence of vascular invasion. Known risk factor such as the tumor size and the tumor distribution within the liver were not found to be significant in our study because there was an unimportant incidence of positive tumor characteristics (tumor < 3 cm, unilobular) in our patients. This could be underlined by the fact that none of our patients was a candidate for liver resection either because of advanced underlying liver disease (child B or C) or because of bilobular or central tumor spread.

Despite these results, many series report occasional long-term survival even of patients with advanced-stage disease. Therefore, it seems that cure is possible, and patients with advanced tumors should not be excluded from transplantation. Instead, attempts at improving therapy should be undertaken. Three recent studies emphasize the use of neoadjuvant treatment besides the surgical option to extend the long-term cure of patients with advanced tumor [8–10]. Three rationales are used to explain its usefulness: control of tumor growth during the waiting period, elimination of tumor cells that are disseminated during the operation, and control of remaining micrometastases postoperatively. In Stone's report 59% of the patients were alive at 3 years with 54% disease-free when concomitant neoadjuvant chemotherapy was used [9]. In over a half of the patients the tumor size was greater than 5 cm. We believe that multimodal treatment is the treatment of the future, and we have therefore started a program of pre-, intra- and postoperative adjuvant chemotherapy at the beginning of this year. So far we have one complete remission, no major side effects, and no recurrence of disease in the first patients treated with this regime. It is reasonable to advocate that tumor patients should continue to receive transplants as long as there is no competition with other patients on the waiting list for benign disease, in the expectation of a cure for some and good long-term palliation in the remainder. Recurrence rates in advanced-stage tumor patients with an actuarial survival figure of under 30 % at 3 years should lead to the decision to give these patients a low priority for transplantation. These recurrence rates illustrate the importance of early diagnosis of tumors in the cirrhotic liver by ultrasound screening of these patients in order to prolong survival after transplantation.

References

1. Iwatsuki S, Shaw BW, Starzl TE, et al (1985) Role of liver transplantation in cancer therapy. Ann Surg 202: 401–407
2. Iwatsuki S, Starzl TE, Sheahan DG, et al (1991) Hepatic resection versus transplantation for hepatocellular carcinoma. Ann Surg 214: 221–229
3. Ringe B, Wittekind C, Bechstein WO, et al (1989) The role of liver transplantation in hepatobiliary malignancy. A retrospective analysis of 95 patients with particular regard to tumor stage and recurrence. Ann Surg 209: 88–98
4. Yokojama I, Todo S, Iwatsuki S, et al (1990) Liver transplantation in the treatment of primary liver cancer. Hepatogastroenterology 37: 188–193
5. Yokojama I, Sheahan DG, Carr B, et al (1991) Clinicopathologic factors affecting patient survival and tumor recurrence after orthotopic liver transplantation for hepatocellular carcinoma. Transplant Proc 223: 2194–2196
6. McPeake JR, O'Grady JG, Zaman S, et al (1993) Liver transplantation for primary hepatocellular carcinoma: tumor size and number determine outcome. J Hepatol 18: 226–234
7. Bismuth H, Chiche L, Adam R, et al (1993) Liver resection versus transplantation for hepatocellular carcinoma in cirrhotic patients. Ann Surg 218: 145–151
8. Cherqui D, Piedbois P, Pierga JY, et al (1994) Multimodal adjuvant treatment and liver transplantation for advanced hepatocellular carcinoma. Cancer 73: 2721–2726
9. Stone MJ, Klintmalm GBG, Polter D, et al (1993) Neoadjuvant chemotherapy and liver transplantation for hepatocellular carcinoma. Gastroenterology 104: 196–202
10. Olthoff KM, Rosove MH, Shackleton CR, et al (1995) Adjuvant chemotherapy improves survival after liver transplantation for hepatocellular carcinoma. Ann Surg 221: 734–743
11. Ringe B, Pichlmayr R, Wittekind C, et al (1991) Surgical treatment of hepatocellular carcinoma: experience with liver resection and transplantation in 198 patients. World J Surg 15: 270–285

Transpl Int (1996) 9 [Suppl 1]: S155–S156
© Springer-Verlag 1996

R. Raakow
W. O. Bechstein
N. Kling
K. John
M. Knoop
H. Keck
P. Neuhaus

The importance of late infections for the long-term outcome after liver transplantation

R. Raakow (✉) · W. O. Bechstein · N. Kling ·
K. John · M. Knoop · H. Keck · P. Neuhaus
Department of Surgery, Virchow Clinic,
Humboldt University,
Augustenburger Platz 1, D-13353 Berlin,
Germany

Abstract We investigated the late infections of 400 consecutive liver transplantations performed in 368 patients. After a mean follow-up of 45 months, a total of 180 late infections occurred in 110 liver recipients. Frequent agents were CMV, enterococcus, candida and staphylococcus. Pneumonia was the most dangerous late infection with a high mortality rate. Late infections were responsible for ten deaths that were all caused by atypical pneumonia. The majority of late infections appeared during the first year after liver transplantation. Thereafter, the risk of infection declined significantly.

Key words Liver transplantation · Late infections · Atypical pneumonia · Long-term outcome

Introduction

Early infections after orthotopic liver transplantation (OLT) represent a significant threat to the success of OLT [1–3]. However, little attention has been focused on the role of infections in the long-term outcome of patients after liver transplantation. For that reason we would like to report on the significance of late infections, based on our patient population in Berlin.

Patients and methods

This analysis investigated the long-term outcome of 400 consecutive liver transplantations performed on a total of 368 patients between September 1988 and July 1993. The mean follow-up was 45 months (range 10 days – 85 months). Infections with bacterial, fungal or viral agents were classified as late infections if they occurred after the primary hospitalization (> 48 days) and required specific therapeutic intervention. Infections were categorized as mild, serious or life-threatening depending on their clinical presentation. Reinfections of the graft with hepatitis were not included in our study. Screening of infectious sites and agents was done according to standard clinical and diagnostic methods.

Results

Currently, 312 patients of the total of 368 are still alive. The 1-year survival rate was 90.2 %. The 5-year survival rate, as calculated according to Kaplan-Meier, was 84.2 %. A total of 180 late infections occurred in 110 liver recipients. Infections were located predominantly (26.7 %) in the lung ($n = 48$). Other frequent locations of late infections were the biliary tract ($n = 34$), the blood ($n = 25$), the urinary tract ($n = 16$), the ear, nose and throat territory ($n = 16$), the liver parenchyma ($n = 11$) and the female genital organs ($n = 9$; Table 1).

As far as the underlying infectious agents are concerned, we found the CMV virus to be the leading cause in 20.6 % of cases. Other common infectious agents were enterococci and *Candida* with 11.7 % each, and staphylococci in 8.3 % of cases. Infections due to *Aspergillus, Pseudomonas, Pneumocystis, Legionella* and tuberculosis were rare by comparison. Exotic culture results were encountered in 7.8 % of cases. In the remaining 40 cases microbiological testing failed to identify a clear pathogen (Table 2).

Infections were categorized as mild if they were amenable to out-patient treatment. More than half of infectious episodes (57.8 %) belonged to this group. Fifty-six (31.1 %) of the 180 late infections were associated with

Table 1 Locations of 180 late infections

Lung	$n = 48$ (26.7 %)
Bile duct	$n = 34$ (18.9 %)
Blood	$n = 25$ (13.9 %)
Urinary tract	$n = 16$ (8.9 %)
ENT	$n = 16$ (8.9 %)
Parenchyma of the liver	$n = 11$ (6.1 %)
Female genital organs	$n = 9$ (5.0 %)
Others	$n = 21$ (11.6 %)

Table 2 Infectious agents of 180 late infections

CMV	$n = 37$ (20.6 %)
Enterococcus	$n = 21$ (11.7 %)
Candida	$n = 21$ (11.7 %)
Staphylococcus	$n = 15$ (8.3 %)
Aspergillus	$n = 9$ (5.0 %)
Pseudomonas	$n = 7$ (3.9 %)
Pneumocystis carnii	$n = 6$ (3.3 %)
Legionella	$n = 6$ (3.3 %)
Tuberculosis	$n = 4$ (2.2 %)
Others	$n = 14$ (7.8 %)
No agent found	$n = 40$ (22.2 %)

Table 3 Cause of death by infectious agents

Pneumocystis pneumonia	$n = 3$
Aspergillus pneumonia	$n = 2$
CMV pneumonia	$n = 2$
Candida pneumonia	$n = 2$
Legionella pneumonia	$n = 1$
	$n = 10$

serious clinical symptoms and ordinary hospital admission. Twenty patients or an equivalent of 11.1 % were in need of aggressive medical intervention in an intensive care unit because of life-threatening late infections.

Of the 368 liver recipients, 40 died during follow-up after primary hospitalization. Late infections were re-

sponsible for ten (25 %) deaths All infections that culminated in a patient's demise were atypical pneumonias. The offending agents were *Pneumocystis carinii* in three, *Aspergillus*, CMV and *Candida* in two cases each and *Legionella* in one patient (Table 3).

Most late infections (71.7 %) appeared during the first year after liver transplantation. It is noteworthy indeed that out of the ten fatal late infections, eight occurred in the first year. After this period the risk of infection declined significantly. Beyond the 2-year mark we havn't observed a single case of death due to late infection.

Discussion

Although great strides have been made in liver transplantation, infection remains a major problem [1, 2]. This concerns early and late infections [4]. However, the impact of late infections of the long-term prognosis after liver transplantation has not been fully recognized.

The risk of infection is greatest during the first year after transplantation [5]. In our patient population the majority of late infections appeared during this period. Life-threatening late infections with a high mortality rate were most frequent after primary hospitalization during the first postoperative year. Pneumonia with high lethality is the most dangerous late infection. Most infectious agents of late pneumonias are atypical organisms like CMV, *Pneumocystis*, *Aspergillus*, *Candida* and *Legionella* [6].

Late infections are important determining factors for the long-term prognosis after liver transplantation. Early signs of infection should be taken seriously by both the patient and the doctor, and comprehensive microbiological screening and effective treatment should be undertaken [6]. This may diminish the morbidity and mortality associated with late infections.

References

1. Colonna JO, Winston DJ, Brill JE, Goldstein LI, Hoff MP, Hiatt JR, Quinones-Baldrich W, Ramming KP, Busuttil RW (1988) Infectious complications in liver transplantation. Arch Surg 123: 360–364
2. Kusne S, Dummer JS, Singh N, Iwatsuki S, Makowka L, Esquivel C, Tzakis AG, Starzl TE, Ho M (1988) Infections after liver transplantation: an analysis of 101 consecutive cases. Medecine 67: 132–143

3. Maddrey WC, Van Thiel DH (1988) Liver transplantation: an overview. Hepatology 8: 948–959
4. Mora NP, Gonwa TA, Goldstein RM, Husberg BS, Klintmalm GB (1992) Risk of postoperative infection after liver transplantation: a univariate and stepwise logistic regression analysis of risk factors in 150 consecutive patients. Clin Transplant 46: 443–449

5. Barkholt L, Ericzon BG, Tollemar J, Malmborg AS, Ehrnst A, Wilczek H, Andersson J (1993) Infections in human liver recipients: different patterns early and late after transplantation. Transplant Int 6: 77–84
6. Afessa B, Gay PC, Plevak DJ, Swensen SJ, Patel HG, Krowka MJ (1993) Pulmonary complications of orthotopic liver transplantation. Mayo Clin Proc 68: 427–434

Transpl Int (1996) 9 [Suppl 1]: S157–S159
© Springer-Verlag 1996

LIVER

S. Uemoto
Y. Inomata
K. Tanaka
N. Ozaki
H. Egawa
H. Okajima
H. Nishizawa
S. Yabe
Y. Yamaoka

Living related liver transplantation in children with hypoxemia related to intrapulmonary shunting

S. Uemoto (✉) · Y. Inomata · K. Tanaka ·
N. Ozaki · H. Egawa · H. Okajima ·
H. Nishizawa · S. Yabe · Y. Yamaoka
The Second Department of Surgery,
Kyoto University Hospital, 54 Kawara-cho,
Shogoin, Sakyo-ku, Kyoto 606, Japan

Abstract Living related liver transplantation (LRLT) was performed in seven children with hypoxemia related to intrapulmonary shunting. Based on the degree of the shunt ratio calculated by technetium ^{99}m macroaggregated albumin (MAA) scintigraphy, the seven patients were classified in the moderate (shunt ratio under 40 %, $n = 4$) or severe group (shunt ratio over 40 %, $n = 3$). While PaO_2 was maintained over 60 mmHg in the moderate group, that in the severe group continued at a low level of under 40 mmHg in the early postoperative period. However, 48 h after surgery the arterial ketone body ratio recovered to a safe level of 1.0 in both groups. Values of aspartate aminotransferase and serum total bilirubin decreased at a constant rate in both groups. Six patients survived, but one died of portal vein thrombosis on the 53rd postoperative day. Five of six surviving patients recovered from hypoxemia. We concluded that the transplanted liver can tolerate the stress of severe hypoxemia after LRLT.

Key words Living related liver · transplantation Hypoxemia · Intrapulmonary shunting

Introduction

Indications for liver transplantation in patients with hypoxemia related to intrapulmonary shunting have been controversial. Some authors consider severe hypoxemia as an absolute contraindication for liver transplantation [1, 2]. In contrast, it has been documented that hypoxemia in patients with cirrhosis may improve after successful liver transplantation [3, 4]. It would be reasonable to speculate that organs other than the transplanted liver can tolerate the stress of hypoxemia even after transplantation because prolonged hypoxemia existed before transplantation. However, the transplanted liver is suddenly exposed to hypoxemia after liver transplantation. Therefore, the success of liver transplantation in patients with hypoxemia may depend on whether the transplanted liver can function well under hypoxic conditions.

Patients and methods

Seven pediatric patients (one male, six female) with a mean age of 9.8 years (2.4–14.4 years) underwent living related liver transplantation (LRLT) between December 1994 and July 1995. The original liver disease was biliary atresia in all cases. All patients had portal hypertension defined by esophageal varices with previous episodes of bleeding or splenomegaly with hypersplenism. Three patients previously underwent partial splenic embolization (two patients) or splenectomy (one patient) for hypersplenism. Three patients previously underwent distal splenorenal shunt (one patient) or endoscopic sclerotherapy (two patients) for esophageal variceal bleeding. Jaundice was less severe (serum total bilirubin under 4 mg/dl) in these six patients compared to nonhypoxic patients with biliary atresia treated during this period. Only one patient had a moderate degree of jaundice (serum total bilirubin: 28.5 mg/dl).

All patients had cyanosis and digital clubbing. Five had dyspnea on effort and three often required oxygen. Table 1 shows the results of preoperative respiratory tests. Patients were divided into two groups according to the degree of the intrapulmonary shunt ratio calculated by technetium ^{99}m macroaggregated albumin scintigraphy (MAA scintigraphy). The severe group consisted

Table 1 Respiratory test prior to living related liver transplantation (LRLT). Values are mean ± SD (*MAA scintigraphy* technetium ^{99}m macroaggregated albumin scintigraphy)

Group	MAA scintigraphy (%)	PaO$_2$ at room air (mmHg)	PaO$_2$ under 100 % O$_2$ (mmHg)
Moderate (n = 4)	25.0 ± 9.4	56.5 ± 4.4	215.9 ± 61.6
Severe (n = 3)	54.1 ± 9.0	40.6 ± 6.5	57.3 ± 12.5

Table 2 Changes in aspartate aminotransferase and serum total bilirubin. Values are mean ± SD (*AST* aspartate aminotransferase, *T-Bil* serum total bilirubin, *POD* postoperative day)

	1	2	3	7	14 (POD)
AST (IU/l)					
Moderate	132 ± 24	120 ± 31	64 ± 12	42 ± 15	48 ± 17
Severe	102 ± 8	113 ± 13	58 ± 2	28 ± 9	25 ± 7
T-Bil (mg/dl)					
Moderate	8.9 ± 3.0	5.8 ± 2.2	5.4 ± 3.2	3.3 ± 2.9	1.8 ± 1.4
Severe	6.0 ± 3.1	3.1 ± 0.7	3.0 ± 0.6	2.2 ± 0.6	1.5 ± 0.8

of three patients with a high shunt ratio of over 40 % (44.0–61.1 %), while the moderate group consisted of four patients with a shunt ratio under 40 % (16.1–35.0 %). Increase in the PaO$_2$ after 100 % oxygen breathing was marked in the moderate group, but the severe group only showed a slight increase.

LRLT was performed electively in all patients. Segmental liver grafts (six left lobe and one lateral segment) were obtained from the patients' parents (three fathers and four mothers). Viability of the liver after transplantation was evaluated by the arterial ketone body ratio (AKBR). As long as the AKBR was maintained over a safety level of 1.0 and vital signs were stable, FiO$_2$ was not increased over 0.6 and positive end-expiratory pressure (PEEP) was maintained at under 2 cm H$_2$O. Patients were extubated as early as possible. Immunosuppressive therapy consisted of Tacrolimus (FK 506) and low dose steroids.

Results

Six patients were extubated on the first postoperative day (1 POD), and one on the 2 POD. Figure 1 shows the changes in PaO$_2$ after transplantation. In the moderate group, PaO$_2$ was maintained over 60 mmHg during the first postoperative week, and none of the patients required any more oxygen 2 weeks after transplantation. In contrast, low PaO$_2$ values (under 40 mmHg) persisted in the severe group. One patient aged 2.4 years in the severe group demonstrated recovery from hypoxemia on the 7 POD, and did not require any more oxygen 2 weeks after transplantation.

Figure 2 shows the changes in the AKBR after transplantation. The AKBR recovered to 1.0 in five patients 12 h after transplantation and remained over 1.0 in all patients 48 h after transplantation. Postoperative peak

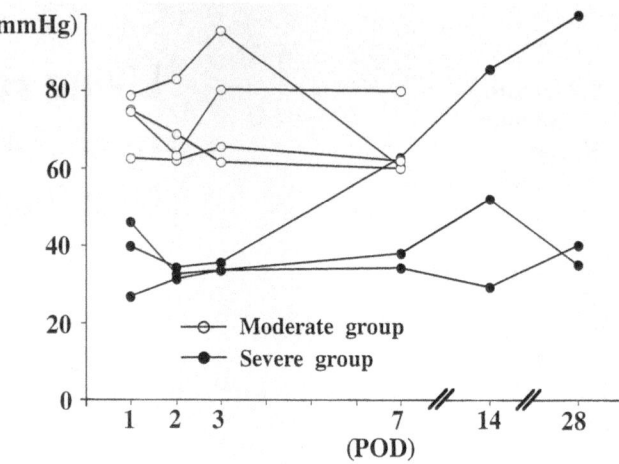

Fig. 1 Changes in PaO$_2$ after transplantation

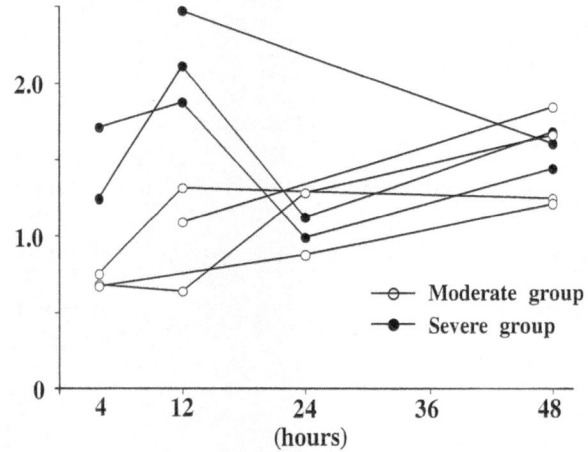

Fig. 2 Changes in arterial ketone body ratio (AKBR) after transplantation

values of aspartate aminotransferase (AST) were minimal (under 200 IU/l) in all cases, and decreased at a constant rate. There was no significant difference between the two groups. Serum total bilirubin also decreased at a constant rate in the two groups (Table 2). The hematocrit in the two patients in the severe group remained elevated (over 40 %); however, the other patients demonstrated a decrease in the hematocrit (29 %) on the 14 POD concomitant with an improvement in hypoxemia.

One patient in the severe group did not recover from hypoxemia, and the elevated hematocrit persisted. This patient developed portal vein thrombosis on the 37 POD and underwent a second operation to remove thrombi from the portal, superior mesenteric, and splenic veins. However, the patient died of hepatic failure on the 53 POD. Six patients survived, with follow-up periods ranging between 3 and 10 months. Five patients recovered from hypoxemia clinically, and demonstrated normal blood gas analysis. Closure of the intrapulmonary shunting on MAA scintigraphy was shown in two patients 3 months after transplantation. Another three patients did not undergo this examination. One patient in the severe group had not recovered from hypoxemia 3 months after transplantation.

Discussion

One of the advantages of LRLT is that highly viable liver grafts can be obtained with shorter cold ischemia compared to that in cadaveric liver transplantation. In this study, the AKBR clearly demonstrated that transplanted segmental liver in LRLT functioned well under severe hypoxemia, even when the PaO_2 was under 40 mmHg. Maintenance of good liver function was confirmed by very low values of AST and a steady decrease in serum total bilirubin after transplantation.

Hobeika et al. reported that of nine pediatric patients with hypoxemia three died from worsening hypoxemia after liver transplantation [5]. However, in our series none of the patients died of respiratory insufficiency and all patients were extubated by the 2 POD. We believe that patients with long-term hypoxemia can survive severe decreases in PaO_2, even under 40 mmHg, and that stress on lungs and heart, such as a high PEEP or high FiO_2, can be prevented as long as patients have stable vital signs and stable liver function.

One patient developed portal vein thrombosis at a relatively late stage. The patient had not recovered from hypoxemia at that time, and polycythemia continued. It was speculated that the portal vein thrombosis was partly attributable to the polycythemia. Long-term anticoagulant treatment might be necessary to prevent thrombus formation until the patient recovers from hypoxemia and polycythemia.

References

1. Van Thiel DH, Schade RR, Gavaler JS, et al (1984) Medical aspects of liver transplantation. Hepatology 4: 79
2. Zitelli B, Malatack JJ, Gartner JC, et al (1986) Evaluation of the pediatric patient for liver transplantation. Pediatrics 78: 559
3. Stoller JK, Moodie D, Schiavone W (1990) Reduction of intrapulmonary shunt and resolution of digital clubbing associated with primary biliary cirrhosis after liver transplantation. Hepatology 11: 54
4. Gunnarsson L, Blomquist BI, Eleborg L (1990) Liver transplantation in hypoxic patients. Transplant Proc 4: 1528
5. Hobeika J, Houssin D, Bernard O, et al. (1994) Orthotopic liver transplantation in children with chronic liver disease and severe hypoxemia. Transplantation 57: 224

Transpl Int (1996) 9 [Suppl 1]: S 160–S 163
© Springer-Verlag 1996

LIVER

Growth and height in children after liver transplantation

P. Jara
M. C. Díaz
L. Hierro
A. de la Vega
C. Camarena
E. Frauca
R. Lama
M. López Santamaría
J. Vázquez
J. Murcia
M. Gámez

P. Jara (✉) · M. C. Díaz · L. Hierro ·
A. de la Vega · C. Camarena · E. Frauca ·
R. Lama · M. López Santamaría ·
J. Vázquez · J. Murcia · M. Gámez
Hepatology Section and Liver Transplant
Unit, Hospital Infantil "La Paz",
Paseo Castellana, 261, 28046 Madrid, Spain
Tel. + 3 43 58 38 35

Abstract To assess the linear growth after liver transplantation, height curves were constructed for 45 children who underwent liver transplantation at the Children's Hospital "La Paz", Madrid, and were followed for more than 2 years. The prednisolone dose was progressively tapered and switched to alternate-day administration at 12 months. Growth was severely impaired during daily steroid therapy but the mean growth rate normalized in the second year and a significant improvement was observed in successive years. Observations over a long period revealed flucting growth rates under stable or decreasing doses of prednisolone on alternate-day administration. Beyond the first year, some annual periods of abnormal growth rate occurred in 57 % of the children. Marginally better posttransplantation growth was observed in children transplanted for intrahepatic cholestatic diseases. The prednisolone dose did not correlate with growth rate. In the long term, short stature was highly prevalent due to an accumulation of factors: previous disease, daily prednisolone period, inconstant growth rate under alternate-day steroid therapy, and pubertal delay.

Key words Statural growth · Liver transplantation

Introduction

Quality of life after liver transplantation during childhood is hampered by the immunosuppressor agents. Their side effects become a main concern when early posttransplantation complications have been successfully overcome and the graft is functioning well. In the long term, infectious diseases and lymphoproliferative disorders are life-threatening but unusual problems. On the contrary, some degree of renal dysfunction and growth impairment occurs in a majority of children. The endocrinological mechanisms underlying the linear growth failure in this population have been poorly studied to date although therapy with glucocorticoids, even in small doses, constitutes an important factor. Knowledge of the features of growth after liver transplantation may lead to a better management of these children.

Methods

Between January 1986 and January 1995, 118 children received a liver graft at the Children's Hospital "La Paz", Madrid, Spain. Forty-five children (27 male and 18 female) were selected for the study of linear growth on the basis of incomplete statural growth at liver transplantation (OLT), absence of vertebral collapse, and a minimum follow-up lasting two years. The mean follow-up was 3.9 ± 1.6 years. Thirty-four children were observed for at least 3 years and 25 patients were followed up for 4 years.

The indications for OLT were biliary atresia in 18 children, intrahepatic cholestasis in 9 (Alagille syndrome $n = 2$, progressive familial cholestasis $n = 4$, neonatal hepatitis $n = 3$), metabolic disease in 13 (alfa 1 antitrypsin deficiency $n = 3$, hereditary tyrosinemia $n = 5$, Wilson's disease $n = 3$, type IV glycogen storage disease $n = 1$, acid lipase deficiency $n = 1$), and other diseases in 5 children (hepatoblastoma $n = 1$, Budd-Chiari $n = 1$, autoimmune hepatitis $n = 1$, acute idiopathic liver failure $n = 1$, cryptogenic cirrhosis $n = 1$). Ten children underwent retransplantation (1 of them twice) for hepatic artery thrombosis ($n = 5$), chronic rejection ($n = 5$), or

Table 1 Prednisolone dose. Values expressed as mg/kg per day. Alternate-day administration beyond 12th month

	6th months	1st year	2nd year	3rd year	4th year
Number of patients	45	45	45	34	25
Mean (± SD)	0.43 (± 0.17)	0.31 (± 0.13)	0.23 (± 0.10)	0.17 (± 0.08)	0.16 (± 0.09)
Range	0.17–1	0.08–0.76	0.05–0.57	0.05–0.5	0.04–0.45

Table 2 Growth velocity after OLT. Values expressed as z score: mean (± SD)

	1st year	2nd year	3rd year	4th year
All	$-2.7 \longleftrightarrow -1.9$		$-0.8 \longleftrightarrow 0.4$	
	(± 2.5)* (± 3.1)		(± 2.7)** (± 2.2)	
Prepubertal age	$-3 \longleftrightarrow -1.6$		$-1 \longleftrightarrow 0.3$	
	(± 1.6)* (± 2.6)		(± 2.5)** (± 1.8)	

* $P < 0.01$ ** $P < 0.05$

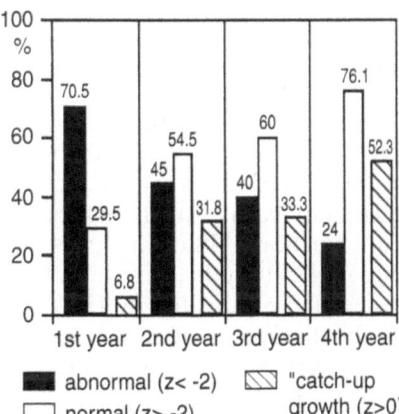

Fig. 1 Patients (%) grouped in categories according to normal (z score > –2) or abnormal (z score < –2) growth velocity after OLT. The *striped column* depicts patients who displayed catch-up growth (z score > 0)

primary non-function ($n = 1$). Their average age at OLT was 6.7 ± 4.2 years, ranging from 6 months to 16 years.

Long-term graft function was normal or showed mild to moderate transaminase elevations, usually linked to chronic HCV hepatitis. Late onset acute rejection episodes occurred in 5 children. Estimated glomerular filtration rate (EGFR) at the end of follow-up was abnormal, range 40–70 ml/min, in 7 patients.

Posttransplant immunosuppression consisted of cyclosporine and prednisolone. Azathioprine was added associated with a lower cyclosporine dose in the 7 cases with compromised renal function. The average cyclosporine dose was 14 mg/kg per day 1 year after OLT and 10.5 mg/kg by the 4th year with mean serum concentrations of 210 and 125 ng/ml (policlonal RIA), respectively. Prednisolone was administered daily during the first postOLT year, at a lower dose during follow-up, and was switched to an alternate-day regime at 12 months. The mean prednisolone dose

(mg/kg per day) is detailed in Table 1. Steroid withdrawal was not attempted.

The patients were seen at our outpatient clinic every 3 months. Length or height were measured in a Harpender infantometer or stadiometer. Linear growth rate was assessed annually. The z scores for growth in height and for linear growth rate were calculated according to the following equation: z score = x–mean value for normal/SD for normal, where x is the value for an individual patient and SD is the standard deviation for the normal population of the same age and gender. The z score indicates the number of SDs above (positive value) or below (negative value) the mean for the normal population. Normal reference values for Spanish children were used.

The Student's t-test was applied to determine the differences in the means of unpaired variables. The correlations were evaluated by regression analysis.

Results

Linear/height growth

Mean z score values for growth rate showed severe deceleration during the first year and a normal rate in the following years (Table 2). A significant improvement occurred in successive years, reaching a value slightly over the mean for normal children 4 years after OLT. Nevertheless, while an increasing proportion of children showed catch-up growth, there was a significant group growing below normal limits at each annual evaluation (Fig. 1).

The observation of the patients over along period showed fluctuations in the rate of statural gain. Beyond the first year, under corticosteroid therapy on alternate-day administration, 57 % of the children had at least one annual period with poor growth (z score below-2).

Growth during prepubertal age

Seven male and six female children could be observed over the period of adolescence and seven cases had a delay in the development of secondary sexual characteristics. That feature conditioned low z scores in growth during the period of growth spurt of normal pubertal children, and high z scores during the period in which normal children have almost completed growth. Other cases with a shorter follow-up, limited to the initial stages of theoretical pubertal development, showed absence of pubertal changes.

To exclude artifacts motivated by pubertal delay, linear growth rate was then assessed excluding all data coming from male children more than 12 years old and female children over 11 years old. Differences were noted when results of prepubertal observations were compared with those coming from the older children. There was a worse growth rate during the 1st year (z score:

−3 ± 1.6) and a better z score in the long term (0.3 ± 1.8). By the 4th year 92.2 % of prepubertal children grew within normal limits.

Prednisolone therapy and growth

Growth rate was markedly lower while on daily steroid administration in comparison to alternate-day administration. There was no correlation between prednisolone dose and growth rate at any time after liver transplantation.

Previous disease and growth

Patients were assigned to major groups of liver disease, biliary atresia (BA), intrahepatic cholestasis (IC), and metabolic diseases (MD). No significant differences in age at the time of liver transplantation were appreciated (BA: 5.9 ± 3.3 years, IC: 5.1 ± 2.3 years, MD: 7.5 ± 5.2 years). There was no correlation between age and z score for height. Height was particularly decreased in children affected by intrahepatic cholestasis. Before liver transplantation, the z score for height in the IC group was −3 ± 1.9, significantly lower than BA patients (−0.4 ± 1.6) and MD patients (0.1 ± 1.4).

After OLT, higher mean values in z score for growth rate were observed in children previously affected by intrahepatic cholestasis, reaching statistical significance 3 years after OLT when compared with the group of patients who underwent transplantation for biliary atresia (Table 3).

Height

Short stature (z score below −2) was present in 23 % of patients at the time of liver transplantation. The height standardized value decreased markedly within the 1st year, 34 % of children had a z score for height lower than −2 at that time. There were no statistically significant differences between the z score 1 year after OLT and the score in subsequent years (Table 4). By the 4th year the height was below normal limits in 52 % of the children (Fig. 2). Only 15 % of the children by the 3rd year and 19 % by the 4th year had maintained or improved the z score for height they had before transplantation.

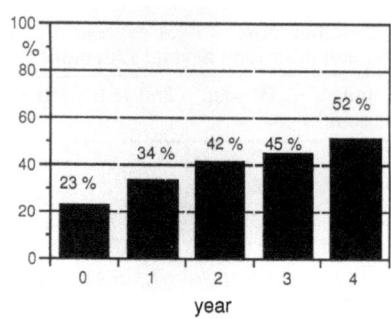

Fig. 2 Patients (%) affected by short stature (z score for height < −2) during follow-up

Discussion

Growth retardation is a sign of malnutrition in children affected by end-stage and cholestatic liver diseases. Short stature before transplantation, as a marker of nutritional derrangement, has been related to higher morbidity and lower patient survival after liver transplantation (4). Recommendations have been made in order to improve nutrition through enteral feeding and to perform OLT at a less-advanced stage of disease. Quality of life in the long term could also be improved by this attitude as features of growth in the present study indicate the difficulty in overcoming a pre-existing statural delay under an immunosuppressor regime including steroids.

Long-term survival is usually associated with satisfactory graft function. Although it was not a requisite for inclusion in the study, liver function tests for our patients were normal or affected by HCV hepatitis without the biochemical signs of choletasis. Rejection episodes had a ready response to treatment. Failure to grow could not be justified by graft dysfunction in any case. Tubular acidosis was detected in 30 % of patients but treatment with bicarbonate was established so that acidosis can be excluded as a contributing factor to

Table 3 Growth velocity after OLT according to previous disease. Values expressed as z score: mean (± SD)

	Biliary atresia (n = 18)	Intrahepatic cholestasis (n = 9)	Metabolic disease (n = 13)
1st year	−2.7 (± 2.5)	−2.8 (± 1.3)	−2.7 (± 1.5)
2nd year	−1.6 (± 3)	−1.9 (± 2.3)	−2.2 (± 2.9)
3rd year	−1.7 (± 2)* ⟷	0.6 (± 2.3)	−0.3 (± 3.4)
4th year	−1 (± 1.9)	0.3 (± 2)	−0.7 (± 2.4)

* $P < 0.05$

Table 4 Z score for height during follow-up

Z score	Pre	1st year	2nd year	3rd year	4th year
Mean	−0.8* ⟷	−1.6 ←n.s.→	−1.9 ←n.s.→	−1.9 ←n.s.→	−2.3
SD	± 2	± 1.7	± 1.6	± 1.4	± 1.2

* $P < 0.05$

growth retardation. Weight for height was preserved in the majority of patients. Prednisolone treatment is, therefore, considered the main responsible factor affecting growth in these children.

Our results show that corticoid administration on an alternate-day regime restores growth rate to normal mean values. Nevertheless, there were children who did not normalize growth and others who showed flucting rates. An explanation for this pattern could not be obtained in view of the absence of correlation between the steroid dose and growth rate. Renal function, assessed by a serum creatinine-based method (Schwartz equation), was no worse in children with growth failure. In some patients, pubertal delay undoubtedly contributed to retarded growth. The cause of the chronic liver disease did not affect postOLT linear growth rate.

Growth was severely impaired in the first postOLT year in this series. Children must grow above normal limits for several years to compensate for this. The achievement of normal growth rate beyond the first year could only maintain the 1-year z score for height.

Cumulated yearly steroid dosage correlated with growth rate scores in the Hannover experience (6). In the experience of the Cochin and Bicetre Hospital, an improvement in the mean z score for height had been achieved 2 years after OLT with respect to the pretransplant value in all the groups of patients established according to previous disease with the exception of the fulminant hepatic failure group (2). Their immunosup-pression protocol included a short period, averaging 7 months, of daily prednisolone, and the duration of continuous steroid therapy was inversely correlated with growth rate scores during the first 3 years after OLT. Catch-up growth and improvement of baseline score for height have also been reported in a large group of biliary atresia patients during the 2nd and 3rd post-OLT years (8). On the contrary, another study which switched to alternate-day steroids at 6 months showed progressive retardation in the children's heights, which was below normal limits in 74 % of patients after a mean follow-up of 28 months, and a significant correlation between the prednisolone dose and growth was not found (7).

Other alternative approaches to ameliorate growth retardation include steroid withdrawal and growth hormone therapy. Rejection while on monotherapy of cyclosporine has ocurred in 11–13 %, but the patients who could be maintained off steroids increased in growth when compared with those on alternate-day steroids (1, 3). The long-term implications of monotherapy are still unknown and further studies are necessary for an appropriate selection of patients. Therapy with growth hormone (GH) could be considered in some patients (8). Reports on the effect of recombinant GH in a short series of children treated with steroids have shown a response inversely related to the amount of prednisone (5).

References

1. Andrews WS, Shimaoka S, Sommerauer J, Moore P, Hudgins P (1994) Steroid withdrawal after pediatric liver transplantation. Transplant Proc 26: 159–160
2. Codoñer-Franch P, Bernard O, Alvarez F (1994) Long-term follow-up of growth in height after successful liver transplantation. J Pediatr 124: 368–373
3. Dunn JP, Falkestein K, Lawrence JP, Meyers R, Vinocur CD, Billmine DF, Weintraub WH (1994) Monotherapy with cyclosporine for chronic immunosuppression in pediatric liver transplant recipients. Transplantation 57: 544–547
4. Mouzarkel AA, Najm I, Vargas J, McDiarmid SV, Busuttil RW, Ament ME (1990) Effect of nutritional status on outcome of orthotopic liver transplantation in pediatric patients. Transplant Proc 22: 1560–1563
5. Rivkees SA, Danon M, Herrin J (1994) Prednisone dose limitation of growth hormone treatment of steroid-induced growth failure. J Pediatr 125: 322–325
6. Rodeck B, Melter M, Hoyer PF, Ringe B, Brodehl J (1994) Growth in long-term survivors after orthotopic liver transplantation in childhood. Transplant Proc 26: 165–166
7. Sarna S, Sipila I, Jalanko H, Laine J, Holmberg C (1994) Factors affecting growth after pediatric liver transplantation. Transplant Proc 26: 161–164
8. Sokal EM (1995) Quality of life after orthotopic liver transplantation in children. An overview of physical, psychological and social outcome. Eur J Pediatr 154: 171–175

Transpl Int (1996) 9 [Suppl 1]: S 164–S 170
© Springer-Verlag 1996

S. Jonas
W. O. Bechstein
S. G. Tullius
Th. Steinmüller
Th. Gamm
P. Neuhaus

Indications for Tacrolimus anti-rejection therapy in liver allograft recipients

S. Jonas · W. O. Bechstein · S. G. Tullius ·
Th. Steinmüller · Th. Gamm · P. Neuhaus
Department of Surgery,
Virchow Klinikum der Humboldt
Universität Berlin, Germany

S. Jonas (✉)
Department of Surgery,
Virchow Klinikum,
Augustenburger Platz 1,
D-13353 Berlin, Germany
FAX: + 49-30-45 05 29 00

Present address
Th. Gamm
Department of Cardiology and Intensive
Care Medicine,
Krankenhaus Neukölln,
D-12351 Berlin, Germany

Abstract We reviewed our experience with conversion to Tacrolimus after 600 liver transplantations, performed from September 1988 to March 1995. Conversion to Tacrolimus as an anti-rejection therapy was implemented in 78 patients because of chronic ductopenic rejection ($n = 9$), early chronic rejection ($n = 5$), OKT3-resistant cellular rejection ($n = 12$), steroid-resistant cellular rejection ($n = 30$), late-onset cellular rejection ($n = 10$), cellular rejection in patients suffering from cyclosporin malabsorption ($n = 5$) and uncomplicated cellular rejection ($n = 7$). Control of rejection was achieved in 72 of 78 patients (92 %); 6 patients (18 %) were non-responsive. Patient and graft survival were 82 % and 77 %, respectively. Fourteen patients died almost exclusively from opportunistic infections. Out of the six patients who did not respond to Tacrolimus treatment, four underwent successful retransplantation and two died from infections associated with a poor graft function. Overall, graft loss with or without patient death occurred in 6 of 9 patients undergoing chronic rejection, in 3 of 12 patients with OKT3-resis-
tant cellular rejection, in 6 of 30 patients suffering from steroid-resistant cellular rejection and in one patient each suffering from late-onset or uncomplicated cellular rejection. In severe steroid-resistant cellular rejection, successful Tacrolimus rescue therapy corresponded to a significantly lower preconversion total serum bilirubin when compared to failures (9.9 ± 6.8 mg % vs. 22.2 ± 7.3 mg %, $P < 0.05$). Conversion to Tacrolimus was a reliable treatment option in liver allograft rejection. However, failures occurred in the OKT3- and steroid-resistant cellular rejection groups, and only in a subgroup of patients suffering from chronic rejection was a permanent benefit observed. Implementation of a conversion early in the course of a rejection episode may result in a further improved outcome. Predictive parameters, e. g. the total serum bilirubin in steroid-resistant cellular rejection, are still needed to select those patients who would profit rather from a retransplantation.

Key words Tacrolimus conversion therapy · Liver allograft rejection · Chronic ductopenic rejection

Introduction

Earlier reports on conversion to Tacrolimus from cyclosporin A (CsA)-based regimens have demonstrated its potency in the treatment of liver allograft rejection [3, 4, 18]. A marked ability of Tacrolimus to reverse ongoing rejection even with evidence of ductopenic changes has been observed in those patients converted for persistent cellular, or during an early stage of chronic rejection [2, 4]. Treatment failures have been reported after conversion during clinically manifest chronic ductopenic rejection and to a lesser extent for steroid-resistant and OKT3-resistant cellular rejections [2, 7, 12]. Prior OKT3 courses and excessive preconversion total serum bilirubin levels were identified as putative risk factors for patient and graft survival. It was concluded that a less stringent selection for rescue therapy, i. e. its implementation early in the course of a rejection episode and prior to an OKT3 application, should result in an improved overall outcome. Herein, we report our experience with 78 patients converted for various types of liver allograft rejection, comprising uncomplicated cellular rejection episodes, as well as patients suffering from vanishing bile duct syndrome (VBDS).

Material and methods

Patient selection

From September 1988 to March 1995, 600 liver transplantations were performed in 546 patients. In 478 transplantations, immunosuppression consisted of cyclosporin-based immunosuppressive regimens. As part of different trials, after a total of 122 transplantations, patients received Tacrolimus in order to evaluate its properties as a primary immunosuppressive agent. After Tacrolimus had become available to our centre in May 1990, it was used as a rescue agent in 78 cases until August 1995. Conversion from cyclosporin-based immunosuppressive regimens to Tacrolimus was implemented after informed consent had been obtained. The course of the patients was followed on an inpatient basis during the first 4 weeks posttransplant, or on a routine clinical and outpatient basis later on.

Liver transplantation

Grafts had been preserved using almost exclusively Belzer's University of Wisconsin solution. In two cases each, Euro Collins' and Bretschneider's HTK solution were applied. The surgical procedure was performed using a standardized technique, comprising a veno-venous bypass and completion of all four vascular anastomoses prior to reperfusion. In all but 53 cases requiring a bilio-digestive anastomosis due to the underlying disease, the biliary reconstruction was performed as a side-to-sidecholedochocholedochostomy [15].

Primary immunosuppression

Primary immunosuppressive protocols consisted either of conventional triple therapy, of our standard quadruple drug induction regimen entailing an antithymocyte or antilymphocyte globulin preparation (ATG; Fresenius, Bad Homburg, Germany) [16], or of another sequential quadruple drug protocol using a monoclonal anti-interleukin 2 receptor antibody (BT563; Biotest GmbH, Dreieich, Germany) [14].

Except for ATG or BT563 treatment, an almost identical immunosuppressive regimen was applied irrespective of the primary protocol group. Cyclosporin was started after surgery as a parenteral dose of 1–2 mg/kg body weight (BW) twice a day. If clinical course and protocol cholangiography on posttransplant day 5 al-

lowed capping the T-tube drainage, cyclosporin was switched to an oral intake of 5 mg/kg BW twice a day. Subsequent dosing was adjusted according to whole blood levels, aiming at 600 and 900 ng/ml as measured by a polyclonal FPIA (TDX-assay, Abbott). Methylprednisolone was given prior to reperfusion and directly after transplantation at a dose of 500 mg i. v. each.

Prednisolone was begun as a single oral dose of 1 mg/kg BW, which was tapered to 20 mg/day during the first month. Parenteral administration of azathioprine was started at 25 mg/day until 1 week after transplantation; on posttransplant day 7 the dosage was increased to 1–2 mg/kg BW orally. Intake was reduced or interrupted according to peripheral white blood counts. ATG was started intra- or postoperatively at a dose of 5 mg/kg BW per day and given for 7 days in a continuous infusion over 6 h. BT563 was administered i. v. for 12 days at a daily dose of 10 mg.

Rejection episodes

Rejection episodes were suspected in cases of scant production of light bile or biochemical graft dysfunction as defined by rising serum levels of bilirubin or hepatic enzymes (> 50 % above initial values) without evidence of mechanical causes or infection [11]. Doppler ultrasonography was done if indicated to rule out hepatic artery or portal vein thrombosis. If suspicion of a vascular complication prevailed, diagnosis had to be confirmed by angiography. Bile leakage or biliary obstruction were excluded by cholangiography. Screening for infectious disorders entailed the collection of routine specimens for culture and microscopy, quantification of fungal and viral titres in blood, direct immunofluorescence for *Legionella* in blood and urine and the search for cytomegalovirus antigen in blood by the polymerase chain reaction [17].

Core liver biopsies were obtained on posttransplant day 7 or when rejection was suspected. The histopathological grading of acute or cellular rejection was classified as listed below:
Mild (grade I): mild periportal mononuclear infiltrate with minimal endothelialitis and focal duct damage involving less than 50 % of the bile ducts
Moderate (grade II): moderate periportal mononuclear infiltrate extending beyond portal field confines, or focal duct damage involving more than 50 % of the bile ducts
Severe (grade III): the same alterations as described for grade II plus severe injuries (arteritis, central ischaemic damage, confluent necroses, paucity of bile ducts)

A diagnosis of chronic or ductopenic rejection relied largely on the evidence of cholestasis with an interlobular and septal duct loss. Other histological criteria were the absence of findings concordant with viral hepatitis, obliterative arteriolar lesions and portal tract fibrosis with linkage between central veins and portal triads. Distinction between early chronic and chronic rejection was based on the extent of lymphocytic bile duct damage or loss. A bile duct loss limited to less than 25 % of the sample triads without cholestasis or lobular changes was categorized as an early chronic rejection. Findings indicative of a chronic rejection were a bile duct loss of 50 % or more, lymphocytic damage in the remaining ducts and hepatocanalicular cholestasis. Corresponding to an onset prior to or after posttransplant day 90, cellular rejection episodes were classified as early- or late-onset rejections, respectively.

Treatment of rejection

Initial therapy consisted of a 3-day course of high-dose steroids, i. e. 500 mg/day methylprednisolone intravenously. Steroid-resistant episodes were treated for another 5–10 days with 5 mg/day of monoclonal OKT3 antibody. Conversion to Tacrolimus was applied in OKT3 non-responders, or as soon as a chronic ductopenic rejection was suspected irrespective of prior OKT3 treatment. A direct switch to Tacrolimus for steroid-resistant cellular rejection was considered in late-onset episodes and in patients with a persistent CsA malabsorption in spite of a capped T-tube drainage. After gaining more experience with Tacrolimus, we were more apt to implement a direct conversion for steroid-resistant or even uncomplicated cellular rejection. Rescue therapy was started with continuation of oral steroids and administration of oral Tacrolimus. Initial dosing ranged from 0.07 to 0.1 mg/kg BW twice a day. Further adjustments were related to toxicity and response or graft function.

Evaluation of outcome

Outcome was evaluated in terms of response or non-response and success or failure. Response was considered positive if a cellular rejection was reversed or if progression of bile duct loss in chronic rejection was at least interrupted, thereby improving liver function. Repeat biopsies were performed unless the clinical course had been unambiguous. Success or failure were determined with regard to both patient and graft survival.

Statistical evaluation

Data were expressed as mean ± standard error of the mean. Comparisons between groups were made by the Wilcoxon rank-sum test for continuous variables and by the chi-square test for categorical variables. Differences were considered statistically significant at $P < 0.05$.

Results

Patient characteristics

Of 600 patients transplanted between September 1988 and March 1995, 78 underwent Tacrolimus rescue therapy after the drug became available to our centre in May 1990. In 478 transplantations, CsA-based regimens had been administered as primary immunosuppression (Table 1). Indications for transplantation in the 78 patients converted to Tacrolimus included 15 patients with hepatitis C virus (HCV) disease, 10 patients with hepatitis B virus (HBV) disease, 7 patients with primary sclerosing cholangitis, 7 patients with primary biliary cirrhosis, 7 patients with Klatskin tumours, 6 patients with fulminant liver failure, 6 patients with alcoholic cirrhosis and 20 patients with various other indications. Forty-one patients were female and 37 were male, with a mean age of 49.1 ± 11.1 years.

Indications for conversion

The secondary diagnoses triggering off rescue therapy are shown in Table 2. The most common indications were chronic ductopenic rejection ($n = 9$), OKT3-resistant cellular rejection ($n = 12$), steroid-resistant cellular

Table 1 Primary immunosuppression in the study population compared to the whole series

Primary immunosuppression	$n = 522$	Tacrolimus rescue $n = 78$
Tacrolimus-based	122 (20.3 %)	
CsA-based	400 (66.6 %)	78 (13.1 %)
Triple	23 (5.7 %)	6 (7.7 %)
Quadruple (ATG/ALG)	234 (58.5 %)	48 (61.5 %)
Quadruple (BT563)	143 (35.8 %)	24 (30.8 %)

Table 2 Indications for conversion to Tacrolimus and outcome in terms of response and survival

Indication for conversion	n	Response		Survival	
		Yes	No	Yes	No
Chronic ductopenic rejection	9	5	4 (3)[a]	6 (3)[a]	3
Early chronic rejection	5	5		5	
OKT3-resistant cellular rejection	12	12		9	3
Steroid-resistant cellular rejection	30	28	2 (1)[a]	24 (1)[a]	6
Late-onset cellular rejection	10	10		9	1
Cellular rejection and CsA malabsorption	5	5		5	
Uncomplicated cellular rejection	7	7		6	1
Overall	78	72 (92 %)	6	64 (82 %)	14

[a] Number of retransplantations

rejection ($n = 30$) and late-onset cellular rejection ($n = 10$). In the group of poor CsA uptake ($n = 5$), three patients had undergone liver transplantation and Whipple's procedure for Klatskin tumours [13]. In two patients, choledochojejunostomy for primary sclerosing cholangitis had been performed. Cycles of OKT3 had already been administered in five patients with chronic rejection and in one patient each of the late-onset and of the early chronic rejection group.

Outcome

After a median follow-up of 2 years (23.3 ± 14.5 months), 72 of 78 patients or 92.3 % were responsive, and six patients or 7.7 % were non-responsive. Patient survival was observed in 64 patients (82.1 %) and graft survival in 60 patients (77.0 %). Non-responsiveness was evident in 4 of 9 patients in the chronic rejection group and in 2 of 30 patients in the steroid-resistant cellular rejection group (Table 2).

There were 14 lethal cases: 3 of 9 patients suffering from chronic ductopenic rejection, 3 of the 12 OKT3 non-responders, 6 of 30 patients in the steroid-resistant cellular rejection group and 1 patient each suffering from an uncomplicated or a late-onset cellular rejection (Table 2). In these patients, the average period of time elapsing from transplantation to the onset of rescue therapy and from the switch to patient death was approximately 4 months (122 ± 150 days; range: 10–454 days) and 3 months (78 ± 151 days; range: 7–526 days), respectively.

Patients died almost exclusively of infectious complications. The most common final diagnoses were *Pneumocystis carinii* and cytomegalovirus (CMV) pneumonia in five and four patients, respectively. Aspergillosis was the cause of death in two patients. One patient each died from recurrent primary disease, an aggravated HCV reinfection and a Klatskin tumour relapse.

Comparing those who, for chronic ductopenic rejection, were converted to Tacrolimus only ($n = 4$) to those who had in addition received at least one prior course of OKT3 ($n = 5$), a rather balanced pattern for the rejection response ($n = 2$ vs. $n = 3$) was found. Looking at the fatalities ($n = 3$), all had undergone a previous course of OKT3 and none had solely been on Tacrolimus. However, neither correlation was statistically significant.

Graft loss that was not related to patient death was observed four times (Table 2). Three patients underwent successful retransplantation for chronic ductopenic rejection and another for a hyperacute rejection in the postoperative course. Chronically rejecting grafts were lost 4–5 months posttransplant or 2–3 months postconversion.

Patients were converted to Tacrolimus on an intent-to-treat basis. Mainly during the earlier phase of our programme, prior to our initial experience with Tacrolimus or its availability, 15 patients received OKT3 alone for treatment of cellular steroid-resistant rejections. Ten patients recovered (67 %), while one patient died and four underwent retransplantation for refractory rejection. A further 19 patients had to be switched to Tacrolimus for progressive rejection after OKT3 therapy.

Adverse events

Adverse events that occurred were mainly infection, renal insufficiency or neurological disorder and were pre-existent in a total of 51 patients (65 %). Their incidence could be split into three categories; those arising de novo, those that were persistent and those improving postconversion (Table 3).

De novo infections were observed in 30 patients (38 %) and nephrotoxic or neurotoxic effects were observed in 18 (23 %) and 22 cases (28 %), respectively. Persistence or even aggravation of pre-existent infectious complications were evident in 6 patients (8 %) and pre-existent renal insufficiency or neurological disorders were evident in 11 (14 %) and 6 patients (8 %), respectively. Improvement of prior disorders occurred in 27 patients (35 %) if they were of infectious nature, and in 10 (13 %) and 11 patients (14 %) if of renal origin or related to a neurological site, respectively.

De novo infection was mostly caused by opportunistic pathogens, i.e. CMV ($n = 13$), *Pneumocystis carinii* ($n = 5$) and *Legionella* ($n = 3$), as well as by fungi ($n = 5$). Aggravation of pre-existent infection after conversion was mainly related to those caused by CMV ($n = 3$). All these took a lethal course, in one patient each suffering from chronic ductopenic, OKT3-resistant cellular or severe steroid-resistant cellular rejection. Five pre-existent CMV infections improved postconversion, and bacterial cholangitis ($n = 12$) was the pre-existent complication improving most often during success-

Table 3 Incidence of adverse events in the study population listed as de novo, persistent or improving in relation to the start of Tacrolimus therapy

Adverse events		De novo n	Persistent n	Improving n
Infections (all)		30	6	27
	CMV (PCR positivity[a])	10	1	4
	CMV pneumonia	3	2	1
	PCP	5		
	Legionella pneumonia	3		
	Fungal infections	5	2	5
	Bacterial cholangitis	5		12
	Urinary tract infection	3		7
	Bacterial pneumonia	3		3
	Peritonitis		1	1
	Tuberculosis	1		
Renal insufficiency (all)		18	11	10
	Serum creatinine > 1.5 mg/dl	12	3	2
	Haemodialysis requirement	6	8	8
Neurological disorders (all)		22	6	11
Minor	Tremor	19	4	5
	Mood changes	2		
	Somnolence	2		
	Headache	3		
	Peripheral neural disorders	1	1	
Major	Organic mental syndrome	4		1
	Psychosis	2		
	Seizures	2	1	
	Encephalopathy			5
	Personality disorder			1
	Dysarthria			2
	Ataxia			1

[a] Polymerase chain reaction (PCR) directed detection of CMV envelope in blood

Table 4 Comparison of preconversion laboratory values as a function of the indication for conversion to Tacrolimus in the groups where failures had occurred

	Bili (mg/dl)	aP (IU/l)	γ-GT (IU/l)	AST (IU/l)	ALT (IU/l)
Chronic ductopenic rejection					
Success	16.6 ± 11.0	727 ± 429	640 ± 195	88 ± 38	194 ± 83
Failure	13.7 ± 4.7	697 ± 444	602 ± 476	61 ± 53	100 ± 67
OKT3-resistant cellular rejection					
Success	12.3 ± 8.1	207 ± 93	320 ± 201	48 ± 35	124 ± 91
Failure	15.9 ± 6.3	263 ± 78	411 ± 237	79 ± 41	137 ± 38
Severe steroid-resistant cellular rejection					
Success	$9.9 \pm 6.8*$	234 ± 147	340 ± 175	70 ± 52	114 ± 41
Failure	$22.2 \pm 7.3*$	139 ± 173	299 ± 261	94 ± 48	147 ± 53

ful rescue therapy irrespective of the secondary diagnosis.

An isolated rise in serum creatinine above 1.5 mg/dl or a requirement for haemodialysis as a complication after the onset of Tacrolimus administration was evident in 12 and 6 patients, respectively. Eight patients undergoing haemodialysis had already done so prior to conversion. In another eight patients, the postconversion kidney function improved to an extent that haemodialysis was no longer necessary. No non-lethal case required haemodialysis for more than 8 weeks. However, renal insufficiency, as measured by a serum creatinine level ranging from 1.6 mg/dl to 3 mg/dl, was persistent in eight patients during long-term follow-up. A further four patients suffering from renal dysfunction were among seven patients (8.9 %) undergoing a reconversion to CsA-based immunosuppression either after dissolution of a rejection episode or after retransplantation due to VBDS ($n = 2$). An improvement in postconversion disorders was observed in six patients after reconversion, while one who reconverted due to an aggravated HCV reinfection died later on.

Neurological disorders were further divided into minor and major disturbances, observed in 22 (28 %) and 8 patients (10 %), respectively. Since the clinical picture was compounded by minor and major manifestations, only 14 patients (18 %) presented solely with minor changes. The most prominent de novo neurological complication after conversion to Tacrolimus was tremor ($n = 19$). It did not display a predilection for any of the secondary diagnoses and occurred in 7 of the 14 lethal cases. However, neurological evaluation in the moribund and critically ill was likely to be impeded by sedation or even relaxation for optimized ventilatory support. Both cases of somnolence were diagnosed in patients dying later of CMV and *Pneumocystis carinii* pneumonia. Among the neurological disorders improving during the rescue therapy, encephalopathy ($n = 5$) was most eminent. Its aetiology was metabolic, and it occurred in two successful rescue cases in the groups of chronic ductopenic and steroid-resistant cellular rejections, as well as in one pa-

tient suffering from cellular rejection in the CsA malabsorption group.

Laboratory findings

Preconversion laboratory parameters in the groups where failures had occurred were checked for a putative predictive potency (Table 4). A significantly elevated total serum bilirubin when comparing failures and the respective successful cases (22.2 ± 7.3 mg/dl vs. 9.9 ± 6.8 mg/dl; $p < 0.05$) was found in the group of steroid-resistant cellular rejection. Prior to conversion in chronic ductopenic rejection, total serum bilirubin levels were rather higher in patients profiting of the rescue therapy. Among OKT3 non-responders, the levels of total serum bilirubin, as well as alkaline phosphatase (aP) and γ-glutamyltransferase (γ-GT) activities had been elevated slightly though not significantly in those where rescue was about to fail.

Discussion

After 2 years of follow-up, patient and graft survival after conversion to Tacrolimus for various types of liver allograft rejection were 82 % and 77 %, respectively, with a response rate of 92 %. These figures exceeded earlier results from the United States multicentre trial, which generated 1-year survival figures of 72 % for patients and 50 % for grafts, as well as our previously reported experience after 33 conversions, where the 2-year data for patient and graft survival were 76 % and 70 %, respectively [7, 12]. While in the United States multicentre trial, patients suffering from chronic or OKT3-resistant cellular rejection had almost exclusively been enrolled, our earlier results have already reflected a more liberal use of conversion therapy. However, it could be concluded from these and other reports that a conversion to Tacrolimus earlier in the course of a rejection episode might be advisable [2]. Therefore, only 33 % of the patients in this study fulfilled the re-

S169

quirements of the United States multicentre trial, while
the remaining were suffering from steroid-resistant and
late-onset cellular rejection, from cellular rejection during inadequate CsA uptake or even from uncomplicated
cellular rejection. The improved outcome was largely
due to a higher share of these less complicated rejection
types, while the survival figures after conversion for
manifest chronic ductopenic rejection, where a restricted impact of rescue therapy is a well-known feature, remained unchanged [2, 4, 8, 9, 19].

Opportunistic infections, i. e. *Pneumocystis carinii*
and CMV pneumonia, account for most of the rescue
failures. Although in 65 % of all cases undergoing conversion to Tacrolimus, many infectious, renal, and neurological complications had already pre-existed, all
Pneumocystis carinii pneumonias were acquired de
novo. It might be worthy of note that four of these five
patients had undergone transplantation prior to a
change in our perioperative prophylaxis from aerosol-
ized Pentamidine to Bactrim. While the incidence of infections was not elevated in primary protocols entailing
Tacrolimus, a rising rate was evident in the same study
among those converted [11]. A distinct risk associated
with conversion was also supplemented by another report indicating a *Pneumocystis carinii* pneumonia incidence of 12 % [8].

In spite of a liberalization of entry criteria, a substantial proportion of the patients were still high-risk cases,
which is reflected by both the 51 patients (65 %) presenting with pre-existent infectious, renal or neurological disorders, and a time interval from onset of Tacrolimus conversion to patient death sometimes being as
short as 1 week. In successfully converted patients, the
benefit applied not only to control of rejection, but also
to these pre-existing disorders. The general improvement might be associated with a gain in liver function
or with previous drug-induced toxicity. Bacterial infections mainly and, herein, cholangitis may have been affected by less impaired non-specific defences and a normalization in bile flow [1, 5]. Kidney function was enhanced to an extent that in eight cases the former requirement for haemodialysis did not persist after con-

version. Neurological disorders that were alleviated after conversion were predominantly metabolic, with a
subsequent gain in liver and kidney function. Conversely, postconversion nephro- and neurotoxicity were
experienced by 23 % and 28 % of the patients, respectively. Possible contributing factors such as infections
or nephrotoxic antibiotics not being taken into account,
the share of patients exhibiting renal dysfunction was
considerably lower than the initial 80–90 % figures of
previous rescue studies [6, 10]. Long-term toxicity was
confined to mild renal insufficiency in eight patients.
However, a reconversion to CsA-based immunosuppression was implemented in a further seven patients
(9 %) mainly for renal dysfunction, resulting in an improved serum creatinine.

In our study, neither the bilirubin level nor serum activities of hepatocellular or canalicular enzymes were
predictive of outcome of conversion in chronic ductopenic and OKT3-resistant cellular rejection. In cellular
steroid-resistant rejection, the preconversion total serum bilirubin was significantly elevated in failures
when compared to the respective successful cases. In all
patients where a biopsy was obtained after conversion,
rejection had resolved completely. In contrast to chronic
rejection, the rise in serum bilirubin was likely to be due
to an impaired hepatocellular function without a significant role of duct loss. Since the predictive potency was
confined to failure and not to non-response, it raises
the question of whether Tacrolimus will be able to overcome a given extent of graft damage only at the expense
of severe overimmunosuppression.

In conclusion, implementation of a conversion to Tacrolimus early in the course of a rejection episode resulted in a further improvement in patient and graft survival. Failures occurred in the groups of OKT3-resistant
and steroid-resistant cellular rejection, and only in a
subgroup of patients suffering from chronic ductopenic
rejection was a permanent benefit observed. Therefore,
predictive parameters, e. g. the total serum bilirubin in
steroid-resistant cellular rejection, are still required to
identify those patients who would profit rather from a
retransplantation.

References

1. Carey M (1982) The enterohepatic circulation. In: Arias I, Popper H, Schach-
ter D, Shafritz DA (eds) The liver: biology and pathobiology. Raven Press,
New York, pp 429–444

2. Demetris AJ, Fung JJ, Todo S, McCauley J, Jain A, Takaya S, Alessiani M,
Abu-Elmagd K, VanThiel DM, Starzl
TE (1992) Conversion of liver allograft
recipients from cyclosporine to FK506
immunosuppressive therapy – a clinicopathologic study of 96 patients. Transplantation 53: 1056–1062

3. Fung JJ, Todo S, Jain A, McCauley J,
Alessiani M, Scotti C, Starzl TE (1990)
Conversion from cyclosporine to FK506
in liver allograft recipients with cy-
closporine-related complications.
Transplant Proc 22: 6–12

4. Fung JJ, Todo S, Tzakis A, Alessiani M,
Abu-Elmagd K, Jain A, Bronster O,
Martin M, Gordon R, Starzl TE (1991)
Current status of FK506 in liver trans-
plantation. Transplant Proc 23: 1902–
1905

5. Gluckman SJ, Dvorak VC, MacGregor RR (1977) Host defences during prolonged alcohol consumption in a controlled environment. Arch Intern Med 137: 1539–1545

6. Hebert MF, Ascher NL, Lake JR, Roberts JP (1991) Efficacy and toxicity of FK506 for the treatment of resistant rejection in liver transplant patients. Transplant Proc 23: 3109–3110

7. Jonas S, Bechstein WO, Lemmens HP, Kling N, Grauhan O, Lobeck H, Neuhaus P (1996) Conversion to Tacrolimus after liver transplantation. Transplant Int 9: 23–31

8. Lewis WD, Jenkins RL, Burke PA, Winn KM, Shaffer D, Lopez R, Monaco AP (1991) FK506 rescue therapy in liver transplant recipients with drug-resistant rejection. Transplant Proc 23: 2989–2991

9. Makowka L, Svanas G, Esquivel C (1986) Effect of cyclosporin on hepatic regeneration. Surg Forum 37: 352–357

10. McCauley J, Fung JJ, Brown H, Deballi P, Jain A, Todo S, Starzl TE (1991) Renal function after conversion from cyclosporine to FK506 in liver transplant patients. Transplant Proc 23: 3148–3149

11. Mor E, Solomon H, Gibbs JF, Holman MJ, Goldstein RM, Husberg BS, Gonwa TA, Klintmalm GB (1992) Acute cellular rejection following liver transplantation: Clinical pathologic features and effect on outcome. Semin Liver Dis 12: 28–40

12. Multicenter FK506 Liver Study Group (1993) Prognostic factors for successful conversion from cyclosporine to FK506-based immunosuppressive therapy for refractory rejection after liver transplantation. Transplant Proc 25: 641–643

13. Neuhaus P, Blumhardt G (1994) Extended bile duct resection – a new oncological approach to the treatment of central bile duct carcinomas? Description of method and early results. Langenbecks Arch Chir 379: 123–128

14. Neuhaus P, Bechstein WO, Blumhardt G, Wiens M, Lemmens P, Langrehr JM, Lohmann R, Steffen R, Schlag H, Slama KJ, Lobeck H (1993) Comparison of quadruple immunosuppression after liver transplantation with ATG or IL-2 receptor antibody. Transplantation 55: 1320–1327

15. Neuhaus P, Blumhardt G, Bechstein WO, Steffen R, Platz KP, Keck H (1994) Technique and results of biliary reconstruction using side-to-side choledochocholedochostomy in 300 orthotopic liver transplants. Ann Surg 219: 426–434

16. Schattenfroh N, Lange D, Bechstein WO, Blumhardt G, Keck H, Langrehr JM, Lohmann R, Neuhaus P (1993) Induction therapy with anti-T-lymphocyte globulin following orthotopic liver transplantation. Transplant Proc 25: 2702

17. Schmidt CA, Oettle H, Neuhaus P, Wiens M, Timm H, Wilborn F, Siegert W (1993) Demonstration of cytomegalovirus by polymerase chain reaction after liver transplantation. Transplantation 56: 872

18. Starzl TE, Todo S, Fung J, Demetris AJ, Venkataramman R, Jain A (1989) FK506 for liver, kidney, and pancreas transplantation. Lancet 2: 1000–1004

19. Winkler M, Ringe B, Gerstenkorn C, Rodeck B, Gubernatis G, Wonigeit K, Pichlmayr R (1991) Use of FK506 for treatment of chronic rejection after liver transplantation. Transplant Proc 23: 2984–2986

Transpl Int (1996) 9 [Suppl 1]: S171–S173
© Springer-Verlag 1996

A. P. van den Berg
I. J. Klompmaker
B. G. Hepkema
A. S. H. Gouw
E. B. Haagsma
S. P. Lems
T. H. The
M. J. H. Slooff

Cytomegalovirus infection does not increase the risk of vanishing bile duct syndrome after liver transplantation

A. P. van den Berg (✉) · T. H. The
Department of Clinical Immunology,
University Hospital Groningen,
P. O. Box 30.001, NL-9700 RB Groningen,
The Netherlands

I. J. Klompmaker · E. B. Haagsma
Department of Gastroenterology and
Hepatology, University Hospital,
P. O. Box 30.001, NL-9700 RB Groningen,
The Netherlands

B. G. Hepkema · S. P. Lems
Department of Transplantation
Immunology, University Hospital,
P. O. Box 30.001, NL-9700 RB Groningen,
The Netherlands

A. S. H. Gouw
Department of Pathology, University
Hospital, P. O. Box 30.001,
NL-9700 RB Groningen, The Netherlands

M. J. H. Slooff
Department of Hepatobiliary and
Pancreatic Surgery, University Hospital,
P. O. Box 30.001, NL-9700 RB Groningen,
The Netherlands

Abstract Cytomegalovirus (CMV) infection and HLA-DR sharing have been reported to be associated with the development of vanishing bile duct syndrome (VBDS) after liver transplantation. We retrospectively analyzed the importance of these risk factors for VBDS in 126 consecutive recipients of a first transplant. In contrast to previous studies, CMV was monitored strictly using the antigenemia assay, a quantitative marker of the viral load. Patient and graft survival were comparable in patients with and without CMV infection. The incidence of VBDS was low, regardless of the CMV infection status or degree of HLA-DR sharing. Improvements in the early diagnosis and treatment of CMV infection may have eliminated its negative influence on graft survival.

Key words Cytomegalovirus · VBDS · HLA-DR · Liver transplantation

Introduction

It has been reported that cytomegalovirus (CMV) infection, in combination with a one or more HLA-DR antigen match between donor and recipient, is associated with a tenfold increase in the relative risk of vanishing bile duct syndrome (VBDS) after orthotopic liver transplantation (OLT) [1]. Others have shown that HLA-DR match increases the incidence of CMV hepatitis, which in its turn increases the risk of VBDS fourfold [2]. Not all groups have been able to confirm these data, however [3].

High-quality virological monitoring is a prerequisite for studies on the relation between CMV infection and specific clinical events. The CMV antigenemia assay that has been developed in our laboratory is a sensitive and specific test to diagnose active CMV infection [4, 5]. It provides a quantitative estimate of the actual viral load, which makes it particularly useful to study the pathogenetic role of CMV on immunological events after transplantation. We analyzed the relation between CMV infection, HLA-DR matching, and VBDS in a cohort of patients who were meticuously monitored for CMV infection.

Materials and methods

Clinical management

A total of 126 consecutive adult recipients of a first OLT and surviving for at least 4 weeks formed the study population. The median duration of follow-up was 30 (range 1–100) months. Immunosuppression consisted of prednisolone, cyclosporin, and azathioprine, with a 1-week induction course of cyclophosphamide [6].

Acute rejections were documented by biopsy and treated with methylprednisolone pulses or a steroid recycle; in cases of steroid resistance, a course of rabbit ATG was given (Bijleveld et al., submitted for publication).

CMV seronegative recipients preferentially received a liver from a seronegative donor. No hyperimmunoglobulin or high-dose acyclovir prophylaxis against CMV were given. Generally, no specific measures were taken in case of asymptomatic CMV infection. When CMV disease occurred, immunosuppression was tapered according to protocol: prednisolone was reduced to 10 mg daily and azathioprine to 50 mg daily, whereas the cyclosporin dosage was kept unchanged. Ganciclovir was started when CMV disease persisted or when organs were involved. Immunosuppression was restored to normal levels when symptoms had subsided, antigenemia had decreased, and an antibody response had occurred.

CMV monitoring

CMV infection was diagnosed by weekly monitoring of antigenemia, viremia, and serology, as previously reported [5]. Biopsies were performed when organ involvement was clinically suspected.

HLA-DR typing

The two-colour fluorescence method using sets of locally obtained, well-characterized allo-antisera was used [7].

Definitions

CMV infection was defined by the detection of antigenemia or viremia, or by demonstration of a significant antibody rise [6]. CMV disease required the presence of laboratory evidence of CMV infection, a compatible clinical syndrome, and the absence of alternative causes of the symptoms. Diagnosis of VBDS required the complete absence of interlobular or small bile ducts in 50 % or more of portal tracts, with or without arteriopathy with intimal proliferation and foamy macrophage infiltration [8].

Statistics

Graft and patient survival rates were calculated using the Kaplan-Meier method, and the log-rank test was used to evaluate statistical significancy. The Wilcoxon rank test for unpaired data and the chi-square test were used where indicated. All tests were performed two-sided, with P values of 0.05 or less being considered as statistically significant. In addition, 95 % confidence interval (CI) levels are given where appropriate.

Results

CMV infection and patient and graft survival

CMV infection occurred in 85 of the 126 patients (67 %). Infection was primary in 14, and secondary in the remaining 71 patients. Clinical manifestations occurred in 61 patients, comprising fever with or without arthralgia, myalgia, and malaise ($n = 48$), fever with biochemical evidence of hepatitis ($n = 11$), or pneumonitis

Table 1 Incidence of vanishing bile duct syndrome (VBDS) in relation to cytomegalovirus (CMV) infection and HLA-DR matching between donor and recipient (*CI* confidence interval)

CMV infection	HLA-DR antigen match	Incidence of VBDS (95 % CI)
No	0	2/22 9 % (1–29)
No	≥ 1	0/19 0 % (0–18)
Yes	0	2/55 4 % (4–13)
Yes	≥ 1	1/30 3 % (0–17)

($n = 2$); 25 patients received ganciclovir because of CMV disease. No patient died as a direct result of CMV infection.

Infection was diagnosed by the presence of antigenemia in 79 patients; a serological response occurred in 82. Antigenemia permitted a presymptomatic diagnosis in the majority of cases and was valuable in the management of infection. Patient and graft survival rates at 2 years were 84 % and 81 %, respectively, and were not different in patients with and without CMV infection.

VBDS

VBDS developed in five (4 %) patients at a median of 3 (range 2–12) months after OLT. Occurrence of VBDS was not related to patient age of sex, cold ischemia time, or operative blood loss. As expected, acute rejection was a risk factor for VBDS [relative risk (RR) 13.4, $P < 0.05$], as was steroid-resistant rejection (RR 12, $P < 0.05$). VBDS occurred in three patients with CMV infection; in all of them, CMV infection preceded VBDS. The RR of VBDS associated with CMV infection therefore was 0.72 (95 % CI 0.13–4.16, $P > 0.1$). VBDS was not related to the maximal CMV load during infection, occurrence of CMV disease, or CMV hepatitis. The risk of VBDS in relation to CMV infection and HLA-DR matching is given in Table 1. No evidence for a pathogenetic role of CMV infection, HLA-DR matching, or their combination was found.

Discussion

These data do not support claims by other groups that CMV infection, alone or in conjunction with a HLA-DR match, is pathogenetically linked to VBDS. Our study was retrospective, but the protocol for CMV monitoring was strict and intensive, and the management of CMV infection and disease was uniform, thus minimizing the potential for bias. It is difficult to explain the conflicting data from Cambridge/King's College [1] and Pittsburgh [2] on the one hand, and those from the Mayo Clinics [3] and our center, on the other. However, VBDS is generally preceded by one or more episodes of acute rejection. More intense immunosuppressive treatment may have promoted the development of CMV infection and facilitated its detection. Thus, CMV infection might just be a reflection of increased alloreactivity. Alternatively, a period of tapering of immunosuppression that was too prolonged might have precipitated the onset of irreversible rejection. Accurate monitoring of viral replication using the antigenemia assay may have prevented undue underimmunosuppression. Finally, antiviral treatment may have limited the amount of damage directly by interruption of the cytopathogenic effects of viral replication, and indirectly, by limiting the cytotoxic T cell response to viral antigens.

References

1. O'Grady JG, Alexander GJM, Sutherland S, et al (1988) Lancet 2: 302–305
2. Manez R, White LT, Linden P, et al (1993) Transplantation 55: 1067–1071
3. Paya CV, Wiesner RH, Hermans PE, et al (1992) Hepatology 16: 66–70
4. Van der Bij W, Torensma R, Van Son WJ, et al (1988) J Med Virol 25: 179–188
5. Van den Berg AP, Klompmaker IJ, Haagsma EB, et al (1991) J Infect Dis 164: 265–270
6. Klompmaker IJ, Haagsma EB, Gouw ASH, et al (1989) Transplantation 48: 814–818
7. Rood van JJ, Leeuwen van A, Ploem JS (1976) Nature 262: 795–797
8. Portmann B, Neuberger J, Williams R (1983) In: Calne RY (ed) Liver transplantation. Grune & Stratton, New York, pp 279–287

Transpl Int (1996) 9 [Suppl 1]: S 174–S 177
© Springer-Verlag 1996

LIVER

A. Tanaka
K. Tanaka
H. Shinohara
E. Hatano
S. Sato
A. Kanazawa
T. Kitai
H. Higashiyama
Y. Nakamura
Y. Yamamoto
H. Okajima
H. Egawa
I. Ikai
S. Uemoto
I. Satomura
N. Ozaki
Y. Inomata
Y. Yamaoka

Extension of the indication for living related liver transplantation from children to adults based on resolution of graft size mismatch in relation to tissue oxygenation and metabolic load: a case report

A. Tanaka (✉) · K. Tanaka · H. Shinohara ·
E. Hatano · S. Sato · A. Kanazawa · T. Kitai ·
H. Higashiyama · Y. Nakamura ·
Y. Yamamoto · H. Okajima · H. Egawa ·
I. Ikai · S. Uemoto · I. Satomura · N. Ozaki ·
Y. Inomata · Y. Yamaoka
Second Department of Surgery,
Faculty of Medicine, Kyoto University,
54 Kawaracho, Shogoin, Sakyoku,
Kyoto 606, Japan
Fax +81-75-751-3551

Abstract We extended the indication for living related partial liver transplantation from pediatric to adult cases. Our first case was a 49-year-old woman with primary biliary cirrhosis. Her sister's left lobe, weighing 280 g, was employed as a graft, and the graft weight/recipient's body weight ratio was calculated as 0.59 %. To decrease the metabolic load to the relatively small graft, the total bilirubin was decreased from a maximum value of 75.0 mg/dl to the most recent preoperative value of 36.2 mg/dl by plasma exchange. Intraoperative recovery of tissue oxygenation and its heterogeneity were satisfactory due to a relatively high blood supply. A postoperative decrease in bilirubin and increase in cholesterol esterification were facilitated, concomitant with regeneration of the graft, which weighed 280 g, to 860 cm^3 at 3 weeks. Linear regression analysis with respect to tissue oxygenation and metabolic capacity obtained in pediatric cases were applied to this adult case.

Key words Graft size mismatch · Living related liver transplantation in an adult · Tissue oxygenation · Metabolic capacity

Introduction

In partial liver transplantation with a living related donor, when the left lateral segment or left lobe is employed as the graft, the graft size and weight are anatomically limited within a narrow range. By contrast, the recipient body size is distributed over a wide range, namely, from infancy to adolescence, as shown in Fig. 1 [4, 6]. It has been reported that normal ratios of whole liver weight relative to body weight (BW) is 2 % in adults. Therefore, the ratio of graft weight to recipient body weight (G/R ratio) is a matter of serious concern in living related liver transplantation (LRLT). In 47 pediatric cases of LRLT, we have shown that the following are affected by the G/R ratio [5]: (1) the tissue oxygenation and synthetic and detoxication capability of the graft, in terms of oxygen saturation of hemoglobin in the liver sinusoid (SO$_2$) and coefficient of variation of SO$_2$ (CV) measured by near-infrared spectroscopy at multiple points, as indices of extracellular oxygenation and its heterogeneity, (2) arterial ketone body ratio (AKBR) as an index of intracellular oxygenation, (3) aspartate aminotransferase as an index of graft injury and, (4) bilirubin clearance, cholesterol esterification [3], and production of total ketone bodies as indices of the metabolic capability of the graft. Based on these results, we started a program of LRLT for adults.

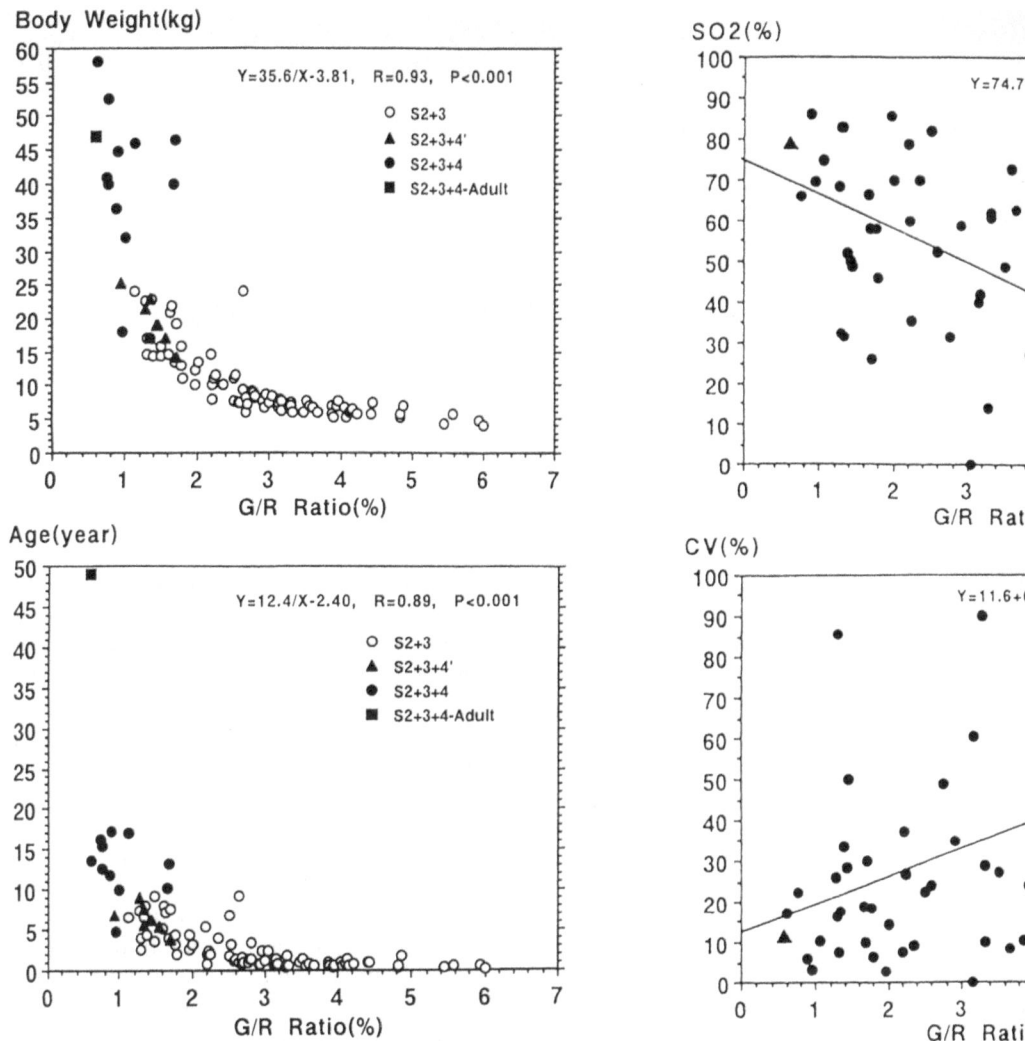

Fig. 1 Hyperbolic correlations among the ratio of graft weight to recipient body weight (G/R ratio), age, and body weight ratio in 100 pediatric cases and 1 adult case

Fig. 2 Fitting of oxygen saturation of hemoglobin in the liver sinusoid (SO_2) and coefficient of variation of SO_2 (CV) after reflow of the portal vein in the adult case to the linear regression analysis obtained in 47 pediatric cases. *Triangle* indicates the adult case

A case report

Our first case was a 49-year-old woman who was suffering from primary biliary cirrhosis with a positive mitochondrial antibody. Ruptured esophageal varices were treated by sclerotherapy, but hepatic coma developed following a catheter infection. The Mayo Clinic risk score was 8.5 and her 1-year survival rate was expected to be less than 50 %. Her sister's left lobe, weighing 280 g, was employed as a graft, and the G/R ratio was calculated to be 0.59 %. To decrease the metabolic load to the relatively small graft, the total bilirubin was decreased from a maximum value of 75.0 mg/dl to a preoperative value of 36.2 mg/dl by plasma exchange on nine occasions. Intraoperative recoveries of SO_2 and its CV were satisfactory due to a relatively high blood supply. The total bilirubin decreased to 2.5 mg/dl and the ester ratio (ER: esterified cholesterol/total cholesterol) increased to 0.643, concomitant with sufficient regeneration of the graft, which weighed 280 g, to 860 cm³ at 3 weeks.

Analysis of the tissue oxygenation and metabolic capacity of the graft in comparison with pediatric cases

Tissue oxygenation and its heterogeneity were assessed by the mean value of SO_2 and its CV at ten different points as measured by near-infrared tissue spectroscopy [2]. Synthetic and detoxication capacity of the graft were assessed by exponential recovery of the ER and exponential decay of total bilirubin (TBIL) as expressed as $\log_e[ER(nPOD)/ER(nPOD)]$ and $\log_e[TBIL(nPOD)/TBIL(nPOD)]$, respectively (POD: postoperative day).

In the present adult case, the SO_2 was 79.8 and 84.1 %, while the CV was 10.9 and 11.0 % after reflow of the portal vein and at the end of the operation, respectively. Figure 2 shows that the values of SO_2 and CV after reflow of the portal vein were nearly on the line obtained by the linear regression analysis of the 47 pediatric cases of our ealier study [5]. $\log_e[TBIL(1POD)/TBIL(preop)]$ and $\log_e[TBIL(14POD)/TBIL(7POD)]$ were −0.882 and −0.257, respectively, while $\log_e[ER(14POD)/ER(preop)]$ and $\log_e[ER(28-$

S176

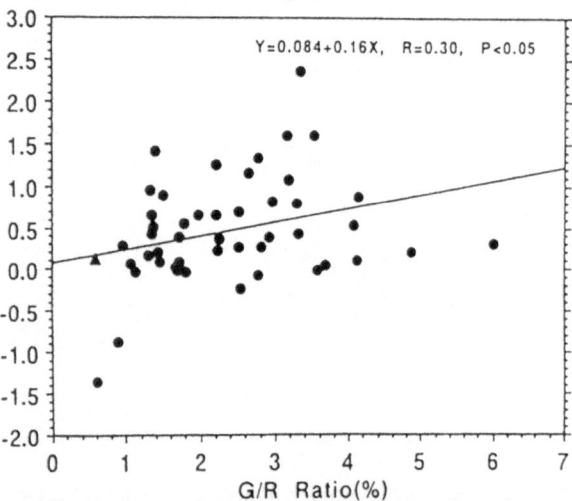

Fig. 3 Fitting of Log$_e$[TBIL(lPOD)/TBIL(preop)] and log$_e$[ER(14POD)/ER(preop)] in the adult case to the linear regression analysis obtained in 47 pediatric cases. *Triangle* indicates the adult case (*TBIL* total bilirubin, *POD* postoperative day, *ER* ester ratio)

POD)/ER(14POD)] were 0.137 and 0.257, respectively. Figure 3 shows that Log$_e$[TBIL(1POD)/TBIL(preop)] and log$_e$[ER(14-POD)/ER(preop)] were also nearly on the line obtained by the linear regression analysis of the 47 pediatric cases.

Discussion

The present study showed that, as compared with small infants with relatively large grafts, intraoperative recovery of tissue oxygenation and its heterogeneity in LRLT for an adult with a relatively small graft were satisfactory even after reflow of the portal vein because of sufficient blood supply. By contrast, both the synthetic capacity of the graft, as assessed by recovery of cholesterol esterification, and detoxication capacity, as assessed by increased bilirubin clearance, were retarded in the postoperative early phase, but were normalized in the late phase. Substantial increases in liver volume (60–200 %) have been reported to occur at 1 month after liver transplantation in cases where the graft liver is smaller than the ideal volume [1]. In our case of LRLT in a 49-year-old woman, the graft regenerated from the initial weight of 280 g to 860 cm^3 at 3 weeks after transplantation. Therefore, early and sufficient regeneration facilitated an increase in metabolic capability.

In the present adult case, the value of the G/R ratio was 0.59 %, which corresponded to 30 % (0.59 %/2.0 %) of the ideal graft volume, since the ideal ratio of liver weight to body weight is 2.0 %. It is known that the normal liver can tolerate right trisegmentectomy with resection of the caudate lobe, which reduces the liver volume by 80 %. Taking disadvantages of procurement, cold preservation, reperfusion, and subsequent immunologic events into consideration, a minimal value of 30 % in LRLT seems to be reasonable.

Since linear regression analysis with respect to tissue oxygenation and metabolic capacity obtained in pediatric cases were applied to this adult case, we concluded that LRLT, using relatively small grafts, can be performed successfully in adults when early regeneration is ensured. These results would suggest that the indication for LRLT can be extended to adult cases.

References

1. Kawasaki S, Makuuchi M, Ishizone S, Matsunami H, Terada M, Kawarazaki H (1992) Liver regeneration in recipients and donors after transplantation. Lancet 339: 580–581

2. Kitai T, Tanaka A, Tokuka A, Tanaka K, Yamaoka Y, Ozawa K, Hirao K (1993) Quantitative detection of hemoglobin saturation in the liver with near-infrared spectroscopy. Hepatology 18: 926–936

3. Sano K, Tanaka A, Uemoto S, Honda K, Tanaka K, Ozawa K (1993) Lipid metabolism after liver transplantation from a living related donor. Clin Sci 85: 83–88

4. Tanaka K, Uemoto S, Tokunaga Y, Fujita S, Sano K, Nishizawa T, Sawada H, Shirahase I, Kim HJ, Yamaoka Y, Ozawa K (1993) Surgical techniques and innovations in living related liver transplantation. Ann Surg 217: 82–91

5. Tanaka A, Tanaka K, Tokuka A, Kitai T, Shinohara H, Hatano E, Sato S, Inomoto T, Takada Y, Higashiyama H, Nakamura Y, Yamamoto Y, Egawa H, Uemoto S, Ikai I, Ozaki N, Inomata Y, Yamaoka Y (1996) Graft size-matching in living related partial liver transplantation in relation to tissue oxygenation and metabolic capacity. Transplant Int 9: 15–22

6. Yamaoka Y, Ozawa K, Tanaka A, Mori K, Morimoto T, Shimahara Y, Zaima M, Tanaka K, Kumada K (1991) New devices for harvesting a hepatic graft from a living donor. Transplantation 52: 157–160

Transpl Int (1996) 9 [Suppl 1]: S178–S181
© Springer-Verlag 1996

LIVER

H. P. Lemmens
U. Neumann
W. O. Bechstein
O. Guckelberger
R. Lüsebrink
S. Jonas
H. Keck
P. Neuhaus

Incidence and outcome of arterial complications after orthotopic liver transplantation

H. P. Lemmens (✉) U. Neumann ·
W. O. Bechstein · O. Guckelberger ·
R. Lüsebrink · S. Jonas · H. Keck ·
P. Neuhaus
Department of Surgery,
Virchow Clinic, Humboldt University,
Augustenburgerplatz 1, D-13353 Berlin,
Germany

Abstract Arterial complications can be a major factor in morbidity and mortality after orthotopic liver transplantation (OLT), as they may cause graft failure, sepsis and complications of the biliary tract. From September 1988 to December 1994, 571 OLT were performed in 529 patients. The follow-up period ranged from 8 to 83 months. Actuarial 1-, 3- and 5-year survival figures were 91 %, 87 % and 85 %, respectively. In 12 cases (2.1 %) complications of the arterial anastomoses were observed. Early arterial complications occurred in eight cases from various causes, while late arterial complications were exclusively thromboses and developed in four patients 8, 12, 26 and 37 months after surgery, respectively. The main clinical course in patients with arterial thromboses was septic cholangitis with destruction of the biliary tree. Although 70 % of the grafts with arterial thrombosis were lost, 30 % could, at least temporarily, be salvaged by other treatment options. Provided adequate treatment is carried out, arterial complications do not affect overall patient survival.

Key words Liver transplantation · Arterial complications · Hepatic artery thrombosis

Introduction

Arterial complications can be a major factor in morbidity and mortality after orthotopic liver transplantation (OLT), as they may cause graft failure, sepsis and complications of the biliary tract [6, 8, 10, 11]. Early thrombosis of the hepatic artery usually necessitates urgent retransplantation; late occlusions have been successfully treated nonoperatively [4, 7]. Meticulous surgical technique is essential to minimize arterial damage, the need for reconstruction and invisible injuries such as intima lesions. It is important to preserve and to reconstruct, if necessary, accessory hepatic arteries to the graft to ensure adequate arterial perfusion after transplantation [5]. The purpose of this study was to examine the incidence and type of arterial complications, their clinical course, the treatment options and the outcome of patients with arterial complications.

Material and methods

From September 1988 to December 1994, 571 OLT were performed in 529 patients, of whom 519 were adults (98.1 %) and 10 were children less than 16 years of age (1.9 %). Recipient age ranged from 2 to 72 years (median 47 years). The indications for OLT are shown in Table 1. The follow-up period ranged from 8 to 83 months (median 37 months). During donor hepatectomy the coeliac axis was taken including an aortic patch. Accessory arteries were preserved. For eventual vascular reconstruction, the iliac vessels (artery and vein) were also routinely taken. OLT was performed according to standard techniques with the routine use of a venovenous bypass. The arterial anastomosis was generally prepared with a 7/0 prolene running suture using a microsurgical technique. Vascular anastomoses were completed before reperfusion of the graft. Intraoperatively and for 3 days postoperatively, aprotinin 100000 U/h was used for prevention of hyperfibrinolysis. Heparin treatment started 48 h after OLT with a dosage of 7500–10000 units per day and was continued until postoperative day 28. In cases of arterial reconstruction of the graft, heparin treatment started 24 h postoperatively at a dose between 7500 and 15000 units per day, and was also continued until day 28. In the perioperative period fresh frozen plasma and AT III were administered in an attempt to correct coagulation abnormalities.

Dicumarol or aspirin were not given for prevention of arterial thrombosis. The patency of the arterial anastomosis was examined during the first 2 weeks daily by duplex ultrasonography, then during the first postoperative year routinely every 3 months and afterwards annually. When there was any evidence of graft dysfunction the patency of the arterial blood supply was tested, and if indicated an additional angio-CT-scan and/or angiography were performed.

Results

Variations of arterial anatomy of the graft

While 87.7 % of the transplanted grafts had a regular arterial anatomy, 12.3 % showed variations of the hepatic artery as demonstrated in Table 2. All accessory right hepatic arteries (4.6 %) were reconstructed on back table by end-to-end anastomosis to the origin of the donor gastroduodenal or splenic artery.

Locations of the arterial anastomoses

At transplantation in 74.3 % of the cases an end-to-side anastomosis between the coeliac axis of the graft and the common hepatic artery of the recipient at the origin of the gastroduodenal (62.7 %) or splenic artery (11.6 %) was chosen. The different locations of the arterial anastomoses are shown in Table 3.

Early complications

Five adult patients (1.0 %) developed arterial thrombosis in the early postoperative phase, one patient 2 weeks, two patients 6 weeks, one patient 8 weeks and one patient 10 weeks after OLT. The clinical course in four patients was associated with fever and septic cholangitis. One patient developed a fulminant graft failure due to early arterial thrombosis and was successfully treated by an urgent retransplantation (re-OLT). At 28 months he was well with normal liver function. Two of the patients with septic cholangitis were treated by early retransplantation. One of these patients had to be retransplanted again 3 months later due to an intractable chronic rejection. At 31 months, he was in good health with normal liver function. The other retransplanted patient died 12 months later due to fulminant sepsis based on ascendent cholangitis. Upon autopsy arterial thrombosis was excluded. One patient with symptoms of septic cholangitis due to destruction of the biliary system mainly of the left liver lobe was treated successfully with a hepaticojejunostomy. At 32 months the liver function was undisturbed with normal serum bilirubin

Table 1 Indications for liver transplantation

	n	%
Postnecrotic cirrhosis	325	56.8
Cholestatic disease	86	15.1
Liver tumour	38	6.6
Acute liver failure	37	6.5
Metabolic disorder	18	3.2
Other	26	4.6
Retransplantation	41	7.2
Total	571	100

Table 2 Variations in the hepatic arteries of the grafts

	n	%
Normal anatomy	501	87.7
Accessory left hepatic artery	41	7.2
Accessory right hepatic artery	17	3
Accessory left and accessory right hepatic arteries	9	1.6
Others	3	0.5

Table 3 Locations of the arterial anastomoses (recipient) with the donor artery

	n	%
Origin of gastroduodenal artery	358	62.7
Origin of splenic artery	66	11.6
Hepatic artery	54	9.5
Coeliac axis	38	6.7
Common hepatic artery	27	4.7
Suprarenal aorta[a]	14	2.5
Infrarenal aorta[a]	14	2.5
Total	571	100

[a] The interposition of a graft (a segment of the donor iliac artery) was necessary for reconstruction in 9/14 and 12/14 cases, respectively

and transaminases. Only the γGT and the alcalic phosphatase (a. p.) were still elevated (γGT 400 U/l; use alk. phos. = alkaline phosphatase 800 U/l).

Another patient with early thrombosis of the hepatic artery and destruction of the left biliary tract was treated initially successfully with a temporary PTCD (**p**ercutaneous **t**ranshepatic **c**holangio-**d**rainage). At 8 months the bilirubin and the cholestatic enzymes were increasing (bilirubin 4 mg/%; γGT 400 U/l; use alk. phos. = alkaline phosphatase 700 U/l), so that a re-OLT may be necessary.

A 2-year-old child developed an arterial thrombosis 11 weeks after segment transplantation (segment II and III). The leading clinical symptoms were severe septic cholangitis with fever and increased cholestatic enzymes, so that re-OLT was inevitable. After re-OLT

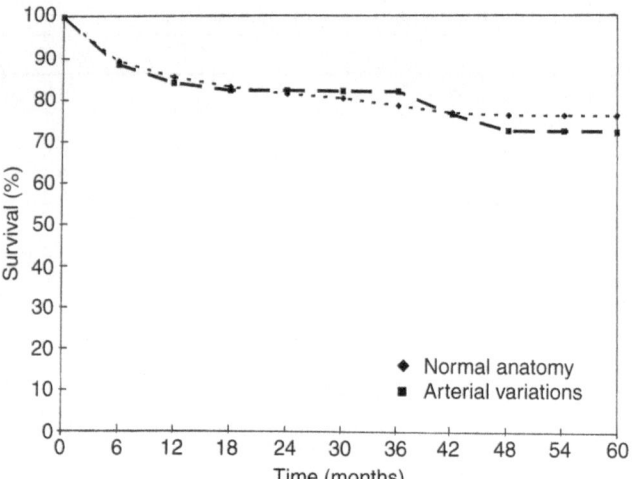

Fig.1 Graft survival according to the arterial anatomy

(also a segment transplantation) the clinical course was uneventful during a follow-up of up to 13 months.

One patient in our series suffered a severe intraabdominal hemorrhage 6 weeks after OLT caused by a mycotic aneurysm of the hepatic artery at the area of anastomosis. The aneurysm was treated by resection and interposition of a venous graft (vena saphena magna). The follow-up (28 months) was undisturbed.

One patient developed a slight elevation of SGOT (200 U/l) and SGPT (230 U/l) 11 weeks after OLT while bilirubin and the synthetic function of the liver were normal. Rejection and infection were ruled out. On angio-CT-scanning a diminished arterial perfusion was seen without perfusion defects. Simultaneously performed coeliacography showed a 70 % stenosis of the arterial anastomosis. As transaminases decreased and liver function was undisturbed, specific treatment was not necessary. This patient was followed up for 38 months.

Late arterial complications

Late arterial complications were exclusively thromboses, and developed in four adult patients 8, 12, 26 and 37 months after surgery, respectively. In two patients septic cholangitis based on an increasing destruction of the biliary system was the leading clinical sign of the arterial thrombosis. These patients were sucessfully retransplanted with normal liver function until the time of writing (47 and 16 months after re-OLT).

One patient developed a temporary dysfunction of the graft 26 months after OLT due to arterial thrombosis with an elevation of SGOT to 2000 U/l and of bilirubin to 6 mg%. As liver function first normalized, no specific treatment was necessary. During more recent months, however, this patient suffered from increased

cholangitis. Destruction of the biliary tree was found on ERC (endoscopic retrograde cholangiography). With decreasing liver function a re-OLT may be necessary in the near future. The fourth patient developed fulminant graft failure with hepatic coma due to a late arterial thrombosis 12 months after OLT. The liver function at this time was reduced due to a HCV (hepatitis c virus) reinfection. The liver function decreased 9 months after an initially successful re-OLT again due to HCV (hepatitis c virus) reinfection (bilirubin 20 mg/%; PT (prothrombine time) 30 %).

Patient and graft survival

Actuarial 1-, 3- and 5-year patient survival figures of all patients were 91 %, 87 % and 85 %, respectively. Patient survival was not different between patients with or without arterial complications. Of 12 patients with arterial thrombosis, 1 (8.3 %) died during the follow-up period. There were also no differences in the survival rates of grafts with or without anatomical variations of the hepatic artery as demonstrated in Fig. 1. Of the 12 patients with arterial complications, 7 (58 %) needed re-OLT, while 5 (42 %) could be at least temporarily salvaged with other treatment options.

Discussion

The incidence of arterial complications after OLT was a significant prognostic factor in the past [2, 4, 6, 8–11]. However, with refinements in surgical technique, arterial complications have become a rare event and have no influence on mortality of the patients. An arterial thrombosis after liver transplantation is usually considered as an indication for urgent retransplantation [10, 11]. Although in our series 3 out of 10 patients with hepatic artery thrombosis could be treated successfully at least temporarily with other options, during follow-up in two patients increased biliary destruction gradually developed. An alternative procedure for the treatment of arterial thrombosis instead of retransplantation can be an urgent revascularization [7, 12]. Recently successful angiographic revascularizations of hepatic artery thromboses after OLT have been described [1, 3].

Prompt surgical revascularization or retransplantation is still the cornerstone of treatment of most cases of hepatic artery thrombosis following OLT to avoid destruction of the biliary tree and septic complications.

References

1. Bjerkvik PS, Vatne K, Mathisen O, Sorlide O (1995) Percutaneous revascularization of postoperativ hepatic artery thrombosis in a liver transplant. Transplantation 59: 1746–1748
2. Blumhardt G, Ringe B, Lauchart W, Burdelski M, Bechstein WO, Pichlmayr R (1987) Vascular problems in liver transplantation. Transplant Proc 19: 2412
3. Figueras J, Busquets J, Dominguez J, Sancho C, Casanovas-Taltavull T, Rafecas A, Fabregat J, Torras J, Jaurrieta E (1995) Intraarterial thrombolysis in the treatment of acute hepatic artery thrombosis after liver transplantation. Transplantation 59: 1356–1357
4. Langnas A, Marujo W, Stratta R, Wood R, Shaw B (1991) Vascular complications after orthotopic liver transplantation. Am J Surg 161: 76–83
5. Lemmens HP, Blumhardt G, Neuhaus P, Keck H, Tsiblaskis N, Rossaint R, Langer R, Steffen R (1992) Technique of arterial anastomosis in liver transplantation, surgical management in routine situations and anatomical variations. Transplant Int 5: 198
6. Lerut J, Gordon R, Iwatsuki S, Starzl TE (1987) Surgical complications in human orthotopic liver transplantation. Acta Chir Belg 87: 193–204
7. Marujo WC, Langnas AN, Wood R, Stratta R, Li S, Shaw B (1991) Vascular complications following orthotopic liver transplantation: outcome and the role of urgent revascularization. Transplant Proc 23: 1484–1486
8. Starzl TE, Demetris A, van Thiel D (1989) Liver transplantation. N Engl J Med 321: 1092–1099
9. Todo S, Makowa L, Tzakis A, Marsh J, Karrer FM, Armany M, Miller C, Tellert M, Esquivel C, Gordon R (1987) Hepatic artery in liver transplantation. Transplant Proc 19: 2406–2411
10. Tzakis A (1985) The dearterialized liver graft. Semin Liver Dis 5: 375–376
11. Tzakis A, Gordon R, Shaw B, Iwatsuki S, Starzl TE (1985) Clinical presentation of hepatic artery thrombosis after liver transplantation in the cyclosporine era. Transplantation 40: 667–671
12. Yanaga K, Lebeau G, Marsh J, Gordon R, Makowa L, Tzakis A, Todo S, Stieber A, Iwatsuki S, Starzl TE (1990) Hepatic artery reconstruction for hepatic artery thrombosis after orthotopic liver transplantation. Arch Surg 125: 628–631

Transpl Int (1996) 9 [Suppl 1]: S182–S184
© Springer-Verlag 1996

LIVER

U. J. Hesse
L. Defreyne
P. Pattyn
I. Kerremans
F. Berrevoet
B. de Hemptinne

Hepato-venous outflow complications following orthotopic liver transplantation with various techniques for hepato-venous reconstruction in adults and children

U. J. Hesse (✉) · L. Defreyne · P. Pattyn ·
I. Kerremans · F. Berrevoet ·
B. de Hemptinne
Department of Surgery and Radiology,
University Hospital Ghent, B-9000 Ghent,
Belgium

Abstract Orthotopic end-to-end cavostomy following liver transplantation was without any complications in 63 cases as compared to latero-lateral cavostomy (14.2 %) and the piggy-back technique of partial liver grafts (14.2 %). Transjugular catheterangioplasty was a practical and successful treatment for the latter, while reoperation for thrombosis in the latero-lateral anastomosis resulted in lethal pulmonary embolism.

Key words Liver transplantation · Complications · Surgical techniques

Introduction

The cavo-caval end-to-end anastomosis in orthotopic liver transplantation is less frequently associated with complications than the arterial or portol-venous anastomosis because of the large size of the anastomosis and the voluminous blood flow. However, with the increasing use of modified liver grafts such as reduced livers or partial livers as obtained from split liver transplantation, modified techniques for the anastomosis of the hepato-venous junction have recently been described [1–5]. Exceptionally, complications with these anastomoses and their treatment have been reported [4, 7]. Our own experience with these techniques regarding the incidence, clinical outcome and morphology of complications, the diagnostic approach and therapy is presented.

Patients and methods

Between May 1991 and December 1994 a total of 110 liver transplants was performed in 76 adults and 34 children. Transplantation was in 75 % ($n = 81$) of cases with a full-size liver (FS), was in 11 % ($n = 12$) of cases a reduced-size liver (RED) in which the vena cava was preserved and in 14 % ($n = 17$) of cases a partial liver (PL) graft in which only the vena hepatica was preserved for the anastomosis (three of these were from living related donors).

Three different techniques were employed to reconstruct the hepato-venous outflow. In the majority of cases ($n = 63$), an orthotopic replacement of the vena cava was performed, with end-to-end anastomosis of the donor vena cava to the recipient vena cava. The so called piggy-back[3] technique was performed in 35 cases, mainly in paediatric patients with an end-to-side hepato-caval, cavo-caval anastomosis or an end-to-end anastomosis of the recipient and the donor hepatic veins, depending on the anatomy of the graft used, i.e. reduced or partial grafts with or without preservation of the donor vena cava, respectively. A latero-lateral cavo-cavostomy [1, 2] was performed in 12 cases.

The use of veno-venous bypass, preservation time in minutes and operating time in minutes during transplantation were registered. The postoperative course and the diagnostic approach in case of complication, including the results of daily ascites production, Doppler sonography and angiography, were analysed.

For transjugular intravascular venoplasty, a number 5 French Cobracatheter was used for cannulation and an Olbert catheter with a 6- to 8-mm balloon was used for dilatation. The patients were followed for a median time of 24 months posttransplantation. For statistical analysis, a Man-Whitney U test was used to compare quantitative differences and a Chi^2 test to compare qualitative differences. Differences were significant when $P < 0.05$.

Results

Veno-venous bypass was used in 39 patients with orthotopic vena cava replacement (62 %) and only in 7 (20 %) patients in whom a piggy-back procedure was performed. When the latero-lateral anastomosis was done, the bypass was never used. The operating time and the preservation time did not differ in the subgroups (Table 1). Regarding the complications relating to graft size and technique applied, there were a total of three

Table 1 Veno-venous bypass, operation time and cold ischaemia time according to the anastomosis used

Anastomosis	Number of patients		Mean operation time (min)	Mean cold ischaemia time (min)
	With bypass	Without bypass		
Orthotopic	39	24	665	798
Piggy-back	7	28	690	875
Latero-lateral	0	12	656	852

arterial thromboses, no portal vein thromboses and three complications (3.4 %) at the hepato-venous reconstruction. The latter complications occurred significantly more frequently with the modified techniques than with orthotopic vena cava replacement ($P = 0.01$) (Table 2).

One adult patient who received a FS liver transplant in which the anastomosis was performed following the technique of Belghiti et al. [1] (latero-lateral cavo-costomy) developed, 7 days posttransplant, a partial thrombosis at the anastomosis. As diagnosed by echography and angiography, two paediatric recipients of partial liver grafts undergoing a piggy-back anastomosis developed a stenosis that could be successfully dilated in one patient at the 63rd and 145th day and in the other at the 56th and 89th day posttransplantation. In the single patient who developed a partial thrombosis in the latero-lateral cavo-cavostomy, reoperation resulted in a lethal lung embolism. Reduced-size liver transplant with preserved donor vena cava did not develop complications at the hepato-venous anastomosis, in common with the full-sized liver with orthotopically replaced vena cava.

Discussion

The orthotopic cavo-caval end-to-end cavostomy following liver transplantation was not associated with complications in this series. In contrast, one patient with a latero-lateral cavo-cavostomy and two patients with the termino-lateral piggy-back technique had to be treated for complications at the anastomosis. Certainly, each of these techniques has its particular indication, regardless of the advantage that veno-venous bypass does not have to be employed during implantation. However, complications at the reconstructed anastomoses have to be anticipated, as was recently reported [5–7]. During piggy-back anastomoses, the vena cava can be stenosed due to the manipulations, which might be treated by additional latero-lateral cavo-cavostomy [6]. The problems with the rotation of liver segments at the hepato-venous anastomoses have been described in particular with reduced-size grafts [4] and preexisting vena cava abnormalities can also cause complications at the anastomosis [7]. The piggy-back anastomosis was stenotic in the two patients who were transplanted with a partial liver graft without preserved donor vena cava, while this complication did not occur in the patients who received a transplant with preserved vena cava of the donor, most certainly due to the larger diameter of the vena cava as compared to that of the hepatic veins. The transjugular catheter angioplasty was useful in the therapy of stenosis in these cases. A similar experience was recently reported in a series using only segmental grafts from living relatives [5]. The partial thrombosis that occurred with the latero-lateral cavo-cavostomy might have been due to the siphon-like blood flow associated with this technique. To our knowledge, no such complication has been reported until now. The face-à-face cavoplasty as described by Bismuth [2] avoids the siphon forming. The preparation of the anastomosis, however, appears to be more difficult than the preparation of the latero-lateral cavo-cavostomy. This particular complication occurred in the early experience with this technique and has to be seen in the context of a learning curve. Nevertheless, its occurrence should be anticipated in order to employ appropriate therapeutic measures.

Table 2 Complications

Anastomosis	Liver size	Arterial thrombosis	Portal vein thrombosis	Hepato-venous reconstruction/ stenosis	Bleeding
Orthotopic $n = 63$	Full size	2	0	0	12
	Reduced	0	0	0	0
	Partial	0	0	0	0
Piggy back $n = 53$	Full size	1	0	0	1
	Reduced	0	0	0	2
	Partial	0	0	2	1
Latero-lateral $n = 7$	Full size	0	0	1	0
	Reduced	0	0	0	0
	Partial	0	0	0	0
Total $n = 110$		3 (3 %)	0	3* (3 %)	3* (3 %)

* $P = 0.01$ for orthotopic versus piggy-back + latero-lateral

References

1. Belghiti J, Panis Y, Sauvanet A, Gayet B, Fékété F (1992) A new technique of side to side caval anastomosis during orthotopic hepatic transplantation without vena caval occlusion. Surg Gynecol Obstet 175: 271–272
2. Bismuth H, Castaing D, Sherlock T (1992) Liver transplantation by 'face-à-face' veno-cavoplasty. Surgery 111: 151–155
3. Calne RY, Williams R (1968) Liver transplantation in man. Br Med J 4: 535–540
4. Emond JC, Heffron TG, Whitington PF, Broelsch CE (1993) Reconstruction of the hepatic vein in reduced size hepatic transplantation. Surg Gynecol Obstet 176: 11–17
5. Fujimoto M, Moriyasu F, Someda H, Nada T, Okuma M, Uemoto S, Inomata Y, Tanaka K, Yamaoka Y, Ozawa K (1995) Recovery of graft circulation following percutaneous transluminal angioplasty for stenotic venous complications in assessment with Doppler ultrasound. Transpl Int 8: 119–125
6. Lerut J, Gertsch P (1993) Side-to-side cavo-cavostomy: a useful aid in "complicated" piggy-back liver transplantation. Transpl Int 6: 299–301
7. Lerut J, Tzakis A, Bron K, Gordon R, Iwatsuki S, Esquivel C, Makowka L, Todo S, Starzl TE (1987) Complications of venous reconstruction in human orthotopic liver transplantation. Ann Surg 205: 404
8. Tzakis A, Todo S, Starzl TE (1989) Orthotopic liver transplantation with preservation of the inferior vena cava. Ann Surg 210: 649–652

Transpl Int (1996) 9 [Suppl 1]: S185–S187
© Springer-Verlag 1996

LIVER

B. H. Ferraz-Neto
D. F. Mirza
B. K. Gunson
T. Ismail
A. D. Mayer
J. A. C. Buckels
P. McMaster

Bile duct splintage in liver transplantation: is it necessary?

B. H. Ferraz-Neto · D. F. Mirza ·
B. K. Gunson · T. Ismail · A. Mayer ·
J. A. C. Buckels · P. McMaster (✉)
The Liver Unit, Queen Elizabeth Hospital,
Edgbaston, Birmingham B 15 2 TH, UK

Abstract The choledochocholedochal (duct-duct, D-D) anastomosis in orthotopic liver transplantation (OLT) is usually splinted by a T-tube to facilitate easy cholangiography, monitor bile quality and allow biliary decompression. T-tubes, however, are a focus for sepsis and sludge deposition, and their removal may result in bile leakage. From January 1993 to December 1994, 199 consecutive adult OLTs in 183 patients (median age 50 years, range 16–69 years, 118 females) with a D-D anastomosis were studied prospectively with a median follow-up of 16 (3–27) months. Of the 199 OLTs, 110 had an 8 Fr T-tube (group 1) and 89 had no T-tube (group 2). The two groups were similar for indication, preservation solution, median cold and warm ischaemia times and early graft function parameters. Biliary complications developed in 26/110 patients, including 10 with bile leaks on T-tube removal in group 1 compared to 10/89 biliary complications in group 2 ($P = 0.024$). The use of T-tubes is associated with increased morbidity and their routine use should be discontinued.

Key words Biliary complications · Liver transplantation · Surgical technique

Introduction

Despite improvements in preservation techniques, bile duct complications continue to be a source of significant posttransplant morbidity, with an incidence ranging from 5 to 25 % [1–4]. Choledochocholedochostomy is the preferred method of biliary reconstruction in orthotopic liver transplantation (OLT) in cases where the recipient common duct is not diseased. Usually this anastomosis is splinted by means of a T-tube, introduced via the recipient duct. The use of a T-tube facilitates easy cholangiography during times of graft dysfunction, achieves biliary decompression during the early postoperative phase and enables monitoring of bile quality. T-tubes, however, act as foreign bodies, predisposing to biliary sludging, and provide a potential route for infection. External bile drainage affects absorption of oral cyclosporin. In addition, T-tube removal is associated with a risk of bile leakage. Because of this increased morbidity, many transplant units have questioned the use of T-tubes. The aim of this study was to analyse the incidence of biliary complications in all adult patients undergoing OLT over a 2-year period with a duct-duct (D-D) anastomosis with or without a T-tube.

Patients and methods

From January 1993 to December 1994, 199 consecutive OLTs with a choledochocholedochal anastomosis were carried out in 183 adult recipients (118 females, 81 males). The median age was 50 years (range 16–69 years), and the median follow-up was 16 months (range 3–27 months). In 110 OLTs the choledochocholedochostomy (D-D) was splinted with an 8 Fr T-tube, introduced via the recipient duct (group 1; D-D with T-tube). In 89 patients the D-D anastomosis was not splinted (group 2; D-D no T-tube). All biliary anastomoses were sutured with a continuous 5/0 PDS suture. The two groups were comparable for indication (Table 1), preservation solution used, median cold and warm ischaemic times and early graft function parameters.

Results

Of the 199 OLTs studied, biliary complications developed in 36. Of 110 patients with a T-tube, 26 (23.6%) developed a biliary complication, compared with 10 of 89 patients (11.2%) without a T-tube ($P < 0.05$; Table 2). Bile leakage after T-tube removal was the most frequent complication observed (10 of 26). Five patients were managed conservatively, and four were treated with nonsurgical intervention (one percutaneous pigtail drain, one ERC with stent, two ERC with stent and pigtail catheter drainage). One patient underwent a laparotomy for biliary peritonitis, and died 28 days postoperatively due to sepsis and multiorgan failure. When patients with leaks following T-tube removal were excluded from the analysis, the difference in the incidence of biliary complications between the two groups was not statistically significant. Five and six patients in group 1 (with T-tube) and group 2 (without T-tube), respectively, underwent biliary reconstruction. Two patients with bile leakage and associated hepatic artery thrombosis, both in group 1, underwent retransplantation. The management of the biliary complications is listed in Table 3.

Discussion

The development of biliary complications after liver transplantation is related to several factors: technical reasons, preservation injury, arterial inflow, rejection and the use of stents [1–4]. The wide variation in rates of biliary complications may be attributed to the use of different classification methods for bile duct complications. This series included all possible biliary problems, including minor bile leaks and abnormalities visualized on routine protocol cholangiography.

The overall incidence of biliary complications was higher in the group with T-tubes, and this was due to the high incidence of leaks following T-tube removal. Most of these patients were managed without surgery, although the one death due to biliary complications was following surgical drainage of an infected bile collection. The rate of biliary reconstructive surgery was similar in both groups (five and six, respectively), suggesting that the use of stents themselves do not influence the development of major complications necessitating reconstructive surgery.

The ability of endoscopists (or interventional radiologists, if required) to obtain good quality biliary imaging in the absence of biliary ductal dilatation even during the early postoperative period may decrease the importance of easy T-tube cholangiography to investigate graft dysfunction [5, 6]. This, along with the high incidence of complications related to the use of T-tubes, is a strong argument in favour of discontinuing their use.

Table 1 Indications for transplantation

Indication	D-D + T-tube	D-D without T-tube
Fulminant hepatic failure	14	13
Primary biliary cirrhosis	48	22
Alcoholic cirrhosis	7	9
Hepatitis C	4	10
Cryptogenic cirrhosis	8	6
Chronic active hepatitis	9	5
Alpha-1-antitrypsin	5	5
Others	8	10
Regrafts	7	9

Table 2 Biliary complications (*HAT* hepatic artery thrombosis)

Complication	D-D + T-tube	D-D without T-tube
Anastomotic strictures	3	5
Sludge syndrome	3	2
Sphincter of Oddi dysfunction	1	0
Cystic duct syndrome	1	0
Anastomotic leaks	8 (2 HAT)	3
Leaks after T-tube removal	10	–
Total	26/110	10/89*

* $P < 0.05$

Table 3 Treatment (*HAT* hepatic artery thrombosis)

Treatment	D-D + T-tube	D-D without T-tube
Conservative	11	2
Radiological/endoscopic	7	2
Pigtail	1	0
ERCP + stent/dilatation	3	1
ERCP + nasobiliartube	0	1
ERCP + stent + pigtail	3	0
Surgical	8	6
Biliary reconstruction	5	6
Laparotomy + drainage	1	0
Regraft (HAT)	2	0

In conclusion, the use of T-tube splintage of the choledochodochal anastomosis is not necessary, and its discontinuation would reduce morbidity in liver transplantation.

References

1. Chardot C, Candinas D, Mirza D et al (1995) Biliary complications after pediatric liver-transplantation – Birmingham's experience. Transplant Int 8: 133
2. Colonna JO, Shaked A, Gomes AS et al (1992) Biliary strictures complicating liver-transplantation. Incidence, pathogenesis, management, and outcome. Ann Surg 216: 344
3. Stratta RJ, Wood RP, Langnas AN et al (1989) Diagnosis and treatment of biliary-tract complications after orthotopic liver transplantation. Surgery 106: 675
4. O'Connor HJ, Lewis WD, Jenkins RL (1995) Biliary-tract complications after liver transplantation. Arch Surg 130: 312
5. Ostroff JW, Roberts JP, Gordon RL et al (1990) The management of T tube leaks in orthotopic liver transplant recipients with endoscopically placed nasobiliary catheters. Transplantation 49: 922
6. Kuo PC, Lewis WD, Stokes K et al (1994) A comparison of operation, endoscopic retrograde cholangiography, and percutaneous transhepatic cholangiography in biliary complications after hepatic transplantation. J Am Coll Surg 179: 177

Transpl Int (1996) 9 [Suppl 1]: S 188–S 190
© Springer-Verlag 1996

Effect of pre-reperfusion portal venous blood flush on early liver transplant function

D. F. Mirza
B. K. Gunson
H. Khalaf
J. W. Freeman
J. A. C. Buckels
P. McMaster
A. D. Mayer

D. F. Mirza · B. K. Gunson · H. Khalaf ·
J. W. Freeman · J. A. C. Buckels ·
P. McMaster · A. D. Mayer
The Liver Unit, Queen Elizabeth Hospital,
Edgbaston, Birmingham B15 2TH, UK

Abstract Portal venous blood for rinsing out the University of Wisconsin solution (UWs) has the advantages of being a physiological fluid, removing acidotic mesenteric venous blood and perhaps resulting in more stable haemodynamic parameters during reperfusion. A group of 209 consecutive adult OLTs carried out between July 1993 and February 1995 were studied prospectively. The UWs was flushed out with 500 ml portal blood in 95 OLTs (group 1) and with 1.0 L 0.5 % dextrose at 37 °C in 114 OLTs (group 2). The median day 1 and peak day 1–5 AST levels were significantly elevated in the 5 % dextrose group: median 755 (118–11090) vs. 546 (121–6150) IU/l

($P = 0.007$, Wilcoxon); and median 1095 (159–11090) vs. 744 (157–7870) IU/l ($p = 0.008$, Wilcoxon), respectively. A median of 5 (0–27) units of blood were transfused in group 1 compared to 4 (0–54) units in group 2 (n. s.). There was no difference in peak bilirubin, lowest day 1–5 PT levels, primary nonfunction, median ITU stay, total inpatient stay and 1-month graft survival between the two groups (89 % vs. 88 %). Pre-reperfusion blood flush may be associated with less hepatocellular damage, without significant additional blood usage.

Key words Early graft function · Liver transplantation · Preservation · Reperfusion injury

Introduction

In orthotopic liver transplantation (OLT), reperfusion of the cold-stored liver allograft is necessary for the expression of preservation-reperfusion injury [1, 2]. Prior to reperfusion, the potassium-rich (120 mmol/l) University of Wisconsin solution (UWs) is rinsed out, usually using a colloid or crystalloid solution. More recently special rinse solutions such as the Carolina rinse solution rich in buffers have been advocated to decrease the extent of preservation-reperfusion injury [3]. The use of portal venous blood as a flushout fluid may have potential advantages: it is physiological, achieves effective prewarming of the graft, and removes acidotic mesenteric venous blood. In addition, its use has been reported to result in more stable haemodynamic parameters and a decreased incidence of post-reperfusion syn-

drome [4]. However, it does add to intraoperative blood losses and may result in increased transfusion requirements. Our aims were to study the effects of a pre-reperfusion portal venous blood flush compared to a 5 % dextrose washout on parameters of early graft function and on intraoperative blood transfusion requirements.

Patients and methods

From July 1993 to February 1995, 209 consecutive adult OLTs were studied prospectively. OLT was performed using standard techniques, and all livers were preserved with UWs. In 95 cases (group 1) the UWs was washed out with portal venous blood, with the first 500 ml of effluent blood drained out via a cannula through the lower caval anastomosis. During this stage 1 unit of blood was rapidly transfused to prevent hypotension. Following this the portal venous clamp was reapplied, and both upper and lower IVC

Table 1 Blood flush vs. 5 % dextrose – demographic data, indications, cold and warm ischaemia. Values are median (range)

	Blood ($n = 95$)	5 % dextrose ($n = 114$)	
Sex (M/F)	46/49	49/65	n.s.
Age (years)	47 (16–68)	52 (17–73)	n.s.
Routine	71	82	n.s.
Urgent	16	19	n.s.
Emergency	8	13	n.s.
Cold ischaemia time (min)	763 (174–1325)	738 (265–1132)	n.s.
Warm ischaemia time (min)	50 (25–102)	49 (30–88)	n.s.
Venovenous bypass	80/15	104/10	n.s.

clamps were released, establishing caval circulation and providing adequate venous return. The portal clamp was then gradually released, carefully monitoring haemodynamic parameters, to establish revascularization of the graft. In the remaining 114 cases (group 2), the UWs was rinsed out with 1000 ml 5 % dextrose at 37° C, the caval clamps released and the graft revascularized with portal venous inflow. The two groups were comparable for age, sex, urgency of indication, use of venovenous bypass, and cold and warm ischaemia times (Table 1).

Results

The early graft function parameters are given in Table 2. The day 1 AST levels and the peak day 1–5 AST levels were significantly higher in group 2 (5 % dextrose washout). There were three cases of primary nonfunction in group 1 (blood flush) compared with one in group 2 ($P = 0.25$, n.s.). There was no significant difference in peak day 1–5 bilirubin levels and lowest day 1–5 prothrombin times. Patients in group 1 received a median of 5 units of blood intraoperatively, and those in group 2 received 4 units (n.s.). The median ITU stay, median total inpatient stay and 1-month graft survival were similar in both groups (Table 2).

Discussion

The degree of preservation-reperfusion injury in liver transplantation depends on several factors [1, 2], including the events prior to reperfusion such as the gradual rewarming during construction of the vascular anastomoses, the time taken to full arterial and venous revascularization of the graft, the nature and temperature of the fluid used to wash out the UWs, and the mode of reperfusion. The use of portal venous blood as a flushout fluid has possible benefits in that it gets rid of acidotic venous blood proximal to the portal venous clamp, utilizes a physiological fluid to washout the liver and achieves more effective prewarming prior to complete revascularization of the graft. There have also been reports of a decreased incidence of postreperfusion haemodynamic syndrome when the first 500 ml of portal venous blood are allowed to drain out [4]. One potential disadvantage is the associated blood loss resulting in an increase in blood transfusion requirements.

The lower transaminase levels (day 1 AST, peak day 1–5 AST) in grafts flushed with blood suggest less hepatocellular damage in this preliminary analysis. The overall incidence of primary nonfunction was low (4 of 209 OLTs, although 3 were washed out with portal venous blood; $P = 0.25$, n.s.). Further studies looking at more sensitive markers of preservation injury such as neutrophil activation and adhesion, platelet adhesion and cytokine release [5, 6] could determine whether grafts flushed out with venous blood do in fact suffer less preservation-reperfusion injury.

The median intraoperative blood transfusion requirements were not significantly increased in group 1 (blood flush) (5 vs. 4, n.s.), although a rapid infusion of 1 unit of blood was required in all cases.

In conclusion, the use of portal venous blood as a flushout fluid may be associated with less hepatocellular damage, without adversely affecting intraoperative transfusion requirements. Further studies looking at more specific features are necessary before its influence on preservation reperfusion injury can be determined.

Table 2 Early graft function parameters and outcome. Values are median (range)

	Blood flush ($n = 95$)	5 % dextrose washout ($n = 114$)	Wilcoxon test
Day 1 AST (IU/l)	546 (121–6150)	755 (118–11090)	p = 0.007
Peak AST (day 1–5) (IU/l)	744 (157–7870)	1095 (159–11090)	p = 0.008
Peak bilirubin (day 1–5) (mmol/L)	152 (29–1540)	170 (32–838)	ns
Lowest prothrombin time (day 1–5) (s)	15 (11–23)	14 (11–22)	ns
Primary nonfunction	3	1	ns
Intraoperative blood (units)	5 (0–27)	4 (0–54)	ns
ITU/inpatient stay (days)	3/14	3/14	ns
1-month graft survival	89 %	88 %	ns

References

1. Clavien PA, Harvey PRC, Strasberg SM (1992) Preservation and reperfusion injuries in liver allografts – an overview and and synthesis of current studies. Transplantation 53: 957–978
2. Chazouilleres O, Calmus Y, Vanbourdolle M, Ballet F (1993) Preservation induced liver injury. Clinical aspects, mechanisms and therapeutic approaches. J Hepatol 18: 123–134
3. Currin RT, Toole JG, Thorman RG, Lemasters JJ (1990) Evidence that Carolina rinse solution protects sinusoidal endothelial cells against reperfusion injury after cold ischaemic storage of rat liver. Transplantation 50: 1076–1078
4. Brems JJ, Takiff H, McHutchinson J, Collins D, Biermann LA, Pockros P (1993) Systemic versus nonsystemic reperfusion of the transplanted liver. Transplantation 55: 527–529
5. Suzuki S, Toledo-Pereyra LH, Rodriguez EJ, Cejalvo D (1993) Neutrophil infiltration as an important factor in liver ischaemia and reperfusion injury – modulating effects effects of FK506 and cyclosporine. Transplantation 55: 1265–1272
6. Nishiyama R, Nakamura S, Suzuki S, Baba S (1993) Platelet activating factor in hepatic ischaemia-reperfusion injury – the effects of a PAF antagonist combined with a prostaglandin I_2 analogue. Transplantation 55: 1261–1265

Transpl Int (1996) 9 [Suppl 1]: S191–S194
© Springer-Verlag 1996

H. Mäkisalo
K. Salmela
H. Isoniemi
E. Tierala
K. Höckerstedt

How to estimate the size of the donor liver

H. Mäkisalo (✉) · K. Salmela ·
H. Isoniemi · K. Höckerstedt
Division of Transplantation,
4th Department of Surgery,
Helsinki University Hospital,
Kasarmikatu 11–13, FIN-00130, Helsinki,
Finland
Tel. +358 0 4718 238;
Fax +358 0 174 975

E. Tierala
Department of Radiology,
Helsinki University Hospital, Helsinki,
Finland

Abstract Of readily available methods to estimate the donor liver size, measurement of the body circumference at the xiphoid level (xiphoid measure) appeared to be the most accurate in the present prospective study of 60 donors and 57 recipients ($r = 0.64$, $P = 0.0001$). The estimated liver volume could be calculated using the equation: bloodless liver volume (l) = 1.44 × xiphoid measure (m). The difference between donor and recipient xiphoid measures was significantly higher in slowly recovering patients than in those recovering uneventfully (7 ± 7 cm vs. -5 ± 8 cm, $P < 0.001$). The bloodless donor liver volume measured by water displacement averaged 1249 ± 230 ml and had increased by 3 weeks post-transplant by 64 ± 28 % as determined using computed tomography. The volume of the liver graft seemed

to adapt to the recipient as it correlated positively with body weight ($r = 0.64$, $P < 0.01$) and negatively with the age of the recipient ($r = -0.42$, $P < 0.01$). The liver graft volume seemed to increase less markedly in patients with a slow recovery than in those with an uncomplicated recovery ($37 \% \pm 15 \%$ vs. $68 \% \pm 24 \%$, $P < 0.001$). We conclude that a simple measurement of the body circumference at the xiphoid level can be used to estimate the donor liver volume. A gross mismatch of this parameter between the donor and the recipient seems to increase the risk of graft dysfunction. We also found that the change in the liver graft volume is influenced by the recipient's age and body weight.

Key words Liver radiography · Liver transplantation · Liver anatomy

Introduction

Liver size disparity is a well-known major problem in pediatric liver transplantation surgery. Accurate size-matching between adult liver donors and recipients is also important because of increased complications after transplanting a disproportionate liver graft. Hepatic artery or portal vein thrombosis may be caused by compression of an oversized graft [8]. Graft dysfunction [9] and increased risk of rejection [11] have been seen when an undersized graft has been used. On the other hand, a larger liver than expected for the donor body size carries a risk of occult liver dis-

ease and especially a risk of advanced alcoholic liver disease [10, 12].

As the most reliable clinical method for assessing the liver size, computed tomography (CT) [3] is usually not available for the donor, so the liver volume is estimated by the donor body size. According to previous findings there is a relationship between the total liver volume and the body surface area (BSA) [5, 6, 13]. However, to calculate the BSA, body height (BH) and weight (BW) have to be estimated by the donor hospital personnel. In addition, the actual size of the organ is usually only approximately estimated by the donor surgeon.

Table 1 Donor and recipient characteristics

	Donors	Recipients
Number	60	57
Sex (male/female)	43/17	24/33
Age (years)	37 ± 11	49 ± 8
Body weight (kg)	70 ± 9	69 ± 13
Body height (cm)	175 ± 7	170 ± 7
Body surface area (m²)	1.84 ± 0.15	1.78 ± 0.19
BMI (kg/m²)	23 ± 2	25 ± 10
Xiphoid measure (cm)	86 ± 6	89 ± 9
Umbilical measure (cm)	78 ± 10	92 ± 12
Liver volume (ml)		
After harvest	1249 ± 230	
3 weeks posttransplant		2036 ± 342

We sought to determine a relationship between easily available body dimensions and the exactly measured liver volume. The other interest was to find factors that determine the change in the size of the liver graft after transplantation.

Materials and methods

This prospective study included 60 consecutive liver donors and 57 adult recipients between September 1992 and August 1995. Recipients receiving reduced liver transplants or imported liver grafts were excluded from the evaluation. Of the 57 transplantations, 44 were performed because of chronic liver disease and 13 because of acute fulminant liver failure. In three cases the procedure was a retransplantation. The recovery of the patients was evaluated against graft function and biliary complications at the end of the first postoperative month and at the end of the follow-up period.

The body circumference at the xiphoid and the umbilical levels of the donor and the recipient were precisely measured by the coordinators of the transplantation centre. The bloodless volume of the donor liver was first measured by water displacement on the back table after harvesting and the perfused liver 3 weeks after the transplantation by CT scanning. CT scans were obtained at 8-mm intervals on a Somatom CR CT. Using a track ball device, the perimeter of each slice of the liver was outlined, and the enclosed area was calculated electronically. The donor BW and BH were provided by the personnel of the donor hospital. BSA was determined from the table of DuBois and DuBois [2] and the body mass index (BMI) was calculated using the standard formula: BW/BH^2.

The data are presented as means ± SD, and the relationship between variables was tested using linear regression. The significance of the regressions was determined using the F-test. The significance of differences between means was determined using the Mann-Whitney U-test for unpaired populations.

Results

The characteristics of the liver donors and recipients and the volumetric data of the livers are given in Table 1. The bloodless liver volume averaged 1249 ±

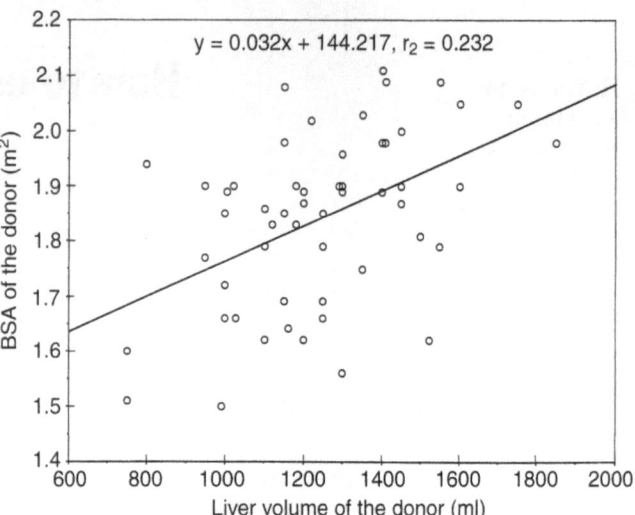

Fig. 1 Correlation between liver volume and the BSA of the donors ($r = 0.48$, $P < 0.001$)

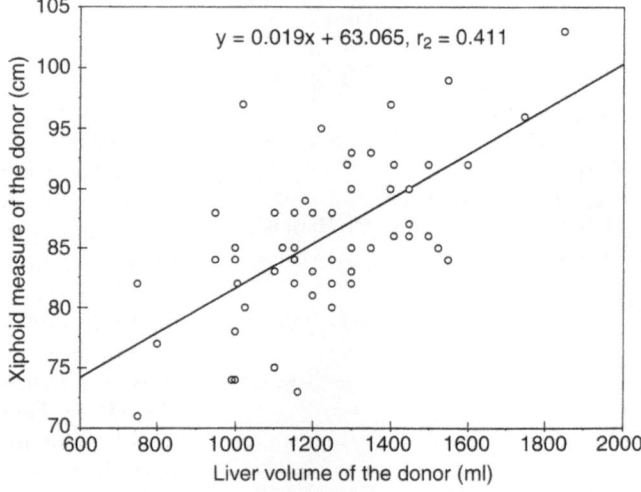

Fig. 2 Correlation between liver volume and the xiphoid measure of the donors ($r = 0.64$, $P = 0.0001$)

230 ml. It correlated with both donor BW and BSA ($r = 0.48$, $P < 0.001$, Fig. 1) and donor BMI ($r = 0.31$, $P < 0.05$). However, a strong correlation was shown only with the xiphoid measure ($r = 0.64$, $P = 0.0001$, Fig. 2), and this was accentuated if the donor was either less than 30 or more than 39 years old ($r = 0.75$, $P = 0.0001$). The ratio between the liver volume (l) and the xiphoid measure (m) was quite constant at 1.44 ± 0.21. Thus the expected liver volume could be calculated from the equation: bloodless liver volume (l) = 1.44 × xiphoid measure (m).

The liver volume increased 3 weeks posttransplant to 2036 ± 342 ml and was correlated with the BW of the recipient ($r = 0.40$, $P < 0.01$), although no correlation was seen between these parameters at the time of transplan-

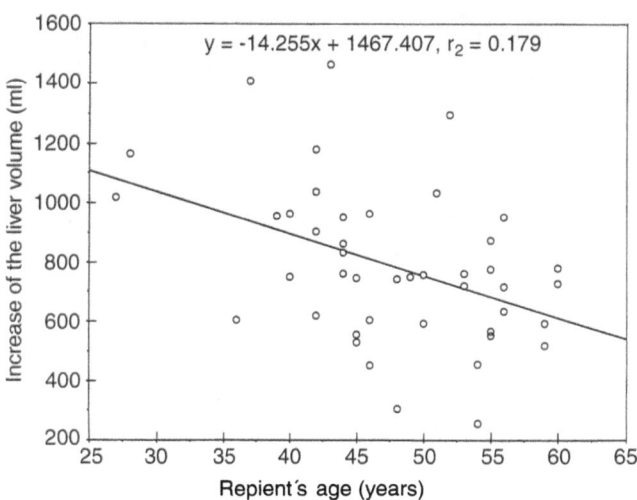

Fig.3 Correlation between recipient's age and increase in liver volume during the 3 weeks following liver transplantation ($r = -0.42$, $P < 0.01$)

tation. The increase in liver graft volume ($64 \pm 28\%$) correlated negatively with advancing age of the recipient ($r = -0.42$, $P < 0.01$, Fig.3).

During the follow-up, nine patients had signs of graft dysfunction leading to slow recovery and infectious complications (Table 2). Biliary stricture led to the loss of one patient. The three other patients died for reasons unrelated to graft function, namely tumour metastases or reactivation of HCV infection. The differences between the xiphoid measures of the donor and recipient were significantly higher in these nine patients than in the patients with an uncomplicated recovery (7 ± 7 cm vs. -5 ± 8 cm, $P < 0.001$, Table 3). In addition, patients with graft dysfunction showed a significantly smaller increase in liver graft volume 3 weeks posttransplant than recipients with an uneventful recovery ($37\% \pm 15\%$ vs. $68\% \pm 24\%$, $P < 0.001$).

Discussion

Our finding of only a comparatively weak correlation between the liver volume and the donor BW or BSA differs from previous studies, in which the association shown in healthy persons was highly significant [5, 6, 13]. Because in the present study the liver volume was accurately measured by water displacement the source of error seems to be the crude estimation of the donor BW and BH by the personnel at the donor hospital. Thus the estimation of the donor liver size based on these measurements may lead to most inconvenient surprises, particularly as one of the main criteria in the selection of the donor is the expected liver size. Our finding of a strong correlation between a simple measurement of the body circumference at the xiphoid level

Table 2 The outcome after the liver transplantation (follow-up 2 months to 2 years)

	1 month posttransplant	End of follow-up
Good liver function	51	52
Biliary stricture	1	
Bile leakage	1	
Liver dysfunction	9	
Prolonged cholestasis	5[a]	
Biliary stricture	2	
Bile leakage	2	
Hepatic arterial thrombosis	1[a]	
Chronic rejection		1
On the list for retransplant		1
Died		4
Biliary strictures		1
Tumour metastases		2
HCV reinfection		1

[a] Three patients retransplanted, bone patient had both prolonged cholestasis and bile leakage

Table 3 Body circumferences at the xiphoid level of donors and recipients in relation to the speed of recovery after transplantation

	Slow recovery ($n = 9$) (cm)	'Normal' recovery ($n = 49$) (cm)
Donor	91 ± 4	85 ± 6*
Recipient	84 ± 8	90 ± 9
Donor – recipient	7 ± 6	-5 ± 8

* $P < 0.05$, ** $P < 0.001$

and the liver volume may be used as a guide for estimation of the liver graft volume. The present results indicate the equation for the estimation of the volume to be: bloodless liver volume (l) = $1.44 \times$ xiphoid measure (m).

The only body dimension of the donor or the recipient predictive of graft dysfunction was also the difference in their xiphoid measures. The difference in favour of the donor was significantly higher in slowly recovering patients than in recipients with an uneventful recovery. In addition, slowly recovering patients seemed to gain significantly less hepatic volume during the first 3 posttransplant weeks. This fact is in agreement with previous findings of a correlation between the hepatic mass and the liver function both in partially hepatectomized patients [15] and patients receiving an undersized liver graft [1].

The significant increase in the liver size after transplantation did not correlate with any body dimension, but was negatively associated with the age of the recipient. This fact may indicate diminishing metabolic demands which have previously been found in elderly patients [7] and is in congruence with a finding of a negative correlation between recipient age and liver volume

[14]. In addition, the host body size seemed to determine, at least in part, the liver graft size because the BW of the recipient correlated with the liver graft volume 3 weeks posttransplant, whereas no correlation between these parameters was seen at the time of transplantation. This result confirms an earlier finding made using a canine model, in which the change in the liver graft volume was determined by the recipient's size [4].

We conclude that measuring the body circumference at the xiphoid level is the simplest and most accurate parameter for the estimation of the donor liver volume. A gross mismatch of this parameter between the donor and the recipient seems to increase the risk of graft dysfunction. We found also that a well-functioning liver graft seems to gain markedly in weight during the first few posttransplant weeks, and the change in the graft volume is influenced by the recipient's age and body size.

References

1. Adam R, Castaing D, Bismuth H (1993) Transplantation of small donor livers in adult recipients. Tranpslant Proc 25: 1105–1106
2. DuBois D, DuBois EF (1916) A formula to estimate the approximate surface area if height and weight be known. Arch Intern Med 17: 863–871
3. Heymsfield SB, Fulenwider T, Nordlinger B, et al (1979) Accurate measurement of liver, kidney, and spleen volume and mass by computerized axial tomography. Ann Intern Med 90: 185–187
4. Kam I, Lynch S, Svanas G, et al (1987) Evidence that host size determines liver size: studies in dogs receiving orthotopic liver transplant. Hepatology 7: 362–366
5. LeLand FH, North WA (1968) Relationship between liver size and body size. Radiology 91: 1195–1198
6. Leung NWY, Farrant P, Peters TJ (1986) Liver volume measurement by ultrasonography in normal subjects and alcoholic patients. J Hepatol 2: 157–164
7. Marchesini G, Bua V, Brunori A (1988) Galactose elimination capacity and liver volume in aging man. Hepatology 8: 1079–1083
8. Payen DM, Fratacci MD, Dupuy P, et al (1990) Portal and hepatic arterial blood flow measurements of human transplanted liver by implanted Doppler probes: interest for early complications and nutrition. Surgery 107: 417–427
9. Ploeg RJ, D'Alassandro AM, Knechtle SJ, et al (1993) Risk factors for primary dysfunction after liver transplantation – a multivariate analysis. Transplantation 55: 807–813
10. Sato H, Takase S, Takada A (1989) Changes in liver and spleen volumes in alcoholic liver disease. J Hepatol 8: 150–157
11. Shiraishi M, Csete ME, Yasunaga C, et al (1994) Regeneration-induced accelerated rejection in reduced-size liver grafts. Transplantation 57: 336–340
12. Tarao K, Hoshino H, Motohashi I (1989) Changes in liver and spleen volume in alcoholic liver fibrosis of man. Hepatology 9: 589–593
13. Urata K, Kawasaki S, Matsunami H, et al (1995) Calculation of child and adult standard liver volume for liver transplantation. Hepatology 21: 1317–1321
14. Wynne HA, Cope LH, Mutch E, et al (1989) The effect of age upon liver volume and apparent liver blood flow in healthy man. Hepatology 9: 297–301
15. Yamanaka N, Okamoto E, Kawamura E, et al (1993) Dynamics of normal and injured human liver regeneration after hepatectomy as assessed on the basis of computed tomography and liver function. Hepatology 18: 79–85

Transpl Int (1996) 9 [Suppl 1]: S195–S197
© Springer-Verlag 1996

LIVER

R. Charco
V. Vargas
H. Allende
A. Edo
J. Balsells
E. Murio
J. L. Lázaro
I. Bilbao
C. Margarit

Is hepatitis C virus recurrence a risk factor for chronic liver allograft rejection?

R. Charco (✉) · V. Vargas · H. Allende ·
A. Edo · J. Balsells · E. Murio · J. L. Lázaro ·
I. Bilbao · C. Margarit
Liver Transplantation Unit,
Hospital General Universitario Vall
d'Hebron, Paseo Vall d'Hebron s/n,
E-08035 Barcelona, Spain
Tel. +34-3-4 18 34 00, ext. 40 46;
Fax +34-3-4 28 14 17

Abstract Several risk factors have been reported that may favour the development of chronic rejection. From October 1988 to December 1993, 97 liver transplants with survival of more than 3 months were included in the study. Fifty-two patients (54.1 %) had chronic hepatitis C virus (HCV) infection before liver transplantation. Immunosuppression consisted of cyclosporine A and prednisone, whereas 14 patients received FK 506 and prednisone. Severe graft HCV reinfection was present in 32 patients (61.5 %) after liver transplantation and chronic graft hepatitis C was found in 26 cases at the end of the study. Chronic rejection occurred in 8 of 97 allografts (8.25 %); 5 presented chronic rejection and concomitant chronic graft hepatitis C. The incidence of chronic rejection in patients with HCV infection before liver transplantation (9.6 %) did not differ when compared with the negative HCV patients (6.6 %). However, when the 26 cases that developed graft dysfunction due to chronic hepatitis C after liver transplantation were considered, 5 presented chronic rejection, a significantly higher incidence than in the remaining patients (3 of 71) (Yates chi-square test: $P < 0.05$). In our experience, there appears to be a relationship between the development of chronic rejection and chronic hepatitis C in the graft after liver transplantation.

Key words Chronic rejection · Hepatitis C virus · Liver transplantation

Introduction

Chronic rejection of liver allograft is generally considered to be an irreversible condition, characterized by immune-mediated destruction of bile ducts and obliterative vasculopathy involving large- and medium-sized arteries [1]. This results in a syndrome of progressive cholestasis, which is usually unresponsive to immunosuppression, leading to graft failure. Several risk factors have been reported that may favour the development of chronic rejection [2].

Hepatitis C infection is a major cause of end-stage liver disease requiring liver transplantation (LTx). The hepatitis C virus (HCV) remains detectable in serum and other tissues after LTx. and leads to recurrence of hepatitis C in many patients [3, 4]. Our aim was to study HCV infection as a predisposing risk factor for chronic rejection.

Patients and methods

From October 1988 to December 1993, 127 liver transplants were performed in 110 adult patients at the Hospital General Universitario Vall d'Hebron, Barcelona. All liver allografts with survival of more than 3 months (97 grafts) were included in the study. Fifty-two patients (54.1 %) had chronic HCV infection before LTx. No patient received AB0 blood-incompatible grafts. In the early years, Eurocollins solution was used. Thereafter, all remaining grafts were preserved with the University of Wisconsin solution. Mean follow-up was 22 months (range: 3–70 months). Minimum follow-up of living patients was 12 months.

Table 1 Incidence of hepatitis C virus *(HCV)* recurrence and chronic rejection. (*PSC* Primary sclerosing cholangitis, *PBC* primary biliary cirrhosis, *HBV* hepatitis B virus, *LTx* liver transplantation)

Diagnosis pre-LTx	Patients	Severe graft HCV reinfection	Chronic graft hepatitis C	Chronic rejection
Cirrhosis-tumour HCV	52	32/52 (61 %)	26/52 (50 %)	5/26 (19 %)
HBV hepatitis	4	–	–	–
PSC, PBC	9	–	–	–
Alcoholic cirrhosis	15	–	–	2/71 (3 %)
Other	17	–	–	1/71 (1 %)
Total	97	32 (33 %)	26 (29 %)	8/97 (8.2 %)

Immunosuppression

Standard postoperative immunosuppression consisted of cyclosporine A (CsA) and prednisone (P), whereas 14 patients received FK 506 and P. Acute rejection episodes were treated with one to three bolus injections of 1 g methylprednisolone. If rejection persisted, a 14-day course of OKT3 5 mg/day was given. When acute rejection episodes recurred or chronic rejection was suspected or confirmed by histology, patients were converted to FK 506.

Chronic rejection

Chronic rejection as diagnosed if hepatic histology showed evidence of interlobar or septal bile duct loss in more than 50 % of portal tracts. Obliterative vasculopathy involving large- and medium-sized arteries was considered a non-obligatory but supportive feature. Arterial lesions were rarely seen in biopsy specimens. At least 20 portal tracts were reviewed in liver biopsy to exclude sampling error and confirm the diagnosis of chronic rejection. Furthermore, chronic rejection was usually confirmed in explanted livers.

HCV infection

Donor and recipient serum samples were obtained immediately before LTx. Recipient samples were also obtained after transplantation during hospitalisation and at outpatient visits. Serum samples were rapidly frozen and stored at –40 °C until analysis.

Donor and recipient pre-transplant and selected post-transplant samples were tested for anti-HCV by second-generation enzyme-linked immunoassay (ELISA II) (Abbott Laboratories, Chicago, Ill.). All positive samples were confirmed by second-generation recombinant immunoblot assay (RIBA 2; Chiron, Emmeryville, Calif.). In patients with more than one serum sample available, the latest sample, at least, was determined for anti-HCV and serum HCV-RNA. HCV-RNA was tested by polymerase chain reaction [5].

Liver biopsies were routinely obtained in HCV-infected patients between 6 and 15 months after transplantation or when graft dysfunction was present, and were evaluated by a single staff pathologist. If more than one liver biopsy was obtained during this period, the latest one was evaluated. Alanine aminotransferase (ALT) levels and clinical evaluation were performed at regular intervals.

Severe graft reinfection was defined by histological findings indicative of hepatitis infection including portal and parenchymal mononuclear infiltrates of varying degrees, acidophilic necrosis and swollen hepatocytes in patients with graft dysfunction (maintained increase in ALT levels for at least 6 weeks). Other common findings included lymphoid aggregates, bile duct damage and fatty changes.

Results

Table 1 shows pretransplant diagnosis and incidence of severe graft HCV reinfection, chronic graft hepatitis C and chronic rejection.

Thirty-two of 52 patients with pretransplant HCV infection developed severe graft reinfection after LTx; 9 of these 32 were treated with alpha-interferon (INF). Chronic graft hepatitis C was found in 26 grafts at the end of the study. Chronic rejection occurred in 8 of 97 allografts (8.25 %); 5 presented chronic rejection and concomitant chronic graft hepatitis C. In seven of eight grafts, chronic rejection or chronic rejection with HCV infection was confirmed in explanted livers. No patients treated primarily with FK 506 had chronic rejection.

The incidence of chronic rejection in patients with HCV infection before LTx (9.6 %) did not differ when compared with negative HCV patients (6.6 %) (Yates' chi-square test: P not significant) However, when the 26 cases that developed graft dysfunction due to chronic hepatitis C after liver transplantation were considered, 5 presented chronic rejection, a significantly higher incidence than the in remaining patients (3 of 71) (Yates' chi-square test: $P < 0.05$). Furthermore, 2 of 9 patients (22 %) treated with INF for HCV recurrence developed chronic hepatitis and concomitant chronic rejection.

Discussion

The incidence of chronic rejection after liver transplantation in our experience was 8.25 %, similar to that of other reports [1]. Our finding of an increased incidence of chronic rejection in patients with HCV reinfection was found only in patients who developed chronic hepatitis C [6]. Five of our patients suffered severe hepatitis C recurrence concomitant with chronic rejection. All these patients developed cholestasic features with duct damage or mixed portal infiltrates and difficulties arose in determining whether chronic rejection or hepatitis was responsible for duct damage [5, 7].

Explanations for the increased incidence of chronic rejection in patients with chronic hepatitis C remain unknown. Viral infections such as cytomegalovirus (CMV) may up-regulate the immune system, and an association between CMV, hepatitis B virus, and HCV infection and both acute and chronic rejection has been reported [8, 9]. HCV reinfection may play a direct role in the pathogenesis of chronic rejection. Immunosuppression permits higher viral replication and, therefore, higher viraemia levels in the liver recipient. This large amount of cytopathological virus and/or specific viral strains could produce a different and more aggressive chronic hepatitis with duct damage in certain transplant recipients [5, 10]. Owing to the lack of satisfactory therapy to eradicate HCV, lower baseline immunosuppression should be considered in patients with severe graft HCV recurrence [6, 8].

In our experience, there appears to be a relationship between the development of chronic rejection and chronic graft hepatitis C after LTx. INF therapy may favour chronic rejection, whereas FK 506 therapy may prevent the evolution of chronic rejection [11].

References

1. Hubscher S, Neuberger J (1993) Chronic rejection of the liver allograft. In: Neuberger J, Adams D (eds) Immunology of liver transplantation. Arnold, London, pp 216–229
2. Demetris AJ, Murase N, Delaney CP, Woan M, Fung JJ, Starzl TE (1995) The liver allograft, chronic (ductopenic) rejection, and microchimerism: what can they teach us? Transplant Proc 27: 67–70
3. Poterucha JJ, Raquela J, Lumeng L, Lee C-H, Taswell HF, Wiesner RH (1992) Diagnosis of chronic hepatitis C after liver transplantation by the detection of viral sequences with polymerase chain reaction. Hepatology 15: 42–45
4. Shah G, Demetris AJ, Gavaler JS, Lewis JH, Todo S, Starzl TE, Van Thiel DH (1992) Incidence, prevalence and clinical course of hepatitis C following liver transplantation. Gastroenterology 103: 323–324
5. Vargas V, Comas P, Casells LL, Quer J, Esteban JI, Allende E, Esteban R, Guardia J, Margarit C (1994) Incidence and outcome of hepatitis C virus after liver transplantation. Transplant Int 7 (Suppl 1): S216–S220
6. Sheiner PA, Schwartz ME, Mor E, Schluger LK, Theise N, Kishikawa K, Koleskinov V, Bodenheimer H, Emre S, Miller CM (1995) Severe or multiple rejection episodes are associated with early recurrence of hepatitis C after orthotopic liver transplantation. Hepatology 21: 30–34
7. Ferrell LD, Wright JR, Roberts J, Ascher N, Lake J (1992) Hepatitis C viral infection in liver transplant recipients. Hepatology 16: 865–876
8. Bronster O, Mañez R, Kusne S, Irish W, Roland A, Jain A, Llull R, Demetris AJ, Starzl TE (1995) Posttransplant B, non-A non-B, and cytomegalovirus hepatitis increase the risk of developing chronic rejection after liver transplantation. Transplant Proc 27: 1206–1207
9. Mañez R, Whitw LT, Linden P, Kusne S, Martin M, Kramer D, Demetris AJ, Van Thiel DH, Starzl TE, Duquesnoy RJ (1993) The influence of HLA matching on cytomegalovirus hepatitis and chronic rejection after liver transplantation. Transplantation 55: 1067–1071
10. Feray C, Gigou M, Samuel D, Paradis V, Mishiro S, Maertens G, Reynes M, Okamoto H, Bismuth H, Brechot C (1995) Influence of the genotypes of hepatitis C virus on the severity of recurrent liver disease after liver transplantation. Gastroenterology 108: 1088–1096
11. Charco R, Ruiz C, Allende E, Balsells J, Lázaro JL, Murio E, Bilbao I, Gifre E, Margarit C (1995) Experience in therapy of chronic liver allograft rejection. Transplant Proc 27: 2018–2019

Transpl Int (1996) 9 [Suppl 1]: S 198–S 201
© Springer-Verlag 1996

K.-P. Platz
A. R. Mueller
R. Neuhaus
H. Keck
P. Lemmens
U. Hopf
P. Neuhaus

Hepatitis C: indication for anti-viral therapy?

K.-P. Platz (✉) · A. R. Mueller ·
R. Neuhaus · H. Keck · P. Lemmens ·
P. Neuhaus
Department of Surgery, Virchow Clinic,
Humboldt University Berlin,
Augustenburger Platz 1, D-13353 Berlin,
Germany
Tel. +49-30-45052001;
fax +49-30-45052900

U. Hopf
Department of Hepatology,
Virchow Clinic,
Humboldt University Berlin,
Germany

Abstract Hepatitis C infection is a frequent indication for liver transplantation. In general, recurrent graft hepatitis is assumed to be mild, but may be the cause of lethal postoperative complications in a small patient population. Out of 500 transplants in 458 patients, 123 patients were transplanted due to hepatitis C infection (26.7 %) between September 1988 and April 1994. Cumulative 1- to 6-year patient survival was similar for patients transplanted due to hepatitis C (87.0 %) and those transplanted for other indications (86.0 %). In patients with hepatitis C virus (HCV), death, in 50 % of the cases, was related to HCV recurrence and chronic rejection. Four patients (25.0 %) died because of severe infection and multiple organ failure syndrome unrelated to HCV recurrence and chronic rejection. The incidence of retransplantation was similar in HCV (9.8 %) and other patients (8.4 %). In HCV patients, 6 of 12 retransplantations (50.0 %) were performed due to HCV recurrence and chronic rejection. Of 123 HCV patients, 45 experienced histologically proven recurrent graft hepatitis between 2 weeks and 5.5 years after transplantation. The incidence of acute rejection was similar in both groups. The incidence of steroid-resistant rejection was, however, higher in HCV patients (29.3 %) than in those transplanted for other indications (14.5 %; $P \leq 0.05$). Furthermore, there was a significant association between acute rejection and the development of recurrent graft hepatitis. In conclusion, patients with hepatitis C may be transplanted with as good patient and graft survival rates as patients transplanted for other indications. However, the combination of recurrent graft hepatitis and chronic rejection remains the most limiting factor for some of these patients, which strengthens the neccessity for a specific anti-viral therapy.

Key words Liver transplantation · Hepatitis C · Acute and chronic rejection

Introduction

Posthepatic cirrhosis and acute liver failure due to hepatitis C and NANBNC infection is a frequent indication for liver transplantation. Currently, no prophylaxis of hepatitis C virus (HCV) recurrence or anti-viral therapy has been established. HCV reinfection or the persistence of the virus, as determined by polymerase chain reaction techniques, was observed in almost all patients (> 90 %) during the first year after liver transplantation [1, 2, 4, 5, 10, 13]. Virus elimination is possible, but rare. Recurrent graft hepatitis occurred in approximately 50 % of patients. In general, recurrent graft hepatitis is assumed to be mild in nature and spontaneously resolves over time [4]. However, in a small group of patients, severe recurrent graft hepatitis was associated with severe immunological or other complications. Therefore, 123 patients transplanted for HCV disease were analyzed and compared with patients transplanted for other indications.

Materials and methods

Patients

Between September 1988 and May 1994, 500 orthotopic liver transplantations (LTX) were performed in 458 patients at the University Clinic Rudolf Virchow. Indications for LTX included 94 patients with hepatitis B virus (HBV) and 118 patients with HCV disease, 79 patients with alcoholic cirrhosis, 45 with primary biliary cirrhosis (PBC), 28 with primary sclerosing cholangitis (PSC), 16 patients with cryptogen cirrhosis, 13 patients with autoimmune cirrhosis, 10 patients with Budd Chiari syndrome, 16 patients with primary bile duct carcinoma, hepatocellular carcinoma (HCC) or other tumors, and 39 patients with various other indications. A further 22 HCC were observed in patients primarily transplanted due to HBV and HCV cirrhosis. A total of 42 retransplantations were performed.

Immunosuppresssion and concomitant treatment

In 61 patients, FK506 was given i. v. for the first 3 days and subsequently oral medication was continued [8]. A total of 44 patients received primarily oral FK506 medication (0.03 mg or 0.05 mg/kg body weight twice daily). Cyclosporine A (CsA) therapy was commenced as quadruple therapy including anti-thymocyte globulin (ATG; Fresenius, Germany) for 1 week in 208 patients or including the interleukin-2 receptor antagonist, BT563 (Biotest, Dreireich, Germany) for 12 days in 145 patients and both groups were subsequently continued on triple therapy [9]. Surgical procedures, aprotinin administration, i. v. antibiotic treatment, selective bowel decontamination and various other prophylaxes were performed perioperatively, as previously described [8, 9].

Clinical and laboratory investigations

Patients were evaluated prior to transplantation by medical history, demographic data, physical examination, and laboratory evaluations. Laboratory investigations, including CsA blood levels (non-specific TDX assay) and whole blood FK506 levels, as well as clinically adverse experiences, were evaluated on a daily basis for the first month, and subsequently, after predefined time intervals. HCV RNA (blood and liver) and second generation anti-HCV enzymëlinked immunosorbent assay (ELISA) [4] were performed at predefined time points pre- and postoperatively, and whenever recurrent graft hepatitis was suspected.

Management of rejection and recurrent graft hepatitis

Diagnosis of acute rejection was based on clinical (fever, change of color, and amount of bile production) and laboratory (aspartate transaminase, alanine transaminase, bilirubin, γGT, and alkaline phosphatase) findings, and was confirmed by histological evaluation of graft biopsies, as previously reported [8]. Patients received methylprednisolone for treatment of acute rejection at a dosage of 500 mg/day for 3 days and either OKT3 monoclonal antibody

Table 1 Cause of death in patients infected with hepatitis C virus (*HCV*). (*CR* Chronic rejection, *MOFS* multiple organ failure syndrome)

Cause of death	n	Percentage
HCV recurrence, CR	8/16	50.0
Severe infection, MOFS	4/16	25.0
Neurological complications	2/16	12.5
Others	2/16	12.5

(Cilag, Sulzbach, Germany) or FK506 (0.1 mg/kg body weight twice daily) or the combination of both immunosuppressive agents for steroid-resistant or severe recurrent rejection [8]. No attempt was made to treat patients with steroid recycles. Criteria for recurrent graft hepatitis were used as previously described [4]. Liver biopsies were routinely performed at postoperative day (POD) 7, and whenever rejection or recurrent hepatitis was suspected.

Statistical analysis

Kaplan Meier estimates, Wilcoxon, chi-square and Kruskal-Wallis tests were used as indicated. Results were expressed as means ± standard error of the mean.

Results

Survival

The cumulative 6-year graft and patient survival was similar in patients transplanted owing to hepatitis C infection and other indications with 78.1 % and 77.2 % for graft survival and 87.0 % and 86.0 % for patients, respectively. Of 123 HCV patients, 16 died. In 50 % of these patients, death was related to chronic rejection or recurrent HCV cirrhosis; predominantly a combination of both complications was observed (Table 1). This was followed by severe infections with multiple organ failure syndrome in 25 % of patients. Patients dying because of HCV recurrence and chronic rejection mostly acquired severe atypical or fungal infections, such as *Pneumocystis carinii* pneumonia and *Aspergillus* sepsis, which prohibited retransplantation in this group of patients.

The incidence of retransplantation was similar in patients transplanted because of hepatitis C disease (9.8 %) or other indications (8.4 %). The main cause of retransplantations in HCV patients was recurrent graft hepatitis and chronic rejection followed by refractory acute rejection and initial non-function (INF). The latter two diagnoses occurred significantly more often in HCV than in other patients (Table 2). INF was observed in 1.3 % and refractory acute rejection in < 0.5 % of all liver transplanted patients. Of the 12 retransplanted patients, 5 (41.7 %) subsequently died, including 3 of 6 patients retransplanted for recurrent graft hepatitis and chronic rejection.

Table 2 Cause of retransplantation in patients infected with hepatitis C virus *(HCV)*. (*CR* Chronic rejection, *INF* initial non-function)

Cause of retransplantation	n	Percentage
HCV recurrence, CR	6/12	50.0
Refractory acute rejection	2/12	16.7*
INF	2/12	16.7*
Others	2/12	16.7

* $P \leq 0.05$ versus patients transplanted for other indications

Table 3 Incidence of acute rejection in patients infected with hepatitis C virus *(HCV patients)*

	HCV patients	Other indications for orthotopic liver transplantation
Acute rejection	58/123 (47.5%)	153/335 (45.7%)
Steroid-resistant rejection	36/123 (29.3%)*	34/335 (10.1%)
Recurrent graft hepatitis	45/123 (36.6%)	–

* $P \leq 0.05$ versus patients transplanted for other indications

Hepatitis C reinfection and rejection

Histologically proven recurrent graft hepatitis was observed in 45 of 123 patients (36.6%) between 2 weeks and 5.5 years after transplantation. The majority of reinfections occurred between 4 and 12 months after transplantation. One or more rejection episodes were observed in 47.5% of HCV patients and 45.8% in patients with other indications. However, the incidence of steroid-resistant rejection requiring FK506 rescue therapy or OKT3 was significantly higher in HCV patients than in patients transplanted for other indications (Table 3).

HCV recurrence was highly associated with acute allograft rejection and anti-rejection therapy. Of 45 patients, 39 (86.7%) experienced one or more acute rejection episodes prior to the onset of recurrent graft hepatitis. The time interval between acute rejection and onset of recurrent graft hepatitis varied considerably between 1 week to 12 months. A further five patients developed acute rejection from 1 week to 6 months after the onset of recurrent graft hepatitis, while one patient developed chronic rejection requiring retransplantation. Only 1 of these 45 patients developed no immunological complications at all.

Discussion

Persistence or early recurrence of hepatitis C viremia has been commonly observed after liver transplantation (> 90% of patients) [1, 2, 4, 5, 10, 13]. Recurrent graft hepatitis has been reported to occur in 14–45% of HCV patients [11, 12]. However, the clinical course varies considerably from being clinically asymptomatic with mild laboratory abnormalities to acute liver failure requiring retransplantation. More than one-third of our HCV patients developed recurrent graft hepatitis to different degrees of severity. More patients may have experienced hepatitis C recurrence, which has not been confirmed as recurrent graft hepatitis by histological studies. Reevaluation of all HCV patients with quantitative HCV RNA determination in serum and blood may more sensitively detect HCV recurrence and increase the number of confirmed recurrent graft hepatitis cases. However, to date, histology in conjunction with abnormalities in liver function tests seems to be most reliable.

An association with acute allograft rejection and augmented immunosuppression has been previously reported [12]. The present data confirm these observations. There was only one patient experiencing recurrent graft hepatitis who never developed acute or chronic rejection. The majority of patients experienced first acute rejection with increased immunosuppressive therapy, which was followed by recurrent graft hepatitis within 1 week to 12 months. In some patients, both events occurred almost simultaneously, while only 5 patients first developed recurrent graft hepatitis and only subsequently acute or chronic rejection.

Although patient and graft survival were similar in HCV patients than in those transplanted for other indications, the predominant life-threatening factor for HCV patients is recurrent graft hepatitis in association with acute and chronic rejection. Others have also observed that the outcome after retransplantation is poor in this small patient population [11, 12]. Since the high incidence of rejection in patients with recurrent graft hepatitis prohibits reduction of immunosuppression, an answer to the current dilemma may only be a prevention of HCV recurrence or treatment with an anti-viral agent.

Of note, furthermore, is the fact that a relatively high number of HCV patients died from neurological complications, which conforms to previous observations [6, 7]. There was also a markedly increased incidence of refractory acute rejection and INF in this group of patients compared with patients transplanted for other indications [3].

In conclusion, we found that hepatitis C is a good indication for liver transplantation with respect to patient and graft survival. However, there was a high association between recurrent graft hepatitis and acute allograft rejection. Furthermore, 50% of these patients died from problems related to recurrent graft hepatitis and chronic rejection. Therefore, the most optimal solution will be the prevention of viral replication and an anti-viral strategy for patients transplanted because of HCV disease.

References

1. Arnold JC, Kraus T, Otto G, et al (1992) Reccurrent hepatitis C virus after liver transplantation. Transplant Proc 24: 2646–2647
2. Feray C, Samuel D, Thiers V, et al (1992) Reinfection of liver graft by hepatitis C virus after liver transplantation. J Clin Invest 89: 1361–1365
3. Haller GW, Langrehr JM, Blumhardt G, et al (1995) Factors relevant to the development of primary dysfunction in liver allograft. Transplant Proc 27: 1192
4. König V, Bauditz J, Lobeck H, et al (1992) Hepatitis C reinfection after orthotopic liver transplantation. Hepatology 16: 1137–1143
5. Lake JR, Wright T, Ferrell L, et al (1993) Hepatitis B and C in liver transplantation. Transplant Proc 25: 2006–2009
6. Mueller AR, Platz K-P, Christe W, et al (1994) Severe neurotoxicity after liver transplantation: association between FK506 therapy and hepatitis C virus disease. Transplant Proc 26: 3131–3132
7. Mueller AR, Platz K-P, Bechstein WO, et al (1995) The optimal immunosuppressant after liver transplantation according to diagnosis: cyclosporine A or FK506. Clin Transpl 9: 176–184
8. Neuhaus P, Bechstein WO, Blumhardt G, et al (1993) Comparison of quadruple immunosuppression after liver transplantation with ATG or IL-2 receptor antibody. Transplantation 55: 1320–1327
9. Neuhaus P, Blumhardt G, Bechstein WO, et al (1995) Comparison of FK506- and cyclosporine A-based immunosuppression in primary orthotopic liver transplantation. A single center experience. Transplantation 59: 31–40
10. Poterucha JJ, Rakela J, Lumeng L, et al (1992) Diagnosis of chronic hepatitis C after liver transplantation by detection of viral sequences with polymerase chain reaction. Hepatology 15: 42–45
11. Shah G, Demetris AJ, Gavaler JS, et al (1992) Incidence, prevalence, and clinical course of hepatitis C following liver transplantation. Gastroenterology 103: 323–324
12. Sheiner PA, Schwartz ME, Mor E, et al (1995) Severe or multiple rejection episodes are associated with early recurrence of hepatitis C after liver transplantation. Hepatology 21: 30–34
13. Wright TL, Donegan E, Hsu HH, et al (1992) Recurrent and acquired hepatitis C viral infection in liver transplant recipients. Gastroenterology 103: 317–322

Transpl Int (1996) 9 [Suppl 1]: S 202–S 203
© Springer-Verlag 1996

LIVER

O. Boillot
F. Berger
E. Rasolofo
F. Mion
P. Chevallier
D. Gille
P. Paliard

Effectiveness of early α-interferon therapy for hepatitis C virus infection recurrence after liver transplantation

O. Boillot (✉) · F. Berger · E. Rasolofo ·
F. Mion · P. Chevallier · D. Gille · P. Paliard
Unité de Transplantation Hépatique,
Pavillon D, Fédération des Spécialités
Digestives, hôpital Edouard Herriot,
F-69003 Lyon, France

Abstract The results in this short series show that early and prolonged α-interferon therapy for hepatitis C virus recurrence after liver transplantation could bring some benefit to the infected liver grafts. The risk of graft rejection was clearly minimised by maintaining immunosuppression at normal levels.

Introduction

Following liver transplantation (LT) for hepatitis C virus (HCV)-related cirrhosis, the risk of HCV infection recurrence on the graft remains high and the long-term progression to chronic hepatitis and cirrhosis seems strongly probable. The use of α-interferon (IFN) for HCV infection in transplanted patients is still controversial because of the risk of graft rejection and of questionable efficacy. Nevertheless, in the aim to preserve viability of the graft, an early treatment in the acute phase of the disease could be justified. We present our series of LT in patients with positive HCV antibodies and the preliminary results of IFN therapy for HCV infection recurrence after LT in 13 patients.

Patients and methods

From October 1990 to February 1995, 40 patients with anti-HCV antibodies detected using a third-generation radioimmunoblotting assay (RIBA), and cirrhosis, had LT. Before LT, six patients had known hepatocellular carcinoma and HCV-RNA was detected in the serum in only 18 patients (46 %) using polymerase chain reaction (PCR) for the 5′ non-coding region. Sera from 35 patients were screened for HCV genotypes using, the inno-lipa technique (Ingen); 23 (65.7 %) were positive for type 1b, 7 (20 %) for 2a, 3 (8.5 %) for 3a and 2 (5.7 %) for 4a. HCV-RNA was found in 71.4 %, 0 %, 33 % and 100 % of patients' sera containing genotypes 1b, 2a, 3a and 4a respectively. Following LT, after a mean study period of 27 ± 20 months (8–100 months), 33 (83 %) patients are alive, 36 remained (100 %) or became (80 %) PCR-positive for HCV, 16 (40 %) developed acute HCV-related hepatitis and 13

(32.5 %) were put under IFN therapy. Concerning the 16 patients who developed hepatitis, genotypes were represented as 50 % of 1b, 42 % of 2a, 33 % of 3a and 50 % of 4a; PCR for HCV was positive in all patients. Indication for IFN therapy was the onset of elevation of serum alanine aminotransferase (ALT) levels (247 ± 200 U/l) and the evidence of histological ongoing features of HCV hepatitis on two consecutive liver biopsies (portal inflammation, lobular mononuclear cell infiltrate, onset of fibrosis, hepatocyte necrosis and steatosis). The time between LT and detection of HCV-RNA in the serum and in the liver of the all 16 patients with HCV-related hepatitis, LT and the rise of ALT, the ALT elevation and the onset of IFN therapy was, respectively, 8 ± 12 weeks, 45 ± 35 weeks and 26 ± 37 weeks. Three patients with mild histological features have not yet been put under IFN therapy. During IFN therapy, the immunosuppressive regimen was maintained at normal levels. IFN (Introna, Shering Plough) therapy was initiated using low doses (1 MU subcutaneously 3 times a week for 2 weeks, 2 MU for the next 2 weeks and 3 MU 3 times a week for the following 20 months). Doses were adjusted (1.5–2 MU) according to leukopenia or thrombocytopenia. Every month, liver blood tests were performed and at 3, 6, 12, 18 and 21 months, PCR and histological evaluations were done.

Results

Four patients had the whole treatment for 21 months, six others are still under IFN therapy after 15–19 months. In three patients, IFN therapy had to stop at 4, 8 and 14 weeks for acute and reversible rejection in two cases and psychiatric complication in one case. Nevertheless, 12 patients were responders, as underlined by normalisation of serum transaminases which occurred 10 ± 12 weeks (2–47) following the beginning of IFN therapy and was maintained during the course of the treatment. From 4 to 12 months after an entire course of IFN, ALT were still at normal levels in three out of four patients; in one patient, C hepatitis recurred and was successfully treated using IFN and ribavirin therapies. After a mean follow-up period of 13 months, four patients under IFN therapy cleaned HCV-RNA from their serum. The liver biopsies were analysed by the same histologist (F.B.). Global histological improvement was seen in the ten patients (77 %) but was more obvious in patients who were under IFN for more than 3 months; in one case, histological features were unchanged and worsened in one other case; in these cases IFN doses were reduced following mild rejection and thrombopenia. Features of mononuclear cell infiltrate, fibrosis, hepatocyte necrosis and steatosis improved, respectively, in 90 %, 72 %, 90 % and 50 % of the cases. No factors (HCV genotype, status of PCR-HCV before LT, age, sex, CMV infection, rejection episodes, early graft function, surgical events) were found to influence significantly the development of posttransplant hepatitis C-related cirrhosis in patients, but hepatitis recurrence was more likely in patients with longer period from LT (37 versus 21 months, $P < 0.05$).

Discussion

The course of HCV infection after LT is not yet well understood, however, the risk of progression to chronic active hepatitis (CAH) seems high, as it has been reported in a series of 79 patients positive for serum HCV antibodies in whom 72 % experienced acute hepatitis progressing to CAH in 61 % of the cases within 3 years [1]. With time, progression to cirrhosis and liver failure seems inescapable and may justify an early and effective treatment in the aim to preserve the viability of the graft. IFN still represents the only effective treatment against HCV infection. In non-transplanted patients with chronic hepatitis, the present tendency is to start early IFN therapy and to maintain it for at least 1 year [2]. In such a way, the rate of responders increased to 71.4 % at the end of treatment and to 57.1 % after 3 years of follow-up [2]. Efficacy of IFN has been underlined y other studies with reduction of liver fibrosis in chronic HCV hepatitis [3]. Progression of the disease in transplanted patients seems accelerated, probably because of immunosuppression [1]. This situation, in our view, could justify the decision of an early treatment against HCV hepatitis with IFN. In fact, Wright et al. [4] have treated 18 patients for HCV infection after LT with IFN (3MU 3 times weekly for 4 months); however, the rate of responders was only 28 %, possibly because of the brevity of treatment duration. In our series, 12 (92.3 %) of 13 patients were responders in terms of normalisation of transaminase blood levels and improvement of histological features; the reasons could be the early onset and prolonged duration of IFN therapy. Chronic rejection was not observed because immunosuppressive therapy was given at upper normal levels and was strictly monitored during the whole course of IFN therapy. According to HCV genotypes, the rate of post-LT HCV infection seemed not significantly different between patients, whatever the HCV genotype.

References

1. Feray C, Gigou M, Samuel D, et al. (1994)Hepatology 20: 1137

2. Sarocco G, Rosina F, Abate ML, et al. (1993) Hepatology 18: 1300

3. Manabe N, Chevallier M, Chossegros P, et al. (1993) Hepatology 18: 1344

4. Wright TL, Coombs C, Kim M, et al. (1994) Hepatology 20: 773

Transpl Int (1996) 9 [Suppl 1]: S 204–S 209
© Springer-Verlag 1996

LIVER

Lucio Caccamo
Bruno Gridelli
Maurizio Sampietro
Ernesto Melada
Maurizio Doglia
Giovanna Lunghi
Noemi Corbetta
Giorgio Rossi
Michele Colledan
Luigi Rainero Fassati
Gemino Fiorelli
Dinangelo Galmarini

Hepatitis C virus Genotypes and reinfection of the graft during long-term follow-up in 35 liver transplant recipients

L. Caccamo (✉) · B. Gridelli · E. Melada ·
M. Doglia · G. Rossi · M. Colledan ·
L. R. Fassati · D. Galmarini
Istituto di Chirurgia Sperimentale
e dei Trapianti, Università di Milano,
Centro Trapianto Fegato,
Ospedale Maggiore IRCCS,
via F. Sforza 35, I-20122 Milan, Italy,
Tel. +39-2-551-81-435/551-92-578

M. Sampietro · N. Corbetta · G. Fiorelli
Istituto di Medicina Interna e
Fisiopatologia Medica,
Università di Milano,
Ospedale Maggiore IRCCS,
via F. Sforza 35, I-20122 Milan, Italy

G. Lunghi
Istituto di Igiene,
Ospedale Maggiore IRCCS,
via F. Sforza 35, I-20122 Milan, Italy

Abstract To understand the clinical outcome of hepatitis C virus (HCV) recurrence, data from 35 liver transplant recipients who survived more than 6 months were reviewed. The presence of HCV-RNA was evaluated and genotyping was performed. On the basis of alanine aminotransferase (ALT) levels, patients were sorted into four groups. In 20 patients, a chronic elevation in ALT was found; HCV-RNA detection was positive in 17/17 and the following genotypes were found in 15 of them: 1b in ten patients, 2a in four patients, and 3a in one patient. In 11 patients, ALT levels remained normal throughout follow-up; in nine of them HCV-RNA was positive; HCV genotyping was available in eight patients and identified type 1b in two, type 2a in five, and type 3a in another patient. In two patients, ALT fluctuated above and below the upper limits of normality; type 1b HCV-RNA was found in one of them. In two patients, after an initial period of normality, ALT levels showed an abrupt rise; HCV-RNA was positive and type 1b was

identified in both patients. Eight patients developed HCV-related deep jaundice and three of them spontaneously recovered. Progressive hepatic injury occurred in eight patients, six with chronic ALT elevation and two showing a late ALT elevation; genotype 1b was present in seven patients while in one, genotype 3a was found; sub-acute graft failure developed in five of them, leading to death in two and retransplantation in the others; the other three patients are alive with recurrent overt cirrhosis. The 1, 3, and 5 year actuarial survivals were 89 %, 79 %, and 63 % respectively. The 1, 3, and 5 year actuarial risks of progressive graft damage were 6 %, 7 %, and 15 %, respectively. In conclusion, HCV reinfection causes a slow decrease in the long-term patients' survival. Persistent elevation of ALT is more frequently observed in patients with genotype 1b infection.

Key words Liver transplantation · Hepatitis C virus · Polymerase chain reaction

Introduction

Liver cirrhosis in patients with hepatitis C virus (HCV) infection is a major indication for orthotopic liver transplantation (OLT) [15, 26]. HCV infection is responsible for a large number of postoperative graft impairments [7, 20]. In pretransplant HCV-positive recipients, a high-

er risk of disease is dependent from the primary infection because, differently from hepatitis B virus (HBV) disease, no prophylaxis is available.

The prevalence and the clinical course of HCV infection after liver transplantation is still not well established [1]. This is partly due to the lack of simple and valid tools for the diagnosis of HCV disease: HCV antibody (anti-HCV) testing seems to be of little use in the follow-up of pretransplant infected patients [7]. Direct detection in serum of the HCV genome (HCV-RNA) by the polymerase chain reaction (PCR) faces an array of technical problems that still prevent it from becoming a routine procedure [19]. HCV-RNA detection with viral genome typing [2, 7] and viremia quantification [4, 8, 17] are currently the only methods that can be used to study the course of HCV infection.

The aim of this retrospective study is to evaluate the role of HCV genotypes in the natural posttransplant history of pretransplant infected recipients and their different impact in longterm patients' and grafts' survival.

Patients and methods

Up to 30 September 1995, 284 liver transplants were performed at our center. HBsAg negative, IgM anti-HBcAg negative patients with a post-transplant follow-up of at least 6 months were selected from our series. Immunosuppressive treatment was based on administration of cyclosporine A or FK506, and low doses of prednisone and azathioprine, when possible on the basis of the white cell count. Administration of steroids was gradually tapered and was finally withdrawn during follow-up. Liver function tests were regularly determined over posttransplant time. Serum alanine aminotransferase (ALT) levels were assumed as expression of functional hepatic injury and patients were sorted according to the course of ALT mean monthly values. In order to enhance the specificity of ALT variations secondary to HCV infection, ALT levels were analyzed from the begining of the second postoperative month to the subsequent follow-up. Therefore, ALT variations due to ischemic or rejection injuries, which more frequently occur in the first postoperative month, were ignored. Functional graft impairment was defined as persistent when abnormal ALT levels lasted longer than 3 months. In the presence of biochemical dysfunction, both biliary and vascular technical complications were ruled out by appropriate diagnostic imaging procedures. Liver biopsy samples, when available, were evaluated for hepatitis. The histological diagnosis of hepatitis required the presence of portal inflammation, lobular mononuclear cell infiltration, and hepatocellular necrosis; the appearance of intralobular bridging fibrosis defined an active evolution. In order to establish the etiology of the allograft damage, causes of hepatitis other than HCV were excluded by serial analysis of patients' serum samples for HBV markers, P65 cytomegalovirus (CMV) antigen and antibodies against CMV, hepatitis A, Epstein-Barr, herpes simplex and herpes zoster viruses. Each liver sample was fixed in buffered formalin and routinely processed. Staining for HBV and in situ hybridization for CMV were performed to definitively rule out these infections. The presence of either histological hepatitis or persistent liver dysfunction together with HCV-RNA positivity and no evidence of other known causes of hepatitis was defined as HCV hepatitis. Usually the diagnosis of viral hepatitis led to a rapid reduction or withdrawal of steroids, while no antiviral therapy was undertaken.

Recipients' sera were tested using a second- or third-generation anti-HCV enzyme-linked immunosorbent assay (ELISA); supplementary testing with a second- or third-generation recombinant immunoblotting assay (RIBA) was performed in all ELISA-positive cases. Both anti-HCV assays were carried out according to the manufacturers' instructions, as described elsewhere [3]. All posttransplant sera were stored at −20 °C before being tested for

Table 1 Data of 35 pretransplant hepatitis C virus (HCV)-positive liver transplant recipients

Sex (male/female)	25/10
Age (years)	
Mean ± SD	39 ± 19
Range	2–63
Primary disease	
Posthepatitis cirrhosis	19
Hepatoma-cirrhosis	9
Primary biliary cirrhosis	3
Metabolic deficiency	2
Biliary atresia	2
Follow-up (months)	
Mean ± SD	41 ± 32
Range	6–118

periods of 1–12 months. RNA extraction was performed with the acid guanidinium thiocyanate-phenol-chloroform method [5] with the addition of 1 μg of glycogen as a carrier prior to isopropanol precipitation. Complementary DNA (cDNA) synthesis (Promega, Madison, USA) was primed from the core region of HCV-RNA. A 267-bp fragment from the 5' untranslated region of the viral genome was amplified by heminested polymerase chain reaction (HNPCR) after cDNA synthesis by reverse transcription (RT). We employed a modification of methods previously described, achieving single-tube RT and amplification of viral sequences [21]. Strict measures to prevent contamination were adopted; reagent-negative, sample-negative, and sample-positive controls were included in each batch of RNA extraction and carried on through PCR. HCV genotyping was performed using a fraction of the PCR products, which was hybridized to oligonucleotides directed against the variable region of 5' untranslated region and immobilized as parallel lines on membrane strips (line probe assay, LIPA, Innogenetics, Gent, Belgium). The reactivity of the amplified fragments with one or more lines in the strip allowed identification of the five major genotypes and their subtypes. Viral genotypes were denominated according to Simmonds [24].

Values were expressed as mean ± standard deviation (SD) and range between minimum and maximum values. Chi-square test and Fischer's exact test were used to analyze differences between groups. A P value less than 0.05 was considered to indicate a significant difference. Actuarial patients' survival and risk of HCV-related graft failure were calculated according to the method of Kaplan-Meir.

Results

Data from 37 pretransplant HCV-positive recipients were reviewed. At the time of the last out-patient control (mean 41 months, SD 32, range 6–119) a biliary complication was found in two recipients, who were excluded from this study. Follow-up data from 35 patients were analyzed and are summarized in Tables 1 and 2. The majority of the patients could be divided into two patterns of follow-up ALT levels (Fig. 1): chronic persistent elevation (20 patients) or sustained normal levels (11 patients). In 16 of the 20 patients showing chronic ALT elevation, histologically acute hepatitis was pre-

Table 2 Sorting of recipients according to the four individualized patterns of posttransplant alanine aminotransferase (ALT) levels. Serum HCV-RNA positivity, HCV genotypes, and occurrence of graft failure due to HCV infection are shown. In the first two groups of patients, the pattern of ALT levels relative to the HCV genotypes (1b versus non-1b) at the Fischer's exact test showed $P = 0.0894$ and relative risk = 1.83, with a 95 % confidence interval between 0.915 and 3.675

Patterns of ALT	Patients	Positive HCV-RNA	Type 1b	Type 2a	Type 3a	Graft failure
Elevated	20	17/17[a]	10	4	1	6
Normal	11	9/11[b]	2	5	1	0
Late elevated	2	2/2	2	0	0	2
Fluctuating	2	1/1	1	0	0	0

[a] Genotyping of two HCV-RNA-positive patients was not available
[b] Genotyping of one HCV-RNA-positive patient was not available; two patients were HCV-RNA-negative

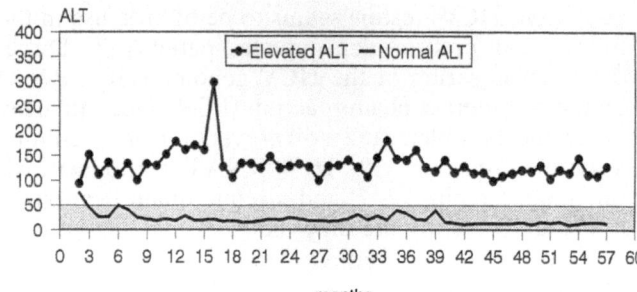

Fig.1 Mean values of serum alanine aminotransferase *(ALT)* after liver transplantation: 20 patients showed chronic ALT elevation and 11 patients showed normal ALT levels

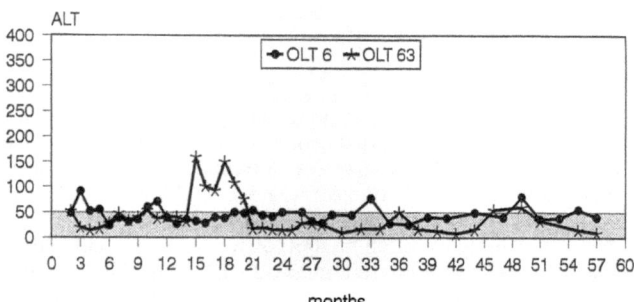

Fig.2 Mean values of serum ALT after liver transplantation in two patients *(OLT6* and *OLT63)* with levels fluctuating above and below the normal limits

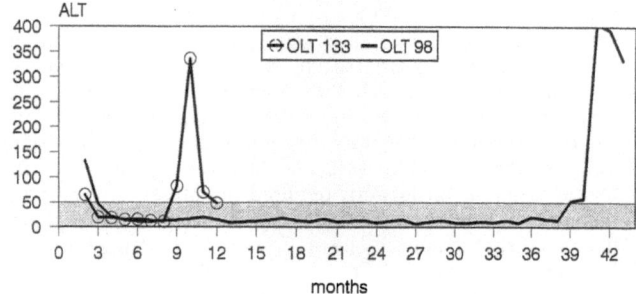

Fig.3 Mean values of serum ALT after liver transplantation in two patients *(OLT98* and *OLT133)* with late elevation and death due to hepatitis C virus (HCV)-related sub-acute graft failure

sent 1 month after surgery; in three others it was recognized during the second and third postoperative months and in the latter after 9 months of follow-up. HCV-RNA detection was positive in 17/17 of them and the following genotypes were identified in 15: 1b in ten patients, 2a in four patients, and 3a in one patient. In the 11 patients who showed normal ALT levels throughout follow-up, a graft biopsy during the long-term follow-up was not available, but in three of them the acute hepatitis had been histologically proven during the first postoperative month. In nine of these 11 patients, HCV-RNA was positive; HCV genotyping identified type 1b in two patients, type 2a in five patients, and type 3a in another patient; genotyping was not available in a HCV-RNA-positive patient. Of the two patients in this group who were HCV-RNA-negative, one was found anti-HCV negative at 69 months after surgery. The four remaining recipients showed two different patterns of presentation: ALT fluctuating above and below the normal limits (two patients) and an abrupt rise in ALT levels after a sustained period of normal values (two patients). In two patients, ALT levels were found fluctuating above and below the upper limits of normality (Fig.2) during a follow-up of 82 and 119 months, respectively (histology not available). HCV-RNA was positive in 1/1 of them and type 1b was identified. In the last two patients, after an initial period of normal liver biochemistry, ALT levels showed an abrupt rise (Fig.3) with rapidly progressive graft failure and death at 11 and 52 months after transplantation; HCV-RNA was found positive and type 1b was identified in both patients. Comparing the first two groups of patients, there was a consistent trend for patients in the group with persistent elevation in ALT to be infected by genotype 1b versus other types in patients in the group with normal ALT

levels. However, the difference was not significant ($P = 0.0894$), maybe owing to the small sample size, even if the relative risk for ALT elevation was almost doubled in the presence of genotype 1b infection.

Eight out of all patients examined developed a deep jaundice episode (serum total bilirubin above 10 mg% for a mean of 4 months, range 2–10); six of them had persistent elevated ALT and the others were the two patients with the late ALT elevation; all these patients were infected by genotype 1b. Five of them developed marked cholestasis as a sign of sub-acute HCV-related

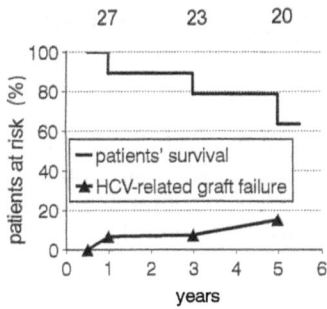

Fig. 4 Actuarial patients' survival curve and risk of HCV-related graft failure after liver transplantation. Data from 32 patients surviving at least 6 months (three deaths for recurrent hepatocarcinoma were excluded)

graft failure, while in three patients jaundice lasted 2, 3, and 10 months, respectively and then spontaneously resolved. After a mean time of 28 months from transplantation (range 1–88), progressive hepatic injury occurred in eight patients, six with chronic ALT elevation and two with the late ALT elevation; the genotype 1b was identified in seven of them and in the remaining patient genotype 3a was present. Sub-acute hepatic failure developed in five recipients after a mean of 12 months (range 3–50) leading to death in two and retransplantation (re-OLT) in the others; re-OLT was performed elsewhere abroad in a patient who died shortly afterwards, and at our center in the remaining two patients (one received her first transplant at another Italian center), who are currently alive 14 and 34 months after re-OLT, respectively, despite a HCV infection in the new liver in both of them. The other three patients have recurrent cirrhosis: one patient was not considered for re-OLT due to her poor respiratory condition, a Le Veen shunt was placed 84 months after surgery and she is now showing a progressively deteriorating condition (follow-up 108 months); another patient improved after medical treatment for ascites, which she had developed 24 months after the transplant (follow-up 35 months); the latter patient spontaneously improved after a hepatic decompensation episode occurred 48 months after surgery and he is stable 79 months after transplantation. Moreover, another patient who has persistent elevated ALT and a genotype 1b infection had been known to have recurrent overt histological cirrhosis but he is still in good general condition with a well-functioning graft 24 months after transplantation.

Fifty-seven graft biopsies from 25 patients were reviewed. Acute hepatitis was found in histological specimens during the early posttransplant period in 21 patients. In five patients the acute phase rapidly progressed to a graft failure with morphological signs of wide disruption of the hepatic structure by marked infiltrates. Subsequent late histology samples were available from eight recipients after a mean time of 10 months after the acute

hepatitis and histological progression to cirrhosis was found in four of them, one of whom remained in good clinical status but expressed repeat marked alteration in ALT levels during 18 months of histological follow-up.

The 1, 3 and 5 year actuarial patients' survival, excluding from the analysis three patients who died of cancer recurrence, were 89 %, 79 % and 63 %, respectively (Fig. 4). The 1, 3, and 5 year actuarial risks of progressive graft decompensation were 6 %, 7 %, and 15 %, respectively (Fig. 4).

Discussion

Hepatitis C virus infection is a well-recognized cause of chronic graft damage in liver transplant recipients [9]. In common with pretransplant HBV-positive liver allograft recipients, pretransplant HCV-positive patients are at high risk of recurrence because of the extra-hepatic sites of viral replication [14]. Differently from HBV disease [22], pretransplant HCV viremia does not seem to be a relevant independent factor for the risk of posttransplant infection [26]. Virtually all patients with pretransplant HCV-related disease develop recurrent viral infection during follow-up, as expressed by the positivity of serum HCV-RNA detection [7, 11]. Moreover, the reappearance of graft dysfunction is common [7, 13, 25] and it occurs soon after transplantation [9, 12, 26], as diagnosed by either histological evidence of hepatitis or persistent elevations in liver enzymes in the absence of other known causes.

In the present study we have described the biochemical appearance and the long-term clinical course of HCV recurrence in 35 pretransplant infected patients. In the majority of patients, two distinct patterns of ALT levels were observed, namely persistent elevation or normal values, whereas in a few patients fluctuating ALT levels above and below the norm and sustained normal ALT levels followed by an abrupt rise associated with graft failure were found. Out of 30 patients in whom HCV-RNA detection was performed, only two were found negative and both had normal ALT levels over time; in one of them, anti-HCV was found negative after the transplant, and we suggest that this patient cleared the viral infection, a rare event that has been reported in the literature [25]. In three patients with long-term normal ALT values, acute hepatitis was found by the end of the first postoperative month. The possibility that normal ALT values do not exclude an underlying hepatitis had been previously reported [11]. However, in our series, no patient having ALT levels within the normal limits showed progressive hepatic damage.

Three different HCV genotypes have been found in 26 patients analyzed and the various types were present both in the elevated and normal ALT level groups of patients. Patients infected by genotype 1b more commonly showed elevated ALT levels, but this finding was not statistically significant. In our patients, regardless of the genotype of the infection, an early recurrent acute hepatitis was the rule. In most patients, the evolution of the acute phase of viral reinfection was favorable, but in rare cases it rapidly worsened, leading to early graft loss. Elevated ALT levels were present in six patients who showed hepatic decompensation; genotype 1b infection was present in all these patients but one, who was infected by type 3a. In the two other patients who experienced HCV-related graft failure, ALT presented a sharp elevation after a long period of normality: a change in the quasispecies mixture of the individual viral population can be hypothesized in these recipients, as recently demonstrated by Gretch et al. [10]. Finally, our data, even without recognizing the genotype 1b infection as a statistically significant negative independent prognostic factor after transplantation [8], showed that the occurrence of HCV-related hepatic decompensation was strikingly linked to this genotype when associated with abnormal ALT levels.

It has been reported that, in some patients, HCV recurrence can cause a marked cholestatic syndrome and this was identified as a negative prognostic factor [25]. Yet, in some series, the occurrence of HCV-associated severe jaundice has been denied [11] or other etiologic factors have been found than the viral infection [23]. In this series a deep jaundice episode appeared in eight patients infected by genotype 1b, and cholestasis spontaneously resolved during a variable length of time in three of them who did not show a rapid deteriorating evolution with loss of hepatic synthesis.

One potential shortcomming of the present study is the lack of sequential histological follow-up in our patients. It is not our policy to perform "protocol" liver biopsies and, therefore, the risk of an underestimation of the HCV recurrent hepatitis may be present in this series. Ferrel et al. [9] showed how difficult it is to achieve a histological diagnosis of HCV hepatitis in grafted patients because of the high frequency of atypical microscopic features, regardless of aspartate aminotransferase levels; in their study the authors emphasized the central role of HCV-RNA positivity in the diagnosis of the cause of liver damage.

HCV infection of the graft has been recognized as a crucial factor affecting the long-term result of liver transplantation [2, 7, 9, 20, 26]. It is known that the clinical evolution of posttransplant HCV disease over time may range from long-term asymptomatic carriers to progressive liver damage [4, 7, 16, 20], even with rapid developing graft failure [6, 17]. In our experience, pretransplant HCV infection commonly led to graft dysfunction and the recurrence of the disease caused a slow decrease in the long-term patients' survival, maybe because of the indolent rate of progression of the graft damage. We believe that although HCV-related graft loss has been rarely reported [1, 2, 6, 12, 26], it is likely to become more prevalent with longer follow-up studies [18]. In this series the risk of graft failure due to HCV disease showed a progressive increase throughout follow-up, leading to death or need for retransplantation. The latter was successful in term of patients' survival, but it was always followed by HCV infection in the new graft, as reported by others [1, 16, 17, 20].

In conclusion, from our results it appears that HCV genotype 1b could have a relevant prognostic role in the posttransplant HCV-recurrent disease. Monitoring long-term postoperative ALT levels is a simple and reliable test in the evaluation of the progression of HCV graft damage. Spontaneous resolution of HCV-related severe cholestatic episodes is possible when hepatic synthesis is maintained. HCV reinfection of the graft seems to affect the long-term survival because of increasing risk of HCV-related graft derangement and failure over time.

Acknowledgements The authors would like to thank Mrs. Laura Vento, Mr. Francesco Cifarelli and Mr. Saverio Di Giuseppe for their excellent technical assistance. The present study was in part supported by a grant from Consiglio Nazionale delle Ricerche con il contributo di ricerca (95.02278.CT04).

References

1. Ascher NL, Lake JR, Emond J, Roberts J (1994) Liver transplantation for hepatitis C virus related cirrhosis. Hepatology 20: 24S–27S
2. Belli LS, Caccamo L, Mazzaferro V, Silini E, Alberti A, Melada E, Regalia E, Gridelli B, Rubino A, Gennari L, Galmarini D, Ideo G, Belli L (1994) Milan multicenter experience in liver transplantation for hepatitis C related cirrhosis: report of 105 cases. Transplant Proc 26: 3582–3584
3. Caccamo L, Colledan M, Gridelli B, Rossi G, Doglia M, Gatti S, Ghidoni P, Lucianetti A, Lunghi G, Maggi G, Paone G, Reggiani P, Galmarini D, Fassati LR (1993) Hepatitis C virus infection in liver allografts recipients. Arch Virol Suppl 8: 291–304
4. Chazouilleres O, Kim M, Combs C, Ferrel L, Bacchetti P, Roberts J, Ascher NL, Neuwald P, Wilber J, Urdea M, Quan S, Sanchez-Pescador R, Wright TL (1994) Quantitation of hepatitis C virus RNA in liver transplant recipients. Gastroenterology 106: 994–999
5. Chomczynski P, Sacchi N (1987) Single-step method of RNA isolation by acid guanidinium-thiocyanate-phenol-chloroform extaction. Anal Biochem 162: 156–169
6. Donataccio M, Lerut J, Ciccarelli O, Comu CH, Laterre PF, Geubel A, Otte JB (1994) Hepatitis C viral infection and adult liver transplantation: a difficult clinical problem. Transplant Proc 26: 3588–3590

7. Feray C, Gigou M, Samuel D, Paradis V, Wilber J, David MF, Urdea M, Reynes M, Brechot C, Bismuth H (1994) The course of hepatitis C virus infection after liver transplantation. Hepatology 20: 1137–1143

8. Feray C, Gigou M, Samuel D, Paradis V, Mishiro S, Maertens G, Reynes M, Okamoto H, Bismuth H, Brechot C (1995) Influence of genotypes of hepatitis C virus on the severity of recurrent liver disease after liver transplantation. Gastroenterology 108: 1088–1096

9. Ferrell LD, Wright TL, Roberts J, Ascher N, Lake J (1992) Hepatitis C viral infection in liver transplant recipients. Hepatology 16: 865–876

10. Gretch DR, Wilson JJ, Faulkner G, Corey L, Perkins J, Carithers RL (1994) Tracking hepatitis C virus quasispecies in liver transplant recipients (abstract). Hepatology 20: 132A

11. Gugenheim J, Baldini E, Mazza D, Fabiani P, St. Paul MC, Goubaux B, Ouzan D, Mouiel J (1994) Recurrence of hepatitis C virus after liver transplantation. Transplant Int 7 (suppl 1): S224–S226

12. Knoop M, Lusebrink R, Langrehr JM, Konig F, Berg T, Wedell A, Hopf U, Neuhaus P (1994) Incidence and clinical relevance of recurrent hepatitis C infection after orthotopic liver transplantation. Transplant Int 7 (suppl 1): S221–S223

13. Konig V, Bauditz J, Lobeck H, Lusebrink R, Neuhaus P, Blumhardt G, Bechstein WO, Neuhaus R, Steffen R, Hopf U (1992) Hepatitis C virus reinfection in allografts after orthotopic liver transplantation. Hepatology 16: 1137–1143

14. Li X, Jeffers L, Reddy R, De Medina M, Parker T, Schiff ER (1992) Detection of HCV-RNA by RT-PCR in lymphocyte subsets (abstract). Gastroenterology 102 (part 2): A842

15. Mateo R, Demetris A, Sico E, Frye C, Wang L-F, El-Sakhawi Y, Reilly M, Ehrlich GD, Cooper D, Fung J (1993) Early detection of de novo hepatitis C infection in patients after liver transplantation by reverse transcriptase polymerase reaction. Surgery 114: 442–448

16. Muller H, Otto G, Goeser T, Arnold J, Pfaff J, Thielmann L (1992) Recurrence of hepatitis C virus infection after orthotopic liver transplantation. Transplantation 54: 743–745

17. Nery J, Esquenazi V, Weppler D, Gomez C, Cirocco R, Gharagozloo H, Zucker K, Reddy R, Casella J, Parker I, Faria W, Jeffers L, Carreno M, Smith J, Markow M, Allouch M, Babischkin S, Bourke G, Hill M, Schiff E, LaRue S, Miller J (1994) Hepatitis C in liver transplantation: preliminary study of prognostic factors. Transplant Int 7 (suppl 1): S229–S231

18. Pappo O, Ramos H, Starzl TE, Fung JJ, Demetris AJ (1995) Structural integrity and identification of causes of liver allograft dysfunction occurring more than 5 years after transplantation. Am J Surg Pathol 19: 192–206

19. Persing DH, Rakela J (1992) Polymerase chain reaction for detection of hepatitis viruses: panacea or purgatory? Gastroenterology 103: 1098–1099

20. Pouterucha JJ, Rakela J, Lumeng L, Lee C-H, Taswell HF, Wiesner RH (1992) Diagnosis of chronic hepatitis C after liver transplantation by detection of viral sequences by polymerase chain reaction. Hepatology 15: 42–45

21. Sampietro M, Salvadori S, Badalamenti S, Graziani G, Fiorelli G (1995) Single tube reverse transcription and heminested polymerase chain reaction of hepatitis C virus RNA to detect viremia in serologically negative hemodialyzed patients. Int J Clin Lab Res 25: 52–54

22. Samuel D, Muller R, Alexander G, Fassati LR, Ducot B, Benhamou J-P, Bismuth H and the investigators of the European Concerted Action on Viral Hepatitis Study (1993) Liver transplantation in European patients with the hepatitis B surface antigen. N Engl J Med 329: 1842–1847

23. Shiffman ML, Contos MJ, Luketic VA, Santal AJ, Purdum PP, Mills AS, Fisher RA, Posner MP (1994) Biochemical and histologic evaluation of recurrent hepatitis C following orthotopic liver transplantation. Transplantation 57: 526–532

24. Simmonds P (1995) Variability of hepatitis C virus. Hepatology 21: 570–583

25. Vargas V, Comas P, Castella LI, Quer J, Esteban JI, Allende E, Esteban R, Guardia J, Margarit C (1994) Incidence and outcome of hepatitis C virus infection after liver transplantation. Transplant Int 7 (suppl 1): S216–S220

26. Wright TL, Donegan E, Hsu HH, Ferrel L, Lake JR, Kim M, Combs C, Fennessy S, Roberts JP, Ascher NL, Greenberg HB (1992) Recurrent and acquired hepatitis C viral infection in liver transplant recipients. Gastroenterology 103: 317–322

Transpl Int (1996) 9 [Suppl 1]: S210–S212
© Springer-Verlag 1996

LIVER

G. W. Haller
W. O. Bechstein
R. Neuhaus
R. Raakow
T. Berg
U. Hopf
P. Neuhaus

Famciclovir therapy for recurrent hepatitis B virus infection after liver transplantation

G. W. Haller (✉) · W. O. Bechstein ·
R. Neuhaus · R. Raakow · P. Neuhaus
Department of Surgery, Virchow Clinic,
Humboldt University of Berlin,
Augustenburger Platz 1, D-13353 Berlin,
Germany

T. Berg · U. Hopf
Department of Internal Medicine,
Virchow Clinic, Humboldt University of
Berlin, Germany

Abstract Between November 1993 and June 1995 18 patients received oral famciclovir (3×500 mg) for treatment of hepatitis B virus (HBV) reinfection after liver transplantation. Reinfection was defined as the reoccurrence of HBsAg in the serum. In the first 15 patients, famciclovir therapy was initiated after clinical signs of graft hepatitis, whereas the last 3 patients received treatment immediately after HBV-DNA was detected. Famciclovir was well-tolerated in all patients. HBV-DNA values were decreased to un- detectable levels in 8 out of 18 patients. Clinical status improved in 7 patients, whereas 5 patients remained unchanged and 6 patients progressed to deteriorating graft function and death. When famciclovir was initiated early after reinfection, a response rate of approximately 66 % was observed. Late onset of therapy in patients with fulminant hepatitis generally failed to provide any clinical benefit.

Key words Liver transplantation · Hepatitis B · Famciclovir

Introduction

Hepatitis B virus (HBV) reinfection is the major cause of fatal outcome after liver transplantation in HBsAg-positive patients. Two-year survival rates are currently estimated at between 50 and 70 % [1–4]. In the case of severe recurrent graft hepatitis, retransplantation is the only treatment option, although associated with disappointing results. Neither short-term immunoprophylaxis, nor interferon treatment have been shown to have a major impact on graft and patient survival. Long-term immunization with anti-HBs hyperimmunoglobulin appears most effective [1–5].

Famciclovir, the oral form of penciclovir, is a novel nucleoside analog with known antiviral effects against herpes simplex and herpes zoster infections. Famciclovir suppresses HBV replication as has been shown in Pekin ducks and humans [6–9]. The results of a phase II trial in patients with chronic hepatitis B seemed promising and may allow expectations for prevention and treatment of HBV recurrence in HBsAg-positive liver transplant patients in the future.

Patients and methods

Patients transplanted because of hepatitis B cirrhosis and acute liver failure due to fulminant hepatitis B, received anti-HBs hyperimmunoglobulin (Hepatect, Biotest Dreieich, Germany) during and after transplantation, commencing on a daily basis and subsequently according to anti-HBs titer [5]. Reinfection was defined by the occurrence of HBsAg after liver transplantation. Between November 1993 and June 1995, 18 patients received famciclovir therapy after reinfection, when HBV-DNA was proven. In the first group of patients ($n = 15$), famciclovir therapy (3×500 mg/day) was initiated after clinical signs of recurrent graft hepatitis. The later group of patients ($n = 3$) received famciclovir treatment immediately after diagnosis of reinfection (HBV-DNA- and HBsAg-positive status). Hyperimmunoglobulin therapy was terminated at the onset of reinfection. HBV-DNA was measured by hybridization assay (Abbott, Wiesbaden, Germany).

Results

Famciclovir therapy was well-tolerated in all patients. HBV-DNA levels were decreased below the detection limit in 8 of 18 patients. In 7 of these patients, clinical

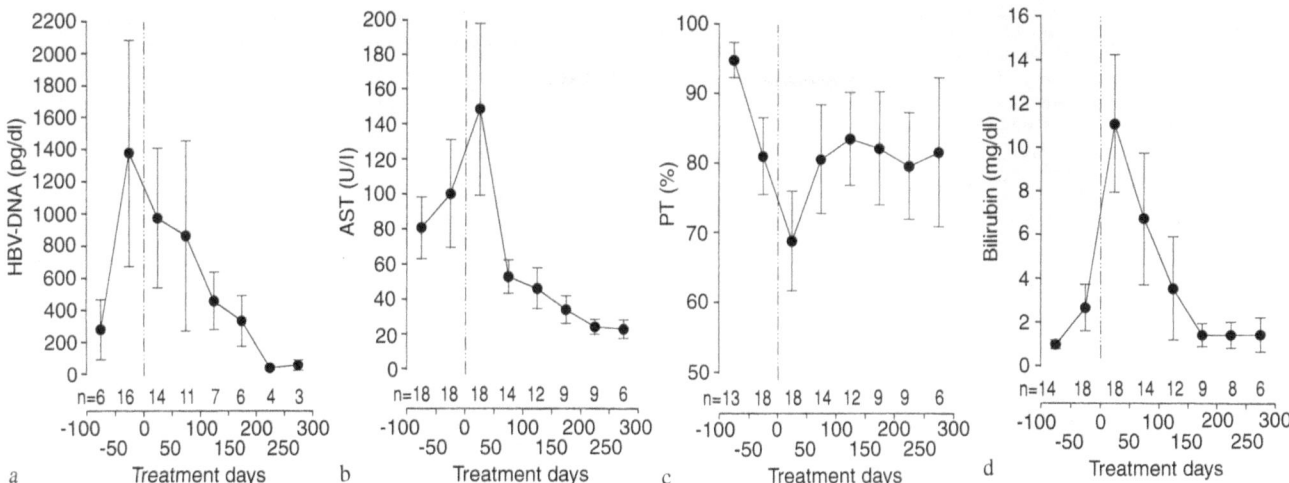

Fig. 1 a Serum hepatitis B virus DNA *(HBV-DNA)*, **b** asparagine transaminase *(AST)*, **c** prothrombin time *(PT)* and, **d** bilirubin during famciclovir treatment. All values are expressed as mean ± SEM

improvement of recurrent graft hepatitis was observed, as reflected by normalization of asparagine transaminase, alanine transaminase, and bilirubin levels, and prothrombin time (Fig. 1). Five patients remained unchanged in clinical status, while in 6 patients a progressive hepatitis with deteriorating graft function occurred. Four of the 6 patients who died had only famciclovir therapy for 8–28 days and were assessed too late for this therapy.

Discussion

When famciclovir first became available, treatment was initiated during the course of recurrent graft hepatitis, irrespective of the time of conversion to HBV-DNA-positive status. Subsequently, treatment was immediately started in all patients proven to be HBV-DNA positive. These differences in therapeutic approach may be responsible for differences in outcome under treatment.

Early treatment of recurrent hepatitis B with famciclovir reduced HBV-DNA levels to virtually zero in 44 % of patients. These patients seemed to profit from famciclovir therapy. However, some patients remained relatively unchanged in clinical status, despite a reduction in HBV-DNA levels.

Success with famciclovir was observed in patients who either developed mild recurrent hepatitis late after reinfection, or in patients treated immediately after they were assessed HBV-DNA-positive, leading to a response rate of approximately 66 %. Furthermore, late onset of famciclovir therapy in patients with fulminant graft hepatitis generally failed to provide any clinical benefit. Therefore, the optimal indication and time point for famciclovir treatment seems to be prophylactic therapy immediately after transplantation. For this purpose, a clinical multicenter study is currently underway.

References

1. Neuhaus P, Steffen R, Blumhardt G, Bechstein WO, Keck H, Lemmens HP, Neuhaus R, Lobeck H, König V, Hopf U (1991) Experience with immunoprophylaxis and interferon therapy after liver transplantation in HBsAg positive patients. Transplant Proc 23: 1522–1524
2. Samuel D, Muller R, Alexander G, Fassati L, Ducot B, Benhamou J-P, Bismuth H (1993) Liver transplantation in European patients with the hepatitis B surface antigen. N Engl J Med 329: 1842–1847
3. Freeman RB, Sanchez H, Lewis WD, Sherburne B, Dzik WH, Khettry U, Hing S, Zeldis JB, Jenkins RL (1991) Serologic and DNA follow-up data from HBsAg-positive patients treated with orthotopic liver transplantation. Transplantation 51: 793–797
4. Lucey MR, Graham DM, Martin P, Di Bisceglie A, Rosenthal S, Waggoner JG, Merion RM, Campbell DA, Nostrant TT, Appelman HD (1992) Recurrence of hepatitis B and delta hepatitis after orthotopic liver transplantation. Gut 33: 1390–1396
5. Müller R, Gubernatis G, Farle M, Niehoff G, Klein H, Wittekind C, Tusch G, Lautz H-U, Böker K, Stangel W, Pichlmayr R (1991) Liver transplantation in HBs antigen (HBsAg) carriers: prevention of hepatitis B virus (HBV) recurrence by passive immunization. J Hepatol 13: 90–96

6. Vere Hodge RA, Sutton D, Boyd MR, Harnden MR, Jarvest RL (1989) Selection of an oral prodrug (BRL 42810; famciclovir) for the anti-herpes virus agent BRL 39123 [9-(4-hydroxy-3-hydroxymethylbut-1-yl)guanine; penciclovir]. Antimicrob Agents Chemother 33: 1765–1773

7. Korba BE, Milman G (1991) A cell culture assay for compounds which inhibit hepatitis B virus replication. Antiviral Res 15: 217–228

8. Tsiquaye KN, Slomka MJ, Maung M (1994) Oral famciclovir against duck hepatitis B virus replication in hepatic and nonhepatic tissues of ducklings infected in vivo. J Med Virol 42: 306–310

9. Böcker KHW, Ringe B, Krüger M, Pichlmayr R, Manns MP (1995) Prostaglandin E plus famciclovir – a new concept for treatment of severe hepatitis B after liver transplantation. Transplantation 57: 1706–1708

Transpl Int (1996) 9 [Suppl 1]: S213–S215
© Springer-Verlag 1996

LIVER

I. Lautenschlager
K. Höckerstedt
E. Taskinen
E. von Willebrand

Expression of adhesion molecules and their ligands in liver allografts during cytomegalovirus (CMV) infection and acute rejection

I. Lautenschlager (✉) · E. Taskinen ·
E. von Willebrand
Laboratory Department,
Helsinki University Central Hospital,
PO Box 21 (Haartmaninkatu 3),
University of Helsinki,
FIN-00014 Helsinki, Finland

K. Höckerstedt
Fouth Department of Surgery,
Helsinki University Central Hospital,
Helsinki, Finland

Abstract Vascular adhesion molecules and their ligands are important in leukocyte-endothelial cell interactions and in T-cell activation of rejection cascade. Also, cytomegalovirus (CMV) infection is suggested to be involved in the mechanisms of rejection. In this study, the expression of vascular adhesion molecules ICAM-1, VCAM-1 and ELAM-1 in the liver allografts, the number of leukocytes positive for their ligands LFA-1, VLA-4 and SLex, and activation markers (class II, IL2-receptor) were investigated in liver allografts during CMV infection and acute rejection and compared to grafts with normal function and histology. The adhesion molecules, their ligands and activation markers were demonstrated from liver biopsy frozen sections by the immunoperoxidase technique and monoclonal antibodies. A significant induction of ICAM-1 and VCAM-1 was seen in vascular and sinusoidal endothelium associated with both CMV and rejection, and induction of ELAM-1 in vascular endothelium in rejection only. In both cases, the number of leukocytes expressing LFA-1 was significantly increased, but VLA-4-positive cells were more characteristic for CMV and SLex-positive cells more for rejection. IL2-receptor positivity was practically seen in rejection only, but class II-expressing cells were increased during both CMV infection and rejection. In conclusion, adhesion molecules were induced and the infiltrating cells expressed their ligands both in liver rejection and during CMV infection, although the expression pattern was slightly different.

Key words Adhesion molecules · Liver transplantation · Cytomegalovirus infection

Introduction

Adhesion molecules and their ligands are important in endothelial cell-leukocyte interactions and in T-cell activation [7]. The expression of cellular adhesion molecules is up-regulated by various cytokines during inflammatory reactions of acute allograft rejection [4, 8]. In addition to rejections, viral infections, e. g. cytomegalovirus (CMV) infections, also common after liver transplantation, may cause inflammatory reactions in the graft [5]. An association between CMV infection and vanishing bile duct syndrome and chronic liver allograft rejection has been suggested [1, 6].

In this study, we have investigated the induction of vascular adhesion molecules, intercellular adhesion molecule-1 (ICAM-1), vascular cell adhesion molecule-1 (VCAM-1), and endothelial leucocyte adhesion molecule-1 (ELAM-1), in the liver allograft, and the expression of their ligands and activation markers in graft-infiltrating leukocytes of patients having CMV infection affecting the liver or undergoing biopsy-confirmed acute rejection. The results are compared to those from patients with normal graft function and histology.

S214

Table 1 The intensity of endothelial adhesion molecule expression and the numbers of graft-infiltrating cells expressing their ligands and activation markers (mean ± SD). (Patient groups: *CMV* posttransplantation with cytomegalovirus infection affecting the liver, *Rx* posttransplantation undergoing acute rejection, *NOR* posttransplantation with normal graft function and histology)

Patient group	ICAM-1		VCAM-1		ELAM-1		LFA-1	VLA-4	SLeX	Class II	IL2-receptor
	Vascular	Sinusoidal	Vascular	Sinusoidal	Vascular	Sinusoidal					
CMV	$1.8 \pm 0.7^*$	$2.6 \pm 0.7^*$	$1.2 \pm 0.6^*$	$1.2 \pm 0.6^*$	0.2 ± 0.4	0 ± 0	$27 \pm 11^*$	$27 \pm 18^*$	7 ± 1	$18 \pm 9^*$	1 ± 2
RX	$1.8 \pm 0.8^*$	$2.3 \pm 0.5^*$	$1.2 \pm 0.8^*$	$1.3 \pm 1.4^*$	$1.3 \pm 0.5^*$	0 ± 0	$35 \pm 6^*$	9 ± 5	$19 \pm 4^*$	$28 \pm 8^*$	$11 \pm 7^*$
NOR	0.8 ± 0.4	1.2 ± 0.4	0.2 ± 0.4	0.4 ± 0.5	0 ± 0	0 ± 0	13 ± 2	4 ± 4	0 ± 0	5 ± 3	1 ± 1

* $P < 0.05$ compared with normal grafts

Patients and methods

The expressions of ICAM-1, VCAM-1 and ELAM-1 in the graft and their ligands LFA-1, VLA-4 and Sialyl Lewis X, and activation markers (class II and IL2-receptor) were examined in 12 liver transplant recipients having CMV infection affecting the liver and in 6 undergoing acute rejection. These results were compared to those from 5 patients with normal graft function and histology.

The diagnosis of CMV infection was based on viral cultures and detection of CMV-specific antigens in blood leukocytes and in liver biopsies. All CMV infections were symptomatic, associated with significant graft dysfunction, and were treated with ganciclovir. All rejections were confirmed by biopsy. The biopsies used for this experiment were obtained before starting anti-rejection treatment. Cases with combined rejection and infection were not included in the study.

Evaluation of adhesion molecule and ligand expression was done from core-needle biopsy frozen sections using indirect immunoperoxidase staining and commercial monoclonal antibodies. The intensity of adhesion molecule expression in vascular and sinusoidal endothelium was semiquantitatively scored from 1 to 3. The numbers of graft-infiltrating cells positive for ligand molecules and activation markers were counted per high power visual field.

Results

Expression of adhesion molecules in various structures of liver allografts during CMV infection, acute rejection and in normal liver grafts without rejection is summarised in Table 1. Compared with normal grafts, a significant up-regulation of ICAM-1 and VCAM-1 in vascular and sinusoidal endothelium was recorded, associated with CMV infection as well as with rejection. The CMV-induced expression pattern of those adhesion molecules was quite similar to that of rejection, but ELAM-1 induction of vascular endothelium was associated with rejection only. ELAM-1 expression was not recorded for sinusoidal endothelium. In addition to endothelial cells, ICAM-1 induction was also seen in hepatocytes and bile duct cells during both CMV infection and rejection. Also, inflammatory cells expressed ICAM-1 and VCAM-1.

The number of LFA-1-positive leukocytes was significantly increased during CMV infection and rejection, but VLA-4-positive cells were mainly associated with CMV and SLex-positive cells with rejection. Increased numbers of class II positive cells were seen in both CMV and rejection, but lymphocytes expressing IL2-receptor in the graft were practically associated only with immunoactivation of acute rejection.

Discussion

Vascular adhesion molecules are involved in the early phase of T-cell activation and leukocyte extravasation in the graft, serving as adhesion receptors for inflammatory cells in the endothelium. The expression of adhesion molecules is up-regulated by various cytokines, such as γ-interferon, IL-1 and TNF-α [2], produced by inflammatory cells during allograft rejection. This was seen in our study, as well as infiltration of inflammatory cells expressing the concomitant ligands.

Increase of vascular adhesion molecule expression in the liver graft was, however, induced also by CMV, and the expression pattern was almost similar to that of acute allograft rejection, but the VCAM-1–VLA-4 pair was more characteristic for CMV and the ELAM-1–SLex pair more for rejection. The inflammatory response against CMV in the graft is also lymphoid cell-dominated [5], and various cytokines, especially g-interferon, produced during the viral infection, may be involved in further immune reactions and increase of MHC-antigens and adhesion molecules in the transplant.

An association between CMV infection and chronic liver allograft rejection has been suggested [1], and some evidence of CMV-induced vascular changes typical of chronic allograft rejection in general has been found in clinical transplantation and in animal models [3]. The early inflammatory events in the graft, MHC-antigen and adhesion molecule expression, T-cell activation and leukocyte extravasation during the viral infection may be involved in the corresponding event of rejection cascade.

Acknowledgements This work was supported by grants from the Finnish Academy of Science, University of Helsinki, Helsinki University Central Hospital (EVO), and the Sigrid Juselius Foundation, Finland.

References

1. Arnold JC, Portman BC, O'Grady JG, Naoumov NV, Alexander GJM, Williams R (1992) Cytomegalovirus infection persists in the liver graft in the vanishing bile duct syndrome. Hepatology 16: 285–292
2. Dustin ML, Stauton DE, Springer TA (1988) Supergene families meet the immune system. Immunol Today 9: 213–215
3. Häyry P, Isoniemi H, Yilmaz S, Mennander A, Lemström K, Räisänen-Sokolowski A, Koskinen P, Ustinov J, Lautenschlager I, Taskinen E, Krogerus L, Aho P, Paavonen T (1993) Chronic allograft rejection. Immunol Rev 134: 33–81
4. Lautenschlager I, Höckerstedt K (1993) ICAM-1 induction on hepatocytes as a marker for immune activation of acute liver allograft rejection. Transplantation 56: 1495–1499
5. Lautenschlager I, Nashan B, Schlitt HJ, Hoshino K, Ringe B, Tillmann HL, Manns M, Wonigeit K, Pichlmayr R (1994) Different cellular patterns associated with hepatitis C reactivation, cytomegalovirus infection and acute rejection in liver transplant patients monitored with transplant aspiration cytology. Transplantation 58: 1339–1345
6. O'Grady JG, Alexander GJ, Sutherland S, Donaldson PT, Harvey FAH, Portman B, Calne RY, Williams R (1988) Cytomegalovirus infection and donor/recipient HLA-antigens: interdependent co-factors in pathogenesis of vanishing bile duct syndrome after liver transplantation. Lancet II: 302–305
7. Springer TA (1990) Adhesion receptors of immune system. Nature 346: 425–434
8. Steinhoff G, Behrend M, Schrader B, Pichlmayr R (1993) Intercellular immune adhesion molecules in human liver transplants: overview on expression patterns of leukocyte receptor and ligand molecules. Hepatology 18: 440–453

Heart/Lung

Transpl Int (1996) 9 [Suppl 1]: S219–S220
© Springer-Verlag 1996

Arrhythmogenic mortality in heart-transplant candidates

H.-G. Fieguth
T. Wahlers
H. J. Trappe
H. G. Borst

H.-G. Fieguth (✉) · T. Wahlers · H. G. Borst
Division of Cardiovascular Surgery,
Hannover Medical School,
D-30623 Hannover, Germany

H. J. Trappe
Division of Cardiology,
Hannover Medical School,
30623 Hannover, Germany

Abstract Sudden cardiac death represents a major problem in patients awaiting heart transplantation (HTx). A retrospective analysis of 1019 patients accepted for HTx revealed a high actuarial risk for sudden death accounting to 14 % after 1 year and 20 % after 2 years waiting time. Unterlying disease and hemodynamic characteristics had no predictive value. The use of implantable cardioverter/defibrillator therapy is discussed.

Key words Heart transplantation · Sudden cardiac death · Myocardial death · Implantable cardioverter/ defibrillator therapy

Introduction

The therapeutic option of heart transplantation (HTx) is limited by the scarcity of donated organs, leading to increasing waiting times for patients in end-stage heart failure. Advances in the medical treatment of congestive heart failure and the broadening acceptance of mechanical support systems have decreased the risk of myocardial death [1]. The incidence of sudden cardiac death in this patient group is, therefore, focusing interest [2].

Patients and methods

For evaluation of the risk of sudden cardiac death in patients awaiting HTx, a retrospective analysis was performed in 1554 patients who were evaluated for HTx at our institution from 1985 through 1994. Of these, 1019 patients were accepted for HTx and entered the study group, while 535 patients were not considered as transplant candidates for medical reasons. Complete follow-up of the study group was accomplished by serial reevaluation via the referring physician and the transplant center. Patient demographics, hemodynamic profile, and follow-up data were stored in a database and analyzed using SPSS software for statistical and actuarial work-up. Values are given as mean ± standard deviation. P values below 0.05 were considered significant.

Results

The mean age of patients entering the study was 45 ± 12 years and of these 608 patients had a dilated cardiomyopathy (DCM), 313 patients revealed an ischemic cardiomyopathy (ICM) due to end-stage coronary disease, and 98 patients suffered from miscellaneous disorders leading to terminal myocardial failure. Of the 1019 patients in the study group, 485 patients were transplanted after a mean waiting period of 13 ± 11 months, 363 patients remained waiting for a mean follow-up of 13 ± 22 months, and 171 patients died after 8 ± 11 months while awaiting HTx. Of these, 69 patients died in hospital and 102 as outpatients. Causes of in-hospital mortality were documented ventricular tachyarrhythmia in 28 patients (40 %) and refractory myocardial failure in 40 patients (59 %); 1 patient sustained a non-cardiac death. Outpatient deaths were sudden in 55 patients (54 %), myocardial in 28 patients (27 %) and not determinable in 19 patients (19 %). Within the whole group, incidence of sudden and myocardial deaths revealed no significant differences with regard to patient hemodynamics including cardiac index (CI) and radionuclide left ventricular ejection fraction (LVEF), as well as with regard to the underlying disease. Interestingly, the incidence of sudden cardiac death rose with increasing waiting periods, thus occurring significantly later than myocardial failure as the

Table 1 Patients characteristics of the study group (*CI* cardiac index, LVEF left ventricular ejection fraction, *DCM* dilated cardiomyopathy, *ICM* ischemic cardiomyopathy)

	Total group	Sudden death	Myocardial death	
CI	1.4 ± 1.0 l/min per m^2	1.7 ± 1.0 l/min per m^2	1.3 ± 1.0 l/min per m^2	n.s.
LVEF	$9.9 \pm 12.9\%$	$16.1 \pm 15.7\%$	$9.1 \pm 12.1\%$	n.s.
DCM	60%	68%	62%	n.s.
ICM	31%	32%	38%	n.s.
Waiting period	12 ± 21 months	13 ± 15 months	6 ± 9 months	$p < 0.05$

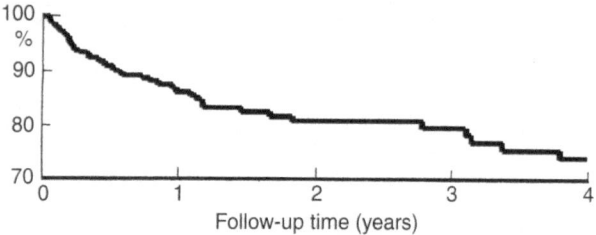

Fig. 1 Actuarial freedom from sudden cardiac death

cause of death in the evaluated population of transplant candidates (Table 1).

Actuarial analysis of survival, according to the Kaplan-Meyer method, was calculated with transplanted patients censored and terminal events grouped as: (1) all deaths, (2) myocardial deaths, and (3) sudden cardiac deaths. This analysis revealed an actuarial survival prior to heart transplantation in the population of accepted candidates of $52.9 \pm 2.7\%$ at 1 year, $47.2 \pm 2.9\%$ at 2 years, and $42.1 \pm 3.1\%$ at 4 years, with 51 of the 1019 patients remaining at risk. Actuarial risk for myocardial death was calculated as $23.4 \pm 2.5\%$ at 1 year, $32.1 \pm 3.2\%$ at 2 years and $39.4 \pm 3.9\%$ at 4 years. Actuarial risk for sudden cardiac death in patients awaiting HTx was predicted as $13.8 \pm 2.1\%$ at 1 year, $19.3 \pm 2.8\%$ at 2 years and $28.1 \pm 3.9\%$ at 4 years (Fig. 1).

Discussion

The results of our retrospective analysis clearly reveal that sudden cardiac death is a major hazard for patients prior to HTx, accounting for 40% of the overall mortality and representing an actuarial risk of 20% within 2 years. Risk of sudden cardiac deaths showed no significant differences with regard to the underlying disease and patient hemodynamics. Thus, especially with regard to the limitations of a retrospective study, it was not possible to define a subgroup of patients, within the whole population of transplant candidates, that is especially at risk. The finding that the underlying disease process has no significant influence on the risk of sudden cardiac death is supported by other large evaluations of patients in severe heart failure [3]. Furthermore, there are currently no established risk factors or diagnostic markers for sudden cardiac death in patients with chronic heart failure, and no correlation between the degree of ventricular arrhythmias and sudden cardiac death could be demonstrated [4]. In contrast, prolonged waiting periods for transplant candidates increase the risk of sudden death significantly. This, together with the advances in the medical treatment of severe heart failure [5], emphasize the need for control of arrhythmogenic mortality in patients considered for heart transplantation [6].

Interventional approaches including implantation of an automatic implantable cardioverter/defibrillator (ICD) should be considered, since pharmacological approaches have proven ineffective or even dangerous [7]. ICD therapy has proven to be the sole effective means of prevention of sudden cardiac death due to ventricular tachyarrhythmias in patients with severe impairment of left ventricular function [8]. Furthermore, the non-thoracotomy approach for ICD implantation represents a safe method with virtually no mortality, that implies no additional risk or operative difficulties at the time of cardiac transplant [9]. To assess the feasibility of this cost-intensive therapeutic "bridging approach" towards cardiac transplantation, a prospective and randomized study is needed for the evaluation of the effect of ICD implantation on the overall outcome in this high risk patient population.

References

1. Goldman S, Johnson G, Cohn J, et al, V-HeFT Cooperative Study Group (1993) Circulation 87 (VI): 24–31
2. Defibrilat Study Group (1991) J Am Coll Cardiol 68: 545–546
3. Stevenson WD, Stevenson LD, Middlekauf HR, Saxon LA (1993) Circulation 88: 6 2953–2961
4. Packer M (1992) Circulation 85: 1 (I): 50–56
5. Loisance DY, Deleuze PH, Houel R, et al (1993) Ann Thorac Surg 55: 310–313
6. Jeevanandam V, Bielefeld M, Auteri J, et al (1992) Circulation 86 (II): 276–279
7. The Cardiac Arrhythmia Suppression Trial (CAST) Investigators (1991) N Engl J Med 324: 781–788
8. Metha D, Saksena S, Krol RB, et al (1993) PACE 16 (II): 179–185
9. Fieguth HG, Wahlers T, Trappe HJ, et al (1993) Cor Europ I: 2 75–77

Transpl Int (1996) 9 [Suppl 1]: S 221–S 222
© Springer-Verlag 1996

Cytomegalovirus infection accelerates obliterative bronchiolitis of rat tracheal allografts

Karl Lemström
Erkki Kallio
Rainer Krebs
Cathrien Bruggeman
Pekka Häyry
Petri Koskinen

K. Lemström (✉) · E. Kallio · R. Krebs ·
P. Häyry · P. Koskinen
Transplantation Laboratory,
P.O. Box 21 (Haartmaninkatu 3),
FIN-00014 University of Helsinki,
Finland
Tel. + 3 58 0 4 34 65 90;
Fax + 3 58 0 24 11 2 27

C. Bruggeman
Department of Medical Microbiology,
University of Limburg, Maastricht,
The Netherlands

Abstract A cascade of inflammation and injury of the airway wall followed by a fibroproliferative process that results in airway obstruction has been suggested as the explanation of the process of obliterative bronchiolitis (OB) in lung allograft recipients. To determine the impact of rat cytomegalovirus (RCMV) infection on the development of OB, heterotopic rat tracheal allografts were transplanted from DA donors to WF recipients immunosuppressed with 2 mg/kg per day cyclosporine A. Chronic RCMV infection was similarly established 8 weeks before transplantation in donors alone (D +/R −), recipients alone (D −/R +), and both donors and recipients (D +/R +). The control rats were left non-infected, but were similarly immunosuppressed. The results of this study demonstrate that both acute and chronic recipient RCMV infection, but not donor infection, amplify the development of experimental OB in the rat and suggest that RCMV infection-associated immune response, rather than the viral load in the graft, is essential for the development of the accelerated form of OB.

Key words Cytomegalovirus · Obliterative bronchiolitis · Lung · Trachea · Rat

Introduction

We have previously demonstrated that non-immunosuppressed tracheal allografts exchanged between major and minor histoincompatible rat strains develop histological changes similar to obliterative bronchiolitis (OB), and that these changes are primarily due to an alloimmune response to epithelium, associated with epithelial damage as well as marked proliferation of inflammatory cells and granulation tissue [1]. Our results further demonstrated that these changes can be inhibited by cyclosporine A (CsA) in a dose-dependent manner [1]. In this study, the impact of rat cytomegalovirus (RCMV) infection on the generation of experimental OB was investigated.

Materials and methods

Heterotopic rat tracheal allografts were transplanted from DA (AG-B4, RT1^a) donors into the omentum of WF (AG-B2, RT1^v) recipients and the recipients were given 2 mg/kg per day of CsA. For acute infection, recipients were inoculated intraperitoneally on the day of transplantation with 10^5 plaque-forming units of RCMV [2]. Chronic RCMV infection was similarly established 8 weeks before transplantation in donors alone, recipients alone, and both donors and recipients. The control rats were left non-infected, but were similarly immunosuppressed.

A segment of graft was fixed in 3 % buffered paraformaldehyde, routinely processed, and embedded in paraffin. The grafts were examined histologically after sectioning and staining with Mayer's hematoxylin-eosin. To determine in vivo cell proliferation, the rats received bromodeoxyuridine by intravenous injection 3 h before sacrifice. Leukocyte subsets and the level of immune activation of inflammatory infiltrate were determined by the indirect immunoperoxidase technique using mouse monoclonal antibodies against rat determinants.

All data are expressed as mean ± SEM. The non-parametric Mann-Whitney U-test was chosen due to the small sample sizes

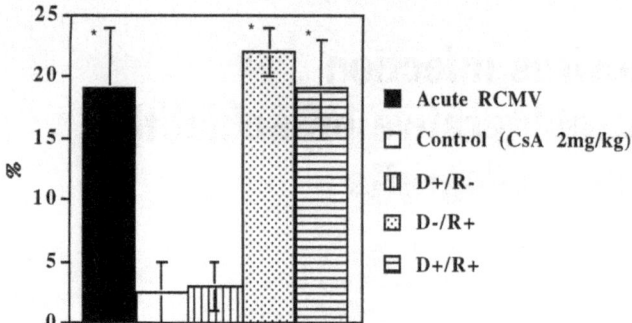

Fig. 1 Impact of acute and chronic RCMV infection in the development of luminal occlusion of tracheal allografts. (* $P < 0.05$, *CsA* cyclosporine A, *D +/R* – chronic RCMV infection in donors only; *D –/R +* chronic RCMV infection in recipients only, *D +/R +* chronic RCMV infection in both donors and recipients, RCMV rat cytomegalovirus)

and the inability to determine if the samples were normally distributed. The total variation between multiple groups was analyzed by the non-parametric Kruskal-Wallis one-way analysis by ranks, followed by the Dunn test for significances. *P* values less than 0.05 were regarded as statistically significant.

Results

RCMV infection significantly enhanced the generation of OB. Firstly, acute RCMV infection was linked to markedly enhanced MHC class II expression on the respiratory epithelium and prominent subepithelial inflammation of helper T cells (W3/25) and macrophages (ED1), with the prominence of lymphoid activation markers, MHC class II (OX 6), ICAM-1 (CD54), and IL-2R (CD25). Secondly acute infection induced a five-fold increase in luminal occlusion of the trachea, due to proliferating inflammatory and alpha-smooth muscle cell actin positive cells (Fig. 1). In chronic infection established in recipients alone, or both recipients and donors, the alterations were quite similar (Fig. 1). Chronic infection in donors alone significantly enhanced peritracheal inflammation, but showed no effect on subepithelial inflammation or luminal occlusion. Immunohistochemistry revealed that RCMV early and late antigen expression was quite similar in acute and chronic infection groups and that it occurred in the peritracheal area.

Discussion

Our results demonstrate that both acute RCMV infection and chronic recipient RCMV infection are significant risk factors for the development of enhanced obliterative changes in rat heterotopic tracheal allografts. Our findings suggest that RCMV replication in the tracheal allografts is unrelated to the development of pathological effects, and that a host immune response against RCMV is required for the enhancement of OB. This implies that either the viral load within the allograft is too low to evoke immune response, or the virus may escape immunocompetent T cells that recognize foreign peptides only in the context of host MHC I and II molecules. Studies determining the impact of RCMV on cytokine and growth factor ligand and receptor expression in the allograft are in progress.

References

1. Koskinen PK, Kallio E, Krebs R, Häyry PJ, Lemström KB (1995) A Dose-Dependent Inhibitory Effect of Cyclosporine A but not of 15-Deoxyspergualin or Mycophenolate Mofetil on Myofibro-proliferation and Luminal Occlusion of Heterotopic Rat Tracheal Allografts (submitted)

2. Lemström KB, Bruning JH, Bruggeman CA, Lautenschlager IT, Häyry PJ (1993) Cytomegalovirus infection enhances smooth muscle cell proliferation and intimal thickening of rat aortic allografts. J Clin Invest 92: 549–558

Transpl Int (1996) 9 [Suppl 1]: S223–S225
© Springer-Verlag 1996

Masayuki Sumitomo
Shoji Sakiyama
Nobuyuki Tanida
Taizo Fukumoto
Yasumasa Monden
Tadashi Uyama

Difference in cytokine production in acute and chronic rejection of rat lung allografts

M. Sumitomo (✉) · S. Sakiyama · N. Tanida
T. Fukumoto · Y. Monden · T. Uyama
Second Department of Surgery,
School of Medicine,
University of Tokushima, Kuramoto-cho 3,
Tokushima 770, Japan

Abstract In Brown Norway to Lewis rat lung transplantation, short-term administration of cyclosporine produces permanent adoption of allografts; however, the adopted grafts show symptoms of chronic rejection. To clarify the difference in cytokine production in acute an chronic rejection of the allografts, an immunohistochemical study was performed. In acute rejection, positive cells for respective cytokines were observed in infiltrating cells, increasing in number as the days after transplantation passed, and reaching a maximum on the fifth day. The strongest reactivity was observed perivenously. In chronic rejection, TNF-α positive cells were observed in the perivascular and peribronchial regions, especially around class II positive epithelia. The number of positive cells was, however, less than that in the vascular phase of acute rejection. Few cells were positive for IL-1β, IFN-γ and, unexpectedly, for IL-4. These facts indicate the functional difference of infiltrating cells between acute and chronic rejection.

Key words Cytokine production · Immunohistochemistry · Lung transplantation

Introduction

Chronic rejection is one of the catastrophic complications in human lung transplantation. Although many studies on human allografts have been published, reports on chronic rejection in animal models have been limited. In Brown Norway (BN) to Lewis (LEW) rat lung transplantation, allografts are indefinitely accepted after administering a short course of cyclosporine A, and the allografts show symptoms of chronic rejection including cellular infiltration reminiscent of the vascular phase of acute rejection [1]. The cellular infiltrates in the accepted allografts decrease gradually, while the damaged airway begins to exhibit bronchiolitis obliterans-like features [2].

In this rat model, we demonstrated a higher ratio of CD4/CD8 and a lower ratio of ED2/ED1 in cyclosporine-treated accepted allografts compared with acutely rejected non-treated allografts [3]. These differences in the subpopulation of lymphocytes and macrophages suggested possible differences in immune response, especially cytokine production in the respective allografts. Moreover, most CD4-positive cells in accepted allografts were negative for CD45RC [4]. This fact suggested the predominance of Th2 cells in accepted allografts and the possible production of IL-4 [5].

In this study, we investigated whether cytokine production in acute and chronic rejection was different. An immunohistochemical examination was performed with antibodies to proinflammatory cytokines (TNF-α, IL-1β), Th1-associated cytokine (IFN-γ), and Th2-associated cytokine (IL-4).

Materials and methods

Male inbred BN (RT1^n) and LEW (RT^1) were obtained from Charles River, Japan. All animals were kept under specific pathogen-free conditions. The left lung was transplanted orthotopically according to the improved technique [6] of Marck. Allogeneic lung transplantation was performed from BN to fully mismatched LEW. In the acute rejection group (AR), no treatment was carried out after transplantation. In the chronic rejection group (CR), cyclosporine A (25 mg/kg) was injected intramuscularly on days 2 and 3 after the operation.

Recipients were sacrificed on days 1, 3, and 5 after the operation in AR, and on days 30, and 90 in CR ($n = 5$, respectively). As a control, syngeneic lung transplantation was performed from BN to BN, and recipients were sacrificed on the same days as in AR ($n = 5$).

Specimens were quickly frozen, processed routinely, and studied histologically and immunohistologically. Subsets of infiltrating lymphocytes and macrophages were identified using a panel of antibodies. This panel included antibodies to TNF-α, IL-1β, IFN-γ, IL-4, OX6 (class II antigens), ED1 and ED2 (macrophages), W3/25 (CD4), and OX8 (CD8).

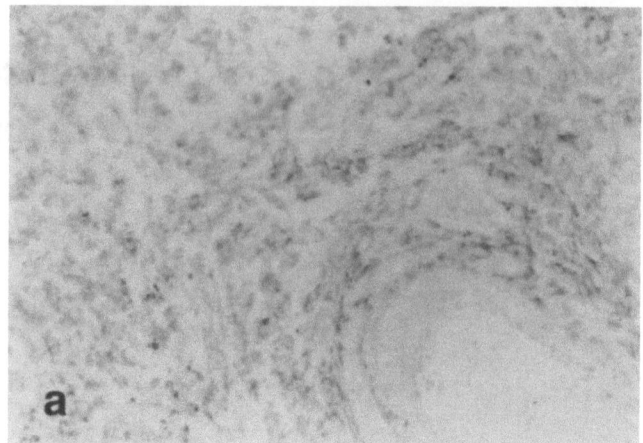

Results

Histologically, AR showed features of latent phase (day 1), vascular phase (day 3), and alveolar phase (day 5), according to Prop's classification [1]. In CR, mononuclear cells (MNCs) infiltrated around the vessels and bronchi, a feature reminiscent of the vascular phase of AR. Infiltrating MNCs were fewer at day 90 than at day 30, however, some large bronchi at day 90 showed protrusion of granulation tissue into their lumens.

Immunohistochemically, TNF-α was detected as early as day 1 in AR. Some MNCs around the venules were positive. The number of positive cells increased as the days progressed, and most MNCs showed positivity to TNF-α on day 5 (Fig. 1a). In CR, some clusters of cells were positive around the bronchi and blood vessels (Fig. 1b). On the sequential sections, bronchial epithelia adjacent to TNF-α positive cells were frequently positive for OX6 (data not shown).

IL-1β positive MNCs were detected around vessels on day 3 in AR, and increased in number on day 5. In CR, only scattered MNCs were positive for IL-1β.

IFN-γ positive cells were found on day 1 in AR, increased as the days progressed, and reached a maximum on day 5. Positive cells were observed in newly infiltrated areas, especially around venules (Fig. 2a) or in the periphery of the lesions. Most MNCs were negative in CR (Fig. 2b).

IL-4 showed similar patterns to those of IL-1β. A moderate number of MNCs were positive on day 5 in AR, but scant in CR. These data are summarized in Table 1.

Discussion

From the present study, the difference in cytokine production in acute and chronic rejection of rat lung allografts was clearly demonstrated. MNCs in AR produced

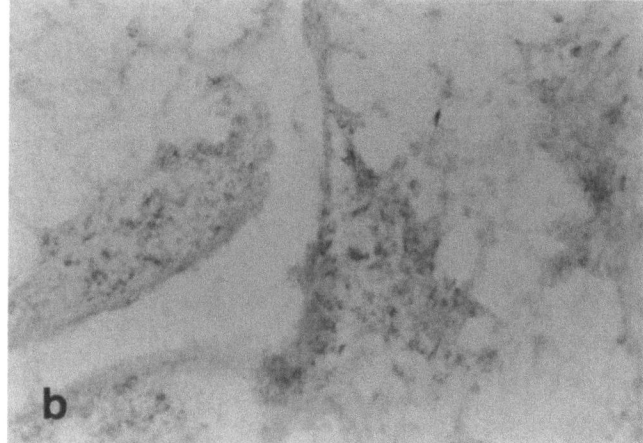

Fig. 1a,b Reactivity for TNF-α is seen on most infiltrates in AR, day 5 (**a**), and on some cells in CR, day 30 (**b**)

every tested cytokine and increased in number as the rejection progressed; however, most MNCs in CR lacked production of IL-1β, IFN-γ, and IL-4. This difference seemed to play an important role in causing the different fates of the allografts, although their histologies are similar.

Recently, we demonstrated that the percentage of CD45RC positive cells in CD4-positive lymphocytes was significantly lower in CR than in AR [4]. CD45RC positive CD4-T cells were postulated as Th1 cells producing IFN-γ, whereas CD45RC negative CD4-T cells were postulated as Th2 cells producing IL-4 [5, 7]. Additionally, in some organs, activation of Th2 cells prevented the accelerated allograft rejection [8]. From these facts, we speculated the predominance of Th1 cells in AR and Th2 cells in CR which resulted in permanent acceptance. Both the considerable number of IFN-γ positive MNCs in AR and the insignificant number in CR were anticipated results, however, the lack of IL-4 positive cells in CR was unexpected. Although the studied cytokines were limited, a more intricate mechanism

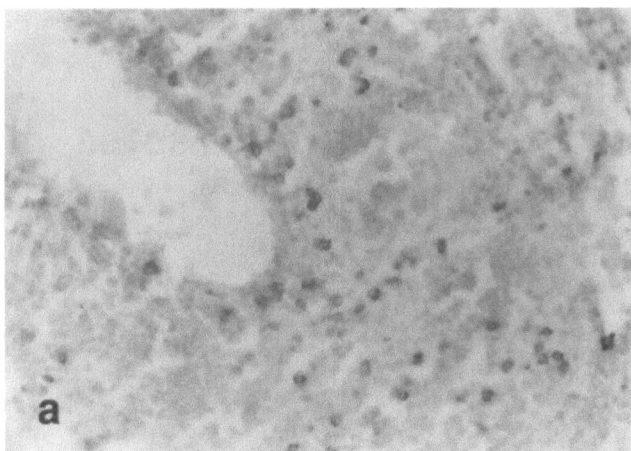

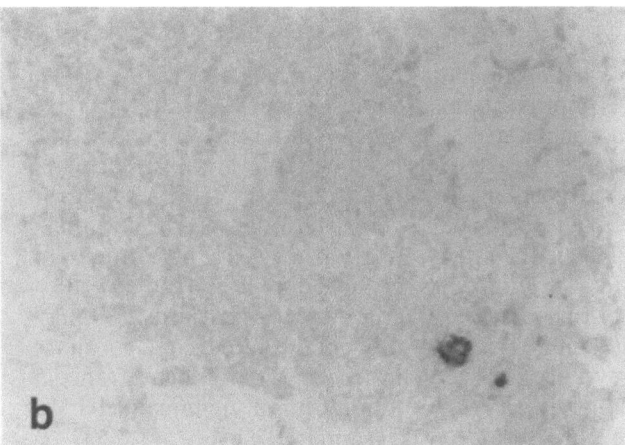

Table 1 Positive cells in the allografts (+/– Few, + some, ++ many, +++ most)

	Acute rejection			Chronic rejection
Day	1	3	5	30–90
TNF-α	+	++	+++	+
IL-1β	+/–	+	+	+/–
IFN-γ	+/–	+	++	+/–
IL-4	+/–	+	++	+/–

Fig. 2 a, b Many infiltrating cells are positive for IFN-γ in AR, day 5 (**a**), while few cells are positive in CR, day 30 (**b**)

than Th2 predominance may be involved in preventing the rejection.

From the standpoint of chronic rejection, cellular production of TNF-α in CR is striking. Reactive cells were often gathered in the bronchial wall, and the bronchial epithelia adjacent to these positive infiltrates frequently expressed class II antigens. These facts may suggest that TNF-α upregulates class II antigens to produce chronic airway damage including bronchiolitis obliterans-like features observed in CR.

To summarize, cytokine production in acute and chronic rejection of rat lung allografts was quite different. Although cytokine production was limited in chronic rejection, Th2 predominance could not be demonstrated.

Acknowledgements This work was supported in part by a grant from the Scientific Research Fund of the Ministry of Education, Japan.

References

1. Tazelaar HD, Prop J, Nieuwenhuis P, Billingham ME, Wildevuur CRH (1988) Airway pathology in the transplanted rat lung. Transplantation 45: 864–869
2. Uyama T, Winter JB, Groen G, Wildevuur CRH, Monden Y, Prop J (1992) Late airway changes caused by chronic rejection in rat lung allografts. Transplantation 54: 809–812
3. Uyama T, Sakiyama S, Monden Y, Prop J (1993) Late airway changes in rat lung allografts: Chronic rejection is a causative factor. Transplant Proc 25: 1169–1171
4. Uyama T, Sakiyama S, Fukumoto T, Tanida N, Tamaki M, Sumitomo M, Monden Y, Prop J (1995) Graft-infiltrating cells in rat lung allograft with late airway damage. Transplant Proc 27: 2118–2119
5. McKnight AJ, Barclay AN, Mason DW (1991) Molecular cloning of rat interleukin 4 cDNA and analysis of the cytokine repertoire of subsets of CD4+ cells. Eur J Immunol 21: 1187–1194
6. Prop J, Ehrie MG, Crapo JD, Nieuwenhuis P, Wildevuur CRH (1984) Reimplantation response in isografted rat lungs. Analysis of causal factors. J Thorac Cardiovasc Surg 87: 702–711
7. Spickett GP, Brandon MR, Mason DW, Willams AF, Woollett GR (1983) MRC OX22, a monoclonal antibody that labels a new subset of T lymphocytes and reacts with the high molecular weight form of the leucocyte-common antigen. J Exp Med 158: 795–810
8. Hancock WW, Sayegh MH, Kwok CA, Weiner HL, Carpenter CB (1993) Oral, but not intravenous, alloantigen prevents accelerated rejection by selective intragraft Th2 cell activation. Transplantation 55: 1112–1118

Transpl Int (1996) 9 [Suppl 1]: S226–S229
© Springer-Verlag 1996

N. Ogawa
I. Koyama
T. Shibata
T. Watanabe
N. Akimoto
Y. Taguchi
N. Shinozuka
R. Omoto

Pravastatin prevents the progression of accelerated coronary artery disease after heart transplantation in a rabbit model

N. Ogawa · I. Koyama (✉) · T. Shibata ·
T. Watanabe · N. Akimoto · Y. Taguchi ·
N. Shinozuka · R. Omoto
Department of Surgery,
Saitama Medical School, 38,
Morohongo, Moroyama-machi, Iruma-gun,
Saitama, Japan, 350-04

Abstract This study was designed to investigate the effects of pravastatin (Pr) on accelerated coronary arteriosclerosis in transplanted hearts. The rabbit hearts were transplanted to the recipients' neck heterotopically, and received FK506. The rabbits in group 1 were fed a normal diet (ND), and cholesterol-rich diet (CD) in group 2 and 3. Pr (10 mg/kg) was given to group 3. They were sacrificed at 4 weeks and the severity of myocardial rejection and arteriosclerosis was assessed and scored histologically. The serum lipid levels were significantly elevated by a CD. However, addition of Pr had no effect on the levels of LDL and total cholesterol (TC). There was no significant difference in myocardial rejection in each group. Transplanted hearts in group 2 showed more severe arteriosclerotic lesions than those in group 1. Pr treatment in group 3 diminished the severity of coronary arteriosclerosis. Pr may prevent the accelerated coronary arteriosclerosis after heart transplantation without significant changes in TC and LDL.

Key words Heart transplantation ·
Coronary arteriosclerosis ·
Pravastatin · FK506

Introduction

The accelerated coronary arteriosclerosis after heart transplantation [7] has been one of the great problems determining long term prognosis [2]. It has been suggested that coronary arteriosclerosis in transplanted hearts may be caused by chronic rejection of the vascular type, but cytomegalovirus infection [8], hypercholesterolemia [6], and toxicity of immunosuppressants [7] have been also considered as other causes. We reported that hypercholesterolemia produced by a cholesterol-rich diet enhanced the progression of coronary arteriosclerosis after heart transplantation [13]. Moreover, it has been reported that coronary arteriosclerosis after heart transplantation was inhibited by the administration of anti-hyperlipidemics such as fish oil [12] and HMG-CoA reductase inhibitor [10]. In this experiment, we studied the effect of the HMG-CoA reductase inhibitor, pravastatin (Pr), on coronary arteriosclerosis after heart transplantation under hyperlipidemia.

Materials and methods

Japanese white male rabbits weighing 3–4 kg were used. After intramuscular injection of ketamine hydrochloride (10 mg/kg) and intravenous injection of sodium pentobarbital (10 mg/kg), thoracotomy of the donors was carried out under anesthesia maintained by 1.5 % halothane. The hearts were excised after cardiac arrest by infusion of cold cardioplegia having added 1000 units of heparin, and were immersed in cold cardioplegic solution. The left carotid artery and vein of the recipients wee exposed and anastomosed to the ascending aorta and pulmonary artery of the grafts, respectively [4]. The total ischemic time of the graft was approximately 60 min. After heart transplantation, the immunosuppressant, FK506 (0.3 mg/kg per day, i. m.), was administered to all rabbits. The antihyperlipidemic, Pr (10 mg/kg per day), was administered orally. Rabbits were fed with a 1 % cholesterol diet (CD) or a normal diet (ND). Both transplanted and native hearts were excised after sacrifice at 4 weeks and were fixed in 10 % buffered formalin solution for histological evaluation. Total cholesterol levels (TC) and LDL-cholesterol levels (LDL) in samples were determined.

S 227

Experimental groups

Recipients were classified into the following three groups: group 1, ND only ($n = 4$), group 2, CD only ($n = 6$), and group 3, CD + Pr ($n = 7$).

Histological staining methods

Four-micron-thick paraffin sections were stained with hematoxylin and eosin (H&E) and Elastica van Gieson (EVG). Also, the ABC method with monoclonal mouse anti-rabbit macrophage (DAKO) or anti-mouse smooth muscle actin antibody (ZYMED) was used for immunohistochemical staining.

Pathological evaluation method

The severity of myocardial rejection after heart transplantation was evaluated by 7 grades of 0, 1A, 1B, 2, 3A, 3B, and 4, and scored to 0.0, 1.0, 1.5, 2, 3.0, 3.5, and 4, respectively, according to the standardized cardiac biopsy grading [3].

All coronary arteries more than 50 μm in diameter were light microscopically studied. According to the references of the standard of Stanford University [12], the severity of arteriosclerosis was judged by the degree of intimal thickening and scored from 0 to 6 points. The mean value of the intimal thickening per blood vessel was used for comparison.

Statistical procedure

The assay of the statistically significant differences was performed by Student's t-test, and the probability rate of the significant difference was defined as < 0.05.

Results

Measurement of serum lipid

The serum lipid level in group 2 was significantly elevated by a 1 % cholesterol diet (TC 1275 ± 51), compared with that in group 1 with a normal diet (TC 50 ± 2, LDL 3.3 ± 6). However, the decrease in serum lipid level was not found in group 3 (TC 1327 ± 354, LDL 1297 ± 9) which was administered Pr as an antihyperlipidemic (Table 1).

Severity of myocardial rejection in transplanted hearts

The pulsation in all transplanted hearts was observed until sacrifice. The severity of the myocardial rejection was 1.0 ± 0.0 in group 1, 2.5 ± 1.56 in group 2, and 1.64 ± 0.37 in group 3. There was no significant difference in the myocardial rejection in each group.

Table 1 Serum cholesterol levels after 4 weeks. Data are expressed as mean ± SD (*ND* normal diet, *CD* cholesterol-rich diet, *Pr* pravastatin, *TC* total cholesterol, *LDL* LDL-cholesterol)

Group	n		TC (mg/dl)	LDL (mg/dl)
1	ND	4	50 ± 32	3.3 ± 2.6
2	CD	6	$1275 \pm 960^*$	$1260 \pm 951^*$
3	CD + Pr	7	$1327 \pm 354^*$	$1297 \pm 49^*$

* $P < 0.05$ vs group 1

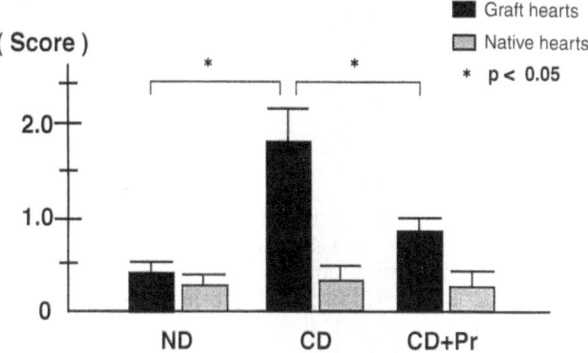

Fig. 1 Coronary arteriosclerosis in grafted and native hearts (*ND* normal diet, *CD* 1 % cholesterol diet, *CD + Pr* 1 % cholesterol diet and added pravastatin)

Severity of coronary arteriosclerosis

The score of the coronary intimal thickening in transplanted hearts in group 1 fed a normal diet was 0.43 ± 0.15. A cholesterol-rich diet enhanced the intimal thickening, which was found in group 2 (1.78 ± 0.45). The severity of coronary intimal thickening was significantly decreased in group 3 (0.80 ± 0.32), suggesting that pravastatin would inhibit the progression of the arteriosclerosis in transplanted hearts (Fig. 1). Moreover, coronary intimal thickening in native hearts in each group was minimum (0.34 ± 0.13 in group 1, 0.36 ± 0.16 in group 2, and 0.25 ± 0.18 in group), indicating that the influence of the hyperlipidemia or pravastatin was not found in native hearts without immunological injury.

When coronary arteries in transplanted hearts were observed light microscopically, foam cells or fibrous thickening was found in the arterial intima (Fig. 2). On the other hand, macrophages and smooth muscle cells in the thickened intima were observed by immunohistochemical stainings with the anti-smooth muscle cell actin and anti-macrophage antibodies (Fig. 3).

Discussion

Various factors are proposed to accelerate coronary arteriosclerosis in transplanted hearts. Hyperlipidemia is considered to be one of these factors. Alonso et al. [1]

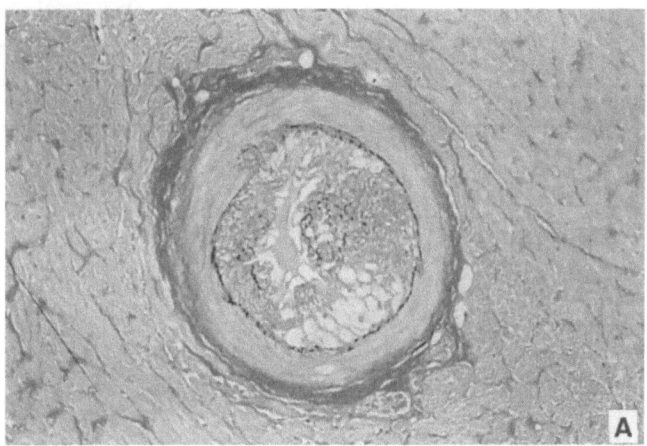
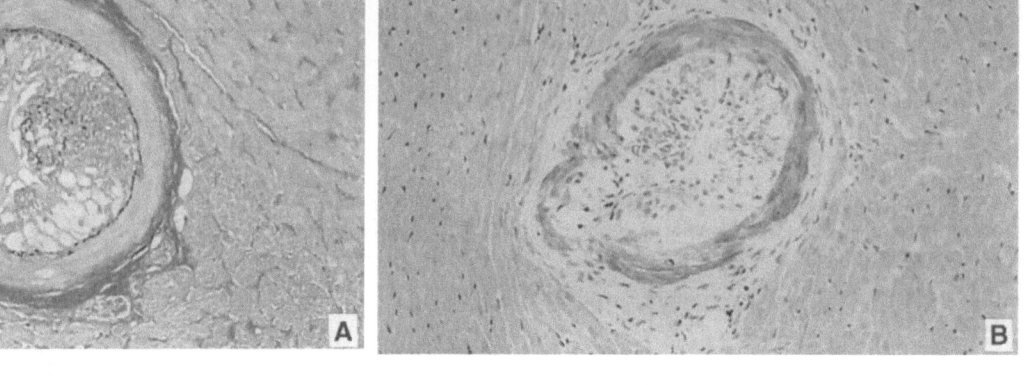

Fig.2 A An intramyocardial branch of the transplanted heart, group 2. The intima is remarkably thickened with numerous foam cells (scored as 6). Elastica van Gieson (EVG) original magnification × 100. **B** Similar artery as in **A** with immunohistochemical staining. It shows the smooth muscle cells stained with anti-actin antibody. There are numerous positive cells in the thickened intima. Anti-actin antibody stain, original magnification × 100

reported that coronary arteriosclerosis in transplanted hearts was rapidly accelerated by the combination of hyperlipidemia and immunological injury. We also reported previously [13] that hyperlipidemia in a heart-transplanted model is an increasing factor in intimal thickening in the coronary artery.

This study was undertaken on the assumption that accelerated coronary arteriosclerosis in transplanted hearts could be inhibited by antihyperlipidemic drugs.

Fig.3 A Main branch of a transplanted heart, group 3. The intima shows slight and patchy thickening (scored as 1). EVG, original magnification × 40. **B** Similar artery as in **A** with immunohistochemical staining with anti-actin antibody. There are positive cells in the thickened intima. Anti-actin antibody stain, original magnification × 40

Sarris et al. [12] reported that fish oil inhibited the coronary arteriosclerosis in transplanted hearts. Meiser et al. [10] demonstrated the beneficial effect of HMG-CoA reductase inhibitor on FK506-induced coronary artery disease using a rat model. But both results showed no changes in serum cholesterol levels despite the use of antihyperlipidemic drugs.

In in vitro experiments, Hidaka et al. [9] reported that HMG-CoA reductase inhibitor inhibited the migration of poricine aortic smooth muscle cells which were stimulated by platelet-derived growth factor. Corisini et al. [5] also demonstrated that the proliferation of smooth muscle cells in rats and humans was inhibited by simvastatin. However, no clinical meaning was indicated because the concentration of simvastatin in those experiments was 100 times higher than the clinical dose. These reports suggested that simvastatin was much more potent than pravastatin in inhibiting the activation of smooth muscle cells. Moreover, Soma et al. [14] showed that HMG-CoA reductase inhibitors inhibited the proliferation of the smooth muscle cells in the intima without decreasing the serum cholesterol level. They reported that the effect of pravastatin was less than other HMG-CoA reductase inhibitors, and the dif-

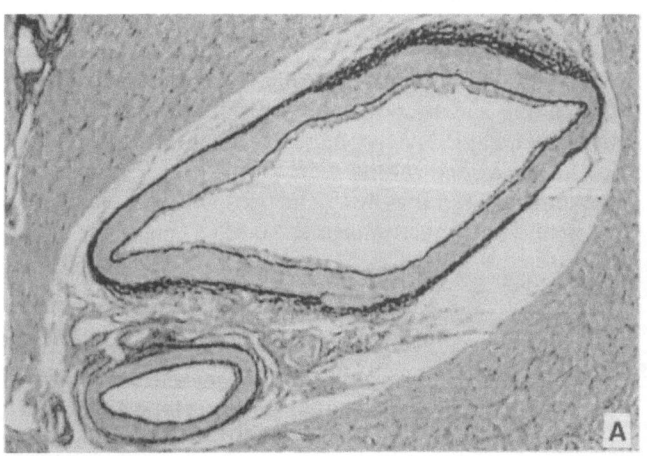
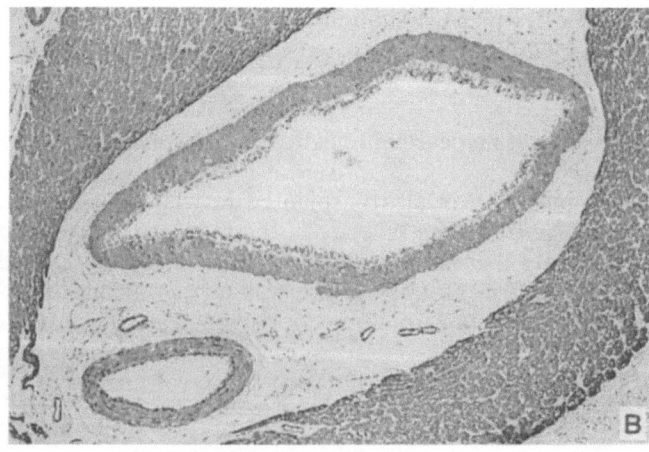

ference among HMG-CoA reductase inhibitors could be caused by the differing permeability of cellular membranes or the effect of enzyme inhibition. However, this experiment demonstrated that pravastatin was effective for coronary arteriosclerosis in transplanted hearts using a rabbit model and a hypercholesterol diet.

Concerning the development of the arteriosclerosis, the "response to injury theory" which was proposed by Ross et al. [11] has been widely cited. In transplanted vessels, arteriosclerosis would be initiated by immunological injury of the endothelium and followed by prolif-

eration and migration of smooth muscle cells. These processes are induced by many growth factors which are secreted from platelets, endothelial cells, or macrophages. It would be presumed that the progression of the arteriosclerosis can be inhibited by suppressing any step from endothelial injury to smooth muscle cell migration. Further investigations are necessary to elucidate the mechanism of the beneficial effect of the HMG-CoA reductase inhibitor, pravastatin, on the inhibition of arterisclerosis.

References

1. Alonso DR, Starek PF, Minick CR (1977) Studies on pathogenesis of atheroarteriosclerosis induced in rabbit cardiac allografts by synergy of graft rejection and hypercholesterolemia. Am J Pathol 87: 415–422
2. Billingham ME (1987) Cardiac transplant atherosclerosis. Transplant Proc 19: 19–25
3. Billingham ME, Cary NRB, Hammond ME, Kemnitz J, Marboe C, McCallister HA, Snovar DC, Winters GL, Zerbe A (1990) A working formulation for the standardization of nomenclature in the diagnosis of heart and lung rejection: heart rejection study group. J Heart Transplant 9: 587–593
4. Carrel A (1907) The surgery of blood vessels, etc. Bull Johns Hobkins Hosp 18: 18
5. Corsini A, Rainteri M, Soma MR, Gabbiani G, Paoletti R (1992) Simvastatin but not pravastatin has a direct inhibitory effect on rat and human myocyte proliferation. Clin Biochem 25: 399–400
6. Eich D, Thompson JA, Ko D, Hatillo A, Lower R, Katz S, Katz M, Hess ML (1991) Hypercholesterolemia in long term survivors of heart transplantation. An early marker of accelerated coronary artery disease. J Heart Lung Transplant 10: 45–49
7. Gao SZ, Schroeder JS, Alderman EL, Hunt SA, Silverman JF, Wiederhold V, Stinson EB (1987) Clinical laboratory correlates of accelerated coronary artery disease in the cardiac transplant patient. Circulation 76: 56–61
8. Grattan MT, Moreno-Cabral CE, Starnes VA, Oyer Pe, Stinson EB, Shumway NE (1989) Cytomegalovirus infection is associated with cardiac allograft rejection and atherosclerosis. J Am Med Assoc 261: 3561–3566
9. Hidaka Y, Eda T, Yonemoto M, Kamei T (1992) Inhibition of cultured vascular smooth muscle cell migration by simvastatin (MK-733). Atherosclerosis 95: 87–94
10. Meiser BM, Wenke K, Thiery J, Wolf S, Devens Ch, Seidel D, Hammer C, Billingham ME, Reichart B (1993) Simvastatin decreases accelerated graft vessel disease after heart transplantation in an animal model. Transplant Proc 25: 2077–2079
11. Ross R (1993) The pathogenesis of atherosclerosis: a perspective for the 1990s. Science 362: 801–809
12. Sarris GE, Mitchell RS, Gillingham ME, Glasson JR, Cahill Pd, Miller DC (1989) Inhibition of accelerated cardiac allograft arteriosclerosis by fish oil. J Thorac Cardiovasc Surg 97: 841–855
13. Shibata T, Ogawa N, Koyama I, Kaneko N, Hokazono K, Omoto R (1993) FK506 accelerates the development of coronary artery disease in the transplanted heart as well as the native heart? Transplant Proc 25: 1145–1148
14. Soma MR, Dometti E, Parolini C, Ferrari G, Fumagalli R, Paoletti R (1993) HMG COA reductase inhibitors – In vivo effects on carotid intimal thickening in normocholesterolemic rabbits. Arterioscler Thromb 13: 266–273

Transpl Int (1996) 9 [Suppl 1]: S 230–S 233
© Springer-Verlag 1996

T. Leivestad
A. Foerster
S. Simonsen
A. Bratlie
E. Thorsby
O. Geiran

HLA-DR matching reduces rejection rate in heart transplantation

T. Leivestad (✉) · A. Bratlie · E. Thorsby
Institute of Transplantation Immunology,
Rikshospitalet, N-0027 Oslo, Norway

A. Foerster
Institute of Pathology, The National
Hospital, Oslo, Norway

S. Simonsen
Medical Department B, The National
Hospital, Oslo, Norway

O. Geiran
Surgical Department A, The National
Hospital, Oslo, Norway

Abstract We have studied the influence of serological matching for ten HLA-DR antigens on the occurrence of acute cellular rejection in heart transplantation by correlating the findings in routine endomyocardial biopsies taken during the first posttransplant year with the results of HLA typing of all recipients of a first cardiac graft and their donors during 1983–1994 at our center. We found that recipients of HLA-DR matched hearts had a lower frequency of acute cellular rejection, especially so for the moderate/severe rejection grades. Also, rejection appeared earlier in the DR-mismatched combinations. Whether the mismatch was for one or two DR antigens did not make a significant difference, neither could we demonstrate any influence of HLA-A or -B mismatches. The survival of DR-matched cardiac grafts tended to be higher at 1 year than DR-mismatched grafts, but the difference did not reach statistical significance.

Key words Cardiac transplantation · Rejection · HLA matching

Introduction

Donor hearts are usually allocated to recipients based on ABO and size match, while matching for HLA is seldom attempted. Due to the polymorphism of the HLA system, and to the logistical problems, only a few recipients obtain a graft fully matched for HLA. Large patient series, as in the Collaborative Transplant Study [7], are required to establish the influence of HLA matching on cardiac graft survival.

Cardiac grafts are usually monitored for rejection by routine endomyocardial biopsies at fixed intervals. The classification systems for the histological diagnosis of rejection have been several, but an international standard was established in 1990 [1]. Several centers including our own [2–4, 8, 9] have earlier reported a correlation between HLA mismatch and the occurrence of early rejection episodes. The present study presents data from 1983–1994, correlating the findings in routine endomyocardial biopsies, revised according to the international standards, to the prospective serological HLA typing of all first cardiac graft recipients and their donors.

Patients and methods

HLA typing

Serological HLA typing and cross-matching based on the immunomagnetic (IM) technique [10] have been used since 1986, some DR typings have also been confirmed genomically. Recipients were typed for "broad" HLA-A and -B specificities and for the HLA-DR antigens 1–10, and tested for the presence of panel-reactive antibodies (PRA) before waiting-list notification. The donors were similarly HLA typed and a microlymphocytotoxic cross-match was performed, in most instances previous to organ harvesting. The transplant was said to be HLA-A, -B, or -DR compatible if there were no detectable mismatches between the donor and recipient in the HLA-A (n = 10), -B (n = 25), or -DR (n = 10) antigens. Organ allocation was, however, mainly based on blood group and body size match. A negative T cell cross-match was required, although sometimes anticipated for logistical reasons in PRA negative patients.

Patients

During 1983–1994, a total of 208 patients received a first cardiac graft from an HLA-typed donor. Median age was 52 years (range 1–62). In 20 patients there was no demonstrable DR mismatch, in

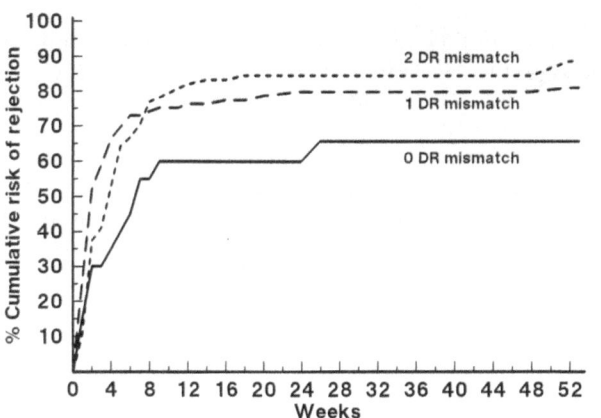

Fig. 1 Cumulative risk of acute cellular rejection (grade 1A–4) during the first posttransplant year in first cardiac graft recipients according to the number of demonstrable HLA-DR mismatches between donor and recipient (Mantel-Haenszel: no DR mismatches vs 1–2 DR mismatches, $P = 0.0389$)

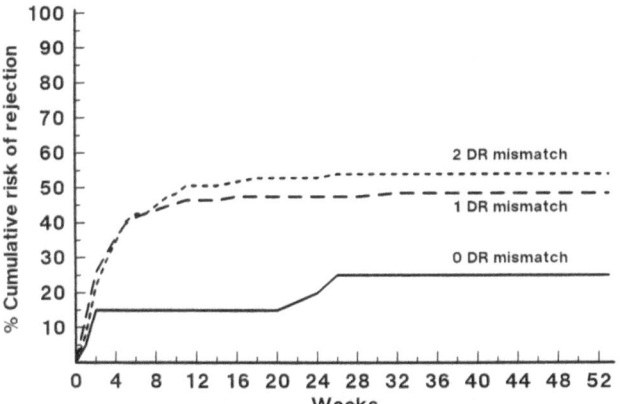

Fig. 2 Cumulative risk of moderate/severe acute cellular rejection (grade 2–4) during the first posttransplant year in first cardiac graft recipients according to the number of demonstrable HLA-DR mismatches between donor and recipient (Mantel-Haenszel: no DR mismatches vs 1–2 DR mismatches, $P = 0.0366$)

101 the donor had one, and in 87 the donor had two mismatched DR antigens. Age distribution was equal in these three groups.

Immunosuppression

Cyclosporine and azathioprine treatment was started preoperatively and corticosteroids peroperatively. Antibodies were not used for basal immunosuppression. Rejection episodes were primarily treated with corticosteroids alone if low grade, or in combination with antithymocyte globulin if moderate or severe.

Biopsies

Transvenous endomyocardial biopsies were taken weekly during the first 2 months after transplantation, then at 2-week intervals until 3 months, at 6 months, and later at each yearly control. Additional biopsies were taken when clinically indicated. All biopsies

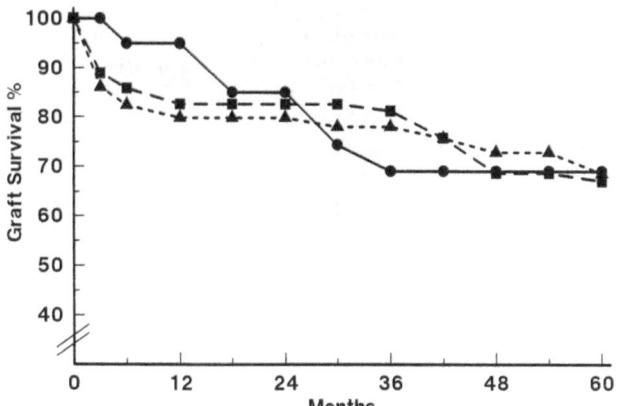

Fig. 3 Survival of first heart grafts according to number of HLA-DR mismatches between donor and recipient (● no DR mismatches, $n = 20$; ■ 1 DR mismatch, $n = 101$; ▲ 2 DR mismatches, $n = 87$)

were classified according to the international classification: 0 = normal; 1A, 1B = degrees of mild rejection; 2, 3A, 3B = degrees of moderate rejection; 4 = severe rejection [1].

Statistics

Group comparisons were done with Fisher's exact test, chi-squared test, or Student's t-test as appropriate. Graft survival, counting death from any cause as graft failure, and time-related risk of rejection were estimated by the Kaplan-Meier method, comparing curves for equality using the Mantel-Haenszel test and testing for the separate influence of HLA-A, -B and, -DR mismatch by the Cox regression.

Results

Incidence of rejection during the first year

Acute cellular rejection (grade 1A–4) was diagnosed in 163 out of 208 patients during the first year. This was observed in 13 (65 %) recipients of DR-compatible grafts, in 77 (76 %) recipients of grafts mismatched for one DR antigen, and 73 (84 %) mismatched for two DR antigens. These differences do not reach statistical significance. Figure 1 shows, however, that acute rejection occurred earlier in recipients of DR-mismatched compared to DR-compatible grafts. The time-related cumulative risk of acute cellular rejection during the first year was significantly lower in recipients of DR-matched grafts.

Risk of moderate/severe acute rejection

Moderate to severe acute rejection (grades 2, 3A, 3B, or 4) was diagnosed in 101 patients during the first year. This was observed in five (25 %) recipients of DR-matched grafts, 49 (49 %) recipients of grafts mismatch-

S 232

ed for one DR antigen, and 47 (54 %) recipients of grafts mismatched for two DR antigens (DR-matched vs DR-mismatched grafts: $P < 0.05$). Figure 2 shows the time-related cumulative risk of such rejection during the first year, confirming a significantly lower risk of moderate to severe acute cellular rejection in recipients of HLA-DR-matched grafts. No further effect of matching for HLA-A, or -B could be detected (data not shown).

Graft survival

There was a trend toward higher graft survival at 1 year for DR-matched grafts, as seen in Fig. 3, but the difference did not reach statistical significance. Nine patients died from acute rejection during the first year, three of these were recipients of a graft mismatched for one DR antigen and six of a graft mismatched for two DR antigens. At 5 years, the survival rate was similar for all groups, but the numbers were quite small.

Discussion

This study confirms that HLA matching influences the posttransplant course in cardiac transplantation. The main difference was seen when comparing the DR-matched grafts with the DR-mismatched grafts. Whether the incompatibility involved one or both DR antigens played a minor role.

Due to short waiting lists and a limited collaboration with other centers, the proportion of HLA well-matched grafts in low. A proportion of nearly 10 % DR-matched combinations, as in our material, is higher than would be expected, even within such a relatively homogeneous population as the Norwegians. We find that the negative influence of a single DR-antigen mismatch, together with the lack of influence by HLA-A, -B mismatch, gives an argument against comparisons using, e.g., 0–2 ABDR mismatch as the "well-matched" group. In our material, such a group will include a number of fully DR-mismatches grafts and exclude most of the DR-matched ones. If analyzed in that way, no significant HLA effect can be found.

Restricting HLA matching to take into account only the "broad" DR1–10 specificities increases the chance of obtaining HLA "matched" combinations. Our results indicate that such a selection would help to avoid acute cellular rejection episodes compared to random allocation. Whether matching for the DR subtypes, such as the serologically definable DR 11–18 antigens or the even more numerous DNA-based DRB1 variants, may add further advantages is still unclear. In renal transplantation we were unable to detect any pronounced effect of genomic DRB1 matching additional to that obtained by Serological matching for the DR antigens 1–10 [5].

A reduced rejection rate would be expected to result in improved long-term graft survival. A trend during the first year was seen (Fig. 3), but the difference did not reach statistical significance. More transplants may be needed to observe an effect. Further, since mortality, especially over long time, will be influenced by many immunological as well as non-immunological factors, a more detailed analysis of such factors is needed. However, a reduced rejection rate alone is valuable since it saves costs in terms of rejection treatment and hospitalization.

To take advantage of the DR-matching effect, a fast and reliable HLA typing technique that can be applied to blood samples drawn prior to organ harvesting is required. With the immunomagnetic technique all necessary typings and cross-matches may be safely performed on peripheral blood samples in less than 2 hours [10]. Compared to results from DNA typing, our routine serological typing has a discrepancy rate of approximately 5 % [5]. With the exception of grafts imported from outside our country, HLA typing and cross-matching have always been completed prior to heart transplantation, even with donors residing 2000 km away. Thus, even with the present 4-h limit to ischemia time, optimalization of HLA typing service and logistics could allow HLA-based organ exchange between centers leading to an increased number of well-matched heart grafts [5, 6]. However, better preservation methods are needed before the potential benefits of HLA matching can be fully utilized.

References

1. Billingham ME, Cary NRB, Hammond ME, Kemnitz J, Marboe C, McCallister HA, Snovar DC, Winters GL, Zerbe A (1990) A working formulation for the standardization of nomenclature in the diagnosis of heart and lung rejection: Heart rejection study group. J Heart Transplant 9: 587–593

2. DeMattos A, Head MA, Everett J, Hosenpud J, Hershberger R, Conaglu A, Ott G, Ratkovec R, Norman DJ (1994) HLA-DR mismatching correlates with early cardiac allograft rejection, incidence, and graft survival when high confidence-level serological DR typing is used. Transplantation 57: 626–630

3. DiSesa VJ, Kuo PC, Horvath KA, Mudge GH, Collins JJ, Cohn LH (1990) HLA histocompatibility affects cardiac transplant rejection and may provide one basis for organ allocation. Ann Thorac Surg 49: 220–224

4. Foerster A, Abdelnoor M, Geiran O, Lindberg H, Simonsen S, Thorsby E, Frøysaker T (1992) Morbidity risk factors in human cardiac transplantation. Histoincompatibility and protracted graft ischemia entail high risk of rejection and infection. Scand J Thorac Cardiovasc Surg 26: 169–176

5. Leivestad T, Spurkland A, Bratlie A, Pfeffer P, Fauchald P, Sødal G, Thorsby E (1994) Does genomic HLA-DR matching further enhance the effects of serologic DR matching in clinical renal transplantation? Transplant Proc 26: 1748–1749

6. Morris PJ (Ed) (1994) HLA matching and cardiac transplantation. N Engl J Med 330: 857–858

7. Opelz G, Wujciak T (1994) The influence of HLA compatibility on graft survival after heart transplantation. N Engl J Med 330: 816–819

8. Pfeffer PF, Foerster A, Frøysaker T, Simonsen S, Thorsby E (1988) HLA-DR mismatch and histologically evaluated rejection episodes in cardiac transplants can be correlated. Transplant Proc 20: 367–368

9. Sheldon S, Hasleton PS, Yonan NA, Rhaman AN, Deiraniya AK, Campbell CS, Brooks NH, Dyer PA (1994) Rejection in heart transplantation strongly correlates with HLA-DR antigen mismatch. Transplantation 58: 719–722

10. Vartdal F, Gaudernack G, Funderud S, Bratlie A, Lea T, Ugelstad J, Thorsby E (1986) HLA class I and II typing using cells positively selected from blood by immunomagnetic isolation – a fast and reliable technique. Tissue Antigens 28: 301–312

Transpl Int (1996) 9 [Suppl 1]: S 234–S 236
© Springer-Verlag 1996

Nicole M. van Besouw
Aggie H. M. M. Balk
Bas Mochtar
Lenard M. B. Vaessen
Willem Weimar

Phenotypic analysis of lymphocytes infiltrating human cardiac allografts during acute rejection and the development of graft vascular disease

N. M. van Besouw (✉) · L. M. B. Vaessen ·
W. Weimar
Department of Internal Medicine I
(Room Bd 299),
University Hospital Rotterdam-Dijkzigt,
Dr Molewaterplein 40,
NL-3015 GD Rotterdam, The Netherlands,
Tel. + 3 11 04 63 54 20; Fax 3 11 04 63 54 30

A. H. M. M. Balk · B. Mochtar
Thorax Center,
University Hospital Rotterdam-Dijkzigt,
Rotterdam, The Netherlands

Abstract Acute rejection (AR) and graft vascular disease (GDV) are processes mediated, at least in part, by cellular processes. Therefore, we cultured graft-infiltrating lymphocytes (GIL) from endomyocardial biopsies (EMB) taken during the first year after transplantation, determined their phenotypic composition, and correlated it to AR and GVD. We observed more often GIL growth from EMB with AR than from non-rejection EMB ($P = 0.02$), but no difference was found between patients with and without GVD 1 year after transplantation. CD4 $^+$ cells were always more numerous than CD8 $^+$ cells, and no difference in phenotypic composition was found between AR and non-rejection EMB nor between EMB derived from patients with or without signs of GVD. In conclusion, AR is correlated with cell growth of EMB, but the development of GVD is not associated with AR, GIL growth from EMB, or their phenotypic composition.

Key words Graft-infiltrating lymphocytes · Acute rejection · Graft vascular disease

Introduction

In several studies, we and others have shown that alloactivated graft-infiltrating lymphocytes (GIL) can be expanded *in vitro* from endomyocardial biopsies (EMB) in IL-2-containing medium [1–3]. This culture system is thought to promote growth from *in vivo* activated GIL only [3]. We also have suggested that the outgrowth of GIL from EMB and their phenotypic composition corresponded with histological findings of acute rejection (AR) [1] and graft vascular disease (GVD) [2]. In the present study, we applied the same method of culturing GIL and studied per patient the proportion of EMB from which GIL could be obtained and their phenotype in three periods during the first year after heart transplantation (HTx) in an attempt to show whether our previous findings in groups of patients could be applied to individual cardiac transplant recipients. We compared these parameters for episodes with and without AR and patients with and without GVD in the first year after HTx.

Patients and methods

We studied 60 cardiac allograft recipients, who were transplanted between March 1991 and September 1993. EMB were taken at regular intervals after HTx and examined histologically. According to the criteria of the International Society of Heart and Lung Transplantation [4], AR was defined as cell infiltrate with myocyte necrosis and anti-rejection therapy was prescribed.

One year after HTx, the diagnosis of GVD was assessed by coronary angiography and scored by one of us (AHMMB). GVD was defined as clinically significant vascular changes including minimal wall irregularities [5]. Twenty of the studied patients did have signs of GVD in their angiography one year after HTx, and 40 patients did not.

Culture method and phenotypic analysis

We received EMB from 49 out of 60 patients taken in the first year after HTx to obtain GIL. GIL were cultured from EMB in IL-2-containing medium as described before [1, 2]. GIL were analyzed by two-colour flow cytometry on a FACScan for the expression of cell surface markers. Initial screening was performed with the combinations WT31 FITC-CD3 PE, CD4 FITC-CD8 PE, and CD16

FITC-CD56 PE. When CD3 $^+$ WT31 $^-$ cells were found, the GIL cultures were stained for T-cells bearing TCR-$\gamma\delta$. WT31 (TCR-$\alpha\beta$) and TCR-$\gamma\delta$ were obtained from Becton Dickinson (San Jose, CA, USA) and the other monoclonal antibodies from Immunotech (Marseille, France).

Statistics

We determined from all individual patients the fraction of EMB in the first year posttransplantation showing signs of AR, the GIL growth from EMB, and their phenotypic composition at fixed periods after HTx. The Mann-Whitney U-test was used to evaluate the differences between the patient groups.

Results

Acute rejection

Most acute rejections occur in the first 3 months after HTx [6]. Therefore, we analyzed the relationship between AR and outgrowth of GIL from EMB and the percentage of phenotypic composition in this period. More outgrowth of GIL from EMB was seen when AR was diagnosed (Table 1). The same quantities of TCR-$\alpha\beta$, TCR-$\gamma\delta$, CD16, CD3, CD4, and CD8 were found in the GIL derived from rejection and non-rejection EMB (Table 1). Significantly more CD4 $^+$ than CD8 $^+$ T lymphocytes were obtained from EMB with and without AR ($P = 0.001$).

Graft vascular disease

We found no correlation between the incidence of AR and GVD (Table 2). The development of GVD in the first year after HTx did not influence the cell growth from EMB (Table 3). No relation was detected in the mean percentage TCR-$\alpha\beta$, TCR-$\gamma\delta$, CD3, CD16, CD4, and CD8 at any time after HTx (Table 4). Again, more CD4 $^+$ than CD8 $^+$ cells were found and this proved to be independent of GVD development.

Discussion

The positive correlation between cell growth from EMB and AR is in agreement with our previous study which described the results per EMB taken from cardiac allograft recipients [1], and can be explained by the higher frequencies of cells infiltrating the rejecting allograft compared to non-rejecting grafts. In the previous study [1] and this report, we found CD4 to be the predominant phenotype in most cultures at any time after transplantation. In contrast, in individual patients we could not confirm that cultures derived from EMB with signs of AR were associated with a higher proportion of CD4-

Table 1 Graft-infiltrating lymphocyte (GIL) outgrowth from endomyocardial biopsies (EMB) and their phenotypic composition of non-rejection and rejection EMB taken from 49 patients in the first 3 months after heart transplantation (HTx)

	Non-rejection (mean %)[a]	Rejection (mean %)[a]	P value
Cell growth	42	61	0.02
TCR-$\alpha\beta$	90	94	0.14
TCR-$\gamma\delta$	2	1	0.74
CD3	92	94	0.37
CD16	8	4	0.14
CD4	57[b]	59[c]	0.57
CD8	32[b]	35[c]	0.64

[a] Mean value of all individual patients
[b, c] Mean percentage CD4 vs CD8 in cultures derived from non-rejection ($P < 0.001$)[b] and rejection ($P = 0.001$)[c] EMB

Table 2 Percentage of EMB with signs of rejection during different periods after transplantation in patients without ($n = 40$) and patients with ($n = 20$) signs of graft vascular disease (GVD) one year after HTx

Months after HTx	Without GVD (mean %)[a]	With GVD (mean %)[a]	P value
0–3	25	26	0.75
3–6	20	17	0.68
6–12	9	8	0.70

[a] Mean value of all individual patients

Table 3 Proportion of GIL growth from EMB during different periods after transplantation in patients without ($n = 30$) and patients with ($n = 18$) signs of GVD one year after HTx

Months after HTx	Without GVD (mean %)[a]	With GVD (mean %)[a]	P value
0–3	43	50	0.30
3–6	32	48	0.20
6–12	28	30	0.67

[a] Mean value of all individual patients

dominated cultures [1]. However, we analyzed the phenotypic composition per patient in fixed periods after transplantation and not individual GIL cultures. Another difference between the earlier report and the present results is that we investigated rejection and non-rejection EMB per individual patient and not EMB derived from groups of patients with and without rejection episodes.

Since GVD was diagnosed by annual angiography, the exact moment of onset of GVD could not be determined. Therefore, we analyzed several parameters after different periods in the first year after HTx and their relationship to GVD. We could not detect any correlation between the development of GVD during the first year after HTx and the number of EMB with signs of AR, growth patterns of GIL, or their phenotype. Recently

Table 4 Mean phenotypic composition of cell growth from EMB during different periods after transplantation in patients without and patients with signs of GVD one year after HTx

	Months after HTx	Without GVD (mean %)[a]	With GVD (mean %)[a]	P value
TCR-$\alpha\beta$	0–3	90	93	0.54
	3–6	97	94	0.38
	6–12	79	88	0.47
TCR-$\gamma\delta$	0–3	1.9	1.6	0.73
	3–6	0.1	0.7	0.66
	6–12	7.4	1.7	0.98
CD3	0–3	93	94	0.68
	3–6	97	95	0.30
	6–12	88	90	0.77
CD16	0–3	7.2	4.3	0.37
	3–6	1.5	4.0	0.60
	6–12	11.3	7.6	0.95
CD4	0–3	54[b]	60[e]	0.46
	3–6	68[c]	66[f]	0.98
	6–12	63[d]	53[g]	0.45
CD8	0–3	35[b]	31[e]	0.53
	3–6	31[c]	33[f]	1.0
	6–12	20[d]	29[g]	0.34

[a] Mean value of all individual patients
[b-g] Mean percentage CD4 vs CD8 in cultures derived from EMB of patients without signs of GVD taken 0–3 $(P < 0.001)$[b], 3–6 $(P = 0.003)$[c], and 6–12 $(P < 0.001)$[d] months after HTx and from EMB of patients with signs of GVD taken 0–3 $(P = 0.002)$[e], 3–6 $(P = 0.01)$[f], and 6–12 $(P = 0.02)$[g] months after HTx

we published that in a different population of cardiac transplant recipients, patients with GVD had a higher percentage of CD8$^+$ T lymphocytes during the first year after transplantation [2]. The discrepancy between this and the previous report is again the difference in analysis: the present study is per individual patient and the previous study per GIL culture.

From the described study, we conclude that AR is positively related to GIL growth from EMB, and there is no relation to the phenotypic composition of the GIL and AR. GVD is not related to AR, and also the GIL growth and their phenotype could not make a distinction between patients who did or did not develop GVD in the first year after transplantation.

Acknowledgements We thank C.C. Baan, C.R. Daane, N.E.M. van Emmerik, and E.H.M. Loonen for technical assistance. Support for this research was provided by grant 92.094 from the Netherlands Heart Foundation.

References

1. Ouwehand AJ, Vaessen LMB, Baan CC, Jutte NHPM, Balk AHMM, Essed CE, Bos E, Claas FHJ, Weimar W (1991) Alloreactive lymphoid infiltrates in human heart transplants. Loss of class II-directed cytotoxicity more than 3 months after transplantation. Hum Immunol 30: 50–59

2. Jutte NHPM, Groeneveld K, Balk AHMM, Ouwehand AJ, Loonen EHM, Van der Linden M, Strikwerda S, Mochtar B, Claas FHJ, Weimar W (1994) The development of transplant coronary artery disease after cardiac transplantation is correlated with a predominance of CD8$^+$ T lymphocytes in endomyocardial biopsy derived cultures. Clin Exp Immunol 98: 158–162

3. Zeevi A, Fung J, Zerbe TR, Kaufman C, Rabin BS, Griffith BP, Hardesty RL, Duquesnoy RJ (1986) Allospecificity of activated T cells grown from endomyocardial biopsies from heart transplant patients. Transplantation 41: 620–626

4. Billingham ME, Cary NRB, Hammond ME, Kemnitz J, Marboe C, McCallister HA, Snovar DC, Winters GL, Zerbe A (1990) A working formulation of nomenclature in the diagnosis of heart and lung rejection: Heart Rejection Study Group. J Heart Transplant 9: 587–593

5. Balk AHMM, Simoons ML, Van de Linden MJMM, De Feyter PJ, Mochtar B, Weimar W, Bos E (1993) Coronary artery disease after heart transplantation: Timing of coronary arteriography. J Heart Lung Transplant 12: 89–99

6. Balk AHMM, Simoons ML, Jutte NHPM, Brouwer ML, Meeter K, Mochtar B, Weimar W (1991) Sequential OKT3 and cyclosporin after heart transplantation: a randomized study with single and cyclic OKT3. Clin Transplant 5: 301–305

Transpl Int (1996) 9 [Suppl 1]: S 237–S 240
© Springer-Verlag 1996

C. C. Baan
N. M. van Besouw
C. R. Daane
A. H. M. M. Balk
B. Mochtar
H. G. M. Niesters
W. Weimar

Patterns in donor-specific mRNA and protein production of Th1 and Th2 cytokines by graft-infiltrating lymphocytes and PBMC after heart transplantation

C. C. Baan (✉) · N. M. van Besouw ·
C. R. Daane · W. Weimar
University Hospital Rotterdam-Dijkzigt,
Internal Medicine I, Room BD 299,
Dr Molewaterplein 40,
NL-3015 GD Rotterdam, The Netherlands
Tel. + 31 10 463 54 20; Fax + 31 10 463 54 30

A. H. M. M. Balk · B. Mochtar
Thorax Center, University Hospital
Rotterdam-Dijkzigt, The Netherlands

H. G. M. Niesters
Diagnostic Institute of Molecular Biology/
Virology, University Hospital Rotterdam-
Dijkzigt, The Netherlands

Abstract We used RT-PCR and ELISA to study the kinetics of IL-2 (Th1) and IL-4 (Th2) both on mRNA and protein level from "naive" PBMC and "primed" graft-infiltrating lymphocytes (GIL) obtained from a heart transplant recipient. For this purpose, these cells were stimulated for 1–48 h with donor and control third-party antigens. Only stimulation of GIL with donor-specific antigen resulted in early detectable IL-2 and IL-4 mRNA and protein levels. Maximal relative IL-2 mRNA levels were significantly higher than maximal relative IL-4 mRNA levels (100-fold) in both GIL and PBMC after donor-specific stimulation. This was accompanied by a maximum protein production of 908 pg/ml IL-2 and 19 pg/ml IL-4 by GIL, and of 82 pg/ml IL-2 and undetectable IL-4 production by PBMC. These results suggest that, after stimulation donor-specific "primed" GIL, and not "naive" PBMC, rapidly produce abundant levels of IL-2 (Th1) and IL-4 (Th2) at both the transcriptional and protein level.

Key words Graft-infiltrating · lymphocytes · PBMC · IL-2 · IL-4 · mRNA

Introduction

Distinct functional T helper (Th) subsets, differing in patterns of cytokine production (Th1: IL-2 and Th2: IL-4), regulate and mediate the immune response after transplantation. We and others found that, in particular, expression of IL-2 mRNA and protein production by graft-infiltrating lymphocytes (GIL) is associated with cardiac graft rejection [1–3]. Furthermore, these GIL produce donor-specific cytokine mRNA and protein patterns in response to in vitro allogeneic stimulation [3, 4]. Also the frequency of IL-2 producing helper T-cells with specificity for donor antigens in the peripheral blood of heart transplant recipients was associated with rejection [5]. In recent studies, we have shown that in vivo maturated, primed, T-cells with specificity for donor antigens home in the allograft, while naive, precursor T-cells are primarily found in the peripheral blood [6]. Nevertheless, the kinetics of the induction of cytokine production by donor-specific in vivo primed T-cells

and naive precursor T-cells is unknown. Moreover, differences in the kinetics between these different cell populations might be helpful in distinguishing precursors from primed T-cells. Therefore, we studied the time course of T-cell activation (i.e., mRNA expression) and subsequent release of IL-2 (Th1) and IL-4 (Th2) in GIL and in simultaneously taken PBMC during cardiac rejection both obtained from the same patient. Gene expression and protein production were measured after stimulation with donor and third-party antigens by semiquantitative RT-PCR and ELISA, respectively.

Material and methods

Patient

Rejection was diagnosed in endomyocardial biopsies by histological criteria according to ISHLT [7]. We analyzed GIL and simultaneously taken PBMC from one heart transplant patient during the first rejection episode at day 15 posttransplant.

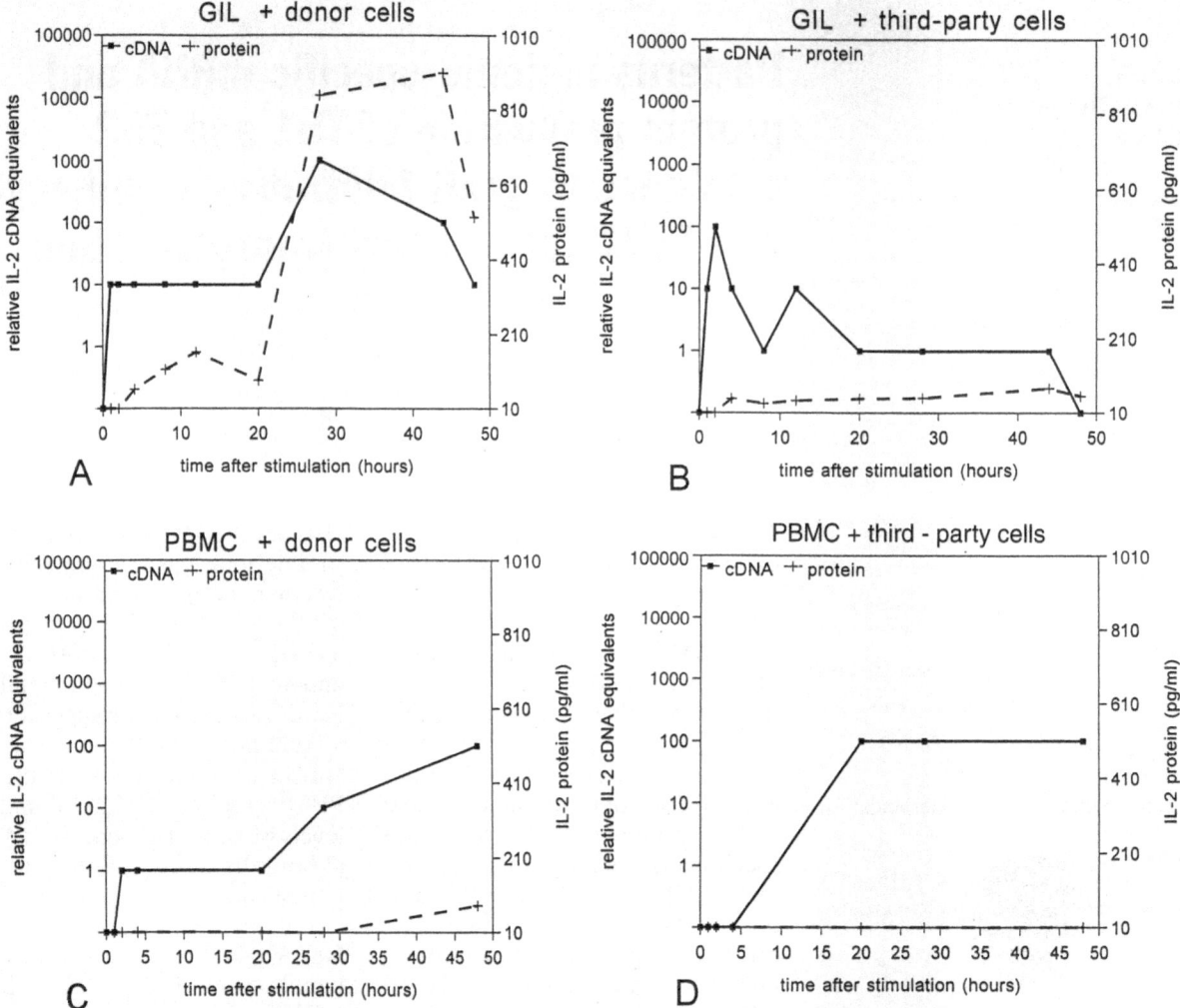

Fig. 1 A–D Time course for induction in "primed" graft-infiltrating lymphocytes (GIL) and "naive" PBMC of IL-2 mRNA and protein by semiquantitative RT-PCR and ELISA, respectively. Kinetics of IL-2 mRNA expression and protein production after stimulation with donor and third-party cells by GIL (**A,B**) and PBMC (**C,D**). After titration, the relative amount of IL-2 cDNA was determined by the highest dilution showing a positive signal. No significant difference in the amount of cDNA for keratin was found between different samples (data not shown)

Cultures

GIL were grown from the endomyocardial biopsy, taken on the day of histological rejection, and expanded in IL-2-containing medium [3]. PBMC were isolated by Ficoll Isopaque ($\delta = 1.077$) density-gradient centrifugation. Before testing, the GIL and PBMC were washed and 5×10^4 cells/well were incubated in IL-2-free medium for 24 h. Thereafter, 5×10^4 irradiated (60 Gy) and washed Epstein-Barr virus-transformed B-cell lines of donor or third-party origin were added. Supernatants and cell pellets were harvested after 1, 2, 4, 8, 12, 20, 28, and 48 h of co-culture and stored at $-80\,^{\circ}$C before analysis of cytokine production.

Total RNA and cDNA preparation

Cell pellets were homogenized in guanidinium isothiocyanate and total RNA was extracted by the phenol/chloroform method in the presence of carrier DNA to improve yields [1]. cDNA was synthesized from the isolated mRNA with random primers. Aliquots were used directly for PCR amplification.

PCR analysis

For semiquantitative analysis, cDNA samples were titrated (tenfold) and aliquots of each dilution were amplified. Samples were amplified using specific primers for IL-2 and IL-4 and were subjected to 40 cycles of denaturation at 94 °C for 1 min, annealing at 60 °C for 2 min, and extension at 72 °C for 3 min. PCR primers detecting transcripts for the house-keeping gene keratin were used as an internal control to confirm successful RNA extraction and cDNA amplification [1]. Verification of an RT-PCR product was achieved by Southern-blot hybridization. After titration, the relative amount of target cDNA was determined by the highest dilution showing a positive signal. To exclude interassay variability, amplification of titrated cDNA of the positive control, cDNA isolated from 10^6 Hut78 cells (ATCC; T-cells with constitutive cytokine mRNA expression), was included in each analysis.

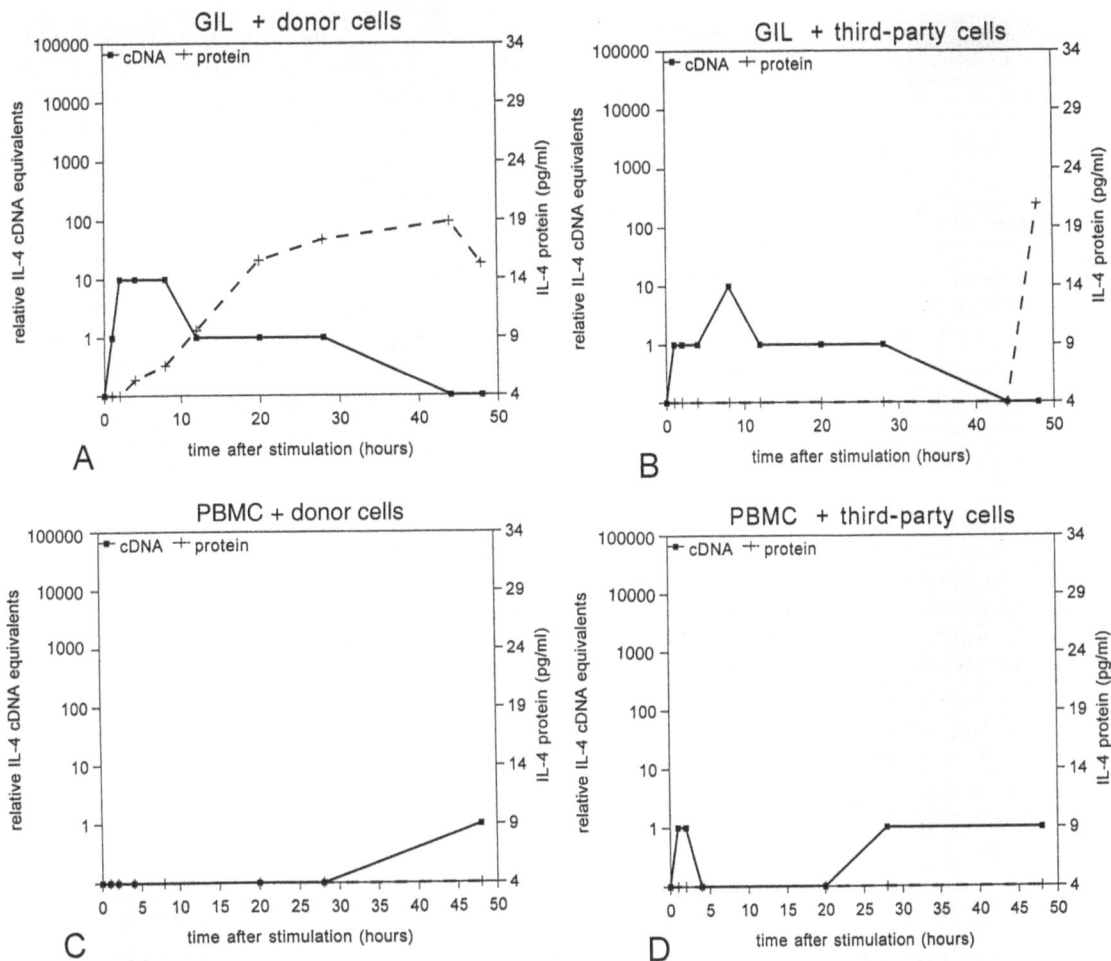

Fig.2A–D Time course for induction in "primed" GIL and "naïve" PBMC of IL-4 mRNA and protein by semiquantitative RT-PCR and ELISA, respectively. Kinetics of IL-4 mRNA expression and protein production after stimulation with donor and third-party cells by GIL (**A,B**) and PBMC (**C,D**). After titration, the relative amount of IL-4 cDNA was determined by the highest dilution showing a positive signal. No significant difference in the amount of cDNA for keratin was found between different samples (data not shown)

Cytokine production

The concentration of IL-2 and IL-4 in the supernatants was determined by ELISA (IL-2, detection range 10–1000 pg/ml, Immunotech, Marseille, France; and IL-4 range 4–450 pg/ml, CLB, Amsterdam, The Netherlands).

Results

Messenger RNA expression and protein production for IL-2 and IL-4 were not measured at detectable levels in unstimulated control GIL and PBMC nor in the irradiated stimulator cells (data not shown). In GIL, messengers coding for IL-2 and IL-4 genes were already detectable 1 h after stimulation with donor and third-party antigens and reached maximum levels within 30 h, while protein production was measurable from 4 h after stimulation with cytokines accumulating at least 48 h after (Fig.1A,B, Fig.2A,B). Both the amounts of IL-2 and IL-4 mRNA and protein were higher after stimulation with donor antigens than after stimulation with third-party antigens. In addition, after stimulation with donor antigens, these GIL produced significantly more IL-2 than IL-4 mRNA (100-fold), which was accompanied with a subsequent maximum production of IL-2 protein (908 pg/ml) and IL-4 protein (19 pg/ml). In PBMC, messengers coding for IL-2 were detectable 2 h, and for IL-4 28 h, after stimulation with donor antigens and 20 h and 1 h, respectively, after stimulation with third-party antigens (Fig.1C,D, Fig.2C,D). Neither the relative IL-2 mRNA level nor the relative IL-4 mRNA level was significantly different between donor and third-party stimulation, but only donor-specific stimulation resulted in measurable IL-2 protein levels at 48 h. Both in GIL and PBMC, the relative maximum donor-specific IL-2 mRNA level was significantly higher compared to the relative donor-specific maximum IL-4 mRNA level (100-fold).

Discussion

After transplantation, it is thought that allogeneic primed T-cells are responsible for the process leading to graft destruction. After allogeneic stimulation these cells produce cytokines. However, the kinetics of donor-specific IL-2 and IL-4 mRNA and the subsequent protein production by these primed, and also by naive T lymphocytes, is not known. Therefore, we have studied the time course for the induction of mRNA and protein for IL-2 and IL-4 in "naive" PBMC and in vivo maturated "primed" GIL after stimulation with either donor or third-party cells. In time, the induction of both mRNA and protein was quicker by GIL than by PBMC. Moreover, in GIL, on both the transcriptional and the protein level the production of IL-2 (Th1) and IL-4 (Th2) was donor specific. These observations suggest that, especially in vivo, primed T-cells with donor specificity mediate early events of the immune response within the transplanted organ. In addition, these results confirm our previously reported data concerning the correlation between cytokine mRNA transcription and protein production by GIL [4]. In contrast, after third-party antigen stimulation even considerable relative mRNA levels did not result in a subsequent high protein production. This could mean that other presently unknown but probably donor-specific posttranscriptional factors are involved in the translation process or that other stimuli might give an additional donor-specific signal. Using limiting dilution analysis, Bishop et al. [8] showed that primed IL-2 producing T-cells could also be measured in the peripheral blood of sponge matrix allografts, whereas conflicting data were reported after clinical transplantation [9, 10]. However, we could not detect these primed T-cells in PBMC on the basis of significant early donor-specific mRNA transcription and subsequent protein production by the highly sensitive RT-PCR and ELISA, respectively. This suggests that alloantigen primed T-cells are not or are below the detection level present in the peripheral blood.

In conclusion, the kinetics of cytokine mRNA and protein production was significantly different between "naive" PBMC and "primed" GIL. We found that only in vivo maturated primed T-cells are capable of secreting IL-2 (Th1) and IL-4 (Th2) immediately upon antigen stimulation.

Acknowledgements This work was supported by grant 92.094 from The Netherlands Heart Foundation.

References

1. Baan CC, van Emmerik NEM, Balk AHMM, Quint WGV, Mochtar B, Jutte NHPM, Niesters HGM, Weimar W (1994) Cytokine mRNA expression in endomyocardial biopsies during acute rejection from human heart transplants. Clin Exp Immunol 97: 293–298
2. Cunningham DA, Dunn MJ, Yacoub MH, Rose ML (1994) Local production of cytokines in the human cardiac allograft. Transplantation 57: 1333–1337
3. Besouw NM van, Daane CR, Vaessen LMB, Balk AHMM, Claas FHJ, Zondervan PE, Jutte NHPM, Weimar W (1995) Different patterns in donor-specific production of helper 1 and 2 cytokines by cells infiltrating the rejecting cardiac allograft. J Heart Lung Transplant (in press)
4. Besouw NM van, Daane CC, Baan CC, Mol WM, Vaessen LMB, Niesters HGM, Weimar W (1995) Concordance of mRNA expression and protein production of IL-2 and IL-4 by human heart graft-infiltrating lymphocytes. Transplant Proc 27: 488
5. Vaessen LMB, Baan CC, Daane CR, Loonen EHM, Balk AHMM, Jutte NHPM, Mochtar B, Claas FHJ, Weimar W (1995) Immunological monitoring in peripheral blood after heart transplantation: frequencies of T-helper cells and precursors of cytotoxic T cells with high avidity for donor antigens correlate with rejection. Transplant Proc 27: 485–488
6. Vaessen LMB, Baan CC, Ouwehand AJ, Jutte NHPM, Balk AHMM, Mochtar B, Claas FHJ, Weimar W (1992) Acute rejection in heart transplant patients is associated with the presence of committed donor-specific cytotoxic lymphocytes in the graft but not in the blood. Clin Exp Immunol 88: 213–219
7. Billingham ME, Path FRC, Cary NRB, Path MRC, Hammond ME, Kemnitz J, Marboe C, McCallister HA, Snovar DC, Winters GL, Zerbe A (1990) A working formulation for the standardization of nomenclature in the diagnosis of heart and lung rejection: Heart rejection study group. J Heart Transplant 9: 587–593
8. Bishop DK, Ferguson RM, Orosz CG (1990) Differential distribution of antigen specific helper T cells and cytotoxic T cells after antigenic stimulation in vivo. Transplantation 144: 1153–1160
9. Schanz U, Roelen DL, Bruning JW, Kardol MJ, Rood JJ van, Claas FHJ (1994) The relative radioresistance of interleukin-2 production by human peripheral blood lymphocytes: consequences for the development of a new limiting dilution assay for the enumeration of helper T lymphocyte precursor frequencies. J Immunol Methods 169: 221–230
10. Deacock S, Scharer A, Batchelor R, Goldman J, Lechler R (1992) A rapid limiting dilution assay for measuring frequencies of alloreactive, interleukin-2 producing T cells in humans. J Immunol Methods 147: 83–88

Transpl Int (1996) 9 [Suppl 1]: S 241–S 242
© Springer-Verlag 1996

C. Decoene
A. Pol
A. Dewilde
P. Wattre
M. C. Coppin
B. Gosselin
C. Stankowiak
H. Warembourg

Relationship between CMV and graft rejection after heart transplantation

C. Decoene (✉) · A. Pol
Service d'Anesthesie-Reanimation
Cardiovasculaire, 3éme Niveau, Bd du
professeur Leclercq, F-59037 Lille, France
Tel. +33 1 20 44 53 52; Fax 20 44 56 61

A. Dewilde · P. Wattre
Department of Virology, Hopital
Cardiologique, Lille, France

M. C. Coppin · B. Gosselin
Department of Anatomy-Pathology,
Hopital Cardiologique, Lille, France

C. Stankowiak · H. Warembourg
Department of Cardiovascular Surgery,
Hopital Cardiologique, Lille, France

Abstract This study, which included 153 heart transplant patients, was designed to determine whether the cytomegalovirus (CMV) status of both donor and recipient may influence graft rejection. The follow-up was 1 year and they all received the same triple-drug immunosuppressive regimen with induction (antilymphocyte serum). There was no difference in the total rejection rate, but an increase in repeated rejection rate was shown in transplant recipients with hearts from CMV seropositive donors ($P < 0.05$).

These data strongly suggest the impact of CMV in enhancement but not in induction of rejection. To prevent iterative rejection in the CMV seropositive donor group, antiviral therapy could be proposed during enhancement of antirejection therapy.

Key words CMV · Graft rejection · Heart transplantation · Antiviral therapy

Introduction

Cytomegalovirus (CMV) is a common infectious agent after heart transplantation and virological signs (viremia, antigenemia) of CMV are frequent during graft rejection, but no study has shown a strong relationship between CMV infection and rejection. The latent state of CMV within the endothelium could lead to a focal reactivation during inflammation and, especially, graft rejection without CMV infection or disease. Focal CMV activation could act as an enhancer of graft rejection leading to repeated rejection and increase in immunosuppressive drugs.

Materials and methods

From 1 January 1989 to 1 January 1994, 153 patients were followed after heart transplantation. These patients were alive 1 month after transplantation and they all received the same immunosuppressive protocol. This protocol consisted of corticosteroids 0.2 mg/kg per day, azathioprine 0.5 mg/kg per day and cyclosporine, according to a first year blood level, between 200 and 300 ng/ml. A 5-day course induction was applied with antilymphocyte serum. Virological screening of both donor and recipient was done twice by IgG serology (ELISA); IgG-positive recipient was called R+, IgG-negative recipient was called R−, IgG-positive donor was called D+, and IgG-negative donor was called D−. According to this screening, four groups of patients have been established: group I, R−/D−; group II, R−/D+; group III, R+/D−; and group IV, R+/D+. Graft rejection was detected by clinical signs, echographical data, and confirmed by endomyocardial biopsy. The biopsies were scheduled as follows: each week for the first 2 months, every 2 weeks for the next 4 months, and then monthly until the end of the first year.

International Heart Transplantation Society Classification [1] was used in order to grade the graft rejection. Positive biopsies per patient during 1 year were classified into two groups: untreated grade IA and treated rejection grade IB or greater. We recorded patients with lethal rejection, repeated rejection, and a group of recipients free of rejection. The chi-squared test was used as the statistical test.

Results

There were no statistical differences in age, sex, and HLA matching in the four groups of patients. The results of the study are summarized in Table 1.

Table 1 Data concerning patients in the study group. Results analysed using chi-squared test. (*CMV* cytomegalovirus, *D* + IgG-positive donor, *D* − IgG-negative donor, *R* + IgG-positive recipient, *R* − IgG-negative recipient)

CMV-matching groups (number)	Grade IA	Grade IB or greater	Repeated rejection	Death-related rejection	Patients free of rejection
Group I, R−/D− (44)	2.44	0.48	0.04	0	0.24
Group II, R−/D+ (19)	2.05	0.57	0.21	1	0.21
Group III, R+/D− (45)	2.2	0.4	0.08	4	0.33
Group IV, R+/D+ (44)	3.22	0.63	0.34	6	0.18

Discussion

This clinical study is a first step toward understanding the relationship between CMV and rejection after heart transplantation. All recipients showed the same rate and grade of first rejection, but for a group of CMV-seropositive donors there were more repeated rejections than for CMV-seronegative donors. No statistical difference was apparent for lethal rejection and rejection-free patients. The hypothesis can be drawn on the statistical relationship between a CMV-seropositive heart donor and repeated rejection. The higher risk of repeated rejection could be explained by focal reactivation of CMV during graft rejection. In seronegative recipients this seems to be the transmission pathway. Changes in the latent state to a replicative state of the virus can be mediated by rejection. An increased immunosuppressive level allows local virus to spread and to enhance inflammation. In seropositive patients, CMV strains of donor and recipient can be different and the immunological host response cannot be sufficient to stop early replication. After replication, CMV induces immunological disorders, such as HLA enhancing, and increases the risk of repeated rejection and resistant rejection. Antiviral treatment should be useful in stopping focal CMV replication and then limiting virologically induced immunological disorders.

In conclusion, these results point out the importance of the CMV donor status. CMV is transmitted to the recipient by the donor heart and focal reactivation of the virus strain could enhance rejection. This data must be taken into account during iterative rejection and an antiviral treatment could be useful. Further studies are needed to evaluate this strategy and to establish a prophylactic regimen against CMV in order to reduce iterative rejections in CMV-seropositive donor hearts.

Reference

1. The International Society for Heart Transplantation, Billingham ME, Cary NR, Hammond ME, et al (1990) A working formulation for the standardization of nomenclature in the diagnosis of heart and lung transplantation: Heart Rejection Study Group. J Heart Transplant 9: 587–593

Transpl Int (1996) 9 [Suppl 1]: S 243–S 246
© Springer-Verlag 1996

Th. Auer
G. Schreier
K. H. Tscheliessnigg
H. Hutten
Th. Allmayr
B. Grasser
A. Wasler
B. Petutschnigg
F. Iberer
M. Schaldach

Evoked epimyocardial electrogram for rejection diagnosis after heart transplantation

Th. Auer (✉) · K. H. Tscheliessnig ·
Th. Allmayr · B. Grasser · A. Wasler ·
B. Petutschnigg · F. Iberer
University of Graz, Department of Surgery,
Auenbruggerplatz 29, A-8036 Graz,
Austria
Tel. + 43 31 63 85 27 30;
Fax + 43 31 63 85 44 46

G. Schreier · H. Hutten
Joanneum Research, Institut für
Medizintechnik, Steyrergasse 17,
A-8010 Graz, Austria

M. Schaldach
University of Erlangen-Nürnberg,
Zentralinstitut für Biomedizinische
Technik, Turnstrasse 5, D-91054 Erlangen,
Germany

Abstract An endomyocardial electrogram (ECG) was reported to be a sensitive and practicable method for rejection monitoring after heart transplantation. Long-term follow up was limited, however, by variations of signals. The repolarization part of ECG signals vary with changes of heart rate. Both can be avoided by using pacemaker-induced signals. For stimulation and sensing of the ventricular-evoked response, a new type of electrode with fractal surface structure was used. Twenty patients undergoing heart transplantation were evaluated. Amplitudes of the depolarization and repolarization part of the ventricular-evoked response signals were analyzed and related to the degree of acute rejection according to histological findings from endomyocardial biopsy. Signals were transferred by Internet and analyzed automatically. In the case of focal moderate rejection (grade 2, International Society for Heart Transplantation grading) and higher degrees of rejection, a significant amplitude decrease was found. This sensitive non-invasive method for rejection monitoring with a high level of reliability provides the possibility of reducing the number of endomyocardial biopsies.

Key words Heart transplantation ·
Epimyocardial electrogram ·
Evoked response · Non-invasive
rejection diagnosis

Introduction

Several studies, using spontaneous electrocardiograms (ECG) from the body surface [6, 10] and from intramyocardial electrodes [9, 12, 13, 15–17], confirm that ECGs, mainly intracardial, are sensitive to rejection. Our previous studies [1, 14], using QRS amplitude changes from spontaneous epimyocardial electrograms (EE), also confirmed the relationship between EE amplitude changes and rejection episodes detected by endomyocardial biopsies (EMB). The recent study, by using pacemaker-induced ECGs, denoted as the ventricular-evoked response (VER), was based on the idea of minimizing signal variations and changes in the long-term, as well as analyzing an additional parameter, the repolarization part of the signals, which is useful only with constant heart rates. Results from VER for rejection monitoring [5] were reported from observations during the early postoperative period. By analyzing evoked T-wave amplitudes, rejection episodes were detected with a high sensitivity. Since an externalized pacing system was used, the observations had to be finished at the time of removal of the epimyocardial leads, 4 weeks postoperatively.

With the option of a new type of electrode with fractal surface structure [4], leading to a minor poststimulus polarization artifact, a simple single-lead system can be used for long-term studies of VER. In the present study we used signals with a constant pacing rate. Our interest was focused on the depolarization as well as on the repolarization phase of VER signals, diagnostic reliability, sensitivity, and specificity of this method in relation to the results of the standard EMB diagnosis.

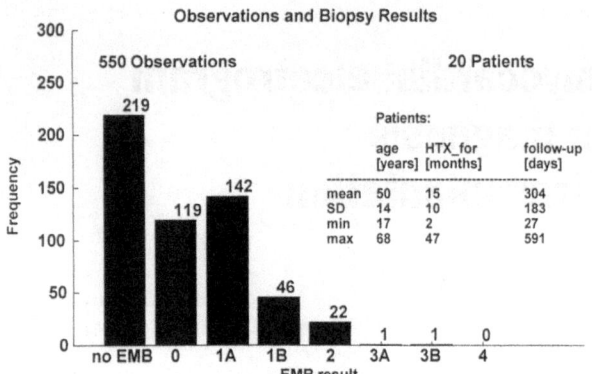

Fig. 1 Number of recordings and associated epimyocardial biopsy *(EMB)* grades, statistics. *(HTX* Heart transplantation)

Methods

Between June 1993 and February 1995, 20 consecutive patients of the heart transplant program at the University of Graz were included in the study. The mean age of patients was 50 years (SD 14 years). The mean observation time was 304 days (SD 183 days). Basic immunosuppression therapy consisted of cyclosporine (serum trough levels of 150–250 ng/ml, determined by high-pressure liquid chromatography) with additional azathioprine (1–2 mg/kg per day) and methylprednisolone (7.5 mg/day). Cytolytic therapy with anti-thymocyte globulin (ATG) was administered postoperatively for 7–14 days. Rejection episodes were treated, beginning with grade 1B [grading of The International Society for Heart Transplantation (ISHT)] [3], with pulses of methylprednisolone. Non-resolving rejections and cases with myocyte necrosis were treated with ATG or with a monoclonal interleukin-2 receptor antibody (BT 563) [8]. EMB were performed weekly during the first 3 months after heart transplantation (HTX). Depending on the patient's course, EMB intervals were extended to every 6 months thereafter. Eight pieces of myocardium were extracted with a number 9 French forceps (Scholten Surgical Instruments, Calif., USA) for each EMB and classified in accordance with the grading system of the ISHT [3].

Equipment

A commercially available VVI pacemaker (PM) with telemetric capabilities and the appropriate telemetry receiver (Mikros-Biogard and Biogard/TM2) were used with an epimyocardial screw-in electrode with fractally coated surface (ELC 54-UP). The PM system was implanted during the transplant operation, placing the electrode at the anterior wall of the right ventricle. The PM was implanted subcutaneously at the left upper abdominal wall. The telemetry system is based on analog frequency modulation and features a band-width from 0.5 to 200 Hz. The PMs were programmed with the appropriate programmer (PMS 600, all appliances mentioned so far: Biotronik, Berlin, Germany). The signals were sampled with 1200 Hz and stored using an adapted, PC-based high resolution ECG system (Predictor I, Corazonix, Okla., USA). Measured data were transferred to a UNIX workstation (DECstation 5000/240, Digital, Mass., USA) for evaluation with specially designed software for serial ECG processing.

Measurement procedure

Recordings were performed under standardized conditions (e.g. rest for 15 min, lying in supine position without moving and talking, at a time period between 2 : 00 and 3 : 00 p.m.).

A 1-min signal sequence of the telemetrically transmitted EE was recorded after the PM had been programmed to a pacing rate of 100 beats/min. Signal recording was started between the 2nd and 7th postoperative day, followed by daily recordings up to the first EMB. Thereafter, EEs were recorded on the days when EMB was scheduled. Additional recordings were taken in case of acute change of the clinical status such as acute rejection (AR) or infection episodes. Signals were recorded and processed without knowledge of the EMB result.

Data transfer

After signal recording, data were transferred to the workstation via Internet data transfer. After signal processing, data were retransferred automatically to the transplant unit within 3–5 min.

Signal processing

VER sequences were automatically processed (beat detection, beat classification, and signal averaging). Two parameters were extracted from the resulting VER sequence:

1. The VER depolarization amplitude (VERDA), defined as the magnitude of the early-negative part of the VER, typically 45 ms poststimulus.
2. The VER repolarization amplitude (VERRA); magnitude of the late-negative part of the VER, typically 350 ms poststimulus.

Statistical methods

All parameter values were expressed as percentages of an individual reference value. The reference value was computed as the mean of the parameter values of all recordings for each patient, independently of the corresponding EMB result. For statistical analysis, the normalized parameter values were grouped according to the associated EMB grades. All rejection grades ≥ 2 were subsumed in one group. For each group means and standard deviations were computed. Differences between the groups were tested via the Wilcoxon-Mann-Whitney two-tailed U-test. The threshold level of significance for the group differences was $P \leq 0.05$.

For diagnostic quality calculation, a single threshold was used as a retrospective diagnosis model. Sensitivity (SENS) and specificity (SPEC) were computed for the threshold that maximized the diagnostic quality index (DQI) for the correlation between the VER and EMB results. DQI was calculated using the following equation:

$$DQI = SENS \cdot SPEC$$

A combination parameter of VERDA and VERRA, denoted VER-AREA, was calculated as the true geometric area of the signal curves in relation to the signal baseline.

Results

Except for two cases of "twiddler syndrome", no severe complications have been observed from the PM-electrode system. In these two cases, epimyocardial elec-

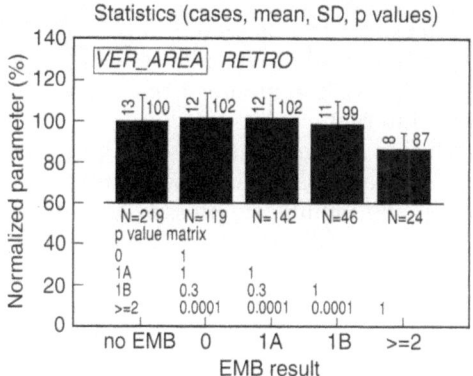

Fig. 2 Normalized parameters (%) and standard deviations of a combination parameter *(VER-AREA)* of the ventricular-evoked response depolarization and repolarization amplitudes. *P* values calculated for EMB grades 0, 1A, and 1B compared with rejection grade ≥ 2

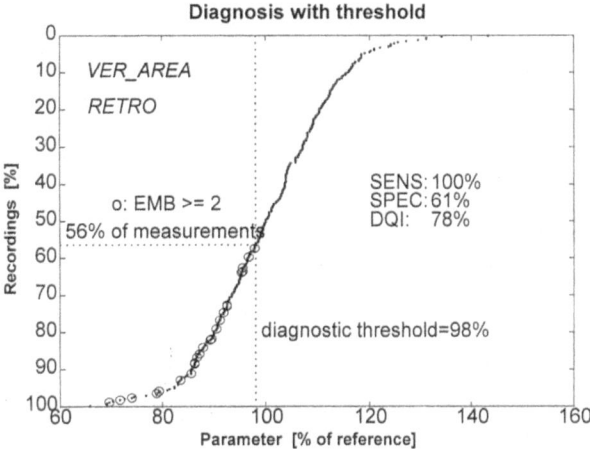

Fig. 3 Example of the application of the diagnosis model on VER-AREA with the threshold of parameter percentage that optimized the diagnostic quality index *(DQI*. The values of all recordings for all patients are plotted in ascending order (beginning in the lower left corner). *Encircled* values represent EMB grades ≥ 2. The values obtained for sensitivity *(SENS)*, specificity *(SPEC)*, and DQI are displayed

trodes have been changed to a transvenous system and the pacemaker fixed. During the investigation period, one patient died because of early graft sclerosis 126 days after HTX. A total of 550 examinations with VER recordings and 331 associated EMBs have been evaluated. Twenty-two acute rejections (ARs) with EMB grade 2, one with grade 3A and one with 3B were observed (Fig. 2).

The VER-AREA parameters did not differ comparing rejection grades 0 to 1B. The values decreased significantly due to rejection episodes of rejection grades ≥ 2 (Fig. 2). The application of the diagnosis model for VER-AREA values is shown in Fig. 3. By using a threshold as previously defined, all grade 2 rejection ep-

isodes and the two grade 3 episodes (3A and 3B) were correctly detected. A SENS of 100 %, SPEC of 61 % resulted in a DQI of 78 %. For optimizing the DQI, the diagnostic threshold was set to 98 % of the reference. In this calculation, 56 % of measurements were obove the diagnostic threshold, with no rejection greater than grade 1B.

Data transfer via Internet was performed by resident doctors trained to use PC applications. After the installation period no problems occurred with data transfer and data processing. Results, with all preceding data and the current in graph form, were available within 3–5 min.

Discussion

This study indicates a significant relationship of VER to rejection, with at least one focus of aggressive infiltration and/or focal myocyte damage as confirmed by EMB.

It has to be emphasized that most rejection episodes detected by VER analysis in this retrospective study were classified as focal moderate. The values of SENS (100 %) and SPEC (61 %) obtained must be regarded in the light of the controversially discussed reliability of EMB itself. Many studies concluded that EMB fails in some cases, at the least, SENS and SPEC do not reach 100 % simultaneously [7, 11, 18].

Since decreasing VER amplitudes were also observed in the case of infection episodes (false-positive diagnoses), additional clinical information can further increase diagnostic reliability. A higher frequency of investigations would allow a more accurate reference value to be obtained. The results of our study, however, have shown a significant accordance with EMB results with regard to the focus of interest in rejection diagnoses, the focal moderate, i.e., grade 2 rejection. Another conclusion of our results is that both pathophysiological and electrophysiological changes are related to AR, although the causal and temporal effects might be different. Longitudinal observations indicate that changes of VER parameters precede histological signs of rejection. After institution of rejection therapy, mainly with the administration of methylprednisolone pulse therapy, VER signal amplitudes increased impressively after 1–3 days; this is earlier than cellular infiltrates are expected to disappear.

Recently, it has been reported that high energy phosphate (ATP) depletion begins when focal moderate degrees of rejection occur [2]. These concordant results could give an estimate of the immunological influence on cellular metabolism and myocyte electrical activity during rejection, independent of or prior to the cellular immune system becoming affected by myocytes. Some cases have been observed in patients with compromised

S246

circulation status, such as dilatation of the ventricles, but in the absence of histological signs of rejection or myocarditis or general infection. VER parameters dropped markedly in these cases and reelevated after reconstitution of the status due to steroid therapy. Had we been confronted with "vascular rejections" in these cases, the method presented would also have been of value.

Data transfer via Internet (during this study between two institutions in the same town) was easy to handle and gives an estimate of the practicality of a multicenter application of the method. Results of the computed data can be available within minutes from every center connected with Internet.

In conclusion, the method gives the option for a noninvasive, easily applicable and inexpensive instrument for rejection and immunosuppressive therapy monitoring which can save 50–60 % of EMBs without exposing patients to a higher risk of undetected rejection.

References

1. Auer T, Schreier G, Hutten H, Schaldach M, Iberer F, Petutschnigg B, Wasler A, Müller H, Allmayer Th, Tscheliessnigg KH (1995) Intramyocardial electrograms for monitoring of allograft rejection after heart transplantation. Transplant Proc 27: 1983–1985
2. Benvenuti Ch, Aptecar E, Deleuze Ph, Benaiem N, Mazzucotelli JP, Charloux C, Castaigne A, Loisance D, Astier A, Paul M (1994) Myocardial high-energy phosphate depletion in allograft rejection after orthotopic human heart transplantation. J Heart Lung Transplant 13: 857–861
3. Billingham ME, Cary NRB, Hammond ME, Kemnitz J, Marboe C, McCallister HA, Snovar DC, Winters GL, Zerbe A (1990) A working formulation for the standardization of nomenclature in the diagnosis of heart and lung rejection: heart rejection study group. J Heart Transplant 9: 587–593
4. Bolz A, Hubmann M, Hardt R, Riedmüller J, Schaldach M (1993) Low polarization pacing leads for detecting the ventricular-evoked response. Med Prog Technol 19: 129–137
5. Grace AA, Newell SA, Cary NRB, Scott JP, Large SR, Wallwork J, Schofield PM (1991) Diagnosis of early cardiac transplant rejection by fall in evoked T wave amplitude measured using an externalized QT driven rate responsive pacemaker. Pacing Clin Electrophysiol 14: 1024–1031
6. Haberl R, Weber M, Reichenspurner H, Kemkes BM, Osterholzer G, Anthuber M, Steinbeck G (1987) Frequency analysis of the surface electrocardiogram for recognition of acute rejection after orthotopic cardiac transplantation in man. Circulation 76: 101–108
7. Hosenpud JD (1992) Noninvasive diagnosis of cardiac allograft rejection. Circulation 85: 368–371
8. Iberer F, Tscheliessnigg K, Freigassner M, Auer T, Kleinert R, Wasler A, Petutschnigg B, Müller H (1994) Clinical experience with a monoclonal interleukin-2-receptor antibody (BT 563) for rejection therapy after orthotopic heart transplantation. Transplant Proc 6: 3237–3239
9. Irvin ED, Bianco RW, Clack R, Grehan J, Slovut DP, Nakhleh R, Bolman M, Shumway SJ (1992) Use of epicardial electrocardiograms for detecting cardiac allograft rejection. Ann Thorac Surg 54: 669–675
10. Keren A, Gillis AM, Freedman A, Baldwin JC, Billingham ME, Sunson EB, Simson MB, Mason JW (1984) Heart transplant rejection monitored by signal-averaged electrocardiography in patients receiving cyclosporine. Circulation [Suppl 1] 70: 124–129
11. Nielsen H, Soerensen FB, Nielsen B, Bagger JP, Thayssen P, Baandrup U (1993) Reproducibility of the acute rejection diagnosis in human cardiac allografts. The Stanford classification and the international grading system. J Heart Lung Transplant 12: 239–243
12. Pirolo JS, Shuman TS, Brunt EM, Liptay MJ, Cox JL, Ferguson TB (1992) Noninvasive detection of cardiac allograft rejection by prospective telemetric monitoring. J Thorac Cardiovasc Surg 103: 969–979
13. Scheuer J, Shaver JA, Harris BC, Leonard JJ, Bahnson HT (1969) Electrocardiographic findings in cardiac transplantation. Circulation 40: 289–296
14. Schreier G, Auer T, Hutten H, Schaldach M (1993) Epicardial electrogram recordings for detection of acute allograft rejection in cardiac transplant recipients. IEEE-EMBS, Proceedings of the 15th Annual International Conference, pp 701–702
15. Sewell DH, Kemp VE, Lower R (1969) Epicardial ECG in monitoring cardiac homograft rejection. Circulation [Suppl 1] 39: 21–25
16. Wahlers Th, Haverich A, Schäfers HJ, Frimpong-Boateng K, Fieguth HG, Herrmann G, Borst HG, Arvanitidou V (1986) Changes of the intramyocardial electrogram after orthotopic heart transplantation. J Heart Transplant 5: 450–454
17. Warnecke H, Müller J, Cohnert T, Hummel M, Spiegelsberger S, Siniawski HK, Lieback E, Hetzer R (1992) Clinical heart transplantation without routine endomyocardial biopsy. J Heart Lung Transplant 11: 1093–1102
18. Zerbe T, Arena V (1988) Diagnostic reliability of endomyocardial biopsy for assessment of cardiac allograft rejection. Hum Pathol 19: 1307–1314

Transpl Int (1996) 9 [Suppl 1]: S247–S248
© Springer-Verlag 1996

Th. Wahlers
J. Albes
K. Pethig
P. Oppelt
H. G. Fieguth
M. Jurmann
B. Hausen
S. Demertzis
H. G. Borst

Valve reconstruction or replacement for long-term biopsy-induced tricuspid regurgitation following heart transplantation

Th. Wahlers (✉) · J. Albes · K. Pethig ·
P. Oppelt · H. G. Fieguth · M. Jurmann ·
B. Hausen · S. Demertzis · H. G. Borst
Department of Cardiothoracic Surgery,
Hannover Medical School,
D-30623 Hannover, Germany
Tel. +49 51 15 32 21 59, 21 98, 22 59;
Fax +49 51 15 32 54 04

Abstract Tricuspid regurgitation following heart transplantation can become a severe problem in a subset of patients, where medical therapy fails. Operative findings are described and results of subsequent results with surgical intervention including repair and replacement are analysed. Although follow-up is short, tricuspid replacement seems superior to reconstruction following heart transplantation.
Best results are obtained, if replacement is performed, before right ventricular function deterioates.

Key words Tricuspid value failure · Valve reconstruction · Valve replacement · Endomyocardial biopsies

Introduction

Tricuspid regurgitation following heart transplantation is a well known entity, which can be demonstrated soon after the primary transplantation in most patients [1, 2, 5]. In some cases, however, progressive deterioration leads to clinical symptoms and the necessity for surgical reintervention if medical therapy fails. The valve insufficiency can be caused by various factors. Apart from the implantation technique used, patient-related factors including rhythm, pulmonary hypertension, cardiac-size matching, pericardial support and the number and size of endomyocardial biopsies have been discussed as causative factors [1, 4, 5]. It was the aim of this retrospective analysis to outline underlying causes and to investigate the results achieved with reinterventions for tricuspid valve failure in cardiac transplant patients.

Patients and methods

From 1983 to 1994, 12 out of 505 patients (2.4 %) following heart transplantation underwent either tricuspid reconstruction ($n = 4$) or replacement ($n = 8$) for severe tricuspid regurgitation, 5.8 ± 2.7 years following cardiac transplantation. The mean age of the patients was 52 ± 10 years and 10 patients were male while 2 patients were female. The underlying diagnosis prior to the initial transplantation was dilative cardiomyopathy in 9 patients and ischemic dis-

ease in 3 patients. All primary transplant operations were performed using standard cardiopulmonary bypass with aortal and bicaval cannulation and hypothermia of $30\,°C$. All donor hearts were preserved with St. Thomas' Hospital solution cardioplegia and anastomosed using the original cuff technique as it was described by Shumway. All patients were on triple-drug immunosuppression including cyclosporine A 3-10 mg/kg azathioprine 1–2.5 mg/kg and prednisolone 0.1–0.5 mg/kg. All patients were monitored by routine endomyocardial biopsy on a scheduled basis. The mean number of biopsies in the first postoperative year was 24 ± 8. The mean total number of biopsies in patients in the study group was 38 ± 20. The status of the heart was assessed by routine echocardiography for cardiac function and valve competence. Apart from applying a four chamber view using transthoracal echocardiography for the verification of right atrial and ventricular enlargement, transoesophageal echocardiography was used on a routine basis [3]. In addition, the diagnosis of right heart failure was also assessed based on clinical symptoms. Liver and renal functional data were analysed on a longitudinal basis throughout the routine outpatient visits. The decision to intervene surgically was made if tricuspid insufficiency was progredient and reaching grade III/IV. Apart from the echocardiographic diagnosis, severe clinical symptoms had to be present which could not be managed by conservative means.

All patients were scheduled for elective reintervention. A CT scan of the thorax was performed to define the distance of the cardiac structures from the sternum. Reoperations were preferably done by resternotomy using bicaval cannulation and moderate hypothermia of $25\,°C$. Valve repair was evaluated in each patient. If no repair was feasable, valve replacement was performed using a bioprosthesis. In these cases, multiple pledgeted sutures of 2/0 dacron with teflon were placed around the valve circumference. Postoperatively, all patients were followed by routine echocardiographic examination and the tricuspid valve function assessed.

Results

All patients survived the reintervention. A total of four reconstructions and eight replacements was performed. Operations were performed without cardioplegia in 9/12 patients. Valve failure, as assessed from the intraoperative findings, included ring dilation in 11/12 patients, ruptured chordae in 6/12 patients and almost no septal leaflet in 3 of 12 patients. One patient received additional coronary and bypass grafting including implantation of the left internal mammaria artery to the LAD. Operative complications included phrenic nerve palsy in 2, one with repair and 1 with replacement, respectively. Atrioventricular block requiring pacemaker therapy occurred in 1 patient following valve replacement. Postoperative intubation was necessary for 1.6 ± 1.2 days. The mean intensive care unit stay of all patients was 6.5 ± 5.5 days. Two patients died within 1 year postoperatively, 10 patients are alive 3–21 months postoperatively. Echocardiographic examination after 1 year showed moderate tricuspid regurgitation grade II/III in 3/4 patients following reconstruction. Adequate valve function was assessed in almost every patient undergoing valve replacement except 2 where a mean gradient of 7 mm Hg was measured across the implanted valve. Excellent remodelling of right ventricular dimensions was observed in all patients following valve replacement. Right ventricular enlargement persisted in the group who underwent valve reconstruction despite clinical improvement.

Discussion

Our experience demonstrates that cardiac reinterventions for tricuspid valve repair or replacement can be performed with a low operative risk after prior transplantation. In most cases a valve replacement seems necessary due to the extensive structural valve failures observed [3, 5]. Injuries by the biopsy forceps have to be suspected as the main cause of the severe changes observed in this small subgroup of patients [4]. In our opinion, valve replacement offers the better causative treatment, since remodelling less frequently achieved good results in the group who underwent reconstruction due to persistent moderate regurgitation. In addition, the life span of modern bioprostheses will probably exceed the possible freedom from transplant vasculopathy in most patients. We, therefore, have adopted replacement as the primary choice of curative treatment in this subgroup of patients.

References

1. Herrman G, Simon R, Haverich A, et al (1989) Left ventricular function, tricuspid incompetence, and incidence of coronary artery disease late after orthotopic heart transplantation. Eur J Cardiothorac Surg 3: 111–117

2. Sievers HH, Weyand M, Kraatz EG, Bernhard A (1991) An alternative technique for orthotopic cardiac transplantation, with preservation of the normal anatomy of the right atrium. Thorac Cardiovasc Surg 39: 70–72

3. Haverich A, Albes JM, Fahrenkamp G, Schäfers HJ, Wahlers T, Heublein B (1991) Intraoperative echocardiography to detect and prevent tricuspid valve regurgitation after heart transplantation. Eur J Cardiothorac Surg 5: 41–45

4. Reddy SC, Rath GA, Zady GM, Matesic C, Kormos R, Tricus R (1993) Tricuspid flail leaflets after orthotopic heart transplant: a new complication of endomyocardial biopsy. J Am Soc Echocardiogr 6: 223–226

5. Suarez JM, Leon CA, Zoghbi WB, et al (1986) Valvular dysfunction in the transplanted heart. J Heart Transplant 5: 392–396

Pancreas

Transpl Int (1996) 9 [Suppl 1]: S 251–S 257
© Springer-Verlag 1996

Rainer W. G. Gruessner
David E. R. Sutherland
Mary Beth Drangstveit
Christoph Troppmann
Angelika C. Gruessner

Use of FK 506 in pancreas transplantation

R. W. G. Gruessner (✉) ·
D. E. R. Sutherland · M. B. Drangstveit ·
C. Troppmann · A. C. Gruessner
University of Minnesota,
Department of Surgery, Box 90 UMHC,
420 Delaware Street S. E.,
Minneapolis, MN 55455, USA
Tel. + 1 612 625 1485; Fax + 1 612 625 9467

Abstract Until recently, FK 506 was used only for rescue therapy after pancreas transplantation. We report our initial experience with FK 506 for 67 pancreas recipients (treated between 1 May 1993 and 30 April 1995). Of these recipients, 49 (73 %) received FK 506 for induction and maintenance therapy, 12 (18 %) for rescue or antirejection therapy, and 6 (9 %) for reasons other than rescue or antirejection therapy. In our induction and maintenance therapy group, 32 recipients (65 %) underwent a simultaneous pancreas-kidney transplant (SPK), 8 (16 %) a pancreas transplant alone (PTA), and 9 (19 %) a pancreas after previous kidney transplant (PAK). Quadruple immunosuppression was used for induction; the median FK 506 starting dose was 4 mg/day p. o. and target levels were 10–20 ng/ml. The most common side effects were nephrotoxicity (16 %) and neurotoxicity (14 %); transient episodes of hyperglycemia were also noted (12 %), in particular in the presence of concurrent rejection and infection episodes. A matched-pair analysis was done to compare graft outcome with FK 506 versus cyclosporin A (CsA). For SPK recipients, pancreas graft survival at 6 months was 79 % with FK 506 versus 65 % with CsA ($P = 0.04$), for PTA, 100 % versus 63 % ($P > 0.35$), and for PAK, 88 % versus 33 % ($P > 0.01$). Pancreas graft loss due to rejection at 6 months posttransplant was lower with FK 506 versus CsA. Two FK 506 recipients died from B-cell lymphomas (Epstein-Barr virus positive) at 6 and 7 months post-transplant. In our rescue or anti-rejection group, 5 recipients underwent SPK, 3 PTA, and 4 PAK. The mean average FK 506 dose was 10 mg/day p. o. and the mean average FK 506 blood level was 11 ng/ml. The most common side effects were nephrotoxicity (33 %) and neurotoxicity (16 %). Two recipients developed hyperglycemic episodes, of whom 1 has remained on insulin with good exocrine pancreas graft function. Graft survival at 6 months after conversion was 75 % for SPK, 67 % for PTA, and 50 % for PAK. Only one graft was lost due to chronic rejection. Our single-center experience shows that FK 506 after pancreas transplantation is associated with: (1) a low rate of graft loss due to rejection when used for induction, in particular for solitary pancreas transplants, (2) a high rate of graft salvage when used for rescue, (3) a 1 % rate of new-onset insulin-dependent diabetes mellitus, and (4) a 3 % rate of posttransplant lymphoma. Further studies are necessary to analyze the long-term impact of FK 506 on pancreas transplant outcome.

Key words Pancreas transplantation · FK 506 · Tacrolimus

Introduction

The use of FK 506 (tacrolimus) for immunosuppression in abdominal solid organ transplantation has been extensively studied in human liver and kidney transplant recipients [5, 8]. But to our knowledge, no information has been published on its use for induction and maintenance therapy in human pancreas transplantation. Previous reports have focused only on rescue therapy in a small number of pancreas transplant recipients [7, 9].

The purpose of this single-center analysis was to study the efficacy and safety of FK 506 for induction and maintenance therapy, as well as for rescue and antirejection therapy, in pancreas transplantation. We studied three groups of FK 506 recipients: (1) those on FK 506 for induction and maintenance therapy, (2) those who convert to FK 506 for rescue or antirejection therapy, and (3) those who convert to FK 506 for reasons other than rescue or antirejection therapy.

Due to our short follow-up time, we report here our 6-month graft and patient survival rates. Matched-pair analysis was done to compare the effect of FK 506 versus cyclosporin A (CsA) for induction and maintenance therapy. An additional purpose of our study was to determine whether FK 506 decreases the incidence of rejection for solitary pancreas transplant recipients, thus improving graft survival. If so, application of this procedure could become more widespread for non-uremic patients with brittle diabetes mellitus.

Materials and methods

Between 1 May 1993 and 5 April 1995, FK 506 was given to 67 pancreas recipients. Of these, 49 (73 %) received FK 506 for induction and maintenance therapy, 12 (18 %) for rescue or antirejection therapy, and 6 (9 %) for reasons other than rescue or antirejection therapy. The three groups were analyzed separately.

1. FK 506 for induction and maintenance therapy

Of 49 recipients, 25 were male and 24 female. The median age was 36 years (range 23–52 years). Pancreas transplants were done in all three recipient categories: 32 patients (65 %) underwent a pancreas-kidney transplant (SPK), 8 (16 %) a pancreas transplant alone (PTA), and 9 (19 %) a pancreas after previous kidney transplant (PAK). The median HLA match was 2. Overall, recipients of solitary pancreas transplants (PTA, PAK) had better matched grafts than SPK recipients (P = 0.001).

For induction therapy, all but 1 recipient received antithymocyte globulin (ATG). The median duration of ATG administration was 10 days (range 5–14 days). All patients received FK 506, prednisone, and azathioprine for induction therapy. FK 506 was given p. o.: the median starting dose was 4 mg/day (range 2–40 mg/day). FK 506 was started in 43 (88 %) of 49 recipients within the first 3 posttransplant days. The median average FK 506 blood level was 12 ng/ml (range 5–30 ng/ml).

The most common side effects attributed to FK 506 were nephrotoxicity – defined as an increase in serum creatinine levels – in 8 (16 %) recipients, neurotoxicity in 7 (14 %) (tremors 7, confusion 1, muscle weakness 1), and gastrointestinal toxicity in 1 (2 %) (diarrhea).

Diabetogenicity – defined by transient hyperglycemia (fasting plasma glucose > 180 mg/dl) or temporary insulin administration – was reported in 6 (12 %) recipients. Hyperglycemic episodes occurred between 28 and 180 days posttransplant and the range of duration was 7–49 days. Of these 6 recipients, 4 experienced concurrent rejection or infection episodes and 1 required gastric tube feeding during treatment of malignancy. In 1 recipient, no cause other than FK 506 administration was held responsible. One recipient converted to CsA, but all 6 became normoglycemic again.

2. Conversion to FK 506 for rescue or antirejection therapy

In all, 12 pancreas recipients converted to FK 506 for rescue or antirejection therapy. Their transplants were done between 29 September 1988 and 19 September 1994. Of these 12 patients, 7 were female and 5 male. The median age at conversion to FK 506 was 37 years (range 11–51 years).

Recipients in all three pancreas transplant categories converted: 5 SPK, 3 PTA, and 4 PAK. There were eight primary transplants and four retransplants. The median HLA match was 2. Overall, recipients of solitary pancreas transplants (PTA, PAK) had better matched grafts than SPK recipients (P = 0.001).

With regard to previous rejection episodes, 6 recipients converted after a first, 3 after a second, 2 after a fourth, and 1 after an eighth rejection episode. Median time interval to FK 506 conversion was 324 days (range 28–2225 days) posttransplant. The median average FK 506 dose was 10 mg/day p. o. (range 2–34 mg/day), divided into two equal doses. The median average FK 506 blood level was 11 ng/ml (range 6–30 ng/ml).

The most common side effects attributed to FK 506 were nephrotoxicity in 4 recipients and neurotoxicity in 2 (tremor 2, headache 1). Diabetogenicity was noted in 2 recipients and both had concurrent rejection episodes. One had transient hyperglycemic episodes over a period of 120 days, remained on FK 506, but became normoglycemic again; the other has remained on insulin, after reversal of his rejection episode, with good exocrine pancreas graft function.

3. Conversion to FK 506 for reasons other than rescue or antirejection therapy

Six pancreas recipients converted to FK 506 for reasons other than rescue or antirejection therapy. Before conversion, all had been on CsA-based triple immunosuppression. The reasons for conversion were CsA side effects in 3 recipients (all neurotoxicity); of the other 3, 1 had memory loss, 1 had hearing loss, and 1 had deterioration of vision. There were 5 female and 1 male recipients and the median age at conversion was 37 years (range 29–48 years). By recipient category, 4 had undergone PTA, 1 SPK, and 1 PAK. The median FK 506 starting dose was 7 mg/day p. o. (range 4–16 mg/day p. o.) and the median average FK 506 level was 12 ng/ml. The most common side effects were nephrotoxicity in 4 recipients and neurotoxicity in 2. Diabetogenicity was not noted in this subgroup.

Statistical analysis

The Kaplan-Meier method was used to calculate patient and graft survival rates as well as the incidence of first reversible rejection episodes and first cytomegalovirus (CMV) infection episodes.

Two different analyses were done. The first analysis considered graft loss due to rejection, technical failure, and death with a functioning graft as graft failure. The second analysis considered only graft loss due to rejection as graft failure (death with a functioning graft and technical failure were censored). In the FK 506 induction and maintenance group, a matched-pair analysis was done to compare the outcome in FK 506 versus CsA recipients. Matching criteria included transplant category, transplant number, recipient and donor age, duct management technique, and HLA type. Outcome between these two subgroups was compared using the generalized Wilcoxon and the log-rank test.

Results

1. FK 506 for induction and maintenance therapy

Patient survival

Overall patient survival at 1, 3, and 6 months posttransplant was 100 %, 100 %, and 93 %. By recipient category, patient survival at 6 months was 89 % for SPK and 100 % for PAK and PTA recipients ($P = 0.8$). Of 49 recipients, 44 are alive. The five deaths were caused by posttransplant lymphoma in 2 recipients (SPK 1, PTA 1), infection in 2 (SPK 2), and hemorrhage in 1 (PTA).

The 2 recipients with posttransplant lymphoma died with functioning grafts at 6 and 7 months posttransplant, respectively. Both had B-cell lymphomas; in situ hybridization and immunoperoxidase stainings were positive for the Epstein-Barr virus (EBV). In both recipients, symptoms were very subtle beginning with diarrhea and a drop in the white blood cell count. Despite alpha-interferon therapy and discontinuation of immunosuppression, they died within several weeks of the diagnosis being made.

Graft survival

Overall pancreas graft survival at 1, 3, and 6 months posttransplant was 96 %, 96 %, and 85 %. For SPK recipients, graft survival at 3 and 6 months was 97 % and 79 %, for PTA recipients, 100 % and 100 %, and for PAK recipients, 100 % and 88 % (Fig. 1). The difference between the three groups was not significant ($P = 0.9$). Of 49 pancreas grafts, 41 are currently functioning and 5 recipients died with a functioning pancreas graft. The graft failed in 3 recipients, due to vascular thrombosis in 2 recipients (SPK 1, PAK 1) and bleeding in 1 (PAK).

Kidney graft survival for SPK recipients at 3 and 6 months posttransplant was 100 % and 89 %. Of 32 SPK grafts, 28 are functioning; 3 recipients died with a functioning kidney graft. The kidney graft failed in 1 recipient, due to infection.

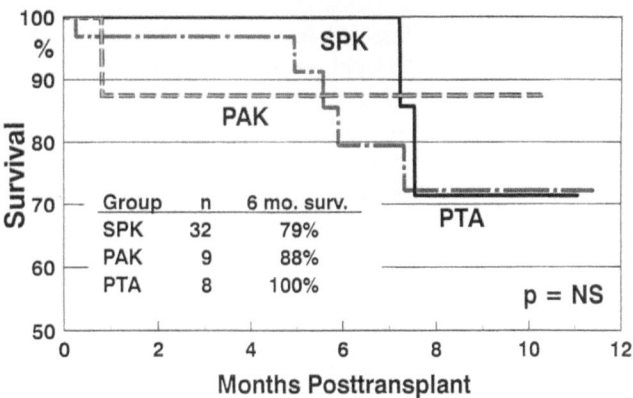

Fig. 1 FK 506 for induction/maintenance therapy. Pancreas graft survival by recipient category

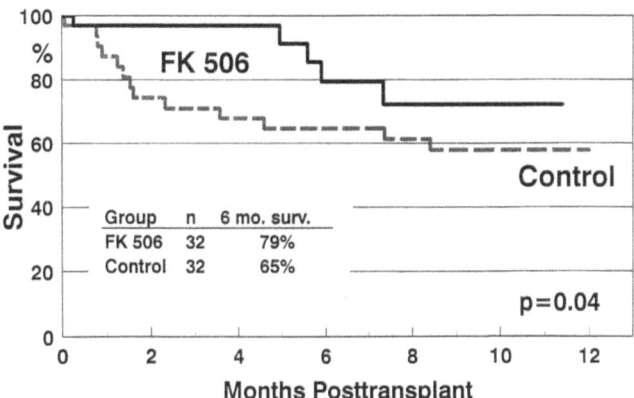

Fig. 2 SPK. Pancreas graft survival with FK 506 versus CsA (induction group)

Matched-pair analysis

For SPK recipients, pancreas graft survival at 3 and 6 months posttransplant was 97 % and 79 % with FK 506 versus 71 % and 65 % with CsA ($P = 0.04$, Wilcoxon test; $P = 0.08$, log-rank test) (Fig. 2). Kidney graft survival at 3 and 6 months posttransplant was 100 % and 89 % with FK 506 versus 78 % and 74 % ($P = 0.04$, Wilcoxon test; $P = 0.01$, log-rank test).

For PTA recipients, pancreas graft survival at 3 and 6 months posttransplant was 100 % and 100 % with FK 506 versus 63 % and 63 % with CsA ($P > 0.35$). When technical failures and deaths with a functioning graft were censored, pancreas graft survival was not statistically significant with FK 506 versus CsA.

For PAK recipients, pancreas graft survival at 3 and 6 months posttransplant was 100 % and 88 % with FK 506 versus 33 % and 33 % with CsA ($P > 0.01$). When technical failures and deaths with a functioning graft were censored, pancreas graft survival was not statistically significant between the FK 506- versus CsA-treated recipients.

Pancreas graft loss due to rejection in the SPK group at 6 months posttransplant was 0 % with FK 506 versus 5 % with CsA ($P = 0.23$), for PTA recipients, 0 % with FK 506 versus 17 % with CsA ($P = 0.19$) (Fig. 3), and for PAK recipients, 0 % with FK 506 versus 30 % with CsA ($P = 0.12$) (Fig. 4).

Rejection episodes

The incidence of first reversible rejection episodes at 3 and 6 months posttransplant for SPK recipients was 29 % and 39 %, for PTA recipients, 25 % and 25 %, and for PAK recipients, 24 % and 24 %. The difference between the three groups was not significant ($P = 0.9$).

Infections

The incidence of first cytomegalovirus (CMV) infection episodes at 6 months posttransplant for SPK recipients was 14 %, for PTA recipients, 0 %, and for PAK recipients, 0 % ($P = 0.7$). Overall, CMV infections were diagnosed in 4 recipients. Posttransplant, six intraabdominal infections and five wound infections developed. Urinary tract infections were noted in 26 recipients. Other types of infections were reported in 7 recipients.

Conversion to cyclosporine

Four recipients converted to cyclosporine: 2 for neurotoxicity, 1 for nephrotoxicity, and 1 for rescue therapy and transient hyperglycemia.

2. Conversion to FK 506 for rescue or antirejection therapy

Patient survival

Overall patient survival at 3 and 6 months after conversion was 92 % and 83 %. For SPK recipients, patient survival at 3 and 6 months was 100 % and 75 %, for PTA recipients, 100 % and 100 %, and for PAK recipients, 100 % and 75 % ($P = 0.7$). Of the 12 recipients, 10 are alive, the two deaths being caused by infections.

Graft survival

Overall pancreas graft survival at 3 and 6 months after conversion was 83 % and 65 %. For SPK recipients, graft survival at 3 and 6 months was 100 % and 75 %, for PTA recipients, 67 % and 67 %, and for PAK recipients, 75 % and 50 % ($P = 0.8$) (Fig. 5). Graft loss from irreversible

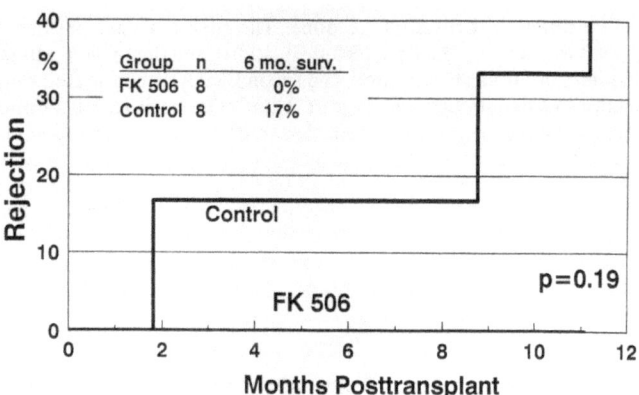

Fig. 3 PTA. Pancreas graft loss from rejection with FK 506 versus CsA (induction group)

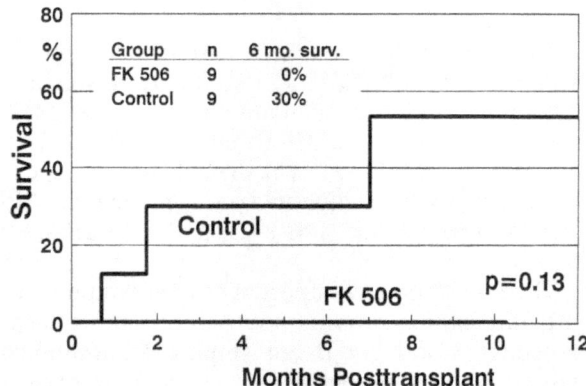

Fig. 4 PAK. Pancreas graft loss from rejection with FK 506 versus CsA (induction group)

rejection for SPK recipients at 6 months after conversion (when technical failures and deaths with a functioning graft were censored) was 0 %, for PTA recipients, 0 %, and for PAK recipients, 33 % ($P = 0.4$). Of 12 grafts, 8 are functioning. Two recipients died with a functioning graft; the pancreas graft failed in 2 recipients, 1 due to chronic rejection (PAK) and the other due to pancreatitis (PTA).

Rejection

The incidence of first reversible rejection episodes for SPK recipients at 3 and 6 months after conversion was 20 % and 47 %, for PTA recipients, 0 % and 0 %, and for PAK recipients, 25 % and 50 % ($P = 0.9$).

Infection

The incidence of first CMV infection episodes at 6 months after conversion for SPK recipients was 20 %,

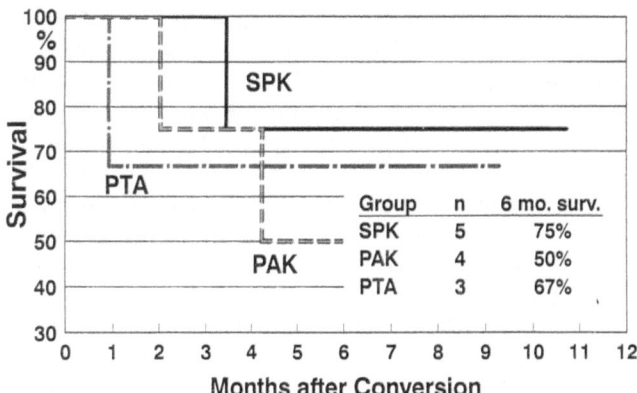

Fig.5 FK 506 for rescue/antirejection therapy. Pancreas graft survival by recipient category

for PTA recipients, 33 %, and for PAK recipients, 0 % ($P = 0.5$). Overall, CMV infections were diagnosed in 2 recipients. After conversion, four intraabdominal infections and seven urinary tract infections developed. Other types of infections were reported in 7 recipients. No lymphomas occurred after conversion.

Reconversion to cyclosporine

Only 1 recipient converted from FK 506 to CsA for transient hyperglycemia. She has remained normoglycemic on CsA.

3. Conversion to FK 506 for reasons other than rescue or antirejection therapy

All 6 recipients who converted to FK 506 for other reasons are alive with functioning pancreas grafts. Two recipients reconverted to CsA 7 and 13 months after conversion to FK 506: 1 due to nephrotoxicity and the other due to neurotoxicity (tremor).

Discussion

Despite the introduction of CsA in the 1980s, rejection has remained a problem after pancreas transplantation. According to the International Pancreas Transplant Registry (IPTR), rejection is the second most common cause of pancreas graft failure in SPK recipients, accounting for 31 % of all their graft losses. It is the most common cause of pancreas graft failure in recipients of solitary pancreas transplants, accounting for 61 % of all graft losses in PTA recipients and 53 % in PAK recipients [2]. Thus, the outcome after pancreas transplantation could be further improved in all three recipient categories (SPK, PTA, and PAK) by decreasing the inci-

dence of rejection as the cause of graft failure. This prospect motivated us to use FK 506 not only for rescue therapy, as previously reported [7, 9], but also for induction and maintenance therapy after pancreas transplantation.

Our single-center study produced encouraging results with the use of FK 506 to prevent rejection and to successfully treat rejection. In our 49 recipients who received FK 506 for induction and maintenance therapy, no pancreas graft was lost within the first 6 months posttransplant due to acute rejection. But eight grafts were lost due to rejection in the matched-pair, CsA group (SPK 2, PTA 3, PAK 3). FK 506 also decreased the incidence of first reversible rejection episodes. At 6 months, the rejection rates were 39 % for SPK, 25 % for PTA, and 24 % for PAK recipients with FK 506 versus 68 %, 85 %, and 65 % with CsA. The results are most striking in our solitary pancreas recipient groups (PTA, PAK), which has prompted us to more intensely promote pancreas transplantation alone for non-uremic patients with brittle diabetes.

The use of FK 506 for rescue or rejection therapy was similarly successful in our study. All 12 recipients who received FK 506 for these reasons had numerous previous rejection episodes (in one case as many as eight) before they converted from CsA to FK 506. Only one graft failed due to chronic rejection. The overall low rate of first reversible rejection episodes after conversion to FK 506 was likewise impressive: at 6 months, 47 % of SPK recipients, 0 % of PTA recipients, and 50 % of PAK recipients had experienced a first reversible rejection episode. Thus, the majority of these recipients, all at high risk for recurrent rejection, did not require additional antirejection therapy within the first 6 months after conversion.

The effect of FK 506 induction and maintenance therapy on pancreas transplant outcome has, to our knowledge, not been reported before. In two previous reports, FK 506 successfully treated relapsing rejection episodes, and was also used for rescue therapy [7, 9]. A third report focused on its successful use in an SPK recipient who developed hemolytic-uremic syndrome while on CsA; conversion to FK 506 normalized kidney function [4]. In all three of these reports, FK 506-induced new-onset diabetes mellitus was not mentioned; in contrast, one group noted normal oral glucose tolerance tests and C-peptide levels 8 months after conversion [7]. Nevertheless, in experimental studies on large and small animals, FK 506 has been shown to cause glucose intolerance, impaired insulin secretion, and decreased insulin release from beta cells [3]. In our study, diabetogenicity was defined by transient hyperglycemia (fasting plasma glucose > 180 mg/dl) or the need for insulin. In our induction and maintenance group, 6 (12 %) recipients seemingly met this definition and in our rescue group, 2 (17 %). However, of these 8 recipients, 6 had concurrent rejection episodes (all reversed) and 1 recipient became hyperglycemic while on gastric tube feedings. All but 1 recipient became normoglycemic again; he converted to FK 506 for rescue therapy and now enjoys excellent exocrine graft function, but has remained on insulin. In addition, 2 recipients successfully converted to CsA without experiencing further hyperglycemic episodes. These findings suggest that impaired glucose metabolism might be associated with FK 506 therapy, particularly in the presence of concurrent rejection or infection episodes. Thus, in our study: (1) new-onset insulin dependent diabetes mellitus was not noted in recipients on FK 506 for induction and maintenance therapy and (2) transient hyperglycemia, if present, was frequently associated with concurrent rejection or infection episodes.

The spectrum of side effects of FK 506, including nephrotoxicity, neurotoxicity, and gastrointestinal toxicity, is similar to CsA. The incidence of nephrotoxicity was 16 % in our induction and maintenance group and 33 % in our rescue and antirejection therapy group. Increases in serum creatinine levels were only transient and controlled by a reduction in the FK 506 dose. The incidence of neurotoxicity was 14 % in our induction and maintenance therapy group and 17 % in our rescue and antirejection therapy group: the most common symptom was tremor, and severe neurologic symptoms were absent. Gastrointestinal toxicity (diarrhea) was noted in 1 recipient only. Most of these FK 506 side effects were dose related and subsided with dose reduction.

Target levels in both our induction and our rescue group were 10–20 ng/ml (median 12 ng/ml) and achieving as well as maintaining target levels with oral dosing was not difficult. FK 506 was given orally to all patients and conversions from CsA were easy to accomplish. Our study also demonstrates that recipients can successfully convert from FK 506 to CsA for rescue therapy or for treatment of transient hyperglycemia.

The spectrum of infectious complications in our FK 506 recipients has, in essence, not been different from our CsA recipients. The most common infections were urinary tract infections and wound infections (including intraabdominal infections in the induction and maintenance group). The incidence of first CMV infection episodes at 6 months posttransplant or after conversion was low, ranging between 0 % and 33 % in the three recipient groups.

Our overall positive impression of FK 506 is tarnished by the occurrence of two lymphomas in our induction group. Two recipients developed B-cell lymphomas, and in situ hybridization or immunoperoxidase stainings were positive for EBV. The diagnosis was made within the first 6 months posttransplant and initial symptoms were subtle. Despite discontinuation of immunosuppressive drugs and alpha-interferon treatment, both recipients died only several weeks after the disease was diagnosed. In contrast, none of the patients in our rescue and antirejection therapy group developed lymphoproliferative disease, even though some had undergone several courses of anti-T-cell therapy. Follow-up studies are necessary to determine whether the incidence of posttransplant lymphoma increases after FK 506 induction therapy and whether this subgroup is at high risk for lymphoma (as with bowel transplant recipients of all ages and liver transplant recipients < 5 years of age) [1, 6].

In conclusion, FK 506 was associated in our study with a low rate of graft loss due to rejection and a low incidence of first reversible rejection episodes in all three pancreas recipient categories. In our induction and maintenance therapy group, the results were better than for CsA recipients, as shown by our matched-pair analysis. In our rescue and antirejection group, only one pancreas graft was lost due to rejection, demonstrating the potent immunosuppressive activity of FK 506. New-onset insulin-dependent diabetes mellitus was not noted in our induction and maintenance group, but several recipients experienced transient hyperglycemia (particularly during the treatment of concurrent rejection or infection episodes). Although the overall rate and the spectrum of infections with FK 506 and CsA appear to be similar, 2 recipients in our FK 506 induction and maintenance group died from EBV-related B-cell lymphomas early posttransplant. FK 506 seems to be a very promising and highly effective drug in pancreas transplantation, but future studies are necessary to determine its optimal use in minimizing the broad spectrum of side effects (including posttransplant lymphomas).

Acknowledgements The authors would like to thank Barbara McDonald for the preparation of the manuscript and Mary Knatterud for editorial assistance.

References

1. Cox KL, Lawrence-Miyaskai LS, Garcia-Kennedy R, et al (1995) An increased incidence of Epstein-Barr virus infection and lymphoproliferative disorder in young children on FK 506 after liver transplantation. Transplantation 59: 425

2. Gruessner RWG, Sutherland DER (1996) Clinical diagnosis in pancreatic allograft rejection. In: Solez K, Racusen LC, Billingham M, Dekker M (eds) Pathology and rejection diagnosis in solid organ transplantation. New York, pp 455–499

3. Hirano Y, Fujihara S, Ohara K, Katsuki S, Noguchi H (1992) Morphological and functional changes of islets of Langerhans in FK 506-treated rats. Transplantation 53: 889

4. Kaufman DC, Kaplan B, Kanwar Y, Abecassis M, Stuart F (1995) The successful use of tacrolimus (FK 506) in a pancreas/kidney transplant recipient with recurrent cyclosporine-associated hemolytic uremic syndrome. Transplantation 59: 1737–1739

5. Klintmalm G (1994) The U.S. Multi-center FK 506 Liver Study Group. A comparison of tacrolimus (FK 506) and cyclosporine for immunosuppression after liver transplantation. N Engl J Med 331: 1110

6. Reyes J, Tzakis AG, Bonet H, et al (1994) Lymphoproliferative disease after intestinal transplantation under primary FK 506 immunosuppression. Transplant Proc 26: 1426

7. Shaffer D, Simpson MA, Conway P, Madras PN, Monaco AP (1995) Normal pancreas allograft function following simultaneous pancreas kidney transplantation after rescue therapy with tacrolimus (FK 506). Transplantation 59: 1063

8. Shapiro R, Jordan ML, Scantlebury VP, et al (1995) A prospective randomized trial of FK 506-based immunosuppression after renal transplantation. Transplantation 59: 485

9. Teraoka S, Babazono T, Koike T, et al (1995) Effect of rescue therapy using FK 506 on relapsing rejection after combined pancreas and kidney transplantation. Transplant Proc 27: 1335

Transpl Int (1996) 9 [Suppl 1]: S 258–S 260
© Springer-Verlag 1996

S. Benz
F. Pfeffer
M. Büsing
M. R. Clemens
A. Waladkhani
H. D. Becker
U. T. Hopt

Liposoluble antioxidants are not consumed in the pancreas after reperfusion in human simultaneous pancreas-kidney transplantation

S. Benz (✉) · U. T. Hopt · F. Pfeffer
Chirurgische Universitätsklinik Rostock,
Schillingallee 35, D-18057 Rostock,
Germany

M. R. Clemens · A. R. Waladkhani
Medizinische Klinik der Universität
Tübingen, Hoppe Seyler Str.,
D-72076 Tübingen, Germany

H. D. Becker
Direktor der Chirurgischen
Universitätsklinik Tübingen,
Hoppe Seyler Str. 3, D-74076 Tübingen,
Germany

M. Büsing
Chirurgische Klinik,
Knappschaftskrankenhaus,
Bochum-Langendreer-Universitätsklinik,
In der Schornau, Bochum, Germany

Abstract There is considerable evidence that under experimental conditions, oxygen free radicals (OFRs) are decisive in the pathogenesis of ischemia-reperfusion injury. Normally OFRs are scavenged by antioxidants such as α-tocopherol. Thus, in the following study we investigated whether antioxidants are consumed locally in human pancreatic grafts after reperfusion. A series of ten patients receiving bladder-drained pancreaticoduodenal and renal allografts were studied. Sequential blood samples were drawn locally from the venous outflow of the graft and simultaneously from the radial artery after reperfusion. α-Tocopherol, retinol, lycopene, and α- and β-carotene levels were determined. After reperfusion these levels remained largely unchanged. Hence, in our study a consumption of antioxidants locally in the pancreatic graft after transplantation was not demonstrated. Therefore, the antioxidant capacity seems not to be exhausted at that time. This suggests that in clinical pancreatic transplantation oxidant stress in the initial reperfusion period might not have the relevance suggested by animal models.

Key words Antioxidants · Tocopherol · Graft pancreatitis · Oxygen free radicals · Pancreatic transplantation

Introduction

Graft pancreatitis is still a major obstacle in pancreas transplantation, causing significant postoperative morbidity [5]. Its pathophysiology is not yet fully understood. It is suspected, however, that ischemia-reperfusion injury is the main pathogenetic factor. Better organ preservation would therefore by highly desirable to improve survival of pancreatic grafts and to reduce postoperative morbidity. During the last few years there has been increasing evidence that oxygen free radicals (OFRs) are instrumental in the development of the ischemia-reperfusion injury of the pancreas. As the main sources of OFR formation, xanthin oxidase, mitochondrial sources, and activated leukocytes have been suggested [4, 8]. Experimental therapy in several animal models with radical scavengers or the administration of allopurinol markedly ameliorates tissue injury [11, 13, 15].

However, these are data from animal models using severly damaged organs under nonsurvival conditions. The mechanisms of ischemia-reperfusion injury in well-preserved organs might, however, differ significantly from these models. There are no conclusive data that scavenger treatment and the use of allopurinol have a significant influence on ischemia-reperfusion injury in human organ transplantation. We therefore conducted a study to assess the extent to which OFRs are involved in ischemia-reperfusion injury in clinical pancreatic transplantation.

Tocopherol is believed to be one of the main antioxidants that is involved in the defence against OFR-induced lipidperoxidation [3]. Like other antioxidants it is consumed in the scavenging process. Therefore, a decrease in an antioxidant in the blood is an indicator of OFR and lipid peroxide formation, and, in particular, tocopherol is considered to be a sensitive parameter to monitor oxidant stress in vivo [12].

Material and methods

A series of ten patients with type I diabetes mellitus and end-stage renal disease receiving bladder-drained pancreaticodoudenal and renal allografts from cadaveric donors were studied. Exclusion criteria for donors were age over 50 years, high-dose catecholamines, and significant abdominal trauma. The grafts were perfused with 2000–3000 ml University of Wisconsin (UW) solution (containing allopurinol at 136 mg/l). Cold ischemia time was 9.6 ± 3.6 h.

Patients had a median age of 39 years and a mean duration of diabetes of 19 years. The only strict contraindication was severe coronary heart disease, proven by coronary angiogram. Quadruple immunosuppression was started in all patients. During the dissection of the graft on the back-table a ch14 catheter was inserted in the distal part of the splenic vein. After reperfusion of the pancreas, sequential blood samples were drawn simultaneously from the venous outflow of the pancreas via the splenic vein of the graft and from the radial artery of the recipient at 0, 1, 2, 5, 10, 30, and 240 min after reperfusion. The samples were immediately put on ice, centrifuged, and stored at − 70 °C. α-Tocopherol, retinol, lycopene, α-carotene, and β-carotene levels were determined simultaneously by high-pressure liquid chromatography (HPLC). Cholesterol levels were determined by the standard CHOD/PAP method on an automatic analyzer. Values are expressed as an antioxidant to total cholesterol ratio (nmol/l antioxidant/mg/dl cholesterol). The degree of graft pancreatitis was assessed by peak C-reactive protein (CRP) levels within the first 24 h after reperfusion. These have previously been shown to correlate closely with the degree of graft pancreatitis. Statistical analysis was performed using linear regression and Student's t-test.

Results

The reperfusion the pancreas was homogeneous in 9 of 10 patients. In all patients slight edema and some fatty necrosis was noted at the end of the operation. Postoperatively in one patient severe graft pancreatitis with partial thrombosis of the splenic vein developed, which required necrectomy and thrombectomy of the pancreas graft. In two patients moderate graft pancreatitis was noted, which necessitated laparotomy in one case. All other patients showed mild signs of graft pancreatitis only. Initial endocrine function of the pancreas and initial renal function was achieved in all patients.

Preoperatively, the mean systemic antioxidant to cholesterol ratios of all antioxidants were close to the levels that are reported in the literature (tocopherol: 134.0 ± 46; retinol: 9.81 ± 2.7; lycopene: 2.2 ± 1.36, α-carotene: 0.4 ± 0.21; β-carotene: 2.6 ± 1.7). No correlation between antioxidant levels at the time of admission and the degree of graft pancreatitis (peak CRP) was found in any of the antioxidants investigated (Fig. 1). In fact, the patient who developed the worst graft pancreatitis had one of the highest preoperative levels of tocopherol (185.4).

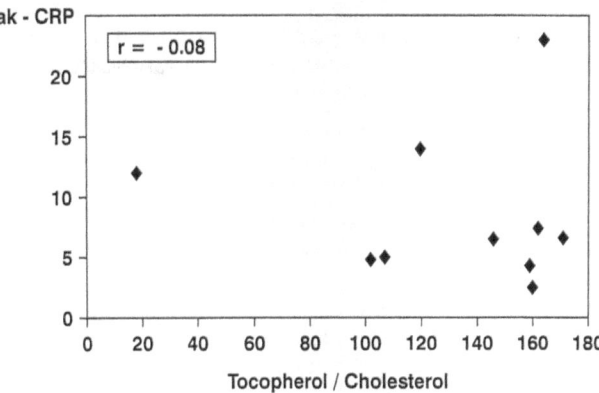

Fig. 1 Lack of correlation between peak CRP levels within the first 24 h after reperfusion of the graft and the α-tocopherol/cholesterol ratio

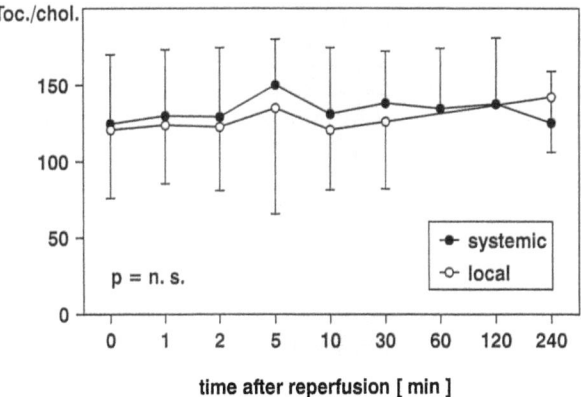

Fig. 2 Local and systemic α-tocopherol levels after reperfusion of the pancreatic graft. There is no significant difference between the systemic and the local levels

After reperfusion antioxidant levels remained largely unchanged, not only in the radial artery, but also in the splenic vein of the graft (Fig. 2). Only α-tocopherol and retinol showed some decrease (8.9 % and 10.4 %, respectively) in the splenic vein compared to the level in the radial artery. These differences, however, were not statistically significant.

Discussion

Serum levels of α-tocopherol have repeatedly been used to demonstrate the involvement of OFRs in ischemia-reperfusion injury. It has been shown several times that serum or tissue levels of α-tocopherol decrease during aortic cross-clamping [10] and in different organs during ischemia and reperfusion [1]. Furthermore, a fall in α-tocopherol serum levels in the systemic circulation after pancreatic ischemia in the rat responding to SOD/catalase treatment has been reported [11]. In addition, after reperfusion of kidney grafts, α-tocopherol has been reported to decrease significantly in the renal vein, as well as in the systemic circulation [14]. Hence, in our study a significant consumption should also have been expected. Suprisingly, in the clinical setting of pancreatic transplantation the levels of α-tocopherol, retinol, α- and β-carotene, and lycopene remained largely unchanged in the systemic circulation after reperfusion of the grafts. Even more striking, however, were our findings that in the venous effluent of the pancreata, no changes in antioxidant levels were found. Thus, our results clearly excluded a significant consumption of liposoluble antioxidants during and early after reperfusion of human pancreats grafts.

It has been demonstrated – at least in the rat liver – that oxidant stress after ischemia and reperfusion is nearly exclusively located extracellularly and for the most part even intravascularly [6, 7]. Hence, in our model significant oxidative stress after reperfusion should have been detected by measuring local antioxidant serum levels. Thus, it is reasonable to assume that the antioxidative capacity in human pancreats grafts is not a limiting factor in respect to the initiation of ischemia-reperfusion injury. This implies, however, that in clinical pancreatic transplantation, mechanisms other than mas-

sive lipidperoxidation by OFRs might be relevant in the development of ischemia-reperfusion injury. One of these mechanisms might be the induction of adhesion molecules on the endothelium by the ischemia itself or by low concentrations of OFRs and radical species that are not capable of lipidperoxidation [16].

Our results don't exclude the possibility that low amounts of OFRs trigger a cascade of noxious events that eventually results in the well-known ischemia-reperfusion injury. It seems unlikely however, that most of the organ damage is mediated by the direct effect of large amounts of OFRs leading to massive lipidperoxidation. This could also explain the finding that in human kidney transplantation treatment with SOD is not able to reduce ischemia-reperfusion injury significantly [2]. Therefore, it seems doubtful that antioxidative therapy will further ameliorate the present standard of human pancreatic graft preservation. Recent evidence that polymorphonuclear neutrophil (PMN) depletion attenuates ischemia-reperfusion injury [9] in different organs rather suggests that prevention of PMN adhesion and activation might be a more promising approach in the treatment of ischemia-reperfusion injury in human pancreats transplantation.

References

1. Abe K, Yoshida S, Watson B, Busto R, Kogure K, Ginsberg MD (1983) Tocopherol and ubichinone in rat brain subjected to decapitation ischemia. Brain Res 273: 166–169
2. Abendroth D, Schneeberger S, Schleibner S, Illner WD, Land W (1992) Stellenwert der Behandlung mit Radikalfängern nach Nieren- und Pankreastransplantation Zentralbl Chir 117: 502–508
3. Burton GW, Joyce A, Ingold KU (1983) Is vitamin E the only lipisoluble chain breaking antioxidant in human blood plasma and erythrocytes membranes? Arch Biochem Biophys 221: 1–10
4. Granger N (1988) The role of xanthine oxidase and granulocytes in ischemia – and reperfusion injury. Am J Physiol 255: 1269–1275
5. Hopt UT, Büsing M, Schareck WD, Becker HD (1992) Management der exocrinen Pankreasekretion. Ein zentrales Problem der allogenen Pankreastransplantation. Chirurg 63: 186–192
6. Jaeschke H (1991) Vascular oxidant stress and hepatic ischemia/reperfusion injury Free Radic Res Commun 12: 737–743
7. Jaeschke HJ (1991) Reactive oxygen and ischemia/reperfusion injury in the rat liver Chem Biol Interact 79: 115–133
8. Jaeschke H, Farhood A, Smith W (1990) Neutrophils contribute to ischemia/reperfusion injury in rat liver in vivo. FASEB J 4: 3355–3359
9. Jaeschke H, Farhood A, Bautista P, Zoltan S, Spitzer J, Smith W (1993) Functional inactivation of neutrophils with a Mac-1 (CD11b/CD18) monoclonal antibody protects against ischemia- and reperfusion injury in rat liver. Hepatology 17: 915–923
10. Murphy ME, Kolvenbach R, Aleksis M, Hansen R, Sies H (1992) Antioxidant depletion in aortic crossclamping ischemia: increase in the plasma level of tocopherol quinone/tocopherol ratio. Free Radic Bio Med 13: 95–100
11. Oda T, Nakai I, Mituo H, Oka T, Yoshikawa T (1992) Role of oxygen free radicals and the synergistic effect of dismutase and catalase on ischemia-reperfusion injury of the rat pancreas. Transplant Proc 24: 797–798
12. Pincemail J, Defraigne JO, Franssen C, Bonnet P, Deby-Dupont G, Pirenne J, Deby C, Lamy M, Limet M, Meurisse M (1993) Evidence for free radical formation during human kindey transplantation. Free Radic Bio Med 15: 343–348
13. Sanfey H, Sarr M, Bulkley G, Cameron J (1986) Oxygen-free radicals and acute pancreatitis. Acta Physiol Scand [Suppl] 548: 109–118
14. Serino F, Citterio F, Lippa S, Oradei A, Agnes S, Nanni G, Pozzetto A, Littarru G, Castagneto M (1990) Coenzyme Q, alpha-tocopherol, and delayed function in human kidney transplantation. Transplant Proc 22: 1375–1378
15. Tamura K, Manabe T, Kyogoku T, Andoh K, Ohshio G, Tobe T (1993) Effect of postischemic reperfusion on the pancreas. Hepatogastroenterology 40: 452–454
16. Welbourn C, Goldmann G, Paterson I, Valeri CR, Shepro D, Hechtmann HB (1991) Pathophysiology of ischemia and reperfusion injury: central role of the neutrophil. Br J Surg 78: 651–655

Small Bowel

Transpl Int (1996) 9 [Suppl 1]: S263–S268
© Springer-Verlag 1996

F. Fändrich
T. Jahnke
J. Peters
B. Exner
A. Papachrysanthou
N. Zavazava

Circumvention of natural killer cell and T-cell mediated allogeneic target killing with tacrolimus (FK 506) in small bowel transplantation related graft-vs-host disease

F. Fändrich (✉) · T. Jahnke · B. Exner ·
A. Papachrysanthou
Department of General and Thoracic
Surgery, University of Kiel,
Arnold-Heller-Strasse 7, D-24105 Kiel,
Germany

J. Peters
Institute of Pathology, University of Kiel,
Kiel, Germany

N. Zavazava
Institute of Immunology, University of
Kiel, Kiel, Germany

Abstract The role of simultaneous donor-specific transfusion of unprocessed cellular bone marrow (BM) together with solid organ transplantation, a postulated concept to achieve long-term graft acceptance, was investigated in an experimental setting of semiallogeneic transplantation of parental small bowel (SBTx) to F1 hybrids. The established graft-vs-host (GvH) model revealed that simultaneous transfer of SB/BM substantially enhanced GvH-mediated immune responses in recipient target organs, e.g. skin, gut, and liver. In comparison to isolated SBTx, animal survival decreased from 16.1($\pm$ 0.9) to 10.1($\pm$ 0.8) days after additional BM transfusion, $P < 0.001$. Severe tissue injury of GvH-susceptible target organs in the setting of simultaneous SB and BMTx was associated with significant changes in recruitment and tissue distribution of NKR-P1$^+$ cells during the GvH-related proliferative immune response. Tacrolimus effectively suppressed these initial events and prevented recipient animals from clinically and histologically observed damage caused by GvH disease.

Key words Small bowel transplantation · Tacrolimus · Microchimerism · Natural killer cells · NKR-P1 receptor

Introduction

After the causal relationship of hematopoietic chimerism to drug-free immunological tolerance had been established by Billingham, Brent, and Medawar [1], their findings were implicated in further experimental [2] and clinical settings [3]. The idea to transplant cells of bone marrow or lymphatic origin and solid organs from the same donor simultaneously was based on the assumption of augmented mutual recognition by two-way migration of "passenger leucocytes" exchanged between graft and host. Besides, the concept was based on the detection of donor-derived cells in tissues of human recipients with functioning kidney [4] and liver [5] grafts, 10–30 years posttransplantation. The chimeric state in these patients had developed, irrespective of the various immunosuppressive protocols applied, while some patients had been off all immunosuppressive medication. In contrast, there is now a large body of evidence from clinical and experimental data which outline the inherent difficulty in separating cause from effect in the framework of cellular chimerism [6–8]. The study of Bushell et al. [7] indicated that the short-term persistence and presentation of donor-derived antigen, rather than the development of microchimerism, is the critical factor in the induction of operational tolerance.

So far not focused on as a relevant subject of discussion in the context of combined bone marrow plus solid organ transplantation is a non-adaptive killing mechanism also designated "allogeneic lymphocyte cytotoxicity" (ALC). ALC is mediated by natural killer (NK) cells (NKR-P1$^+$, CD3$^-$ cells) and characterized as allospecific lysis of lymphocytes and cells of hematopoietic origin. After allogeneic challenge of an MHC-disparate host with either one of these cells, host NK cells eliminate the non-self target cells within 6 to 12 h and without the need for a prior antigen-specific sensitization step [9, 10]. Activation of the host NK cell population is associated with increased release of important cytokines, such as γ-IFN, TNF-α, and IL-2 [11, 12]. Early NK cell production of IFN-γ is necessary to promote MHC class II antigen processing and presentation by macrophages and the development of Th1 T cells [13]. This experimental study was designed to investigate the impact of coincidentally administered donor bone marrow (BM) in a graft-vs-host (GvH) model of small bowel transplantation (SBTx) on: (1) the clinical course and histological grade of graft-vs-host disease (GvHD) in lymphatic and non-lymphatic targets, (2) the migration and tissue distribution of NK cells, (3) the immunoregulatory role of NK cells on T-cell proliferation during the initial recipient immune response, and (4) the T-cell-mediated immune responses of F1 recipients under immunsuppressive treatment with tacrolimus.

Material and methods

Animal groups

A GvH model was established by heterotopic transplantation of male DA[Rt1^{aaavl}] parental small bowel on F1 hybrids, a crossing between male DA and female LEW[Rt1^l] inbred rats weighing between 160 and 250 g. Animals were raised and maintained under conventional animal facilities and screened routinely for common rat pathogens. Heterotopic SBTx was performed as previously reported [14]. Bone marrow cells were obtained from femurs, tibiae, and humeri of sacrified donor strain (DA) rats. After flushing the bones through a 100 µg Nytex filter with a sterile needle and Hank's balanced salt solution (HBSS) cells were washed three times and counted. T-cells were not depleted. After suspension of 5×10^7 bone marrow cells in 1 ml of HBSS, the transplant was infused into the penile vein of the F1 recipient rat. The following experimental groups ($n = 6$) were included into this study: (1) DA(SB)>F1, no treatment (NT), (2) DA(SB + 5×10^7 BM cells) > F1, (3) DA(SB) > F1, FK 506, 1 mg/kg body weight, day 0–14, i.m., and (4) F1(SB) > F1, NT.

Histology

Tissue specimens were harvested on postoperative days (POD) 3, 7, 10, and 14 after HSBTx. Note, however, that in group II only two animals lived for 12 days and one animal for 14 days. These animals were pooled for histological comparison at POD 14. Tissue specimens were sliced into small pieces, either snap-frozen in liquid nitrogen and stored at –80 °C or subjected to 10 % buffered formaldehyde, embedded in paraffin, cut into 4 µm sections, and stained with hematoxylin and eosin. Immunohistological analysis was performed using an indirect APAAP-staining technique. Histological evaluation of the tissue specimens was performed by two observers who had not been informed of the experimental group by grading six different sections of each specimen. Hereby, the number of positive staining cells were counted in serial tissue sections using the photographic view finder of a Zeiss Photomicroscope at 630× magnification under oil immersion (area = 0.030 mm²) and were expressed as numbers of positive cells per

Table 1 Degree of graft-vs-host disease according to clinical and autoptic findings following heterotopic small bowel transplantation. For appropriate classification, each animal had to demonstrate at least three of the listed items for grades I, II, or III. Animals which demonstrated two features of two different columns were assigned to the appropriate grade of GvH according to the histological pattern of tissue lesions (*MLN* mesenteric lymph nodes)

	Grade I	Grade II	Grade III
Weight loss	0–10 %	10–20 %	> 20 %
Appearance	Redness of eyes paws, snout, diarrhea	Piloerection	Listlessness, hunched posture
Spleen index	1–2	2–5	> 5
Volume of MLN	1–1.5	1.5–3	> 3

unit tissue area. Conventional criteria were used to diagnose four different grades of GvHD: (1) grade 0 (none), (2) grade I (moderate); (3) grade II (acute), and (4) grade III (severe), as outlined in Tables 1, 2.

Preparation of splenocytes and mesenteric lymph nodes

Donor and recipient mesenteric lymph nodes and recipient spleens were excised, minced, and pressed gently through a 60-gauge-mesh stainless steal screen into HBSS. Lymph node lymphocytes and splenocytes were obtained by centrifugation on Ficoll-Hypaque gradients (density = 1.077) at 300 × g for 20 min at room temperature. After collection of the mononuclear cells from the gradient interface they were resuspended in RPMI-FBS, washed three times, and immediately used in the experiments described.

Mixed Lymphocyte Reaction

Freshly isolated spleen cells from control and experimental rats of groups 1 to 4 were cultured in triplicate in 0.2 ml complete medium at a concentration of 1×10^5 cells/well in the presence or absence of phytohemagglutinin (PHA) in 96-well flat-bottomed microplates together with 3×10^5 irradiated (2000 rad) stimulator cells. After 96 h of incubation at 37 °C in 5 % CO$_2$/95 % air, cells were pulsed with 1 µCi of [³H]thymidine and subsequently harvested for measurement of radioactivity in a liquid-scintillation spectrometer 18 h later.

Statistics

Animal survival rates were calculated according to Kaplan-Meier life-table analysis using the statistical program package of Astute Module 1, Statistics Add-in for Microsoft Excel, University of Leeds, UK. Differences in survival between the various groups were assessed using the generalized Savage (Mantel-Cox) logrank test. Deaths secondary to technical complications (with functioning grafts) were censored. The F-test was used to test for equality of the variances of the two samples to be compared. Depending on the results of the F-test, Student's *t*-test for equal or unequal variances was used for further analysis.

Table 2 Degree of graft-vs-host disease according to histological findings following heterotopic small bowel transplantation. Each animal was classified histologically according to histological evaluation of eight different specimen, small bowels *(SB)*, mesenteric lymph nodes *(MLN)*, and peyer patches *(PP)* of donor and recipient origin and skin and liver of the host. Grade I, II, or III was diagnosed, if in four of the eight analyzed specimen the designated histological features were present

	Grade I	Grade II	Grade III
SB mucosa	Reduction of villus height, mononuclear cellular infiltrate of lamina propria	Crypt necrosis, clubbing of villi, sloughing of villi, apoptotic cells 2–4/6 crypts	Necrotizing enteritis, epithelial replacement with granulation tissue, apoptotic cells > 4/6 crypts
MLN, PP, spleen	Appearance of histocytoid cells, plasma cells, immunoblasts	Immunoplastic proliferation, circumscribed lymphoid depletion	Loss of follicular architecture, stromal fibrosis, necrosis, depletion of lymphocytes
Skin	Spongiosis and vacuolation of upper dermis	Cell necrosis (apoptosis), lymphocytic infiltration	Polymophonuclear cell infiltration
Liver	Mild portal tract infiltration with mononuclear cells (< 10)	Enhanced infiltration of portal fields with mononuclear cells (10–20)	Liver parenchyma and portal fields are infiltrated, bile duct lesions, endothelialitis of central veins

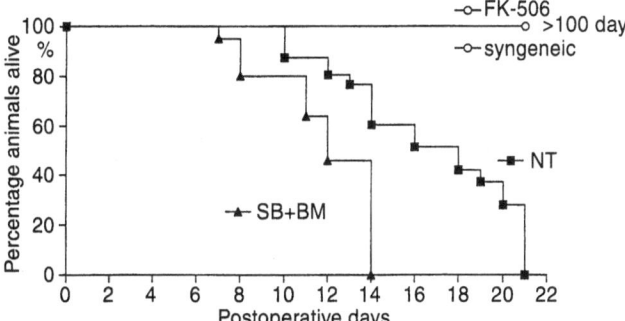

Fig. 1 Survival after DA-parental SBTx of untreated (NT; *n* = 24), DA small bowel plus bone marrow transplanted (SB + BM; *n* = 9), tacrolimus (FK 506; *n* = 10) immunosuppressed, and F1 small bowel transplanted F1 recipient animals (syngeneic; *n* = 10) is depicted. Simultaneous transplantation of parental DA small bowel and 5×10^7 bone marrow cells significantly decreased the mean survival of 16.1 ($\pm$ 0.9) days in group I to 10.1 ($\pm$ 0.8) days, *P* > 0.001. Median survival was determined by the method of Kaplan and Meier. Univariate comparisons of survival was calculated with the log-rank test

Results

Simultaneous transplantation of unprocessed DA-parental BM plus SB into F1 recipients severely impaired the hosts immune response to cope with GvH-related donor immunogenicity. As Fig. 1 illustrates, mean survival of F1 hybrids was significantly reduced to 10.1 ($\pm$ 0.8) days in comparison to 16.1 ($\pm$ 0.9) days after isolated SBTx. Individual survival of the four different investigated groups is summarized in Table 3. Three F1 animals which received combined DA BM/SB were immunsuppressed with FK 506 according to the protocol of group III. Similar to F1 hybrids of groups III and IV, these animals did not suffer from GvHD and showed long-term graft acceptance > 100 days (data not shown). Beside the observed decrease in life ex-

pectancy, animals of group II presented with significantly higher grades of GvHD and a more rapid onset and clinical progression of GvHD including severe diarrhea, weight loss, hunched posture, and massive enlargement of the spleen and MLNs, as catagorized in Tables 1, 2. In conjuction with BMTx, non-lymphatic target tissues, such as recipient gut, skin, and liver, were profoundly impaired as GvHD progressed. Skin lesions included vast damage to epidermis and upper dermis with concomitant infiltration of mononuclear and polymorphonuclear cells. Liver injury related to the donor-derived cytotoxic immune attack showed characteristic features of mononuclear cell infiltration of portal fields, bile duct lesions, and, in some cases, substantial damage to vessel endothelium. Table 4 summarizes the most important data on clinical and histological changes gathered from animals which succumbed to GvHD.

Immunohistochemical analysis of NKR-P1$^+$ cells by use of 3.2.3-mAb in various splenic compartments at POD 3 and 10 was performed to investigate cell frequency, distribution, and migration pattern of this cellular lymphocyte subset. Autographic studies from [^{3}H]-uridine-labeled T- and B cells have traced these lymphocytes for a 24 h period after i. v. injection and revealed that allogeneic lymphocytes had been destroyed within the T-cell areas of both the lymph nodes and the spleen white pulp at 3 h after injection. Fragments of the destroyed cells could be detected inside large non-lymphoid cells of the lymph node paracortex and spleen periarteriolar lymphocyte sheath (PALS) and not in the marginal zone and red pulp of the spleen, where NK cells normally reside [15, 16]. Therefore, our interest was focused on the distribution pattern of NKR-P1$^+$ cells within various, functionally distinguishable, splenic compartments in the four different experimental settings as summarized in Fig. 2 A, B. At POD 14, groups I and II differed significantly from groups III and IV in

Table 3 Survival after small bowel transplantation from DA to F1 (DA × LEW) rats

Group	Donor	Recipient	Treatment	Number	Survival (days × number)	Mean ± SEM
I	DA	F1	SB	24	10 × 4, 12 × 2, 13 × 1, 14 × 4, 16 × 2, 18 × 2, 19 × 1, 20 × 2, 21 × 6	16.1 ± 0.9
II	DA	F1[a]	SB + BM	9	7 × 1, 8 × 3, 11 × 2, 12 × 2, 14 × 1	10.1 ± 0.8[b]
III	DA	F1[c]	SB + FK 506	10	> 100 × 10	> 100
IV	F1	F1	SB	10	> 100 × 10	> 100

[a] F1 recipients received DA-parental small bowel and 5×10^7 unprocessed bone marrow cells, i. v.
[b] P > 0.001 for group I vs group II (according to Mantel-Cox log-rank test)
[c] F1 recipients received DA-parental small bowel and were immunosuppressed with 1 mg FK 506/kg body weight, i. m. from day 0 to day 14

Table 4 Effect of simultaneous SB/BMTx on the grade and clinical course of GvHD

Experimental group n (%)	Clinical and histological grade of GvHD				First signs of GvHD (day ± SD)	Duration of GvHD (days ± SD)
	None	I	II	III		
No treatment (n = 24)	5 (20.8)[a]	6 (25)	6 (25)	7 (29.2)	10.2 (± 1.2)	7.3 (± 2.4)
DA(SB + BM) (n = 9)	None	1 (11)	2 (22)	6 (67)	5.7 (± 0.7)[b]	3.75 (± 0.7)[c]

[a] These 5 animals without signs of GvHD suffered and died from peritonitis and sepsis due to a paradoxical immune response with substantial injury of their parental small bowel grafts and mesenteric lymph nodes
[b] Combined SB + BMTx treated animals suffered from more severe and progressive GvHD with significant earlier appearance of GvHD symptoms as compared to host animals without additional transfer of DA-parental bone marrow cells (P < 0.001)
[c] The enhanced severity of GvHD in F1 hosts after simulaneous SB + BMTx was also mirrored in a shorter clinical course of GvHD until death in these animals as compared to untreated animals (P < 0.0001)

NK cell density, both in the area around the central artery of germinal follicles and in the area of the PALS. There is indirect evidence that in the BM/SB group high numbers of these NK cells are of F1 origin since flow cytometric analysis showed that 35 % of the gated F1 splenocytes were OX-3[+], a LEW MHC class II antigen specific marker which does not cross-react with DA epitopes. Among the OX-3[+] cells, 20 % were NKR-P1[+]/OX-3[+] and 9 % NKR-P1[+]/OX-3[−], in contrast to group I animals were no NKR-R1[+]/OX-3[+] double-positive cells were detected among the 18.6 % OX-3[+] lymphocytes, data not shown. Altogether, NKR-P1[+] cells comprised 15.9 %(± 2.4) of gated splenocytes in group II in contrast to 12.3 %(± 9.9) NK cells in group I. This clearly indicates that additional transfer of donor-specific bone marrow increases the percentage of F1 NK cells and stimulates the upregulation of MHC class II molecules on the surface of these cells. The large amount of NK cells entering the spleen at POD 14 via the central artery (Fig. 2 A), basically homed to the red pulp medullary areas in the spleen. Conversely, at POD 3, high numbers of NK cells were recognized within the marginal zone in all allogeneic groups (I–III) and apparently differed from syngeneic animals where NK cells basically resided in the red pulp. The fact that high densities of NK cells were found in those areas where recirculating lymphocytes normally pass during the initial "proliferative" phase of GvHD (marginal zones of lymph nodes and spleen) emphasize findings of others [15] that lymphocyte killing on one side and cell fragmentation and antigen presentation on the other side might not be spatially and temporally coinciding events. Immunosuppressive treatment of F1 recipients efficiently inhibited NK cell activity and proliferation, as mirrored in Fig. 2 A, B which demonstrate that the migration pattern and distribution within the spleen of FK-treated rats is very similar to syngeneically transplanted animals.

In addition to these findings, T-cell-mediated proliferation responses of freshly harvested F1 splenocytes to F1 syngeneic responder cells was investigated using one-way mixed lymphocyte cultures. Figure 3 gives evidence that combined SB/BMTx led to increased anti-F1 responses, as early as 3 days after transplantation of DA-parental grafts. These results are consistent with the early onset and rapid progression of GvHD in this group, as described above. The increasing percentage of DA immunocompetent cells among recipient splenocytes, hence, considerably enhanced the T-cell response against host stimulator cells at POD 10. Tacrolimus treatment significantly decreased anti-host-directed T-cell activity after DA-parental SBTx. However, whereas

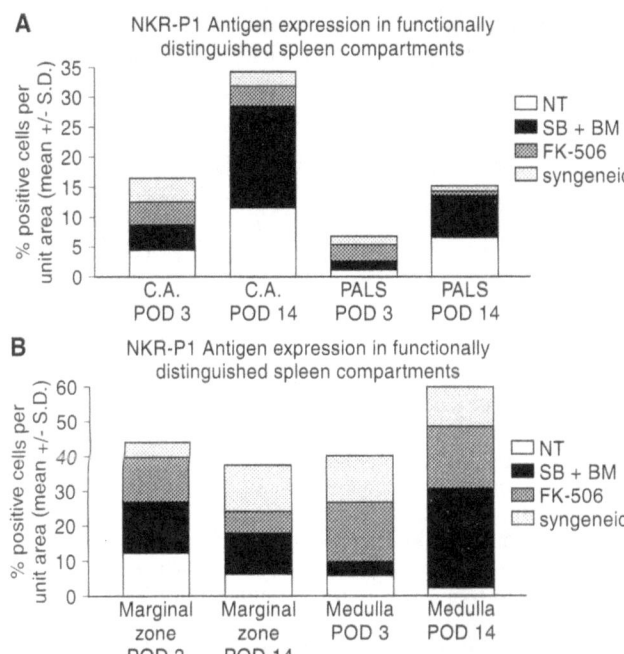

Fig. 2 A, B Four, anatomically and functionally distinguishable compartments within the spleen of F1 recipients were analyzed and evaluated independently by two observers without knowledge of the experimental groups. Each column presents the mean of six different areas of 0.030 mm² for each designated structural unit, using a Zeiss photomicroscope at 630 × magnification under oil immersion. Values of six animals per group have been averaged and are expressed as numbers of positive cells per unit tissue. (*C. A.* Central artery of a germinal follicle, *PALS* periarteriolar lymphocyte sheath)

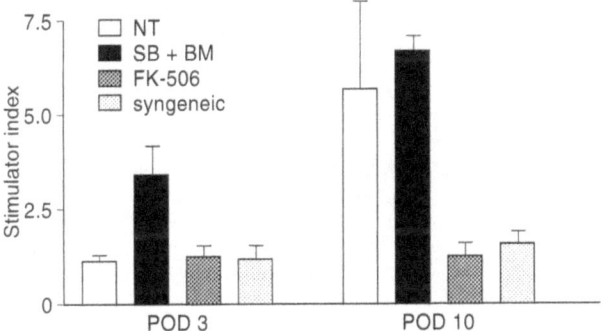

Fig. 3 [³H]Thymidine incorporation assays were performed. One-way MLR was performed with freshly isolated F1 splenocytes used as responder cells and co-cultured with DA or F1 irridiated (2000 rad) stimulator cells. Varying numbers of stimulator cells were mixed in triplicate with F1 responder cells. Columns represent the mean of 6–10 experiments consisting of two pooled rats per experiment. Stimulator index was calculated as E/C, where E = cpm of [³H]thymidine-treated responder cells cocultured with irridiated stimulator cells and C = cpm of [³H]thymidine-treated responder cells not cocultered with stimulator cells. Notice the increased anti-F1 proliferation response in group II animals at POD 3 and 10

splenocytes from F1 recipients of the syngeneic group were still able to proliferate in response to third party stimulator cells, this response was suppressed in FK 506 treated animals (not shown).

Discussion

Coutinho [17] and Cohen [18] have outlined the importance of sustained lymphocyte activity in complex communicating networks as a prerequisite to acquiring transplantation tolerance at a postthymic peripheral level. According to their views, the immunological step for "self"-recognition is linked more to activation of "connected" lymphocytes than to suppression of alloreactive clones. In this framework of operating immune networks, successful transfer of network components, defined by the donor, is required to assure donor-specific tolerance to the graft. According to Starzl et al. [5] this might be achieved by augmentation of cell chimerism in conjunction with non-specific immunosuppression. He speculates that unspecific immunosuppressive drugs exert a "permissive" effect, allowing for mutual recognition, activation and, finally, non-reactivity of engaging donor and recipient derived immunocompetent cells. In this context, the herein presented study explored the significance of increased graft immunogenicity by additional donor-specific BMTx on non-adaptive and cell-mediated immune response patterns in a GvH model of SBTx. NK cells, by virtue of their ability to elicit ALC and various cytokines, function as regulators of myeloid precursor cells and of extramedullary myelopoiesis in the spleen [19]. In fact, we were able to demonstrate that additional transfer of donor-derived BM significantly increased the percentage and density of NKR-P1⁺ cells at sites of antigen recognition (marginal zones, PALS) in close vicinity to interdigitating dendritic cells, concomitant with MHC class II antigen upregulation on NK cells, at POD 10 and later. Besides, BMTx stimulated "homing" mechanisms of NK cells to the medullary areas of recipient spleens via the central follicle arteries. The strategic position of NK cells close to or within the vascular network implicates a high statistical probalility of encountering donor-specific allografted BM and stem cells, which both have been demonstrated to be susceptible to NK cell killing [20]. Our own observations conclusively showed that the initial host NK cell activity following an allogeneic challenge strictly correlated with the degree of GvHD, with F1 host survival, and with anti-parental T-cell responses (submitted for publication). Conversely, BMTx coincided with increased levels of anti-host T-cell activity, suppressed under FK 506 treatment. Whether activation of host activity by BMTx is related to augmented long-term chimerism cannot be answered with this study. However, higher initial lysis of alloantigeneic cells generated by host NK cells led to high levels of processed alloantigen, a crucial factor in the induction of operational tolerance [7].

Acknowledgements The work reported herein was supported, in part, by the Deutsche Forschungsgemeinschaft (DFG), Bonn, Germany, grant code: Fa 295/1–1.

References

1. Billingham RE, Brent L, Medawar P (1956) Quantitative studies on tissue transplantation immunity. III. Actively acquired tolerance. Philos Trans R Soc London SerB 239: 357–412
2. Slavin S, Strober S, Fuks Z, Kaplan HS (1977) Induction of specific tissue transplantation tolerance using fractionated total lymphoid irradiation in adult mice. Long-term survival of allogeneic bone marrow and skin grafts. J Exp Med 146: 34–48
3. Starzl TE, Demetris AJ, Trucco M, Ramos H, Zeevi A, Rudert WA, Kocova M, Ricordi C, Ildstad S, Murase N (1992) Systemic chimerism in human female recipients of male livers. Lancet 340: 876–877
4. Starzl TE, Demetris AJ, Trucco M, Zeevi A, Ramos H, Terasaki P, Rudert WA, Kocova M, Ricordi C, Ildstad S, Murase N (1993) Chimerism and donor-specific nonreactivity 27 to 29 years after kidney allotransplantation. Transplantation 55: 1272–1277
5. Starzl TE, Demetris AJ, Trucco M, Murase N, Ricordi C, Ildstad S, Ramos H, Todo S, Tzakis A, Fung JJ, Nalesnik M, Zeevi A, Rudert WA, Kocova M Cell migration and chimerism after whole organ transplantation: the basis of graft acceptance. Hepatology 17: 1127–1152
6. Lechler RI, Batchelor JR (1982) Restoration of immunogenicity to passenger cell-depleted kidney allografts by the addition of donor-strain dendritic cells. J Exp Med 155: 31–41
7. Bushell A, Pearson TC, Morris PJ, Wood KJ (1995) Donor-recipient microchimerism is not required for tolerance induction following recipient pretreatment with donor-specific transfusion and anti-CD 4 antibody: Evidence of a clear role for short-term antigen persistence. Transplantation 59: 1367–1371
8. Schlitt HJ, Hundrieser J, Ringe B, Pichlmayr R (1994) Donor-type microchimerism associated with graft rejection eight years after liver transplantation. N Eng J Med 330: 646–647
9. Naper C, Vaage JT, Lambracht D, Lovik G, Butcher GW, Wonigeit K, Rolstad B (1995) Alloreactive natural killer cells in the rat: complex genetics of major histocompatibility complex control. Eur J Immunol 25: 1249–1256
10. Rolstad B, Fossum S, Bazin H, Kimber I, Marshall J, Sparshott SM, Ford WL (1985) The rapid rejection of allogeneic lymphocytes by a non-adaptive, cell-mediated mechanism (NK activity). Immunology 54: 127–138
11. Biassoni R, Ferrini S, Prigione I, Pelak VS, Sekaly RP, Long EO (1991) Activated CD3 CD16 + natural killer cells express a subset of the lymphokine genes induced in activated $\alpha \beta^+$ and $\gamma \delta^+$ T cells. Scand J Immunol 33: 247–252
12. Bankhurst AD, Imir T (1989) The mechanisms involved in the activation of human natural killer cells by staphylococcal enterotoxin β. Cell Immunol 122: 108–122
13. Manetti R, Parronchi P, Giudizi MG, Piccinni MP, Maggi E, Trinchieri G, Romagnani S (1993) Natural killer cell stimulatory factor (interleukin 12[IL-12]) induces T helper type 1 (TH1)-specific immune responses and inhibits the development of IL-4 producing cells. J Exp Med 177: 1199–1204
14. Fändrich F, Waaga AM, Schröder J, Schweizer E, Schroeder P (1994) Tissue dependent alteration of the MHC-I and -II expression after the use of deoxyspergualin for suppression of the graft-versus-host disease in small bowel transplantation. Transplant Proc 26: 1592–1593
15. Fossum S, Rolstad B (1986) The roles of interdigitating cells (IDC) and natural killer (NK) cells in the rapid rejection of allogeneic lymphocytes. Eur J Immunol 16: 440–450
16. Rolstad B, Herberman RB, Reynolds CW (1986) Natural killer cell activity in the rat. V. The circulation patterns and tissue localization of peripheral blood large granular lymphocytes (LGL). J Immunol 136: 2800–2809
17. Coutinho A (1989) Beyond clonal selection and network. Immunol Rev 110: 63–87
18. Cohen IR (1992) The cognitive paradigm and the immunological homunculus. Immunol Today 13: 490–492
19. Hansson M, Petersson M, Koo GC, Wigzell H, Kiessling R (1988) In vivo function of natural killer cells as regulators of myeloid precursor cells in the spleen. Eur J Immunol 18: 485–488
20. Murphy WJ, Kumar V, Bennett M (1987) Acute rejection of murine bone marrow allografts by natural killer cells and T cells. J Exp Med 166: 1499–1509

Transpl Int (1996) 9 [Suppl 1]: S 269–S 274
© Springer-Verlag 1996

R. E. Nakhleh
A. C. Gruessner
J. Pirenne
E. Benedetti
C. Troppmann
R. W. G. Gruessner

Colon vs small bowel rejection after total bowel transplantation in a pig model

R. E. Nakhleh
Department of Pathology, Henry Ford
Hospital, Detroit, MI 48202, USA

A. C. Gruessner · J. Pirenne · E. Benedetti ·
C. Troppmann · R. W. G. Gruessner (✉)
Department of Surgery, Box 90 UMHC,
University of Minnesota, Minneapolis,
MN 55455, USA

Abstract With the advent of
FK506, small bowel transplantation
has become clinically feasible. Both
clinically and experimentally, jejunal and ileal biopsies are used for
early diagnosis of rejection. More
recently, the colon, in addition to the
small bowel, has been transplanted
to decrease the high incidence of diarrhea after small bowel transplantation. A Bishop-Koop ileostomy
allows biopsies on a regular basis,
but the diagnosis of rejection remains a problem after takedown of
the ileostomy. Rejection of the ileum is more frequent and more severe than rejection of the jejunum or
the colon. Colon biopsy after ileostomy takedown would not rule out
rejection of the ileum.

Key words Small bowel · Rejection
· Transplantation · Colon · FK 506

Introduction

The advent of FK506 has made small bowel transplantation a clinical reality [1]. Nevertheless, immunologic problems (e. g., rejection, graft-vs-host disease
[GvHD], lymphoma) and infections continue to compli-
cate the posttransplant course of small bowel recipients.
An additional difficulty is the development of posttransplant diarrhea, frequently requiring hospitalization secondary to dehydration. In an attempt to decrease stomal
output and prolong intestinal transit time, the ileocecal
valve and the colon have been added to the small bowel
graft [2]. However, the increased lymphatic mass associated with a total bowel (vs small bowel alone) transplant
might increase the risk of rejection.

Diagnosing rejection in bowel recipients has been
difficult due to the lack of suitable laboratory parameters. In most bowel transplant recipients, an ileostomy
is created at the time of transplant, in order to do posttransplant biopsies to monitor rejection. But very little
is known about the hierarchy of rejection between the
jejunum, ileum, and colon after total bowel transplantation. We studied in a preclinical model the incidence of
rejection in all three grafts to determine: (1) which portion of the intestine was most prone to rejection and
(2) whether reliable monitoring of rejection after ileostomy takedown was possible by obtaining endoscopic
biopsies from the jejunum or colon.

Material and methods

For this experiment, 70 outbred Yorkshire Landrace pigs were randomized as donors or recipients. Five total bowel transplant recipient groups were included: cyclosporin A (CsA) treated pigs
($n = 7$), FK506 treated pigs ($n = 5$), combined bone marrow and total bowel transplant pigs ($n = 8$), bone marrow and total bowel
transplant pigs treated with FK506 pigs ($n = 11$), and combined
liver and total bowel transplant ($n = 4$). For premedication, atropine (0.2 mg/kg intramuscularly) and thiopental sodium (30 mg/kg
intravenously) were used. General anesthesia was maintained
with 3 % isoflurane. Donor pigs were fasted for 72 h before procurement. Magnesium citrate was given for bowel preparation,
and bowel decontamination was not done. Recipient pigs were
fasted for 24 h pretransplant.

Donor operation

Through a midline incision, the portal vein was dissected free from
below the uncinate process up to the level of the liver hilum. The
pancreas was divided anterior to the portal vein, the splenic vein
was ligated and cut, and all pancreaticoduodenal veins were di-

vided. The small bowel was divided proximally (third portion of the duodenum) and the large bowel was divided at the sigmoid colon. The superior mesenteric artery was then identified at its takeoff from the aorta. An aortic tube was dissected free that contained the celiac trunk, which was then ligated. The distal aorta was looped and made ready for perfusion with University of Wisconsin organ preservation solution. Venous drainage was through the distal vena cava. Benchwork preparation of the graft consisted of ligation of the posterior lumbar arteries, then closure with Prolene 5/0 continuous suture of the aortic stump distal to the takeoff of the superior mesenteric artery.

Recipient operation

Total bowel transplantation

The native small and the native large bowel were completely resected, from the third portion of the duodenum up to the sigmoid colon. A Kocher maneuver exposed the recipient portal vein. After systemic heparinization (3 000 units), the infrarenal aorta was clamped and the end-to-side anastomosis of the donor aortic tube to the recipient aorta was done using Prolene 5/0 continuous suture. The recipient portal vein was clamped longitudinally and the donor portal vein was anastomosed to the recipient portal vein, in a piggyback fashion, with Prolene 6/0 continuous suture. Mannitol, bicarbonate, and complementary intravenous fluid were given immediately before graft reperfusion. Graft cold ischemic time never exceeded 45 min. An end-to-end duodenoduodenostomy was followed by an end-to-side anastomosis between the donor sigmoid colon and the recipient sigmoid colon. Finally, a Bishop-Koop ileostomy was constructed about 20 cm proximal to the ileocecal valve. All intestinal anastomoses were done with a two-layer technique [3].

Combined liver and total bowel transplantation

After resection of the native small and the native large bowel, the common bile duct and the left and right hepatic arteries were ligated and divided. Before the recipient hepatectomy was begun, a venovenous bypass was begun under systemic heparinization (100 U/kg). The inferior vena cava was cannulated via the right external iliac vein, the portal vein was ligated at the hepatic hilum and cannulated distally, and the venous return cannula was inserted into the right internal jugular vein. The hepatectomy was done, and the en bloc liver-bowel graft was brought into the field. The suprahepatic followed by the infrahepatic caval anastomoses were done first and a 3 cm segment of the infrahepatic caval anastomosis was left open as a vent. The donor aortic conduit was anastomosed end-to-side to the infrarenal aorta and the recipient portal vein was anastomosed in a piggyback fashion to the donor portal vein. To decrease portal clamping time, most of this latter anastomosis was done with the portal cannula still in place. The aortic conduit and the portal vein were unclamped and the graft was revascularized. The donor common bile duct was ligated and the proximal end of the donor small bowel was anastomosed side-to-side to the recipient gall bladder. The recipient duodenum was anastomosed end-to-side to the donor jejunum 60 cm distal to the biliary anastomosis [4].

Immunosuppression

CsA pigs received quadruple immunosuppression for induction: horse antipig thymocyte globulin (ATG, 10 mg/kg for 10 days),

CsA (3 mg/kg per day), prednisone (2 mg/kg per day), and azathioprine (2.5 mg/kg per day). Prednisone and azathioprine were reduced by 50 % at 8 days and again at 15 days posttransplant. CsA whole blood concentrations, as determined by high-pressure liquid chromatography (HPLC), were maintained > 400 ng/ml for the first 7 days posttransplant, then between 200 and 400 ng/ml thereafter.

FK506 pigs received FK506 (0.2 mg/kg per day) and prednisone (2 mg/kg per day) for induction and maintenance. Prednisone was reduced by 50 % at 8 days and again at 15 days posttransplant. FK506 trough levels, as determined by a microparticle enzyme immunoassay (ABBOTT IMX®), were maintained between 10 and 35 ng/ml posttransplant.

All immunosuppressive regimens were given intravenously. ATG and FK506 were infused daily over a 3-h period; CsA, prednisone, and azathioprine were given daily as single injections. Rejection episodes were not treated in any group.

Preparation of immunosuppressants

ATG

Polyclonal horse ATG was produced by immunizing a horse with 3.4×10^9 fresh pig thymocytes in complete Freund's adjuvant on days 0 and 14. The horse underwent plasmapheresis starting at 21 days, on a 3-day schedule for a total of 15 bleeds. Plasma from each plasmapheresis was stored at $-20\,°C$ until pooled for final fractionation. An equal volume of each bleed was then pooled, adsorbed with human red blood cell membranes (stroma), then adsorbed with pig red blood cell stroma. The plasma was stabilized with SiO_2, and the biologically active horse IgG was isolated by OAE chromatography. The final product was filtered and bottled at a protein concentration of 50 mg/ml. Horse ATG (POT 100) was stored at $-20\,°C$ until used [5].

CsA

The CsA (100 mg/ml) for intravenous injection was prepared from CsA powder (50 g) added to ethanol (250 ml). Then, a sufficient quantity of sterile water was added to obtain a final volume of 500 ml for injection. The final solution was passed through a 0.22 μm filter placed in sterile vials.

Bone marrow preparation

Fresh donor bone marrow was obtained from the exsanguinated donor at the time of procurement. Bilateral long bones (tibiae, femora, and humeri) served as donor bones for marrow collection. Bone marrow cells were immediately processed, using a method identical to our clinical bone marrow transplant program. First, bone debris and fragments were removed and single cell suspensions were prepared. Stroma cells were removed and bone marrow cells were then isolated from neutrophils and red blood cells by density gradient separations. Trypan blue exclusion tests, done on the final cell preparation, indicated more than 95 % cell viability. Fresh bone marrow cells were then infused intravenously a few hours posttransplant. Two doses of DSBMT were tested, low dose (5×10^7 bone marrow cells/kg) and high dose (5×10^8 bone marrow cells/kg).

Fig. 1a Mild to moderate rejection of the colon; there is an increase of inflammatory infiltrate in the mucosa and submucosa (H&E). **b** A higher magnification shows prominents intraepithelial lymphocytes and occasional epithelial cell necrosis (H&E)

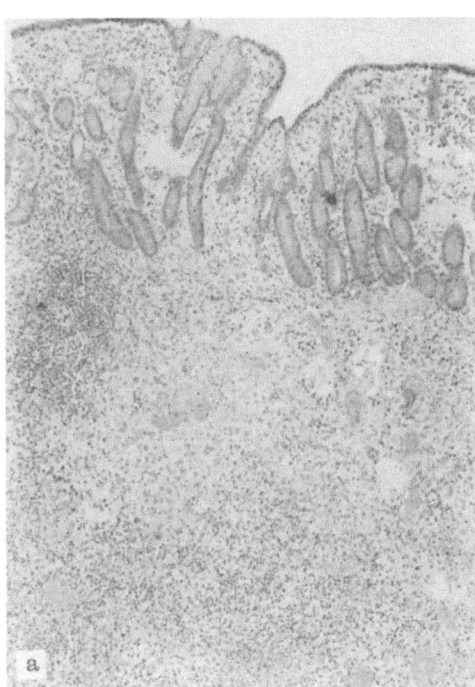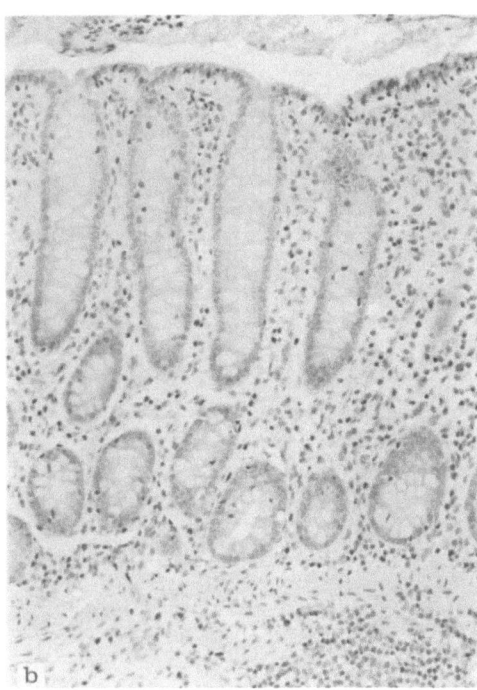

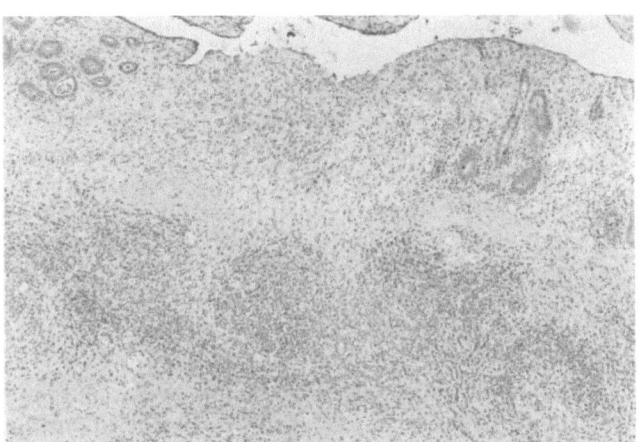

Fig. 2 Severe rejection of the colon shows extensive epithelial loss with increased lamina propria and submucosal inflammation (H&E)

Postoperative care

Recipient pigs received Ringer's lactate with D5W for the first 2 days posttransplant, via a central line placed in the left internal jugular vein. Clear liquids were started on day 3 and normal diet was resumed on day 4. Buprenorphine hydrochloride was given for analgesia (0.3 mg/ml q 6 h). Pigs received the following antibiotic coverage for 7 days: cephalothin (500 mg/ml qd), ticarcillin (1 g b.i.d), and metronidazole (250 mg qd). After 7 days, we did not attempt to treat infectious episodes. Pigs losing more than 30 % of their initial body weight were killed according to the guidelines of the University of Minnesota's Research Animal Resources Committee.

Pathologic evaluation

Pigs survived 3–81 days posttransplant. Of the 35 pigs, 3 % died before 7 days posttransplant, 46 % between 7 and 14 days, 3 % between 14 and 28 days, and 48 % after 28 days. Deaths were due to three main reasons: rejection, GvHD, and infection. At the time of death, tissue sections were taken from the jejunum, ileum, and colon. The sections were fixed in 10 % buffered formalin, paraffin embedded, sectioned at 4 μm intervals, and stained with hematoxylin and eosin. One pathologist (REN) reviewed all the material without knowledge at the experimental groups.

Tissue rejection was evaluated using a previously published grading scheme for interstitial and vascular rejection of small bowel [5]. This grading scheme was modified slightly for colonic mucosa since the colon does not have a villous architecture. Mild interstitial rejection of the colon was defined as mildly increased lymphoplasma cellular infiltrate within the lamina propria and increased intraepithelial lymphocytes with goblet cell loss and occasional epithelial cell necrosis (Fig. 1 a, b). Moderate interstitial rejection of the colon was defined as moderately increased lymphoplasma cellular infiltrate within the lamina propria and increased intraepithelial lymphocytes with goblet cell loss and easily identifiable epithelial cell necrosis. Severe interstitial rejection of the colon was defined as extensive epithelial necrosis with increased lymphoplasma cellular lamina propria infiltrate (Fig. 2). Interstitial rejection of the small bowel was defined very similarly, but with the added feature of mild, moderate, and severe villous blunting (Figs. 3, 4). Vascular rejection was defined as mild, moderate, and severe with the presence of endothelialitis, vasculitis, and vasculitis with fibrinoid necrosis, respectively.

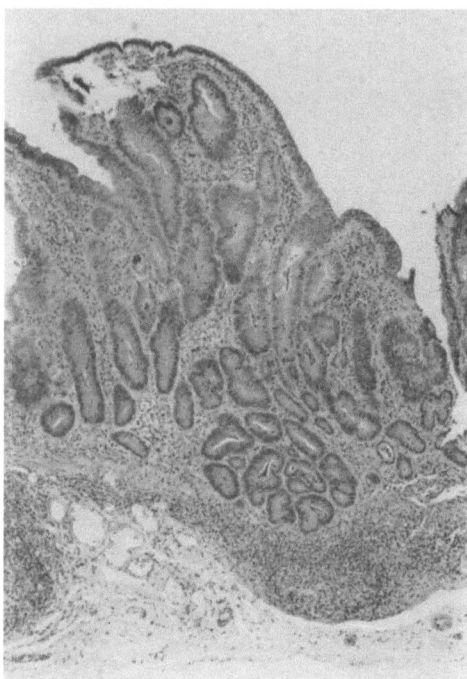

Fig. 3 Moderate rejection of the ileum. There is moderate villous blunting with increased lamina propria inflammation and epithelial cell necrosis (H&E)

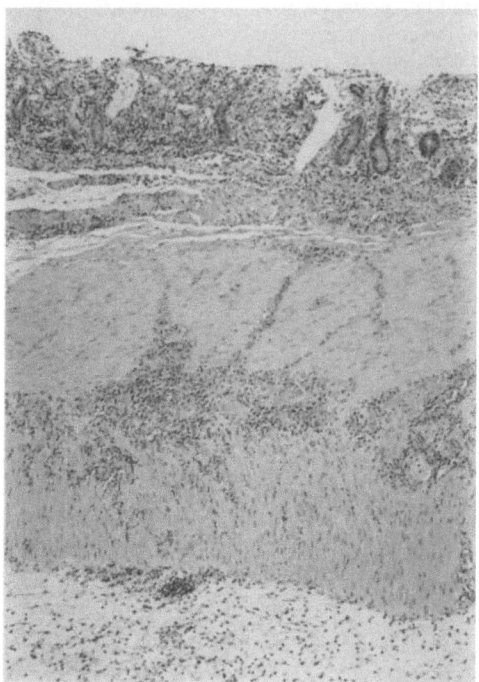

Fig. 4 Severe rejection of the ileum. There is extensive epithelial necrosis with complete blunting of the villi. The infiltrate involves the mucosa, submucosa, muscularis propria, and subserosa (H&E)

Results

Ileum vs colon (Table 1)

Of the 35 pigs, 16 (46 %) had morphologically normal tissue in the ileum and colon, 4 (12 %) had necrotic bowel wall in both grafts, and 6 (18 %) had rejection in both grafts. Five pigs (14 %) had rejection of the ileum, but normal colon morphology. None of the pigs had rejection of the colon without rejection of the ileum, but 1 pig (3 %) showed rejection of the ileum with pseudomembranous colitis of the colon, 1 (3 %) showed fungal infection of the colon with normal ileal morphology, 1 (3 %) showed necrosis of the ileum with a normal colon, and 1 (3 %) showed necrosis of the ileum with rejection of the colon.

Of those pigs with discrepant diagnoses, 2 showed moderate interstitial rejection and 3 showed mild interstitial rejection, while the colons were normal. Of the 6 pigs with rejection in both grafts, 3 had identical rejection grades; in the other 3, rejection was more severe in the ileum than in the colon.

Ileum vs jejunum (Table 2)

Of the 35 pigs described above, 32 also had jejunal tissue sections taken. Of those, 16 (49 %) pigs had normal jejunal and ileal tissue. However, 5 pigs (15 %) showed rejection of the jejunum and the ileum and another 5 (15 %) showed necrosis of the jejunum and ileum. In 4 (12 %) pigs rejection was seen in the ileum but not the jejunum, in 1 (3 %) pig the ileum showed necrosis with rejection of the jejunum, and in 1 (3 %) pig the ileum was normal with necrosis of the jejunum. None of the pigs had rejection of the jejunum without rejection of the ileum.

In pigs with rejection of both the jejunum and the ileum, interstitial rejection was worse in the ileum than in the jejunum. In 2 pigs endothelialitis was seen in the jejunum but not in the ileum; in another 2 pigs endothelialitis was seen in the ileum but not in the jejunum.

Jejunum vs colon (Table 1)

Of the 32 pigs from which tissue sections of the jejunum and colon were taken, 17 (51 %) were normal, 5 (15 %) showed rejection of both grafts, and 4 (12 %) showed necrosis of both grafts. In 2 (6 %) pigs there were discrepancies with regard to rejection; one each of the grafts showed rejection while the other did not. In 4 (12 %) pigs four other discrepancies were noted in the following jejunum/colon combinations: one necrosis/rejection, one necrosis/normal, one normal/fungal infection, one normal/pseudomembraneous colitis.

Table 1 Findings in the colon vs the ileum and the jejunum

		Colon				
		Normal	Rejection	Necrosis	Fungal infection	Pseudomem-branous colitis
Ileum (n = 35)	Normal	16	–	–	1	–
	Rejection	5	6	–	–	1
	Necrosis	1	1	4	–	–
Jejunum (n = 32)	Normal	17	1	–	1	1
	Rejection	1	5	–	–	–
	Necrosis	1	1	4	–	–

Table 2 Findings in the jejunum vs the ileum

Ileum	Jejunum		
	Normal	Rejection	Necrosis
Normal	16	–1	
Rejection	4	5	–
Necrosis	–	1	5

Discussion

Total bowel transplantation offers the opportunity when the ileostomy is eventually taken down to biopsy the colon to monitor for rejection. An abundance of literature addresses small bowel rejection in animal models with an expanding body of literature on human small bowel transplantation. However, little information exists on colon transplantation. The colon is functionally, architecturally, and morphologically different from the small bowel. Therefore, we can expect that the rate and susceptibility of colon rejection may be different from the small bowel. From prior experience with multiple organ transplantation, we know that different organs reject at different rates [6, 7]. Moreover, transplantation of multiple organs may show a different rate of rejection than if the same organs were transplanted individually [7].

In this study, we examined the occurrence of rejection in the colon vs the small bowel. Although five different treatment groups were included, our comparisons were not made in aggregate, but rather for each recipient. The efficacy of the five different treatments will be commented on elsewhere.

While 46 % of pigs did not show rejection of either graft, five more pigs showed rejection in the ileum than in the colon. Furthermore, in several pigs, rejection was more severe in the ileum than in the colon. Therefore, the morphologic manifestations of rejection either occur earlier or are more prominent in the ileum. Either way, the small bowel is a better source of biopsy tissue or specimens for detection of rejection. Similar findings have been reported in a mouse model and in a small series of human small bowel and colon transplants. Simeoni et al. [8] noted that small intestinal biopsy specimens were more informative than colon specimens. Plapler and Cohen [9] suggested that in rats colon allograft rejection was not as severe as small bowel rejection. Clinical incidents of normal colon tissue with advanced ileal rejection have also been reported [2]. From a practical perspective, the ileum seems to be the better organ to biopsy, since colon rejection was not seen without rejection of the small bowel. Therefore, ileostomy takedown should not be done until the risk of rejection is minimal. We found that rejection also occurs at a higher rate in the ileum than in the jejunum. In several pigs, rejection was more severe in the ileum than in the jejunum. These findings justify the use of a Bishop-Koop ileostomy for monitoring rejection.

The features of rejection are similar in the colon and in the small bowel. A notable difference is based on the microanatomy of the small bowel in the presence of villi. Villous blunting, although nonspecific, may provide a very early sign of rejection or be the clue to look for other features. One of the earliest detectable features of rejection in the colon is an increase in intraepithelial lymphocytes with goblet cell loss and possible epithelial cell necrosis. Intraepithelial lymphocytes stand out more notably in the colon and more notably than increased lamina propria inflammation. Rejection progresses with further increases in lamina propria inflammation and increases in epithelial necrosis. Vascular changes, such as endothelialitis and vasculitis, are also identified in the colon. While the primary reason for colon transplantation is to prevent or help control diarrhea, other severe diseases are also seen in the colon (as demonstrated by this study) such as pseudomembranous colitis and fungal infection.

In summary, our study shows that: (1) rejection affects the small bowel more frequently than the colon, (2) colon rejection correlates with small bowel rejection, but a normal colon biopsy may not indicate a normal small bowel, and (3) rejection is more frequent and more advanced in the ileum than in the jejunum. Thus, if only one bowel segment is to be biopsied, the ileum should be chosen. Consequently, ileostomy takedown should not be done unless the risk of rejection appears to be minimal, since biopsies of the jejunum or colon that are obtained via upper or lower endoscopy might miss rejection of the ileum 10–15 % of the time.

References

1. Todo S, Reyes J, Furukawa H, Abu-El-magd K, Lee R, Tzakis A, Rao A, Phil D, Starzl TE (1995) Outcome analysis of 71 clinical intestinal transplantations. Ann Surg 222: 270–282
2. Todo S, Tzakis A, Reyes J, Abu-Elmagd K, Furukawa H, Nour B, Casavilla A, Nakamura K, Fung J, Demetris AJ, Starzl T (1994) Small intestinal transplantation in humans with or without the colon. Transplantation 57 (6): 840–848
3. Pirenne J, Benedetti E, Troppmann C, Moon C, Fryer J, Gruessner RWG (1996) Porcine model of combined small and large bowel transplantation: surgical aspects. Transplant Proc (in press).
4. Benedetti E, Pirenne J, Moon C, Fryer J, Fasola C, Hakim N, Troppmann C, Beebe D, Carr R, Belani K, Gruessner RWG (1995). Simultaneous en bloc transplantation of liver, small bowel and large bowel in pigs: technical aspects. Transplant Proc 27: 341–343
5. Gruessner RWG, Fryer J, Fasola C, Nakhleh RE, Gruessner AC, Kim S, Dunn DL, Pirenne J, Benedetti E, Najarian JS (1995) A prospective study of FK506 versus CSA and pig ATG in a porcine model of small bowel transplantation. Transplantation 59: 164–171
6. Gruessner RWG, Nakhleh RE, Tzardis P, Schechner R, Platt JL, Gruessner A, Tomadze G, Najarian JS, Sutherland DER (1994) Differences in rejection grading after simultaneous pancreas and kidney transplantation in pigs. Transplantation 57 (7): 1021–1027
7. Gruessner RWG, Nakhleh RE, Tzardis P, Platt JL, Schechner R, Gruessner A, Tomadze G, Matas A, Najarian JS, Sutherland DER (1993) Rejection in single versus combined pancreas and kidney transplantation in pigs. Transplantation 56 (5): 1053–1062
8. Simeoni U, Boudjema K, Chenard M-P, Desprez S, Geiss F, Becmeur F, Bientz J, Fischbach M, Wolf P, Odeh M, Ellero B, Jaeck D, Cinqualbre J, Sauvage P, Geisert J (1993) Functional and histological evolution of the grafts after pediatric multiple abdominal visceral transplantation. Transplant Proc 25: 1371–1373
9. Plapler H, Cohen Z (1993) Colon transplantation: a new microvascular technique. Microsurgery 14: 211

Transpl Int (1996) 9 [Suppl 1]: S275–S280
© Springer-Verlag 1996

F. Fändrich
B. Exner
A. Papachrysanthou
X. Zhu
T. Jahnke
W. H. Chambers
N. Zavazava

In vivo depletion of NKR-P1 positive cells in the recipient prior to small bowel transplantation enhances graft-versus-host disease (GvHD) in the rat

F. Fändrich (✉) · B. Exner ·
A. Papachrysanthou · X. Zhou · T. Jahnke
Department of General and Thoracic
Surgery, University of Kiel,
Arnold-Heller-Strasse 7, D-24105 Kiel,
Germany

W. H. Chambers
Pittsburgh Cancer Institute, University of
Pittsburgh, Pittsburgh, USA

N. Zavazava
Institute of Immunology, University of
Kiel, Kiel, Germany

Abstract Recent evidence for major histocompatibility complex (MHC) class I antigen-directed recognition mechanisms of natural killer cells (NKs) have revived interests in investigating non-adaptive immune responses in the framework of solid organ transplantation. A semi-allogeneic rat model of heterotopic small bowel transplantation (HSBTx) from male DA parental to male F1 hybrid rats (DA × LEW) was established to investigate the role of host NKs to attenuate graft-versus-host (GvH)-mediated immunosuppression and tissue injury. By use of anti-NKR-P1 monoclonal antibody (mAb) 3.2.3, host NKs were depleted effectively in vivo after triple intraperitoneal injection prior to HSBTx. In contrast to non-depleted animals, an initial lack of NK activity in F1 hosts significantly decreased the mean survival ($P < 0.01$) and substantially enhanced graft-versus-host disease (GvHD)-related damage to lymphoid and non-lymphoid target organs. These findings emphasize the important immunoregulatory role of host NKs during the early onset of GvHD.

Key words Graft-versus-host disease (GvHD) · Allogeneic lymphocyte cytotoxicity · Natural killer cells · Small bowel transplantation · Major histocompatibility complex (MHC)

Introduction

Natural killer cells (NKs) are endowed with clonally distributed surface receptors which recognize major histocompatibility complex (MHC) class I alleles on potential targets such as tumor cells, virally infected cells, and allogeneic lymphocytes [1–5]. Two genetically distinct NK cell receptor-like molecules have been cloned and categorized and were designated as belonging to the NKR-P1 and Ly-49 murine gene families [6, 7]. Functionally, both receptor molecules were found to deliver opposing signals, with activation of NK cells by NKR-P1 engagement and suppression of NK-mediated killing after encounter of Ly-49 molecules with specific MHC class I epitopes on target cells [6, 8]. In the context of allograft rejection, it is important to note that rapid elimination of MHC-disparate lymphocytes in unsensitized recipient animals, i.e., allogeneic lymphocyte cytotoxicity (ALC), was shown to be conferred by NKs and thus reveals an important mechanism of the non-adaptive immune response to recognize and defeat allogeneic target cells [9, 10]. Independent studies in the mouse have described elimination of parental target cells by F1 hybrids, aligning ALC with "hybrid resistance" against parental allogeneic bone marrow cell grafts [11, 12]. The large amount of lymphatic tissues together with the high frequency of immunocompetent cells transferred in small bowel transplantation bears a potential risk of inducing graft-versus-host disease (GvHD) in the recipient organism. It was a major objective of this experimental study to investigate the immunoregulatory role of the host's initial NK activity as a first line barrier defense directed against donor-specific lymphocytes invading recipient tissues after heterotopic small bowel transplantation (HSBTx). By use of the highly specific monoclonal antibody (mAb) 3.2.3, which engages with the lectin-binding protein NKR-P1 on rat NK cells [13], in vivo depletion of the host NK population can efficiently be achieved [14]. The lack of initial host NK activity, in conjunction with donor-imposed graft-versus-host (GvH)-related immunosuppression and subsequent tissue injuries in the framework of semi-allogeneic HSBTx are described and analyzed immunofunctionally.

Materials and methods

Animals and transplant procedures

Male DA (RT1.^{aaav1}) and male F1 hybrids, a crossing between male DA and female LEW (RT1.^{1}) inbred rats, weighing 160–250 g were raised and maintained at the Institute of Immunology, University of Kiel, Germany and kept under conventional animal facilities. Animals were routinely screened for common rat pathogens and given water and rat chow ad libitum. The experimental protocol was approved by the Ministry of Nature, Environment and Country Development, Schleswig-Holstein, Germany. HSBTx was performed as described previously [15].

Animal groups and experimental points

HSBTx was performed between male DA and male F1 hybrid rats in the following groups: (1) DA > F1, no other treatment (NT), $n = 24$; (2) DA > F1, pretreated with ascites mAb 3.2.3, 50 µl intraperitoneally (i.p.), at days -2, -1, and 0, $n = 10$; and (3) F1 > F1, syngeneic control, $n = 10$. Intestine graft survival was considered synonymous with recipient death or sacrifice before then because of a moribund state. In addition, six animals in each group were sacrificed selectively at postoperative days (POD) 3, 7, 10, and 14 and analyzed histologically. Flow cytometric analysis, cytotoxicity assays, and MLRs were performed from animals sacrificed selectively at POD 3 and 10 after HSBTx. Control experiments included triple injection of an irrelevant isotype-matched mAb prior to HSBTx of F1 hosts and in vivo depletion with mAb 3.2.3 and sham operation of F1 recipients (data not shown).

Histology

Conventional criteria were used to diagnose GvHD and rejection by use of paraffin-embedded tissue specimens, cut at 4 µm, and stained with hematoxylin and eosin (H&E).

Preparation of splenocytes and mesenteric lymph nodes

Donor and recipient mesenteric lymph nodes and recipient spleens were excised, minced, and pressed gently through a 60-gauge mesh stainless steel screen into Hank's balanced salt solution (HBSS). Lymph node lymphocytes and splenocytes were obtained by centrifugation on Ficoll-Hypaque gradients (density = 1.077 g/ml) at 300 g for 20 min at room temperature. After collection of the mononuclear cells from the gradient interface they were resuspended in RPMI-FBS, washed 3 times, and immediately used in the experiments described.

Flow cytometric analysis

Cell populations of recipient spleens and peripheral blood leukocytes were prepared for fluorescence-activated cell sorter (FACS) analysis. Directly conjugated antibodies were matched with an irrelevant, non-reactive isotype-matched control with the same fluorescent tag. Monoclonal antibodies used in cell sorting experiments were all directly labeled. Cells (1×10^6/ml) were preincubated for 10 min with saturating concentrations of anti-Fcγ receptor to block unspecific Fc receptor binding. Incubation with fluorescein isothiocyanate (FITC)-coupled monoclonal antibodies for 30 min followed. After a double washing step in FACS medium, cells were incubated with PE-labeled monoclonal antibodies at saturating concentrations if double staining was performed, washed twice, and mounted in phosphate-buffered saline (PBS) for cytofluorometric analysis. Staining was assessed using a FACStar/Plus flow cytometer (Becton Dickinson, Mountain View, Calif.).

Pretreatment of F1 animals with mAb 3.2.3 (anti-NKR-P1)

Ascites fluid was produced in Balb/c mice bearing the hybridoma 3.2.3 as a source of anti-NKR-P1 mAb. Aliquots of 50 µl of ascites fluid in 0.5 ml HBSS were used on 3 consecutive days for suppression of NK activity in recipient rats, as determined by Yac-1 target cell lysis. mAb 3.2.3 contained 10 mg/ml protein, of which 30% was analyzed to be monoclonal IgG1.

Target cell preparation

To assess target cell lysis in cell-mediated cytotoxicity assays, the rat NK-sensitive Moloney virus-induced lymphoma cell line YAC-1 of A/Sn mouse origin was used. This cell line was maintained in suspension culture in RPMI 1640 and contained 10% (v/v) fetal calf serum, 100 U/ml penicillin, and 100 µg/ml streptomycin (Sigma, Darmstadt, Germany). Target cells were labeled by incubating 1×10^6 cells in 0.2 ml medium with 200 µCi $Na_2^{51}CrO_4$ for 60 min at 37 °C for 1 h.

Cell-mediated cytotoxicity assays

Variable numbers of effector cells were added at five different effector to target cell ratios ranging from 50:1 to 3.125:1 to 10^4 labeled target cells in U-bottomed, 96-well plates in a final volume of 0.2 ml complete medium. The plates were centrifuged at 40 g for 3 min and then incubated at 37 °C in a humidified chamber containing 5% CO_2. After 4 h the plates were centrifuged at 400 g for 5 min, and 0.1 ml of supernatant was collected and radioactivity estimated in an autogamma counter. Spontaneous ^{51}Cr release was determined by incubation of target cells with medium alone. The percentage of specific lysis was calculated as 100 (E − S/T − S) where E is the experimental ^{51}Cr release, S is the spontaneous release, and T is the total incorporated counts.

Mixed lymphocyte reaction

Responder spleen cells (1×10^5) from control, NK-depleted or non-depleted rats were cultured in triplicate in 0.2 ml complete medium together with 3×10^5 irradiated stimulator cells (2000 rad) in the presence or absence of phytohemagglutinin (PHA) in 96-well flat-bottomed microplates. After 96 h of incubation of 37 °C in 5% CO_2/95% air, cells were pulsed with 1 µCi of

Table 1 Effect of monoclonal antibody *(mAb)* 3.2.3 pretreatment on progression and extent of clinical graft-versus-host disease (GvHD)

	DA (SB) > F1 (no treatment)	DA (SB) > F1 (mAb 3.2.3 pretreatment)	Level of significance (*P* values)
First signs of GvHD (days)	10.2 (± 1.2)	7.2 (± 1.8)[a]	< 0.001
Mean duration of GvHD (days)	7.3 (± 2.4)	4.3 (± 0.8)[b]	< 0.0001

[a] Suppression of host natural killer cell *(NK)* activity with mAb 3.2.3 enhanced the development of GvHD in recipient animals with significant earlier onset

[b] Aggrevated GvHD resulted in significant reduction of the mean time period between the first signs of GvHD until death in NK-depleted animals

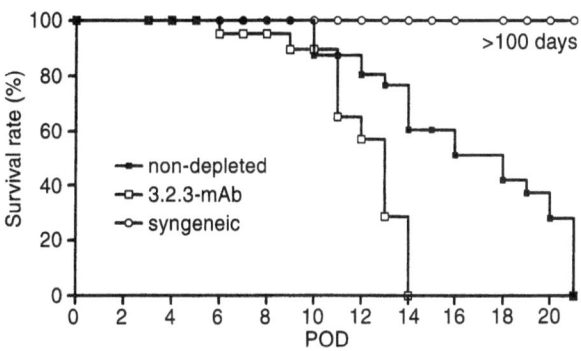

Fig. 1 Survival of monoclonal antibody (mAb) 3.2.3-treated *(3.2.3-mAb)*, n = 10; non-depleted, n = 24; and syngeneic F1 recipient animals, n = 10, after semiallogeneic heterotopic small bowel transplantation *(HSBTx)* of parental small bowel from DA rats is presented. mAb 3.2.3 pretreatment of F1 hybrid rats included triple intraperitoneal injection of 50 μl ascites of the highly specific anti-NKR-P1 monoclonal antibody 3.2.3 on days – 2, – 1, and 0 prior to transplantation. Kaplan-Meier curves were generated and statistical analysis with the Savage (Mantel-Cox) log-rank test showed a significant difference in survival (*P* < 0.01) between natural killer cell (NK) depleted and non-depleted animals

[³H]thymidine, 18 h before harvesting for measurement of radioactivity in a scintillation counter.

Statistics

Animal survival rates were calculated according to Kaplan-Meier life-table analysis using the statistical program package of Astute Module 1, Statistics Add-in for Microsoft Excel, University of Leeds, UK. Difference in survival between the various groups was assessed using the generalized Savage (Mantel-Cox) log-rank test. Deaths secondary to technical complications (with functioning grafts) were censored. The F-test was used to test for equality of the variances of the two samples to be compared. Depending on the results of the F-test, Student's *t* test for equal or unequal variances was used for further analysis.

Results

For depletion of host NKs, F1 hybrid rats received a triple i.p. injection of mAb 3.2.3 prior to HSBTx, as outlined above. F1 recipients lacking NKs suffered from GvH-mediated manifestations far earlier and to a greater extent. In comparison to non-depleted F1 hybrids, which did not suffer from GvHD until POD 10.2 (± 1.2), appearance of the first GvHD symptoms was already evident at POD 7.2 (± 1.8), *P* < 0.001. Thus, the mean time period between the first demonstration of clinical GvHD and death comprised 4.3 (± 0.82) days versus 7.3 (± 2.34) days (*P* < 0.0001) in mAb 3.2.3-pretreated and untreated recipients (Table 1). The fact that F1 hosts lacking their initial NK activity are subject to more advanced and extensive GvHD was also mirrored in life expectancy and survival of mAb 3.2.3-depleted animals. Figure 1 shows the survival of mAb 3.2.3-treated and non-treated F1 hybrid rats which received a parental DA small bowel in comparison to syngeneic F1 control animals which were given a F1 small bowel transplant. The mAb 3.2.3-mediated elimination of NKR-P1⁺ cells led to a significantly shorter survival in comparison to non-depleted animals [Savage (Mantel-Cox) log-rank test, *P* < 0.01]. Whereas non-depleted animals had an average life expectancy of 16.1 (± 0.9) days, mAb 3.2.3-treated hosts surrendered to GvHD after a mean survival time of 11.4 (0.8) days. Table 2 illus-

Table 2 Survival after small bowel transplantation from DA to F1 hybrid rats

Group	Donor	Recipient	Treatment	n	Survival (days)	Mean ± SD (days)
I	DA	F1	None	24	10 × 4; 12 × 2; 13; 14 × 4; 16 × 2; 18 × 2; 19; 20 × 2; 21 × 6	16.1 ± 0.9
II	DA	F1[a]	mAb 3.2.3	10	6; 9; 11 × 3; 12; 13 × 2; 14 × 2	11.4 ± 0.8[b]
III	F1	F1	None	10	> 100 × 10	> 100

[a] F1 recipients were administered 50 μl of anti-NKR-P1 mAb 3.2.3 at days – 2, – 1, and 0 prior to small bowel transplantation

[b] *P* > 0.01 for group I versus group II

Table 3 Flow cytometric analysis of T-lymphocyte subsets in spleen and mesenteric lymph nodes following semiallogeneic parental heterotopic small bowel transplantation. One- and two-color flow cytometric analysis of fresh spleen cells from control, syngeneic, mAb 3.2.3-pretreated, and non-depleted F1 hybrid rats was performed. Splenocytes from six animals in each group were harvested at postoperative day *(POD)* 3 and 10 and submitted to flow cytometric analysis. Results are expressed as mean ± SD of six experiments. Markers were set so that the percentages of PE$^+$ or FITC$^+$ cells in the isotype controls were < 1 %

Spleen (% positive cells)	DA > F^1 (untreated)		DA > F^1 (mAb 3.2.3 pretreated)		F^1 > F^1 (untreated)		F^1 control (untreated)
	POD 3	POD 10	POD 3	POD 10	POD 3	POD 10	
CD4$^+$	35.0 (± 2.19)	19.0 (± 3.74)	32.0 (± 4.33)	12.8** (± 4.40)	34.8 (± 2.04)	31.5 (± 3.08)	36.3 (± 4.92)
CD8$^+$	19.6 (± 6.53)	22.8 (± 8.95)	17.8 (± 1.94)	7.3*** (± 1.96)	16.1 (± 2.48)	15.1 (± 2.04)	16.0 (± 3.16)
CD3$^+$	49.8 (± 4.62)	37.0 (± 13.17)	46.3 (± 4.84)	24.5 (± 2.07)	49.5 (± 2.58)	45.0 (± 5.17)	51.6 (± 10.21)
NKR-P1$^+$	9.8 (± 1.72)	12.3 (± 9.97)	3.0* (± 0.89)	5.5 (± 2.66)	8.8 (± 2.04)	7.0 (± 1.54)	8.6 (± 2.50)
OX-3$^+$	40.2 (± 4.53)	18.6 (± 10.09)	42.0 (± 10.11)	33.6*** (± 4.67)	27.5 (± 2.16)	29.8 (± 2.85)	24.3 (± 8.63)
CD3$^+$/ NKR-P1$^+$	4.8 (± 0.98)	1.2 (± 1.5)	1.1* (± 0.75)	1.0 (± 0.89)	4.2 (± 0.75)	2.8 (± 0.75)	4.5 (± 1.05)
CD4$^+$/ CD8$^+$ ratio	2.0 (± 0.7)	0.9 (± 0.3)	1.8 (± 0.2)	1.8*** (± 0.6)	2.2 (± 0.34)	2.1 (± 0.5)	2.3 (± 0.3)

Comparisons between mAb 3.2.3-pretreated and untreated animals were highly significant for:
* the percentage of NKR-P1$^+$ and NKR-P1$^+$/CD3$^+$ double-positive lymphocytes, at POD 3, $P > 0.0001$; ** the percentage of CD4$^+$ lymphocytes at POD 10, $P < 0.05$; and *** the percentage of CD8$^+$, OX-3$^+$, and CD4$^+$/CD8$^+$ ratios, at POD 10, $P < 0.01$

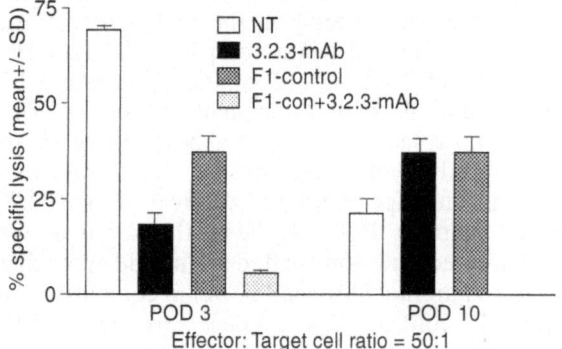

Fig. 2 NK activity of DA small bowel transplanted untreated *(NT)* and mAb 3.2-3-pretreated *(3.2.3-mAB)* F1 hybrid rats and F1 control, and F1 control mAb 3.2.3-pretreated rats was compared and functional assessment was determined as lytic activity of freshly isolated spleenocytes against Yac-1 targets at an effector to target cell ratio of 50:1 at postoperative day (POD) 3 and 10. Each column represents mean NK activity ± SD of four experiments in each group, consisting of two pooled rats per experiment. Assays were performed in three replicates. At POD 3, specific lysis of Yac-1 targets from the untreated F1 host significantly exceeded NK-depleted F1 host activity $(P < 0.001)$

trates the individual survival of each animal in the three different experimental groups. The selective depletion of NK activity in mAb 3.2.3-treated rats strongly affected the cell surface markers associated with NKR-P1$^+$ cells, CD4$^+$, CD8$^+$, OX-3$^+$, and CD3$^+$/NKR-P1$^+$ (double-positive), after HSBTx. Table 3 summarizes the main significant changes of these T-cell subsets evaluated for recipient spleens. At POD 3, the percentage of NKR-P1$^+$ and NKR-P1$^+$/CD3$^+$ double-positive cells was significantly reduced in mAb 3.2.3-pretreated animals, $(P < 0.0001)$. NK cell depletion also affected CD4$^+$ and CD8$^+$ T-cell subsets of mAb 3.2.3-treated animals, which both were significantly diminished compared to non-depleted recipients $(P < 0.05$ and $P < 0.01$, at POD 10, respectively). At this time, the amount of F1-specific OX-3$^+$ cells was profoundly increased following NK cell depletion, consistent with the findings of others that advanced GvHD mediates the upregulation of MHC class II antigen expression on host target cells [16]. Further evidence for advanced clinical progression of GvHD in these animals was gained by calculating the CD4$^+$/CD8$^+$ ratios within the lymphocyte population of freshly harvested spleen cells from F1 hybrid animals. GvH-mediated immunosuppression is a common sequel in host lymphoid organs and correlates with CD4$^+$/CD8$^+$ ratios which, initially, are decreased during the "proliferation phase", characterized by clonally expanding CD8$^+$ T-lymphocyte subsets [17]. Whereas non-depleted animals still demonstrated inverse CD4$^+$/CD8$^+$ ratios of 0.9 (± 0.3) at POD 10 after HSBTx, mAb 3.2.3-treated recipients revealed a mean ratio of 1.8 (± 0.6) due to substantial depletion of both CD4$^+$ and CD8$^+$ lymphocytes, consistent with severely progressed GvHD.

Beside the finding of significant differences in lymphocyte population characteristics of recipient spleens for mAb 3.2.3-pretreated and untreated F1 hybrid rats,

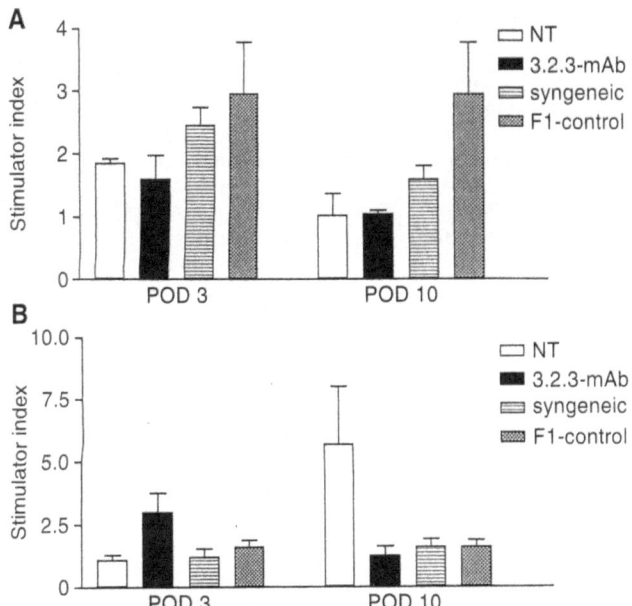

Fig. 3 A, B MLC-Response **A** against DA-stimulator cells and **B** against F1-stimulator cells. One-way MLR was performed with freshly isolated F1 splenocytes used as responder cells and co-cultured with DA or F1 irradiated (200 rad) stimulator cells. Varying numbers of stimulator cells were mixed in triplicate with F1 responder cells. Columns represent the mean of 6 to 10 experiments consisting of two pooled rats per experiment. The stimulator index was calculated as E/C, where E = cpm of [^{3}H]thymidine-treated responder cells co-cultured with irradiated stimulator cells, and C = cpm of [^{3}H]thymidine-treated responder cells not co-cultured with stimulator cells. Notice the increased anti-F1 proliferation response in mAb 3.2.3-pretreated animals at POD 3

the immunofunctional status as determined by Yac-1 target cell lysis and the mixed lymphocyte culture (MLC) response of splenocytes from these animals differed strongly. Figure 2 illustrates the NK activity of both groups ad POD 3 and 10 in comparison to syngeneic and F1 control animals at POD 3 and 10 after HSBTx. Obviously, NK depletion efficiently inhibited the lysis rate of Yac-1 target cells determined in splenocytes harvested at POD 3 ($P < 0.001$) compared to non-depleted animals. Conversely, at POD 10, splenocytes from NK-depleted animals yielded higher NK activity (37.75 % ± 7.5 versus 21.5 % ± 6.7 specific lysis from non-depleted F1 animals, $P < 0.05$). In order to investigate the impact of NK cell depletion on T-cell proliferation, DA and F1 stimulator cells were cultured together with [^{3}H]thymidine-pulsed F1 effector T-cells from mAb 3.2.3-treated and untreated F1 hosts. All experimental groups showed reduced proliferation responses to DA stimulator cells compared to control F1 animals without reaching a level of significance. Interestingly, at POD 3 after HSBTx, splenocytes from NK-depleted recipients responded more strongly to F1 stimulator cells than did undepleted splenic lymphocytes ($P = 0.052$). Besides, lack of host NK activity

was correlated with a stronger anti-F1 response, which exceeded the proliferation rate of F1 host cells in response to parental T-cells (Fig. 3). At POD 10, an opposite picture was observed due to the advanced GvHD status of NK-depleted animals, characterized by severe depletion of CD4$^+$ and CD8$^+$ T-cell subsets and concomitant immunosuppression.

Discussion

The major findings of this experimental approach, designed to delineate the role of NK cell-mediated ALC in semiallogeneic solid organ transplantation, give rise to the conclusion that the initial host NK activity plays an important role as a first line defense barrier for allogeneic targets by initiating effective immunoregulatory signals within the afferent sensitization circuit of the host's immune response to the GvH-related immune attack. Animals lacking NK activity after mAb 3.2.3-pretreatment suffered from and succumbed to far more advanced GvHD than did F1 hosts with, initially, activated levels of NK-mediated lysis (Fig. 2). The inherent nonadaptive response and defense mechanisms of NKs appear to be especially important in MHC-disparate models by virtue of their capability to discriminate allogeneic MHC class I specificities [2–5]. In vitro assays for NK alloreactivity by use of an enlarged panel of intra-MHC recombinant rat strains permitted the comparison of different MHC regions and outlined the importance of non-classical MHC class I molecules encoded by the RT1.C region to elicit efficient NK susceptibility [4, 5]. Thus, early events following NK cell activation in the course of ALC can be initiated by non-classical MHC class I cell surface antigens and include: (1) recognition and elimination of allogeneic target cells within hours following graft reperfusion; (2) release of various cytokines, e. g., γ-interferon, tumor necrosis factor-α, and interleukin-2; and (3) selective enhancement of Th1 clones with concomitant downregulation of Th2 clones [18]. Thus, an anti-parental stimulus of the host's immune response is transiently initiated to balance the donor-derived immunogenicity in the course of GvHD. Host NK cell depletion prior to parental HSBTx obviated this important defense mechanism, with a concomitant decrease of the mean survival time. Our results underline the important role of NK-mediated ALC in the framework of solid organ transplantation. The exact role of non-classical MHC class I-encoded cell surface antigens as triggering structures for NK cell engagement and NK target susceptibility are the subject of forthcoming experiments in the experimental setting of solid organ transplantation.

Acknowledgement This work was supported by the Deutsche Forschungsgemeinschaft Bonn, Germany, grant code: Fa 295/1-1.

References

1. Trinchieri G (1990) Biology of natural killer cells. Adv Immunol 47: 187–376
2. Colonna M, Brooks EG, Falco M, Ferrara GB, Strominger JL (1993) Generation of allospecific natural killer cells by stimulation across a polymorphism of HLA-C. Science 260: 1121–1124
3. Moretta L, Ciccone E, Mingari MC, Biassoni R, Moretta A (1994) Human natural killer cells: origin, clonality, specificity and receptors. Adv Immunol 55: 341–380
4. Vaage JT, Naper C, Lovik G, Lambracht D, Rehm A, Hedrich HJ, Wonigeit K, Rolstad B (1994) Control of rat natural killer cell-mediated allorecognition by a major histocompatibility complex region encoding nonclassical class I antigens. J Exp Med 180: 641–651
5. Naper C, Vaage JT, Lambracht D, Lovik G, Butcher GW, Wonigeit K, Rolstad B (1995) Alloreactive natural killer cells in the rat: complex genetics of major histocompatibility complex control. Eur J Immunol 25: 1249–1256
6. Yokoyama WM, Seaman WE (1993) The Ly-49 and NKR-P1 gene families encoding lectin-like receptors on natural killer cells: the NK gene complex. Annu Rev Immunol 11: 613–635
7. Chambers WH, Adamkiewicz T, Houchins JP (1993) Type II integral membrane proteins with characteristics of C-type animal lectins expressed by natural killer (NK) cells. Glycobiology 3: 9–14
8. Karlhofer FM, Ribaudo RK, Yokoyama WM (1992) MHC class I alloantigen specificity of Ly-49$^+$ IL-2-activated natural killer cells. Nature 358: 66–70
9. Ford WL, Rolstad B, Fossum S (1984) The elimination of allogeneic lymphocytes: a useful model of natural killer cell activity in vivo? Immunol Today 5: 227–228
10. Rolstad B, Fossum S, Bazin H, Kimber I, Marshall J, Sparshott SM, Ford WL (1985) The rapid rejection of allogeneic lymphocytes by a non-adaptive, cell-mediated mechanism (NK activity). Immunology 54: 127–138
11. Kiessling R, Hochman PS, Haller O, Shearer GM, Wigzell H, Cudkowicz G (1977) Evidence for a similar or common mechanism for natural killer cell activity and resistance to hemopoietic grafts. Eur J Immunol 7: 655–663
12. Cudkowicz G, Stimpfling JH (1964) Deficient growth of C57BL marrow cells transplanted in F^1 hybrid mice. Association with the histocompatibility-2 locus. Immunology 7: 291–306
13. Chambers WH, Vujanovic NL, DeLeo AB, Olszowy MW, Herberman RB, Hiserodt JC (1989) Monoclonal antibody to a triggering structure expressed on rat natural killer cells and adherent lymphokine-activated killer cells. J Exp Med 169: 1373–1389
14. Van den Brink MRM, Hunt LE, Hiserodt JC (1990) In vivo treatment with monoclonal antibody 3.2.3 selectively eliminates natural killer cells in rats. J Exp Med 171: 197–210
15. Fändrich F, Waaga AM, Schröder J, Schweizer E, Schroeder P (1994) Tissue dependent alteration of the MHC-I and -II. Expression after the use of deoxyspergualin for suppression of the graft-versus-host disease in small bowel transplantation. Transplant Proc 26: 1592–1593
16. Sviland L, Pearson ADJ, Green MA, Eastham EJ, Malcolm AJ, Proctor SJ, Hamilton PJ, and the Newcastle Bone Marrow Transplant Group (1989) Expression of MHC class I and II antigens by keratinocytes and enterocytes in acute graft-versus-host disease. Bone Marrow Transplant 4: 233–238
17. Hakim FT, Sharrow SO, Payne S, Shearer GM (1991) Repopulation of host lymphohematopoietic systems by donor cells during graft-versus-host reaction in unirradiated adult F1 mice injected with parental lymphocytes. J Immunol 146: 2108–2115
18. Romagnani S (1992) Induction of Th1 and Th2 responses: a key role for the "natural" immune response? Immunol Today 13: 379–381

Transpl Int (1996) 9 [Suppl 1]: S 281–S 285
© Springer-Verlag 1996

M. Navarro-Zorraquino
A. Güemes
R. Lozano
L. Larrad
M. J. Morandeira
J. C. Salinas
C. Pastor

Changes in blood lymphocyte populations in experimental bowel allograft rejection

M. Navarro-Zorraquino · A. Güemes ·
R. Lozano · L. Larrad · M. J. Morandeira ·
J. C. Salinas · C. Pastor
Department of Surgery, University of
Zaragoza, C/Domingo Miral s/n, Zaragoza,
Spain

M. Navarro-Zorraquino (✉)
Capitán Portolés, 7, E-50004 Zaragoza,
Spain

Abstract The aim of this study is to measure percentages of lymphocyte populations and IL-2R cellular expression in peripheral blood during the rejection of a small bowel allograft (SBA) in the rat. Thirty rats were allotted to three groups: A, control, no transplantation (Tx); B, rats receiving an orthotopic SBA; C, similar SBA but with thymostimulin (TP-1) administered before Tx, aimed at increasing the intensity of and accelerating rejection. The percentages of CD19, CD5, CD4 and CD8 cells and of IL-2R were determined when rejection was present. Rejection appeared in rats in group B between days 11 and 26 post-Tx and in group C between days 6 and 7 post-Tx ($P < 0.001$). In both B and C groups, CD5 and CD4 cells decreased ($P < 0.005$) and CD8 cells increased ($P < 0.001$). A correlation between CD8 and IL-2R content was found ($P < 0.05$). In group C, earliness of rejection correlated with the percentage of CD8 cells ($P < 0.05$) and the intensity of rejection with numbers of CD8 and CD19 cells ($P < 0.05$).

Key words Lymphocyte · populations · IL-2R · Rejection · Bowel allograft

Introduction

Until recently, the immune response in allograft transplantation, particularly in bowel allograft transplantation, has not been understood because of its complexity. It is well known that thymus-derived lymphocytes (T-cells) play a major role in transplant rejection; in small intestine allografts the large quantity of lymphoid tissue may stimulate a vigorous rejection from the recipient, and may also induce graft-versus-host disease (GVHD) from the graft. At present it is known that many immunosuppressive regimens to prevent either rejection or GVHD, among these cyclosporin and FK506, work by inhibiting IL-2 mRNA synthesis, blocking early lymphocyte activation. Dynamic lymphocyte population changes and the expression of IL-2 receptors by lymphocyte subsets during the rejection are, however, still not fully understood. The aim of the present study is to ascertain the percentage changes of lymphocyte population and subpopulations and the expression of IL-2R on them, in peripheral blood, during the rejection of an orthotopic small bowel allograft.

Materials and methods

Animals

Wistar Furth rats were allotted to three groups: group A (10 rats), control group without transplantation (Tx); group B (10 rats) received an orthotopic small bowel allograft (SBA); group C (10 rats) received an orthotopic SBA and a thymic hormone [thymostimulin (TP-1) 2 mg/kg i.m.] for 3 days before Tx, aimed at increasing the intensity of and accelerating the rejection. Inbred Fisher male rats were employed as donors and Wistar Furth male rats as recipients; this endogamic strain of rats is directed to produce a single form of rejection. The rats weighed between 200 and 350 g. All the animals were delivered by a laboratory (IFFA, Lyon, France) under standard conditions. All rats were kept under the same conditions in metabolic cages and received paired feeding.

Table 1 Number of rats in groups B and C according to the intensity and earliness of the rejection

	Rejection intensity (pathological criteria)		Maximal clinical signs of rejection			
	(++)	(+++)	6th day	7th day	11th–17th day	17th–26th day
Group B	6	4	0	0	6	4
Group C	8	2	2	8	0	0

Table 2 Preoperative values of CD5, CD4, CD8, CD19 und IL-2R (1 week before transplantation: groups A, B, C; on the day of surgery: group A)

	CD5 (%)	CD4 (%)	CD8 (%)	CD19 (%)	IL-2R (%)
Group A	71.7 ± 1.49	43.5 ± 2.39	23.5 ± 1.91	18.1 ± 1.43	1.7 ± 3.3
Group B	70.5 ± 2.10	42.6 ± 1.17	24.3 ± 2.10	16.4 ± 1.57	1.3 ± 3.4
Group C	72.3 ± 1.23	45.7 ± 2.80	23.8 ± 2.60	15.7 ± 1.36	1.7 ± 2.9
Group A (surgery day)	71.9 ± 1.45	44.9 ± 2.30	22.9 ± 1.80	17.2 ± 1.30	1.9 ± 3.1

Operative procedures

Donors were fasted for 24 h with water ad libitum. All procedures were performed under anaesthesia using an i.m. dose (2 ml/kg) of a mixture of ketamine (0.5 mg/ml), diazepine (2 mg/ml) and atropine (0.1 mg/ml). After anaesthesia, rats received one dose of 1000 IU penicillin-G and 0.5 mg of gentamicin, undergoing surgery according to an experimental model previously described by our team [8] based on an experimental small bowel orthotopic transplant technique described by Monchick and Russell in 1971 [13]. In the donor, the small bowel was dissected from the colonic and vascular attachments and the graft removed with an aortic cuff joined to the superior mesenteric artery. As the warm ischemia time was very short the graft was not perfused before the extraction. After removing the graft it was perfused ex vivo with cold Ringer lactate solution through the aortic cuff. Vascular end-to-side porta-caval and mesenteric-aortic anasthomoses were carried out using a double-running 9/0 monofilament suture. Once the vascular clamp was removed and revascularisation of the graft considered to be correct, the recipient's small bowel was removed and a double intestinal anasthomosis, an end-to-end running everting suture using 7/0 silk, was performed, placing the graft orthotopically.

After anaesthesia, rats received one dose of 1000 IU penicillin-G and 0.5 mg of gentamicin. After operation the rats received a normal diet and water ad libitum and they received no antibiotics in the postoperative period. The rats were weighed 6 times a week, and were sacrified when they showed the clinical signs of rejection described by Schraut and Lee [20]: weight loss, profuse diarrhoea and lack of redding of nose, ears and feet. A histological study of the grafts was carried out by a pathologist who was unaware of the origin of the samples and the results were graded as: (i) incipient rejection (+): normal appearance of villi and moderate mononuclear cell infiltration; (ii) moderate rejection (++): great mononuclear cell infiltration but moderate destruction of villi; or (iii) massive rejection (+++): total destruction of villi and great mononuclear cell infiltration.

One week before the surgical procedures, blood was drawn from a rat tail incision by pressing out the blood. On the day of surgery a blood sample was obtained from one rat of the control group, but no blood was obtained from animals undergoing surgery to avoid lymphocyte changes due to blood loss. In addition, blood samples were obtained from rats of groups B and C on the day of sacrifice. In blood samples, CD5+, CD4+, CD8+ and CD19+ cell percentages and IL-2R percentages on the cellular surface were

determined by flow cytometry (FACS, Becton-Dickinson) using monoclonal antibodies (mAb; anti-rat CD5, CD4, CD8, CD19, and IL-2R provided by Sera-lab): A 100-μl sample of blood with heparin was incubated with 10 μl of the corresponding mAb for 10 min at 10°C. Subsequently, cells were lysed by means of Immunopred (phormic acid, sodium carbonate, paraformaldehyde solution) and were fixed and identified by flow cytometry.

Statistical analysis

Results are expressed as mean ± standard error of the mean (SEM). Cell and IL-2R percentages were compared 1 week before the surgical procedure between groups A (control), B and C; on the day of surgery between the control group and samples from groups B and C obtained 1 week before; and on the day of sacrifice, between groups A (control), B and C (rejection). Data were analysed by means of Student's and ANOVA tests. Regression and Kendall correlation tests were used to study any relationship between variables, as well as between variables and the precocity and intensity of the rejection. Differences and correlation were considered significant at the $P < 0.05$ level.

Results

Rejection appeared in rats in group B between the 1st and 26th post-transplantation days ($\bar{x} = 17.7 \pm 1.8$) and in group C between days 6 and 7 ($\bar{x} = 6.7 \pm 0.1$); this difference was statistically significant ($P < 0.001$). The intensity of rejection was moderate (++) or massive (+++) in all cases. Table 1 shows the number of rats in each group with (++) or (+++) intensity and the time of rejection. No rats showed GVHD.

No differences were found between the percentages of CD5, CD4, CD8 or CD19 cells nor IL-2R from the control and groups B and C obtained 1 week before the surgical procedure as well as between those samples and the sample obtained from the control group on the day of surgery (Table 2). CD5 and CD4 cell percentages decreased in groups B and C when rejection was present

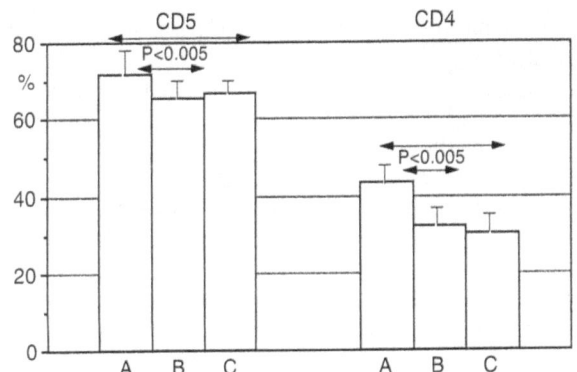

Fig. 1 CD5 and CD4 cell percentage variations in small bowel allograft rejection. Differences between control (group A), transplantation (group B) and transplantation plus thymostimulin (group C)

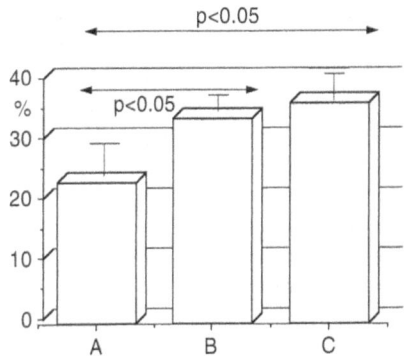

Fig. 2 CD8 cell percentage variations in small bowel allograft rejection. Differences between control (group A), transplantation (group B) and transplantation plus thymostimulin (group C)

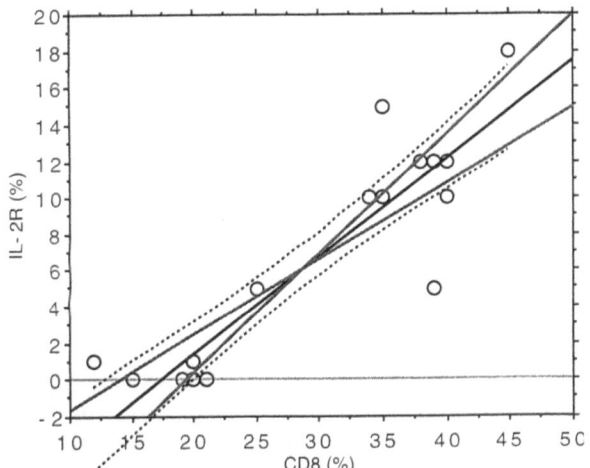

Fig. 3 Correlation between CD8 cell percentage and IL-2R expression

(Fig. 1), whereas CD8 cell percentages increased at the same time (Fig. 2).

The IL-2R percentage increased in both B and C groups on rejection, but in group C the increase was greater (Table 3). CD8 cell and IL-2R percentages showed a significant correlation (Fig. 3). The IL-2R percentage also showed a relationship with that of CD19 (correlation coefficient = 0.623; $P = 0.05$; Kendall test), however, the CD19 variation was not statistically significant in groups during rejection. In group C, the earliness and the intensity of rejection were directly correlated with activated CD8 and CD19 cell percentages (Table 4).

Discussion

Because it is known that antigens from the allograft are presented to the CD4+/T-helper cells by means of antigen-presenting cells, it is believed that the recipient immune response starts with the host T-helper cells against graft passenger leucocytes which express high levels of major histocompatibility complex (MHC) class II [12]. The antigen-presenting cell, in addition to processing the antigen, secretes IL-1, which is essential for T-cell proliferation. IL-1 has pro-inflammatory effects: promoting B-cell growth and differentiation, a synergic effect with IL-4 and IL-6, increasing the cytotoxicity of natural killer cells, increasing the elaboration of platelet activation factor by macrophages and also chemotactic effects on macrophages [4, 9, 19]. The activated T-helper cell releases IL-2 (previously called T-cell growth factor). Until recently, IL-2 has been considered as the main cytokine in rejection because it stimulates the differentiation and proliferation of T cytotoxic cells (CD8+ cells), which are the main effector cells in rejection. In addition, however, IL-2 has an autocrine effect of augmenting, IL-2 and other lymphokine production by activated T-helper cells. IL-2 also has the effect of promoting the recruitment and proliferation of new CD4+ cells and activation factors (such as IL-4 and IL-6). In addition, IL-2 promotes the release of gamma interferon as well as tumour necrosis factor and other cytokines [5, 10, 11, 16]. The increase of IL-2 receptor percentages has been reported during the rejection of different organs [3, 18] and the measurement of soluble IL-2R has been proposed as an indicator of liver allograft rejection [12].

Our results show an important increase in IL-2R when clinical signs of rejection are present and, in addition, show an increase of CD8 cells and also an increase of IL-2 receptors.

CD8 is expressed by cytotoxic/suppressor cells which preferentially respond to antigens presented in conjunction with MHC class I molecules. Activation of CD8+ specific cytotoxic T-lymphocytes by allogenic class I

Table 3 Pre- and posttransplantation values of IL-2R

	Pretransplantation (%)	Posttransplantation (%)
Group A	1.7 ± 3.3	———
Group B	1.3 ± 3.4	8.8 ± 2.5 ($P < 0.05$)
Group C	1.7 ± 2.9	10.7 ± 1.7 ($P < 0.001$)
Group A (surgery day)	1.9 ± 3.1	——

Table 4 Correlation between the intensity and earliness of the rejection and the increase of CD8 and CD19 cells in group C (Kendall correlation coefficient)

Intensity of rejection	CD8 $P = 0.0199$
Intensity of rejection	CD19 $P = 0.0223$
Earliness of rejection	CD8 $P = 0.0199$
Earliness of rejection	CD19 $P = 0.0223$

and their stimulation by IL-2 causes direct specific foreign cell lysis [2], perhaps through direct contact by means of perforin [21].

This study also demonstrates a correlation between activated CD8 cells and the intensity and precocity of rejection when the host immune response is stimulated by means of a thymic hormone [thymostimulin (TP-1)]. Previous studies showed that thymostimulin was able to inhibit the decrease of the immune response induced by both anaesthesia and surgical trauma in the rat [6, 15], by increasing the CD4 cell percentage and inhibiting the increase of the CD8 cell percentage. However, when rats receiving thymostimulin also underwent transplantation of a small bowel allograft, we observed an increase of CD8 cell content in the spleen, thymus and intestinal lymphatic nodes, a decrease of CD4 cells in the spleen and an accelerated rejection [7]. The importance of CD8 cell changes during cardiac allograft rejection has been exposed by Carlquist et al. [1] in three murine experimental models. These authors found a significantly increased percentage of CD4 and a significantly decreased percentage of CD8 cells infiltrating grafts when allografts had a long survival but, in contrast, an increase of CD8 and a decrease of CD4 infiltrating graft cells when allografts were rejected in a short posttransplantation period. In the small bowel rejection of a fully allogeneic graft in rats, Oberhuber et al. [7] found intraepithelial lymphocytes. Among these, 45 % were neither CD4+ nor CD8+, 46.4 % were CD8+ cells, 8 % were CD4+ cells and 23 % were infiltrating host lymphocytes. This observation may be important in the consideration of the role of CD8 lymphocyte subsets in small bowel allograft rejection, especially with regard to passenger leucocytes from the graft.

In our study, in the group with thymostimulin treatment, a relationship was found between the percentage of activated CD19 cells and the intensity of rejection. B-cells are also activated by cytokines produced by T-cells (IL-3, IL-4, IL-6, IL-7, IL-13, BCDF, BCAF, BCSF) [16] in the presence of the antigen to produce high levels of anti-class I antibodies. Even though this is not very important in acute rejection [14], it has an important role in accelerating vascular rejection [2].

We believe that our paper shows the importance of CD8 cells in the rejection phenomenon, particularly in small bowel transplantation. In addition, the increases of CD8 cells and IL-2R in peripheral blood should be considered as a diagnosis of rejection. Finally, we agree with P. J. Morris [14] in believing that therapeutic options, including monoclonal antibodies against the IL-2 receptor, may be the future to controlling small bowel allograft rejection.

Acknowledgements This study was supported by a grant from the Fondo de Investigaciones Sanitarias de la Seguridad Social of Spain.

References

1. Carlquist IF, Shelby J, Hammond EH, et al (1994) Histocompatibility-associated differences in the phenotypes of murine cardiac allograft infiltrating T cells. Immunology 82: 149–153
2. Chandler Ch, Passaro E (1993) Transplant rejection. Mechanisms and treatment. Arch Surg 128: 279–283
3. Cornaby A, Simpson MA, Van Rice R, et al (1988) Interleukin-2 production in plasma and urine, plasma interleukin-2 receptor levels, and urine cytology as a means of monitoring renal allograft recipients. Transplant Proc 20 (Suppl 1): 108
4. Dinarello C (1993) Inflammatory cytokines. In: Neuberger J, Adams D (eds) Immunology of liver transplantation. Arnold, London, pp 57–83
5. Fong Y, Moldawer L, Shires GT, Lowry S (1990) The biologic characteristics of cytokines and their implication in surgical injury. Surg Gynecol Obstet 170: 363–378
6. García-Lechuz JM, Navarro M, Morandeira MJ, et al (1993) Immunorestorative effect of thymostimulin on surgery immunodepression: experimental model. Eur Surg Res 25: 74–82
7. Güemes A, Navarro-Zorraquino M, Lozano R, et al (1994) The role of the spleen and thymus in rat bowel transplantation. Eur Surg Res 26 (S1): 104
8. Güemes A, Navarro M, Sousa R, et al (1994) Técnica simplificada de trasplante de intestino delgado en la rata. Cir Esp 56 (S1): 103
9. Holloran PF, Cockfield SM, Madrenas J (1989) The mediators of inflammation (interleukin 1, interferon-gamma, and tumor necrosis factor) and their relevance to rejection. Transplant Proc 21: 26–30

10. Howard M, Matis L, Malek TR, et al (1983) Interleukin 2 induces antigen-reactive T cell line to secrete BCGF-1. J Exp Med 158: 2024–2039

11. Inaba K, Granelli-Piperno A, Steiman RM (1983) Dendritic cells induce T lymphocytes to release B-cell-stimulating factors by an interleukin-2 dependent mechanism. J Exp Med 158: 2040–2057

12. Larsen CP, Austyn JM, Phil D, Morris PJ (1990) The role of the graft-derived dendritic lymphocytes in the rejection of vascularized organ allografts. Ann Surg 212: 308–317

13. Monchick GJ, Russell PS (1971) Transplantation of the small bowel in the rat: technical and immunological considerations. Surgery 70: 693–720

14. Morris PJ (1990) Rejection: unanswered questions. Hum Immunol 28: 104–111

15. Navarro M, Román A, Lozano R, et al (1991) Prophylasis of the immunodepressive effect of anaesthesia using thymostimulin in an experimental model. Res Surg 3: 236–240

16. Navarro Zorraquino M (1995) Biological response modifiers in the small bowel allograft rejection. Nutr Hosp 10: 1–6

17. Oberhuber G, Schmid Th, Thaler W, et al (1993) Increase in intraepithelial lymphocytes as an early marker of rejection in a fully allogeneic rat small bowel transplantation model. Eur Surg Res 25: 310–315

18. Perkins JD, Nelson DL, Rakela J, et al (1989) Soluble interleukin-2 receptor level as an indicator of liver allograft rejection. Transplantation 47: 77–81

19. Roitt IM, Brostoff J, Male DK (1994) In: Masson-Salvat (ed) Inmunología, 3rd edn. Barcelona, pp 7–10

20. Schraut WH, Lee KKW (1985) Clinico-pathologic differentiation of rejection vs host disease following small bowel transplantation. In: Delz E, Thiede A, Hamelman H (eds) Small bowel transplantation, experimental and clinical fundaments. Springer, Berlin Heidelberg New York, pp 89–115

21. Shinkai Y, Takio K, Okumura K (1993) Homology of perforin to the ninth component of complement (C9). Nature 334: 525–527

Transpl Int (1996) 9 [Suppl 1]: S286–S289
© Springer-Verlag 1996

T. P. Szymula von Richter
R. G. H. Baumeister
C. Hammer

Microsurgical reconstruction of the lymphatic and nerve system in small bowel transplantation: the rat model, first results

T. P. Szymula von Richter
Amalienstrasse 89, D-80799 Munich,
Germany

R. G. H. Baumeister (✉)
Division of Micro-, Hand and
Reconstructive Surgery, Klinikum
Grosshadern,
University of Munich,
Marchioninistrasse 15,
D-81377 Munich, Germany

C. Hammer
ICF, University of Munich,
Marchioninistrasse 15,
D-81377 Munich, Germany

Abstract The goal in tissue transplantation is the restoration of all natural (physiological) communication pathways between the host and the graft. To this end, the effects of microsurgical reconstruction of artery, vein, lymphatic vessel, and nerve during grafting were investigated. Allogenic (MHC class II incompatible) and isogenic orthotopic (graft in functional continuity) small bowel recipients with immediate microsurgical lymphatic and nerve anastomosis were observed clinically as well as by immunological and histological examination. To explain the influence of the lymphatic system in allograft survival, short-term therapy was applied with the immunosuppressant cyclosporin A (10 mg/kg i.m.) for only 5 postoperative days. Average allograft survival ended in the control group after 10 days without any therapy, increased up to 20 days after immunosuppressive therapy (in both groups acute rejection and graft-versus-host disease were seen) and increased further to more than 200 days following lymphatic connection of the host and the graft during allografting. In this group no lymphatic edema of the graft was seen. To determine the optimal location of nerve anastomoses between the host and the graft without irritating the host nerve system, isografts in the same model were investigated. No paralysis of graft neighboring tissues was seen when the last ganglion function, and its following nerve plexus, of the host is saved. Nerve reconstruction must be undertaken after this last crossing of regional nerve fibers before entering the organ. The same rule is effective for organ explantation.

Key words Rat small bowel transplantation · Graft rejection · Lymphatic system · Nerve system · Microsurgical anastomoses

Introduction

Today, the importance of the lymphatic system in immunology is understood, although it has been known for 30 years that the lymphatic vessels are pathways of immunological cells [1]. The importance of the nerve system in immunology was proved a few years ago and the peripheral nerves have been known as pathways of information to innervated tissue since the early days of anatomy [2]. Clinically, microsurgeons have reconstructed lymphatic vessels for the last 15 years and nerves for the last 25 years knowing that these pathways regenerate with time [3, 4]. Our initial inspiration for this study comes from the history of human transplantation investigated originally by plastic surgeons [5–10].

Embryologically, the skin and gastrointestinal tract have the same origin, which makes them difficult to transplant allogenically. Both have close associations with the immune system. The goal of understanding this physiological phenomenon is the knowledge that those particular organs are more frequently circulated by immunological cells than others. High levels of po-

S 287

tential immunosuppressants are needed to allow the allogenic transplantation of these tissues [11].

In this study we used today's most sophisticated microsurgical reconstruction for transplantation, revealing results of interest to immunologists [12].

Materials and methods

Animals

Young female Brown Norway rats as donors [BN (RT1^n) $\times$ LEW (RT^l)] and young male Lewis rats as recipients were transplanted allogenically. Young male Lewis rats were used for the isogenic study. The average weight was 200 g.

Explantation

An orthotopic small bowel transplantation model was used, based on the microsurgical experimental methods of Olszewski and Acland [13, 14], the clinical experience of Buncke and Harii [15] for blood vessels, of Millesi [4] for nerves and of Baumeister for lymphatic vessels [3]. Consequently, a less invasive approach and minimal damage to the graft was possible. Whole explantation was done under the microscope. Only 95 % of the donor small bowel was explanted due to the fact that, during transplantation, the remaining 5 % of the explanted host small bowel must remain to preserve the ileo-caecal valve function of the host. After cutting of the portal vein and perfusion with body temperature isotonic solution, the small bowel was explanted with a 2-mm aorta abdominalis stump, to avoid damage of cysterna chyli.

Preparation of the lymphatic system

Careful preparation allowed damage-free lymphatic grafting. At the end of lymphatic preparation, the lymphatic flow of the small bowel led into the cysterna chyli and the following ductus thoracicus only.

Preparation of the nerve system

Thin intestinal nerves lie after the last ganglion and the following nerve plexus and pursue the lymphatic vessels of the mesenteric lymph nodes; thick intestinal nerves are located before the last ganglion.

Allogenic transplantation with lymphatic system reconstruction

The whole operation of allogenic orthotopic small bowel transplantation with ($n = 10$) and without ($n = 10$) microsurgical lymphatic anastomosis was performed under the operating microscope. First, the aorta of the graft was anastomosed with 10-0 sutures end-to-side to the host aorta abdominalis. Cuff techniques that would need an additional kidney explantation, and which may have influenced the host's condition for long-term results, were not employed. Porto-portal anastomoses would damage connections between liver and host cysterna chyli. Therefore, the venous anastomosis was performed between the graft portal vein and the host vene cava inferior with 10-0 sutures end-to-side. Then lymphatic anastomosis was added end-to-side with 12-0 su-

tures between the graft ductus thoracicus, which remained connected to the graft and the host cysterna chyli during explantation.

Immunological therapy

Allogenic orthotopic small bowel recipients with and without microsurgical lymphatic anastomosis were treated with cyclosporine A (CsA; 10 mg/kg i.m. diluted in 0.3 ml Intralipid) for 5 postoperative days only.

Isogenic transplantation with nerve system reconstruction

Isogenic orthotopic small bowel transplantation with microsurgical nerve anastomoses before ($n = 5$) and after the last ganglion ($n = 5$) were also performed under the operating microscope. In this study, the reconstruction of the intestinal nerves was done end-to-end with 12-0 sutures between the prepared intestinal nerves of the graft and the host. To study the importance of the location for nerve repair, the nerve anastomoses were designed in five animals after and in five animals before the donor's and the host's last ganglions.

Transplantation long-term follow-up

The outcome of grafts was studied up to 1 year by clinical observation, including weight measurements as well as histological studies. In the allogenic group, cytoimmunological monitoring was added.

Results

First, the lymphatic anastomosis prolongs allograft survival after only 5 days immunosuppression with 10 mg/kg i.m. cyclosporin (Fig. 1). The average small bowel survival was more than 200 days when lymphatic anastomosis was added during transplantation, compared with 20 days of average allograft survival in animals without this microsurgical technique. When immunosuppressant was not used, all participants bearing MHC class II incompatibility of the small bowel died, on average, at day 10 after grafting due to rejection, showing weight loss from day one. Animals receiving allogenic organ transplantation with lymphatic repair showed no signs of acute rejection after 5 days immunosuppressive therapy compared to those undergoing allografting without lymphatic anastomosis.

Second, in the isogenic model, transections of recipient intestinal nerves caused no paralysis of the remaining recipient gastrointestinal tract if placed after the last ganglion. The optimal position for the intestinal nerve anastomoses between the graft and the host, therefore, was found to be after the last ganglion.

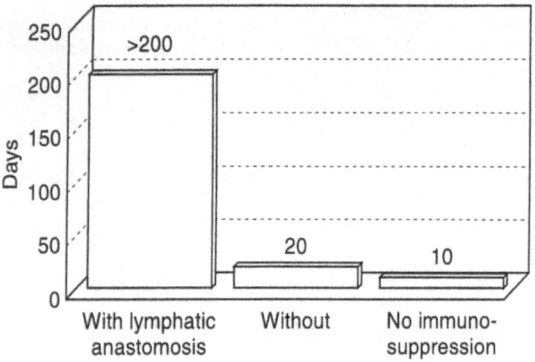

Fig. 1 Average allograft survival after only 5 days of immunosuppressive therapy in orthotopic small bowel transplantation in the rat

Discussion

In discussing the lymphatic influence in allografting, it is of great importance to understand that allogenic sensitization occurs primarily in draining lymph nodes and, in keeping with the principles of fundamental immunology, that naive T-cells are kept within the lymphatic tissue before any kind of rejection starts and that only activated or memory cells are allowed to circulate into peripheral tissue [16]. Since most sensation occurs in the peripheral tissue of the host, the early cell-mediated response via the lymphatic vessels of the graft into the host lymphatic system with the repair of lymphatic vessels makes sense. Most donor cell traffic leaves the allograft directly through the veins and lymphatic vessels in our model. In former models, without lymphatic vessel repair, this traffic occurred at the outset through the vein and tissue connections between the edemic graft and the host. The inflammation which followed may have been due to lymphatic tissue edema that occurs after invasion of immunological cells stimulated by the MHC incompatibility. Lymphoid and dendritic cell replacement may, therefore start, earlier in our lymphatic model, because of the earlier two-way immunological cell migration between the graft and the host [17].

Moreover, the fat-soluble immunosuppressive drug, CsA, may be able to recirculate into the recipient lymphatic system after being eliminated into the gastrointestinal tract, because lymphatic vessels transport long-chain fatty acids that contain CsA transport molecules. Hence, the highest body concentration of CsA is located in the thoracic duct. This may explain the 1-year survival of one participant in the MHC class II incompatible model who showed no histological signs of rejection after only 5 days of CsA therapy.

The future problem in transplantation of some organs may be the nerve regulation of transplanted tissue successful long-term survival, with the goal of maximal original function of the graft [18]. Since it is known that postganglionic parasympathetic nerves survive in the allograft, evidenced by histological studies of postganglionic autonomic nerve fibers, surgical reinnervation after transplantation is the next step to be investigated [17]. Grafting with microsurgical nerve anastomoses allows host nerve axons to grow into the graft using the original nerve pathways. To study the behavior of nerve anastomoses during grafting, and to demonstrate nerve regeneration in organ transplantation, isogenic investigations were first planned. Experimental grafting in plastic surgery suggests that nerve axons find the position of their original nerve synapses after correct nerve anastomoses. Less nerve regeneration time is needed in comparison to incorrect nerve restoration. The more exact the anastomosis is, the better functional results can be achieved.

We therefore think that realisation of primary lymphatic anastomoses during allogenic transplantation could lower immunosuppressive drug consumption and their side-effects as well as prolong graft survival. Concerning the long-term function of grafts, correct nerve reconstruction may also be of importance for integration into the host nerve system. The microsurgical reconstruction of the natural communication pathways of the organ, the arterial, vein, lymphatic, and nerve system, is now approaching reality and should be taken into consideration in transplantation surgery in the future.

References

1. Sprent J (1974) Migration and lifespan of circulating B lymphocytes of nude (nu/nu) mice. In: Rygaard J, Povlsen CO (eds) Proceedings of the first international workshop on nude mice. Gustav Fischer, Stuttgart, pp 11–22
2. Ader R, Felten DL, Cohen N (1990) Psychoneuroimmunology. Academic Press, San Diego
3. Baumeister RGH, Siuda S (1990) Treatment of lymphedemas by microsurgical lymphatic grafting: what is proved? Plast Reconstr Surg 85: 213–216
4. Millesi H (1992) Chirurgie peripherer Nerven. Urban & Schwarzenberg, Wien
5. Dieffenbach JF (1882) Nonulla de regeneratione et transplantatione. Dissertatio Inauguralis, Berlin
6. Lexer E (1911) Über freie Transplantationen. Arch Klin Chir 95: 827
7. Converse JM, Rogers BO (1954–1962) Symposia of the 1st, 2nd, 3rd, 4th, 5th and 6th international tissue homotransplantation research conference at New York Academy of Sciences. Ann NY Acad Sci 5: 277; 64: 735; 73: 539; 87: 1; 99: 335; 162: 64
8. White RJ (1968) Experimental transplantation of the brain. In: Rapaport FT, Dausset J (eds) Human transplantation. Grune and Stratton, New York

9. Murray JE (1976) Transplantation biology – an overview. In: Krizek TJ, Hoopes JE (eds) Symposium on basic sciences in plastic surgery. CV Mosby, Saint Louis
10. Converse JM (1977) Reconstructive plastic surgery, 2nd edn. WB Saunders, Philadelphia, pp 126–151
11. Todo S, Tzakis A, Reye J, Abu-Elmagd K, Casavilla A, Fung JJ, Starzl TE (1993) Intestinal transplantation on humans under FK 506. Transplant Proc 25: 1198–1199
12. Szymula von Richter TP, Baumeister RGH (1995) Does the microsurgical reconstruction of the lymphatic system influence allograft survival? In: Harii K (ed) Transactions of the 11th congress of the international confederation of plastic, reconstructive and aesthetic surgery, Yokohama, Japan. Kugler, Amsterdam, p 65
13. Olszewski WL (1984) Handbook of microsurgery. CRC Press, Boca Raton, Florida
14. Acland RD, Smith P (1979) Experimental lymphatico-lymphatic anastomoses. In: Abstract book of the VIIth international congress of lymphology, Florence
15. Harii K (1983) Microvascular tissue transfer. Fundamental techniques and clinical applications. Igakushon, Tokyo
16. Paul WE (1993) Fundamental immunology, 3rd edn. Raven Press, New York
17. Shumway SJ, Shumway NE (1995) Thoracic transplantation. Blackwell Science, Cambridge, pp 327; 452–470
18. Grant DR, Wood RFM (1994) Small bowel transplantation. Edward Arnold, London

Lung

Transpl Int (1996) 9 [Suppl 1]: S 293–S 295
© Springer-Verlag 1996

Takeshi Hirabayashi
S. Demertzis
J. Schäfers
Ken Hoshino
Björn Nashan

Chronic rejection in lung allografts: immunohistological analysis of fibrogenesis

T. Hirabayashi · B. Nashan (✉)
Klinik für Abdominal- und
Transplantationschirurgie,
Medizinische Hochschule Hannover,
Konstanty-Gutschow-Strasse 8,
D-30625 Hannover, Germany

S. Demertzis · J. Schäfers
Klinik für Herz-, Thorax-, Gefässchirurgie,
Medizinische Hochschule Hannover,
Konstanty-Gutschow-Strasse 8,
D-30625 Hannover, Germany

K. Hoshino
Department of Surgery,
School of Medicine, Keio University,
Shinanomachi 35, Shinjuku, 160,
Tokyo, Japan

Abstract In ongoing chronic rejection after lung transplantation, alveolar interstitial fibrosis develops. However, little is known about the mechanisms involved. In order to investigate these mechanisms, expression of extracellular matrix molecules (ECM) (undulin, decorin, tenascin, laminin, and fibronectin) and cytokines [transforming growth factor(TGF)-β1, TGF-β3, platelet-derived growth factor(PDGF), and PDGF receptor] were semiquantitatively evaluated in chronically rejected lung allografts, using standard immunohistochemical techniques. Additionally, the presence of macrophages was analysed. The present study demonstrates an increased infiltration of macrophages with a concomitant upregulation of cytokines (TGF-β1, TGF-β3, and PDGF) and an increased deposition of ECM in chronic lung rejection. These cytokines have an important role in the stimulation of fibroblasts which are a major source of ECM. Upregulated expression of ECM in the alveolar interstitial space leads to alveolar malfunction by thickening of the wall and, thus, is one of the causative factors of respiratory dysfunction in chronic lung graft rejection.

Key words Chronic rejection · Alveolar interstitial fibrosis · Extracellular matrix · TGF-β · PDGF

Introduction

Alveolar interstitial fibrosis develops in ongoing rejection of lung allografts [1, 2] and is assumed to be a causative factor of respiratory dysfunction. In idiopathic pulmonary fibrosis and animal models of pulmonary fibrosis, alveolar interstitial fibrosis is characterized by an increase in extracellular matrix and cytokines, secreted from alveolar macrophages, i. e., TGF-β and PDGF. Particularly, these cytokines are presumed to have a potent role in the production of extracellular matrix molecules [3]. According to the results of previous studies, upregulated expression of PDGF-mRNA and PDGF were found in macrophages in chronically rejected lungs [4]. It is thought that the interstitial fibrotic change in chronically rejected lungs is immunohistochemically similar to that in idiopathic pulmonary fibropsis [5]. Yet, the mechanism of fibrotic change remains unclear. In order to investigate the process of chronic graft rejection in lungs, we analysed immunohistochemically the expression of ECM, infiltrated macrophages, and cytokines in this setting.

Patients and methods

Seven lung specimens from six patients retransplanted for chronic rejection of lung allografts were obtained at the time of retransplantation and cryopreserved. Patients' clinical data are shown in Table 1. Histological evaluation demonstrated alveolar interstitial fibrosis in all specimens. As controls, five lung specimens were obtained from donors before transplantation. All specimens were immediately frozen in liquid nitrogen and then stored in a deep freezer at − 80 °C until preparation. For immunohistochemical analysis, cryostat sections, 7 μm thick, were obtained. Using standard immu-

Table 1 Clinical data for patients with chronic rejection after lung transplantation (*CF* Cryptogenic fibrosis, *LF* lung fibrosis, *PPHT* primary pulmonary hypertension)

Chronic rejection	Sex	Age (years)	Primary disease	Time since TX
1	Female	22	PPHT	2 months
2	Female	46	LF	11 days
3	Male	27	CF	2 months
4	Male	34	CF	19 months
5	Female	33	CF	48 months
6	Female	53	CF	18 days

Table 2 Expression of extracellular matrix in the alveolar area (− Negative staining, ± weakly positive staining or few positively stained cells, + moderately positive staining or some positively stained cells, ++ strongly positive staining or high number of positively stained cells, +++ very strongly positive staining or very high number of positively stained cells, *ND* not done)

Chronic rejection	Fibronectin	Tenascin	Undulin	Decorin
1a	+++	++	+++	+++
1b	+++	++	+	+~++
2	+~++	++~+++	+~++	+~++
3	+±	++	+~++	+
4	+	±~+	±	±,~+±
5	ND	+±	−~,±	+±
6	+	+±+±,~+	+~+±	
Normal control n = 5	±,~+	±,~+±	−~,±	+~+±

Table 3 Expression of cytokines on the alveolar area

Chronic rejection	TGF-β1 Macrophage	TGF-β3 Macrophage	PDGF Macrophage	PDGF Pneumocyte	PDGFr Interstitium
1a	++	+++	++	++	+++
1b	+±	+++	+++	+++	++
2	++	+++	+~++	+++	±
3	+++	+++	+	+	
4	+~++	+~++	±	±~+	±
5	ND	+~++	−	−	±
6	+	++~+++			+~++
Normal control n = 5	−	±~++	±,~++	−~+	±,~++

nohistochemical techniques previously described [6], expression of ECM molecules (undulin, decorin, tenascin, laminin, and fibronectin), cytokines (TGF-β1, TGF-β3, PDGF, and PDGF receptor) and the macrophage marker (27E10) were semiquantitatively evaluated.

Results

The results of ECM and cytokine expression are shown in Tables 2, 3. In comparison to normal controls, a marked increase in ECM deposition, except for laminin, was observed in expanded alveolar interstitial tissue in chronic lung rejection. The number of infiltrated macrophages in the alveolar space and the alveolar interstitial tissue increased. A concomitant upregulation of TGF-β1, TGF-β3, and PDGF was found on alveolar macrophages in the alveolar area. Expression of PDGF was also found on alveolar epithelial cells and alveolar hyaline membrane, and PDGFr was expressed on the alveolar interstitial tissue.

Discussion

In idiopathic pulmonary fibrosis, TGF-β and PDGF are secreted from activated alveolar macrophages. It is assumed that upon this stimulatory event, lung fibroblasts are activated and produce ECM [3]. In the present study, an increased infiltration of macrophages that stained positive for these cytokines could be demonstrated. Furthermore, severe accumulation of ECM in the interstitial space could be shown. These findings indicate that fibrogenesis is enhanced in chronic lung graft rejection. There is still debate about the cells responsible for the ECM production. From these experiments, we can conclude that cells residing in the interalveolar space demonstrated expression of PDGFr. As these cells are not macrophages, they are most likely to be fibrocytes which are known to be PDGFr positive. These data are in accordance with findings in chronic inflammation in different tissues [8]. Although the biological function of PDGFr in the lung is still debated [7], there is evidence for its pivotal role in fibrogenesis [4].

In conclusion, the present study demonstrates an increased infiltration of macrophages with a concomitant upregulation of cytokines and an increased deposition of ECM in chronically rejected lungs. These cytokines probably have an important role in the stimulation of ECM in the alveolar interstitial space which might lead to alveolar malfunction and, thus, could be one of the causative factors of respiratory dysfunction in chronic lung graft rejection.

References

1. Tazzeler HD, Yousem SA (1988) The pathology of combined heart-lung transplantation: An autopsy study. Hum Pathol 19: 1403–1418
2. Couch E (1990) Pathobiology of pulmonary fibrosis. Am J Physiol 259: L159–L184
3. Gauldie J, Jordana M, Cox G (1993) Cytokines and pulmonary fibrosis. Thorax 48: 931–935
4. Hertz MI, Henke CA, Nakhleh RE, et al (1992) Obliterative bronchiolitis after lung transplantation. A fibroproliferative disorder associated with platelet-derived growth factor. Proc Natl Acad Sci USA 89: 10385–10389
5. Yousem SA, Sucan SR, Ohori NP, et al (1992) Architectural remodeling of lung allografts in acute and chronic rejection. Arch Pathol Lab Med 116: 1175–1180
6. Steinhoff G, Wonigeit K, Pichlmayr R (1988) Analysis of segmental changes in major histocompatibility complex expression in human liver allografts after liver transplantation. Transplantation 45: 394–401
7. Rubin K, Terracio L, Rönnstrand L, et al (1988) Expression of platelet-derived growth factor receptor is induced on connected tissue cells during chronic synovial inflammation. Scan J Immunol 27: 285–294
8. Aubert JD, Hayashi S, Hards J, et al (1994) Platelet-derived growth factor and its receptor in lungs from patients with asthma and chronic air flow obstruction. Am J Physiol 266: L655–663

Transpl Int (1996) 9 [Suppl 1]: S296–S298
© Springer-Verlag 1996

LUNG

Andrés Varela
Carlos Montero
Mar Córdoba
Santiago Serrano-Fiz
Raúl Burgos
Juan Carlos Téllez
Eduardo Tebar
Gabriél Téllez
Juan Ugarte

Clinical experience with retrograde lung preservation

A. Varela (✉) · C. Montero · M. Córdoba ·
S. Serrano-Fiz · R. Burgos · J. C. Téllez ·
E. Tebar · G. Téllez · J. Ugarte
Division of Thoracic and
Cardiovascular Surgery,
Puerta de Hierro Hospital,
c/San Martín de Porres 4,
E-28035 Madrid, Spain

Abstract Previous reports and our own experimental work suggest increased vascularity of the tracheobronchial wall when retrograde lung preservation is used. This principle was clinically applied in 21 consecutive lung transplant recipients (10 single and 11 bilateral). Lung preservation was achieved via the left atrial appendage and drainage was obtained through the pulmonary artery. Pneumoplegic preservation was achieved with modified Euro-Collins solution. Cardioplegia was induced by the standard method and the heart, harvested by different teams, did not exhibit left ventricular dilatation. Thirty-two bronchial anastomoses without wrapping were performed. No primary lung graft failure was documented. Cardiopulmonary bypass was instituted in three cases of pulmonary hypertension; however, this was deemed unnecessary in the remainder of the cases of bilateral transplantation while the second organ was being implanted. All bronchial anastomoses were followed between 2 and 28 months. A single instance of bronchial anastomosis dehiscence was observed on the 30th postoperative day. However, no stents were employed in this series, and no strictures or anastomotic granulomas have been reported so far. All the hearts could be used satisfactorily except for one primary graft failure. In conclusion, retrograde lung preservation is feasible in clinical lung transplantation, with simultaneous harvesting of the heart. The impact of retrograde lung preservation on the late clinical outcome remains to be seen.

Key words Retrograde lung · preservation · Left atrial appendage · Intraparenchymal bronchial circulation

Introduction

The success of clinical lung transplantation represents new prospects for the treatment of the increasing number of patients with end-stage lung disease. However, the number of such operations currently being done is limited, mainly due to the scarcity of donors. This shortage has led to the development of a variety of lung preservation techniques, which are of particular value when an organ must be transported from a distant donation site to the transplantation center [3, 5, 8].

Different techniques have been designed to provide adequate lung preservation by antegrade pulmonary artery flushing (PAF) with a preservation solution, generally modified Euro-Collins solution (EC) or University of Winconsin organ preservation (UW). Yet, despite these pharmacological advances, early allograft dysfunction remains a problem. An entirely new concepts is represented by the retrograde instillation of preservation solution through the left atrial appendage (RELA), using the pulmonary artery for outflow. The first report in three cases of human heart-lung transplantation was done by Sarsam [10].

Antegrade lung preservation

Retrograde lung preservation

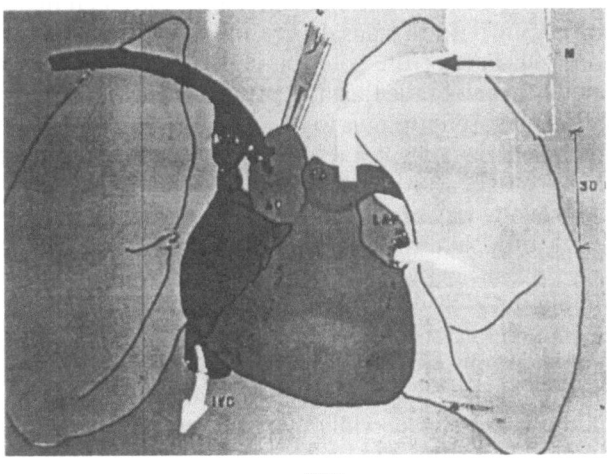

a   PAF

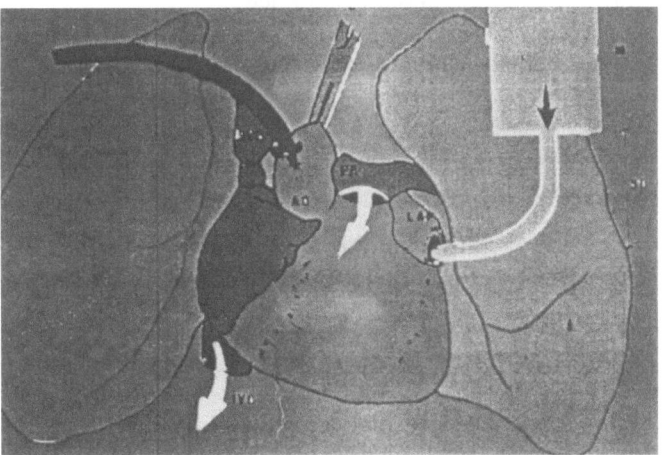

b   RELA

Fig. 1 a *PAF* Pulmonary artery flush. **b** *RELA* Retrograde left atrium flush

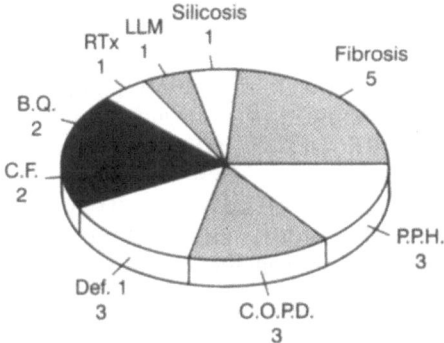

Fig. 2 Clinical experience with retrograde lung preservation. Diagnoses: *PPH* primary pulmonary hypertension, *COPD* chronic obstructive pulmonary disease, *DEF1* deficit and 1 antitrypsin, *CF* cystic fibrosis, *BQ* bronchiectasis, *RTx* retransplantation, *LLM* lymphangioleiomyomatosis

This original approach has been successfully employed in our laboratory and in 21 consecutive lung transplantation procedures. The observations and direct implications derived from this limited experience constitute the basis for the present report. The purpose of this analysis is to: (a) describe the advantages of RELA over PAF and (b) hypothesize on the role of intraparenchymal bronchial circulation in lung graft preservation.

Material and methods

Twenty-one consecutive lung transplantation procedures (10 unilateral and 11 bilateral) were carried out after lung preservation by the "retrograde technique" (Figs. 1, 2). This was accomplished using a short-tipped William Harvey cannula (Bard and William Harvey, Santa Ana, California, USA) for instillation of the pneumoplegic solution with modified EC (Laboratorios Esteve, Barcelona, Spain) through the left atrial appendage (retrograde), with outflow through the pulmonary artery (RELA).

Cardioplegia was induced previously with 1 l of a crystalloid solution instilled into the aortic root. A 14–16 cannula was positioned in the left atrial appendage for retropneumoplegia. A single bolus of prostaglandin E1 (500 mg) was injected into the pulmonary artery prior to pulmonary flushing with normothermic (1000 ml) and later cold (3000 ml, 4 °C) pneumoplegic solution. The effort was made to keep the solution 30 cm above table level to prevent pulmonary edema. The time taken for this technique is usually about 5 min. Left ventricular distension was prevented by venting the pneumoplegic solution through the anterior aspect of the pulmonary artery. Both pleural cavities were opened and irrigated with continuous cold saline slush to further enhance graft preservation. The heart was removed and the double-lung block excised adequately and immersed in a cold solution for transport.

The procedure in the recipient was performed via lateral thoracotomy for unilateral lung transplants or the "clam-shell" incision for bilateral lung transplants with or without cardiopulmonary bypass. The native lung(s) was (were) excised and the appropriate stumps created for the bronchial airway and vascular pedicles.

The airway anastomoses were done with a running 4-0 PDS (posterior row) and single-interrupted stitches (anterior row). The telescope technique was only employed when obvious disparity existed between donor and recipient bronchi. Otherwise, no attempts were made to wrap the anastomoses.

Results

No primary graft failure was detected in this limited series. Gas exchange was satisfactory in all cases, and extubation was carried out within the first 48 h in most patients. Chest X-rays were mostly within normal limits.

No strictures nor granulomas have been observed to date during a mean follow-up period of 2–28 months. One case of airway dehiscence was observed 30 days after the operation, and this was the only case requiring retransplantation in our experience.

All the hearts harvested in the above manner could be used immediately. Graft failure (hyperacute rejection?) occurred in only one case.

Discussion

Clinical lung transplantation has been impeded by inadequate graft preservation and subsequent allograft dysfunction, thus limiting the number and quality of procedures worldwide. Initially, lungs were harvested in situ and transplanted immediately in an effort to minimize organ injury [1]. Different protocols were subsequently established to preserve lung allograft function, including donor-core cooling [6, 13] and PAF with either modified EC [11] or UW [4]. Both gained wide acceptance when associated with a single intravenous prostaglandin bolus for pulmonary vasodilation. This resulted in superior lung preservation but, as a preservation strategy, it ignores the bronchial circulation. RELA flushing of the preservation solution was introduced to address this problem.

The pulmonary venous circulation is a low-resistance high-capacity system. Flushing of preservation fluid through this system is straightforward and results in rapid and uniform distribution of the solution [9]. Timing for administration of the pneumoplegic solution does not hamper delivery of the cardioplegia, and both can be flushed at the same time or once the heart is arrested, since most RELA drainage exits through the anterior aspect of the pulmonary artery.

Furthermore, it has been shown in three cases of heart-lung transplantation that no left ventricular dilatation occurs despite transatrial cannulation for preservation [10]. Part of the solution exits through the aortic valve as in antegrade flushing, returning via the coronary aorta and coronary sinus to the right atrium, from where it is expelled via the venae cavae when these are transected prior to heart removal. Neither EC nor UW solution alters in any way the coronary artery endothelium [12].

The bronchial circulation is also known as the pulmonary systemic network and supplies not only the extra/intrapulmonary airway system, but the neurovascular bundles, lymphoid structures, and visceral pleura, as well [2]. Bronchial veins from the upper airway (especially the extrapulmonary veins) drain into the right heart chambers via the venae cavae, while those arising from the intrapulmonary airway and parenchymal systems drain into the left heart via the pulmonary veins. The latter constitutes the so-called "pulmonary collateral", "bronchopulmonary anastomotic," or "bronchial-pulmonary systemic" blood flow, the role of which has been well defined by Lo Cicero et al. [7]. They demonstrated the architecture of the bronchial circulation, in a rather complex but conclusive manner, by perfusing a closed segment of the mid descending thoracic aorta and collecting the resultant solution in the left atrial appendage. However, the real implications of bronchial-pulmonary preservation are still unclear and remain to be elucidated. Another point that deserves further discussion is that of the revascularization of the bronchial circulation and its impact on medium-term function of the graft, as well as the development of bronchiolitis obliterans.

References

1. Cooley DA, Bloodwell RD, Hallman GL, Nora JJ, Harrison GM, Leachman RD (1969) Organ transplantation for advanced cardiopulmonary disease. Ann Thorac Surg 8: 30–46
2. Deffebach ME, Charan NB, Lakshminarayan S, Butler J (1987) The bronchial circulation. Small, but a vital attribute of the lung. Am Rev Respir Dis 135: 463–481
3. Haverich A, Scott WC, Jamieson SW (1985) Twenty years of lung preservation a review. J Heart Transplant 4: 234–240
4. Hirt SW, Wahlers T, Jurmann MJ, et al (1992) University of Winconsin versus modified Euro-Collins solution for lung preservation. Ann Thorac Surg 53: 74–79
5. Kirk AJB, Colquhoun IW, Dark JH (1993) Lung preservation: A review of current and future directions. Ann Thorac Surg 56: 990–1000

6. Kontos GJ Jr, Adachi H, Borkon MA, et al (1987) A no-flush, core cooling technique for successful cardiopulmonary preservation in heart-lung transplantation. J Thorac Cardiovasc Surg 94: 836–842
7. Lo Cicero J, Massad M, Matano J, Greene R, Dunn H, Michaelis LL (1991) Contribution of the bronchial circulation to lung preservation. J Thorac Cardiovasc Surg 101: 807–815
8. Novick RJ, Menkis AH, McKenzie FN (1992) New trends in lung preservation: A collective review. J Heart Lung Transplant 11: 377–392
9. Sánchez de León R, Orchard CH, Chakrabarti M, Sykes MK (1982) Effect of hypoxia on fluid filtration rate during forward and reverse perfusion of isolated rabbit lungs. Cardiovasc Res 16: 711–714

10. Sarsam MAI, Yonan NA, Deiraniya AK, Rahman AN (1993) Retrograde pulmonaryplegia for lung preservation in clinical transplantation: A new technique. J Heart Lung Transplant 12: 494–498
11. Stuart RS, Monte S, Baumgartner WA, et al (1984) Successful 4 hour hypothermic lung storage with Euro-Collins solution: A simplified model assessing preservation. J Heart Transplant 3: 346–351
12. Swanson DK, Pasaoglu I, Berkoff HA, Southard JA, Hegge JO (1988) Improved heart preservation with UW preservation solution. J Heart Transplant 7: 456–467
13. Yacoub MH, Khaghani A, Banner N, Tajkarimi S, Fitzgerald M (1989) Distant organ procurement for heart and lung transplantation. Transplant Proc 21: 2548–2550

Transpl Int (1996) 9 [Suppl 1]: S299–S302
© Springer-Verlag 1996

Michael Tamm
Linda Sharples
Tim Higenbottam
Susan Stewart
John Wallwork

Bronchiolitis obliterans syndrome (BOS) following heart-lung transplantation

M. Tamm · L. Sharples ·
T. Higenbottam (✉) · S. Stewart ·
J. Wallwork
Transplant Unit, Research and
Development Unit, Laboratory for
Respiratory Physiology, Department of
Pathology, Papworth Hospital,
Papworth Everard,
CBS 8RE Cambridge, UK

Abstract With the increasing number of successfully performed lung transplants and a longer follow up of patients, there is an interest in the analysis of long-term complications and their impact on patient survival. Heart-lung transplantation was performed in 157 patients with 126 patients surviving at least 6 months. Early death was mainly caused by bacterial and viral infection. Long-term patient survival was decisively influenced by obliterative bronchiolitis. With the new international definition of bronchiolitis obliterans syndrome (BOS) based on an irreversible decline of FEV1 from baseline values, it became possible to analyse the incidence of BOS and the impact on patient mortality in long-term survivors. FEV1 reached a peak value of 102 % predicted at a median of 219 days. In 106 of 126 patients (84 %), FEV1 showed no decline within the first year. A total of 60 patients (47.6 %) developed BOS grade 1 with progression to BOS grade 2 in 85 % of these patients. The incidence of BOS was 12.6 % at 1 year increasing to more than 50 % 5 years after transplantation. Patient mortality due to obliterative bronchiolitis increased from 1 % at 1 year to 18 % more than 5 years after transplantation. Almost all deaths (86 %; 32/37) more than 1 year after HLT were associated with bronchiolitis obliterans. In summary, bronchiolitis obliterans decisively contributes to long-term patient morbidity and mortality after heart-lung transplantation. Clinical and research efforts should be directed towards avoiding this important complication.

Key words Bronchiolitis obliterans syndrome · Lung transplantation

Introduction

Lung transplantation has become a therapeutic option for patients with end-stage lung diseases associated with a poor prognosis. Patient mortality following lung transplantation can be attributed to typical short-term and long-term complications. Short-term complications include primary organ failure, pleural bleeding, anastomotic stenosis or dehiscence, acute rejection and infection. Long-term survival and quality of life is mainly affected by obliterative bronchiolitis. As early as 1984, obliterative bronchiolitis was described in a considerable number of heart-lung transplant recipients [1]. Obliterative bronchiolitis was defined as an irreversible severe air flow obstruction as measured by lung function in the absence of acute rejection or infection. Autopsy in patients affected by obliterative bronchiolitis showed bronchiectasis, obliteration of the small airways, interstitial and pleural fibrosis, and accelerated arterial and venous arteriosclerosis. Early reports found obliterative bronchiolitis in around 50 % of patients surviving the first year after surgery [2]. One of the problems associated with earlier reports is that no universally accepted definition of obliterative bronchiolitis was available,

S 300

and, therefore, the definition of the time to develop this complication was not standard between transplant centres. The working formulation for the standardisation of nomenclature of bronchiolitis obliterans syndrome (BOS) as defined by an international working group has recently established a clinical definition [3]. The definition of BOS using lung volumes is very helpful because obliterative bronchiolitis can not often be found in transbronchial biopsies and the efficacy of biopsies in the diagnosis varies between centres [4–6]. After heart-lung transplantation, lung volumes return to the predicted values of the recipient [7] in contrast to single lung transplantation. However, using the decline in FEV1 from baseline values for the definition of BOS, it is now possible to classify patients according to the international grading system and to compare the incidence of BOS between different centres using different immunosuppressive regimens in single, bilateral and heart-lung transplant recipients.

With the increasing number of patients undergoing successful heart-lung transplantation and with a longer follow up, we could study the incidence of BOS up to more than 5 years after transplantation and the impact on patient mortality.

Patients and methods

Patients

Between 1984 and 31 December 1993, 157 patients underwent heart-lung transplantation. The underlying diseases were: 56 cystic fibrosis, 34 Eisenmenger's syndrome, 18 primary pulmonary hypertension, 16 emphysema, 10 bronchiectasis, 5 sarcoidosis and 18 others.

Immunosuppression

Equine anti-lymphocyte globulin (ATG) was given for the first 3 days. Intraoperatively, 1000 mg of methylprednisolone was given followed by three doses of 125 mg during the first postoperative day. Cyclosporin A was given from the first day onwards to achieve whole blood levels between 300 and 600 ng/ml for the first few months and the daily azothioprine dose consisted of 2 mg/kg. Acute rejection was treated with 500–1000 mg methylprednisolone followed by oral prednisone (1 mg/kg) decreasing the dose over 10 days. In patients with repeated rejection episodes, triple therapy with cyclosporin A, azathioprine and prednisone was maintained. Steroids were only withdrawn if lung function remained stable and if there were no signs of rejection in the following 3 months.

Lung function

Routine lung function measurements included FEV1, vital capacity, total lung capacity and diffusion capacity, and were taken at 1, 3, 6, 9 and 12 months after transplantation and thereafter at 3–6 month intervals. In addition, measurements were taken if patients developed symptoms or signs of pulmonary rejection or infection or had radiological abnormalities. Patients performed daily home spirometry and returned to hospital for full lung function tests if a decline of at least 5 % was observed. If a deterioration in lung function was confirmed, bronchoscopy with bronchoalveolar lavage and transbronchial biopsy was performed to detect rejection or infection.

Bronchiolitis obliterans syndrome (BOS)

BOS was defined as an irreversible decline in FEV1 of at least 20 % of the individual baseline values and graded according to the recommendations of an international study group [3]. Baseline was determined as the maximum FEV1, taken at least 30 days apart in the first year after transplantation. Acute rejection and infection were excluded by bronchoalveolar lavage and transbronchial biopsy. Irreversible decline of FEV1 was graded as follows: BOS grade 0, FEV1 at least 80 % of baseline; BOS grade 1, FEV1 between 66 % and 80 % of baseline; BOS grade 2, FEV1 between 51 % and 65 % of baseline; BOS grade 3, FEV1 between 0 % and 50 % of baseline.

Statistics

Kaplan-Meier methods were used to describe the actuarial survival time and time to development of BOS grades.

Results

Between 1984 and December 1993, 157 patients underwent heart-lung transplantation. Overall patient mortality dropped from 9 % (14 of 157) in the first postoperative month to 4 % (6 of 143) in the second and 4 % (5 of 137) in the third. Infection was the most common cause of death, occurring in 18 of the 31 patients (58 %) who died within the first 6 months after surgery. Eleven patients died with bacterial infection including empyema (3) and pneumonia (3). There were 5 cases of fatal CMV pneumonitis, 4 of them involved seronegative recipients of organs from seropositive donors. Three of these occurred before ganciclovir treatment for CMV became available. Non-infective causes of death include primary graft failure (4), tracheal dehiscence (2), cerebrovascular event (1), gastrointestinal bleeding (1) and lymphoproliferative disorder (2). Postoperative bleeding was a frequent complication requiring reoperation in 34 (22 %) patients. There were no deaths as a result of pleural bleeding but reoperation was often associated with secondary complications, especially infection. Acute rejection was very common, occurring in 141 of 157 patients (90 %) within 3 months of transplantation. Rejection was successfully treated in all but 1 patient. One patient died in the second postoperative month with severe graft versus host disease.

Patients surviving at least 6 months were included for analysis of BOS because they were at risk of developing this complication. From these 126 patients, 5 died within the second 6 months after surgery reflecting the consid-

Actuarial survival for 157 recipients of heart-lung transplantation (95% confidence interval)

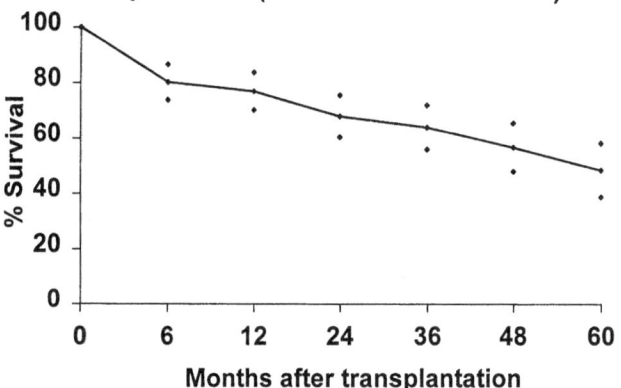

Fig. 1 Actuarial survival for 157 recipients of heart-lung transplantation

erable drop in mortality in the second half of the first year. Only 1 of 36 patients who died within the first year had obliterative bronchiolitis as an underlying complication. Graft survival, which was similar to patient survival, is shown on Fig. 1.

After surgery, FEV1 steadily increased and reached a peak value of 102 % (SD 22.6 %) predicted for the 126 heart-lung transplant recipients surviving at least 6 months. Peak FEV1 was reached at a median of 219 days (interquartile range 140–303 days) after transplantation. FEV1 above 80 % predicted was achieved by 105 patients at a median of 46 days (interquartile range 24–125 days). Using the grading system for BOS as described above, a total of 60 patients (47.6 %) developed BOS grade 1, 51 patients BOS grade 2 and 36 patients BOS grade 3. Table 1 shows the worst BOS grade achieved by patients who survived 6 months, for each year after transplantation. Between 7 and 12 months after surgery, 106 (84 %) patients showed no deterioration of lung function, reflecting an incidence of BOS of 13 %. The number of patients free of any functional deterioration had declined from 84 % at the end of the first year to 61 % at 3 years and 45 % at 5 years. At the final mea-

surement before analysis, 39 % of patients transplanted longer than 5 years still had normal lung volumes. On the other hand, the number of patients developing BOS increased steadily each year to 55 % at 5 years. At the time of reporting, only 15 % (9/60) of patients with BOS grade 1 have failed to develop BOS grade 2 indicating a rapid deterioration of lung volumes in patients with BOS. Median survival time from the time of development of BOS grade 1 was 948 days (interquartile range 306–2039). The percentage of patients who died with obliterative bronchiolitis increased from 1 % (1/126) at 1 year to 18 % (6/33) more than 5 years after transplantation. More than 1 year after transplantation, death was associated with bronchiolitis obliterans in 86 % of patients (32/37). A total of 27 of 60 patients with BOS (45 %) were alive at a median of 2.6 years after the diagnosis of BOS grade 1. There were 9 deaths more than 6 months after transplantation which were not associated with obliterative bronchiolitis (cerebrovascular accident; malignancy; graft versus host disease; renal failure complicated by infection; aeroplane accident; drug overdose; bronchial stenosis).

In summary, almost all patients surviving 6 months achieved predicted lung volumes within the first year after transplantation. Afterwards, the percentage of patients developing BOS steadily increased over the years. Deaths occurring more than 6 months after transplantation are mainly influenced by the occurrence of bronchiolitis obliterans.

Discussion

Early mortality following heart-lung transplantation is mainly due to infection whereas long-term survival is decisively influenced by bronchiolitis obliterans. The new definition of BOS allows the comparison of the incidence of obliterative bronchiolitis between different centres. Given the importance of this long-term complication, much effort should be directed to the prevention of obliterative bronchiolitis.

Table 1 Patients surviving at least 6 months after heart-lung transplantation broken down by the worst grade of bronchiolitis obliterans syndrome *(BOS)* observed in each period *(OB* obliterative bronchiolitis)

BOS grade	Months after transplantation					
	7–12 n (%)	13–24 n (%)	25–36 n (%)	37–48 n (%)	49–60 n (%)	> 60 n (%)
0	106 (84)	80 (70)	57 (61)	36 (51)	21 (45)	13 (39)
I	1 (1)	8 (7)	8 (9)	8 (11)	4 (9)	1 (3)
II	9 (7)	5 (4)	7 (8)	6 (9)	6 (13)	4 (12)
III	5 (4)	9 (8)	16 (17)	13 (19)	10 (21)	9 (27)
Death with OB	1 (1)	10 (9)	4 (4)	6 (9)	6 (13)	6 (18)
Death without OB	4 (3)	3 (3)	1 (1)	1 (1)	0 (0)	0 (0)
Number alive at start of period	126 (100)	115 (100)	93 (100)	70 (100)	47 (100)	33 (100)

References

1. Burke CM, Theodore J, Dawkins KD, Yousem SA, Blank N, Billingham ME, VanKessel A, Jamieson SW, Oyer PE, Balwin JC (1984) Post transplant obliterative bronchiolitis and other late sequelae in human heart-lung transplantation. Chest 86: 824–829
2. Burke CM, Theodore J, Baldwin JC, Tazelaar HD, Morris AJ, McGregor C, Shumway NE, Robin ED, Jamieson SW (1986) Twenty-eight cases of human heart-lung transplantation. Lancet 333: 517–519
3. International society for heart and lung transplantation (1993) A working formulation for the standardisation of nomenclature and for clinical staging of chronic dysfunction in lung allografts. J Heart Lung Transplant 12: 713–716
4. Scott JP, Higenbottam TW, Sharples L, Clelland CA, Smyth RL, Stewart S, Wallwork J (1991) Risk factors for obliterative bronchiolitis in heart-lung transplant recipients. Transplantation 51: 813–817
5. Kramer MR, Stoehr C, Whang JL, Berry GJ, Sibley R, Marshall SE, Patterson GM, Starnes VA, Theodore J (1993) The diagnosis of obliterative bronchiolitis after heart-lung and lung transplantation: low yield of transbronchial biopsy. J Heart Lung Transplant 12: 675–681
6. Yousem SA, Paradis IL, Dauber JH, Griffith BP (1989) Efficacy of transbronchial lung biopsy in the diagnosis of bronchiolitis obliterans in heart-lung transplant recipients. Transplantation 47: 893–895
7. Tamm M, Higenbottam T, Dennis C, Sharples L, Wallwork J (1994) Donor and recipient predicted lung volume and lung size after heart-lung transplantation. Am Rev Respir Dis 150: 403–407

Immunosupression

Transpl Int (1996) 9 [Suppl 1]: S 305–S 307
© Springer-Verlag 1996

A. Johnston
J. M. Kovarik
E. A. Mueller
D. W. Holt

Predicting patients' exposure to cyclosporin

A. Johnston (✉)
Clinical Pharmacology,
St Bartholomew's Hospital,
London EC1A 7BE, UK

J. M. Kovarik · E. A. Mueller
Sandoz Pharma AG, CH-4002 Basel,
Switzerland

D. W. Holt
The Analytical Unit,
St George's Hospital Medical School,
London SW17 0RE, UK

Abstract The introduction of a new formulation of cyclosporin, Neoral, has reduced pharmacokinetic variability and it may be possible to simplify area-under-curve (AUC) measurements using a limited sampling strategy. We have examined the timing of blood samples necessary to obtain accurate AUC predictions for cyclosporin using limited data from stable renal transplant patients dosed twice daily with Neoral. Best subset regression of blood concentration profile data obtained from ten patients at steady state indicated that two samples, timed at 2 and 8 h post-dose, accounted for 97 % of the variance in AUC. The accuracy of this prediction was tested using profile data collected in a further 36 patients on three occasions separated by 4 and 44 weeks. Using the regression, AUC = 1.96 × [2 h] + 11.5 × [8 h] + 355.2, the mean (95 % CI) prediction errors of the three occasions were 1.7 % (− 2.1–5.4 %), 3.3 % (− 2.6–9.2 %) and 0.4 % (− 3.4–4.2 %). Data are presented that suggest AUC monitoring with a single blood sample could be feasible in a clinical setting.

Key words Cyclosporin AUC · Therapeutic drug monitoring · Blood concentration

Introduction

Pre-dose or trough blood cyclosporin concentration is routinely monitored and the result used to alter patients' drug dosing. However, patients with identical pre-dose blood concentrations may have very different systemic exposure to the drug as measured by area under the cyclosporin blood concentration curve (AUC). For this reason it has been suggested that controlling cyclosporin drug dose and therapy would be better achieved by measuring individual patients' AUC rather than trough concentration [7]. Although AUC monitoring is undertaken in some centres, most believe that the variability in cyclosporin pharmacokinetics, together with the increased cost and complexity, make AUC monitoring impractical in a routine clinical setting.

It has been known for some time that two or three blood samples can be use to determine accurately a patient's AUC [4]. However, because of the variability in cyclosporin absorption following Sandimmun administration, the required blood samples must be drawn at very specific times and this makes the practical implementation of abbreviated or limited sampling AUC difficult [1, 4]. The introduction of a new formulation of cyclosporin, Neoral, has improved the drug's absorption and reduced the within- and between-variability in patients' pharmacokinetics [2, 3]. Since the drug's pharmacokinetics are more predictable following Neoral administration, it is probable that AUC could be estimated using a wider range of sampling times than has been possible for Sandimmun. Therefore, it may be possible to simplify AUC measurement using a limited sampling strategy which is more flexible and clinically practical than those previously suggested for Sandimmun. This paper describes such a strategy.

Materials and methods

Patients

During the clinical testing of Neoral, cyclosporin blood concentration profiles were measured in a group of 46 stable renal transplant patients at 8, 12 and 52 weeks after conversion from Sandimmun. On each occasion, blood was taken at 0, 0.5, 1, 1.5, 2, 2.5, 3, 3.5, 4, 4.5, 5, 6, 8, 10 and 12 h after drug administration. The samples were taken into tubes containing EDTA anticoagulant and blood cyclosporin concentration was measured using a specific radioimmunoassay.

Statistical procedures

The AUC of each profile was calculated using the linear trapezoidal method.

The patients were arbitrarily split into two groups. The first consisted of the initial ten patients while the remaining 36 were allocated to the second group. The data from the first group of patients were used to determine the relationship between AUC and blood concentration using multiple linear regression. AUC was taken as the dependent variable and the independent variables were the blood concentrations grouped by time. Stepwise linear regression was used to determine the combination of time points that were most highly correlated with AUC. Predictive equations were derived for all time points individually and for the time points selected by the stepwise regression procedure. These equations were then used to predict the AUC values of the remaining 36 patients and these data from the second group of patients were used to determine the accuracy and precision of the predictions. The agreement between the predicted and measured AUC was examined and the prediction error calculated as shown in Eq. 1.

$$\% \text{ Prediction error} = \frac{\text{Predicted AUC} - \text{Measured AUC}}{\text{Measured AUC}} \times 100 \quad (1)$$

Results

The stepwise linear regression procedure indicated that only two points were needed to account for 97 % of the variance in AUC in the first group of patients. These time points were 2 and 8 h post-dose. Using the derived regression equation (Eq. 2) to predict the AUC values for cyclosporin after Neoral in the remaining 36 patients at 8, 12 and 52 weeks following conversion from Sandimmun resulted in highly accurate predictions. The mean (95 % CI) prediction error of the three occasions were 1.7 % (−2.1–5.4 %), 3.3 % (−2.6–9.2 %) and 0.4 %(−3.4–4.2 %), respectively. These data are shown in Fig. 1.

$$\text{AUC} = 1.96 \times [2 \text{ h}] + 11.5 \times [8 \text{ h}] + 355.2 \quad (2)$$

The variance in AUC explained by cyclosporin concentrations at individual time points varied between 18 % and 85 %. Using the regression equations derived for all time points individually in the first group

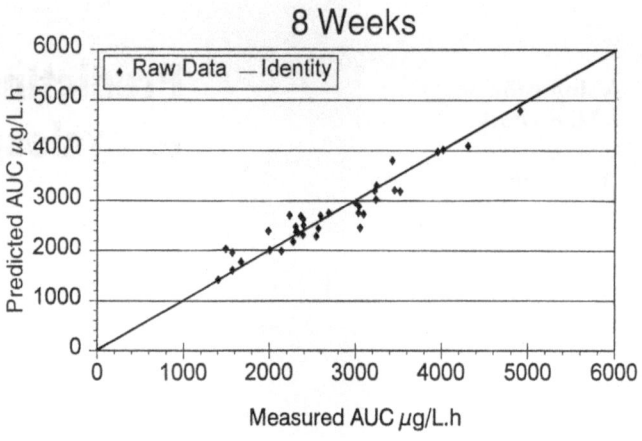

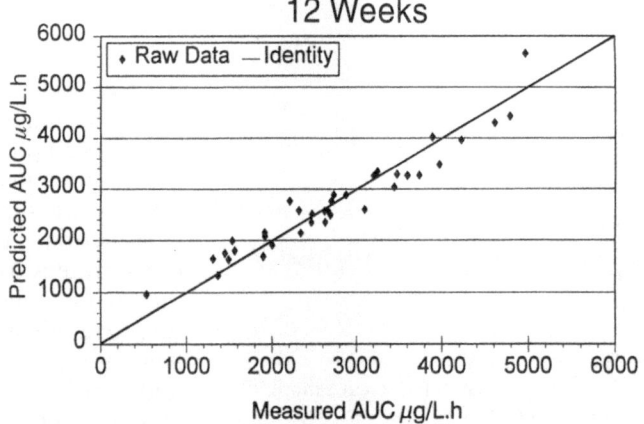

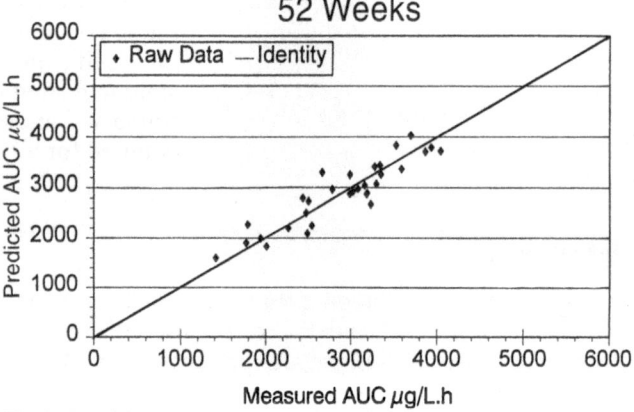

Fig. 1 Predicted area-under-curve *(AUC)* versus measured AUC at 8, 12 and 52 weeks in 36 patients after conversion from Sandimmun to Neoral. The predictions were made using Eq. 2. The raw data are plotted as a *filled diamond* and the line is the line of identity, i.e. one-to-one agreement

of patients to predict the AUC in the second group resulted in a minimum mean predictive error of 0.4 % and a maximum of 35.7 %. The coefficient of determination (r^2), the mean and standard deviation of the prediction error at each time point are shown in Fig. 2.

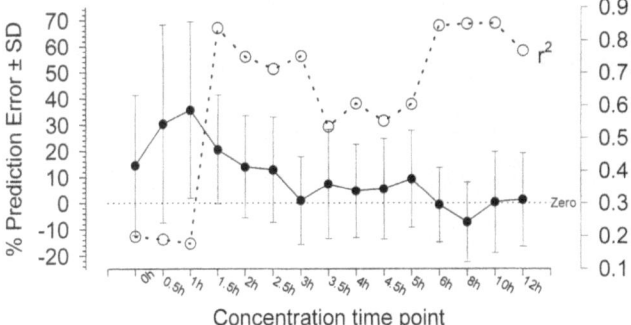

Fig. 2 The mean ± standard deviation of prediction error after using the regression equations derived for all time points individually in the first group of patients to predict the AUC in the second group (*filled circles* and *error bars, left-hand y*-axis scale). The corresponding coefficients of determination (r^2) at each time point are shown as *open circles (right-hand y*-axis scale)

Discussion

It is clear from the results of this study that cyclosporin AUC after Neoral can be determined with a high degree of accuracy and precision with only two concentration measurements in renal patients. The choice of blood concentrations at 2 and 8 h post-dose was made for statistical reasons rather than clinical utility and with other data sets different authors have shown similar correlations with 2 and 6 h [5] and with 0 and 2 h post-dose [6]. Following Neoral administration, AUC prediction error is smaller, less variable and requires one less concentra-

tion measurement than that shown previously for Sandimmun [4]. However, the use of two accurately timed blood samples would still present practical difficulties in many clinical setting.

A more practical method would be to use only one sample which could be taken at any of a given range of time after dosing. The data shown in Fig. 2 suggest that this approach would be feasible since prediction error falls to less than 10 % when blood cyclosporin concentrations measured in samples between 3 and 12 h are used to predict AUC. Thus, a series of equations could be derived to calculate AUC from a single, timed, blood cyclosporin concentration measurement. This could be further simplified for clinical use by using a programmable calculator or by means of a graphical display from which AUC could be read given a cyclosporin concentration measured at a specific time.

Using this approach, it would be possible to use a less restrictive range of blood sampling times and this would allow AUC estimation in routine clinical settings. It would also overcome some of the problems associated with trough concentration measurement when the times of medical out-patient clinics do not correspond with the start or end of patients' cyclosporin dosing regimens. However, it is obvious that before this method could be introduced it would require further testing to confirm its accuracy in a wider range of patients and cyclosporin indications. It is also likely that the derived equations would be unique to Neoral due to the particularly good absorption characteristics of that formulation coupled with its low within- and between-patient variability.

References

1. Grevel J, Kahan BD (1991) Abbreviated kinetic profiles in area-under-the-curve monitoring of cyclosporin therapy. Clin Chem 37: 1905–1909
2. Holt DW, Mueller EA, Kovarik JM, Bree JB van, Kutz K (1994) The pharmacokinetics of Sandimmun Neoral: a new formulation of cyclosporine. Transplant Proc 26: 2935–2939
3. Holt DW, Mueller EA, Kovarik JM, Bree JB van, Richard F, Kutz K (1995) Sandimmun Neoral pharmacokinetics: impact of the new oral formulation. Transplant Proc 27: 1434–1437
4. Johnston A, Sketris I, Marsden JT, Galustian CG, Fashola T, Taube D, Pepper J, Holt DW (1990) A limited sampling strategy for the measurement of cyclosporine AUC. Transplant Proc 22: 1345–1346
5. Kahan BD, Dunn J, Fitts C, Buren D van, Wombolt D, Pollak R, Carson R, Alexander JW, Choc M, Wong R, Hwang DS (1995) Reduced inter- and intrasubject variability in cyclosporine pharmacokinetics in renal transplant recipients treated with a microemulsion formulation in conjunction with fasting, low-fat meals or high-fat meals. Transplantation 59: 505–511
6. Keown PA (1995) Pharmacokinetic, economic, and pharmacoepidemiological analysis of Neoral in renal transplantation in Canada. In: Neoral. The new microemulsion formulation of cyclosporine. World Medical Press, Cedar Knolls, New Jersey, USA
7. Lindholm A, Kahan BD (1993) Influence of cyclosporin pharmacokinetics, trough concentration, and AUC monitoring on outcome of kidney transplantation. Clin Pharmacol Ther 54: 205–217

Transpl Int (1996) 9 [Suppl 1]: S308–S310
© Springer-Verlag 1996

IMMUNOSUPPRESSION

B. Zanker
S. Schleibner
H. Schneeberger
M. Krauss
W. Land

Mycophenolate mofetil in patients with acute renal failure: evidence of metabolite (MPAG) accumulation and removal by dialysis

B. Zanker (✉) · S. Schleibner ·
H. Schneeberger · M. Krauss · W. Land
Division of Transplant Surgery,
Department of Surgery,
Klinikum Grosshadern,
Ludwig-Maximilians-University,
Marchioninistrasse 15, D-81377 Munich,
Germany

Abstract Pharmacokinetics of mycophenolic acid (MPA) was analyzed in eight patients with post-transplant acute renal failure. Furthermore, the effect of hemodialysis upon blood levels of MPA and its major metabolite, MPA glucuronide (MPAG), was determined. The mean duration of the posttransplant renal failure was 18 days, but renal function resumed in all patients eventually. The patients were treated with 3 g/day of mycophenolate mofetil for 28 consecutive days combined with cyclosporine A, methylprednisolone, and ATG for induction therapy. In all patients, accumulation of MPAG but not of MPA was observed. MPA trough levels were in the range between 0.5 µg/ml at day 2 and 2.3 µg/ml at the end of the study period. However, this concentration difference did not reach statistical significance. Trough levels of MPAG accumulated, reaching levels as high as 358 µg/ml. However, with increasing recovery of renal function, MPAG levels fell to a median trough concentration of 141 µg/ml. MPAG, but not MPA, could partially be removed from the circulation by hemodialysis treatment.

Key words Immunosuppression · Drug accumulation · Renal failure · Hemodialysis

Introduction

Mycophenolic acid (MPA) is a powerful new immunosuppressive drug. MPA is a non-nucleotide inhibitor of the type 2 isoform of inosine monophosphate dehydrogenase (IMPDH), a key enzyme of guanosine nucleotide metabolism in activated lymphocytes [1–3]. Stimulation of T- and B-lymphocytes increases the de novo synthesis of guanosine nucleotides as a prerequisite for DNA synthesis. Most eukaryotic cells can use two major pathways of purine nucleotide synthesis, but lymphocytes are totally dependent upon IMPDH-catalyzed de novo synthesis. MPA is a potent inhibitor of IMPDH type 2, blocking the de novo synthesis of guanosine nucleotides by 40–80%. In contrast to other cell types, lymphocytes lack the salvage pathway of purine synthesis. For this reason, actively dividing lymphocytes of T- and B-lineage are highly susceptible to MPA. Mycophe-nolate mofetil (MMF) is the ester prodrug of the active moiety, MPA. After oral administration, MMF is extensively absorbed and undergoes a presystemic metabolism to MPA, which is the active compound. The major metabolite of MPA is MPA glucuronide (MPAG). This metabolite is inactive and is mainly eliminated via urinary secretion and, to some extent, into the feces. The efficacy, safety, and tolerability of MMF as an immuno-suppressant have been demonstrated in a variety of clinical studies [4]. However, the potential clinical impact and pharmacokinetics of repeated dosing of MMF in patients with renal insufficiency are not completely established. Single-dose administration of MMF to patients with severe chronic renal insufficiency yielded an increase of the area under the curve (AUC) compared to that of healthy individuals and the AUC of MPAG was increased up to sixfold. Therefore, we aimed to analyze the pharmacokinetics of MPA and its major metabolite,

MPAG, in patients receiving multiple dosing of MMF in the setting of posttransplant acute renal failure and hemodialysis treatment.

Patients and methods

After written informed consent, eight patients with acute renal failure of the cadaver renal allograft were studied. In all patients, renal function eventually resumed after a mean duration time of 18 days (6–39 days) posttransplantation. The immunosuppressive induction treatment consisted of ATG (Fresenius, Bad Homburg), 4 mg/kg body weight for 7 days; cyclosporine A (Sandimmun; Sandoz, Nürnberg) 6 mg/kg body weight/day; methylprednisolone (Urbason; Hoechst, Hoechst) 20 mg/day; MMF 1.5 g twice daily, kindly provided by Syntex, given orally for 28 consecutive days. Trough blood levels of MPA and MPAG were determined by means of high-pressure liquid chromatography (HPLC; Medeval, USA). In addition, 12 h profiles of plasma concentrations were performed at days 1, 7, 14, 21, and 28 of MMF treatment. In patients requiring hemodialysis, the blood levels of MPA and MPAG were also determined during dialysis treatment.

Results

MPA and MPAG levels were determined in eight patients with acute posttransplant renal failure (ARF). The duration of ARF was a mean time of 18 days (range 6–39 days). The patients were treated with 3 g MMF daily for 28 consecutive days according to our protocol. Median values of MPA trough levels were found in the range between 0.6 µg/ml ± 0.42 µg/ml at day 2 and 2.35 µg/ml ± 1.1 µg/ml at day 28 of the study period (Table 1). Concomitantly, MPAG accumulated, starting from a median value of trough levels between 59.5 ± 85.55 µg/ml at day 2 and reaching a plateau of 358 ± 117.35 µg/ml between day 10 and day 16. With increasing recovery of renal function, indicated by a constant fall of the serum creatinine and a glomerular filtration rate (GFR) exceeding 20 ml/min, the median trough levels of MPAG decreased to 141 ± 43.8 µg/ml, indicating renal excretion of MPAG (Table 2).

In patients undergoing hemodialysis therapy, plasma levels of MPA and MPAG were determined. After 1 h of hemodialysis, blood samples were drawn simultaneously from the afferent arterial (input coil) and the efferent venous (output coil) bloodstream. Under these conditions, MPA mean concentration in the input coil was 2.55 µg/ml and in the output coil 2.49 µg/ml, indicating that MPA was not substantially removed by hemodialysis. In contrast, the mean concentration of MPAG decreased from 118.7 µg/ml in the input coil to 101 µg/ml in the output coil. The amount of MPAG removed from the circulation through dialysis was dependent upon the blood concentration. Starting with mean blood concentrations of MPAG of 80 µg/ml in the input coil, the mean concentration found in the output coil was es-

Table 1 Mycophenolic acid *(MPA)* trough levels from eight patients treated with 3 g mycophenolate mofetil (MMF) daily. All patients suffered from acute posttransplant renal failure. This increase of MPA levels during the study period of 28 days did not reach statistical significance

Day	Median MPA concentration (µg/ml)	SD	95 % confidence
2	0.6	0.42	0.309
4	1.05	0.96	0.665
6	2.1	3.46	2.401
8	1.95	1.20	0.834
10	1.85	1.84	1.272
12	1.35	1.71	1.186
14	2.5	2.42	2.125
16	1.6	0.80	0.591
18	1.65	1.37	1.097
20	2.1	1.97	1.458
23	3.25	2.47	2.425
28	2.35	1.10	0.760

Table 2 Mycophenolic acid glucuronide *(MPAG)* trough blood levels from eight patients treated with 3 g MMF daily. All patients suffered from acute posttransplant renal failure. The accumulation of MPAG resolved with recovery of renal function. MPAG concentrations are given as median values from eight patients

Day	Median MPAG concentration (µg/ml)	SD	95 % confidence
2	59.5	85.55	59.28
4	115	85.57	63.39
6	192	140.18	97.14
8	200	146.26	108.35
10	331	144.93	107.36
12	358	117.35	81.32
16	343	71.58	53.03
18	217	85.31	63.20
20	200.5	50.50	69.99
21	148	47.47	41.61
23	149	78.49	76.92
28	141.5	43.80	30.35

sentially the same. In subjects with a mean concentration of MPAG of 188 µg/ml in the input coil, the mean concentration of MPAG was decreased to 137 µg/ml in the output coil.

Discussion

The efficacy, safety, and tolerability of MMF as an immunosuppressant have been demonstrated in a variety of clinical studies [4]. However, the potential clinical impact and pharmacokinetics of repeated dosing of MMF in patients with renal insufficiency has not been completely established. Therefore, this small study was undertaken in order to gain more insight into the pharmacokinetics of MPA and its major metabolite, MPAG, in patients receiving multiple dosing of MMF in the setting of posttransplant acute renal failure and hemodialysis treatment. After oral administration, the ester prodrug, MMF, is converted into the active immunosuppressant, MPA. More than 99% of the MPA is bound to plasma proteins and is rapidly metabolised into the functionally inactive compound, MPAG. In eight patients treated with 1.5 g of MMF twice daily, the 12-h trough levels of MPA and MPAG were determined every other day by means of HPLC. After 4 days, the median concentrations of MPA from the eight patients were in the range of 2 µg/ml and there was no further increase reaching statistical significance. In contrast, trough levels of MPAG accumulated over time, but resolved with recovery of renal function. Protein binding of MPAG varies and the bound fraction reaches 82%. However, with renal failure, the protein-bound fraction can decrease to 60%. Only the free fraction of MPAG can be removed from the plasma by means of dialysis. These preliminary data reveal that dose adjustment of MMF according to the renal function or substitution after hemodialysis are not required, as deduced from this small single-centre study. However, with prolonged renal failure, patients should be monitored carefully for symptoms of drug toxicity and over-immunosuppression.

References

1. Allison AC, Eugui EM (1993) Mycophenolate mofetil, a rationally designed immunosuppressive drug. Clin Transpl 7: 96–112
2. Eugui EM, Almquist SJ, Muller CD, Allison AC (1991) Lymphocyte-selective cytostatic and immunosuppressive effects of mycophenolic acid in vitro: role of deoxyguanosine nucleotide depletion. Scand J Immunol 33: 161–173
3. Eugui EM, Mirkovich A, Allison AC (1991) Lymphocyte-selective antiproliferative and immunosuppressive effects of mycophenolic acid in mice. Scand J Immunol 33: 175–183
4. Sollinger HW, Belzer FO, Deierhoi MH, Diethelm AG, Gonwa TA, Kauffman RS, Klintmalm GB, McDiarmid SV, Roberts J, Rosenthal JT, Tomlanovich SJ (1992) RS-61443 (mycophenolate mofetil): a multicenter study for refractory kidney transplant rejection. Ann Surg 216: 513–519

Transpl Int (1996) 9 [Suppl 1]: S 311–S 313
© Springer-Verlag 1996

R. H. Moore
The UK Neoral Study Group

UK multicentre study to assess the safety and tolerability of Neoral in stable renal transplant patients

R. H. Moore (✉)
Cardiff Royal Infirmary, Newport Road,
Cardiff CF2 1SZ, UK

Abstract The safety and tolerability of transferring maintained renal transplant patients from Sandimmun to Neoral is being assessed in a multicentre, open-label, single-arm study. A total of 250 patients has been enrolled and results are available from 75 patients up to 12 months post-transfer. A slight trend to higher mean cyclosporin trough levels was seen in this cohort, but trough levels were unchanged in the sub-group receiving ≥ 1 dose changes. The mean dose fell by 13 %. Creatinine levels showed a slight overall upward trend. Blood pressure and uric acid were unchanged and adverse events were typical of those seen with Sandimmun. Neoral was well-tolerated. Data from the full cohort of 250 patients up to 3 months post-transfer support these findings. These results indicate that transfer from Sandimmun to Neoral is safe and well-tolerated and provides appropriate immunosuppression at a lower average dose than Sandimmun. The Neoral dose should be adjusted promptly, as required, to maintain the target trough level.

Key words Cyclosporin · Neoral · Immunosuppression

Introduction

Since its introduction in the early 1980s, cyclosporin has become the cornerstone of rejection prophylaxis in solid organ transplantation. It has improved survival rates significantly: for example, survival of renal allografts has increased from around 65 % 1 year after transplantation in the pre-cyclosporin era to up to 90 % now [3].

Cyclosporin is, however, a highly lipophilic molecule. The conventional formulation of cyclosporin, Sandimmun, forms a coarse emulsion in water which rapidly precipitates, leading to poor and unpredictable absorption from the gut. In contrast, Neoral forms a very fine emulsion of tiny droplets less than 100 nm in diameter. As a result, Neoral provides a significantly more predictable, consistent and rapid absorption of cyclosporin from the upper gastrointestinal tract than does Sandimmun [1].

Pharmacokinetic comparisons in renal patients have demonstrated that the improved absorption of cyclosporin using Neoral provides a number of benefits compared to Sandimmun [2]:
1. More predictable blood levels of cyclosporin.
2. Reduction in intrapatient pharmacokinetic variability.
3. An increase in area under the curve (AUC) of 29 %.
4. Trough cyclosporin levels become a more meaningful clinical measurement. Neoral shows a markedly improved correlation between trough levels and drug exposure (correlation coefficient of approximately 0.8 in renal transplant patients given Neoral versus approximately 0.5 with Sandimmun).

A number of international trials have demonstrated that transferring renal transplant patients from the Sandimmun formulation to the Neoral formulation of cyclosporin is both safe and well-tolerated. A multicentre UK trial of 250 stable renal allograft recipients (NEO 001) is further assessing the pharmacokinetic and clinical impact to transfer to the new formulation.

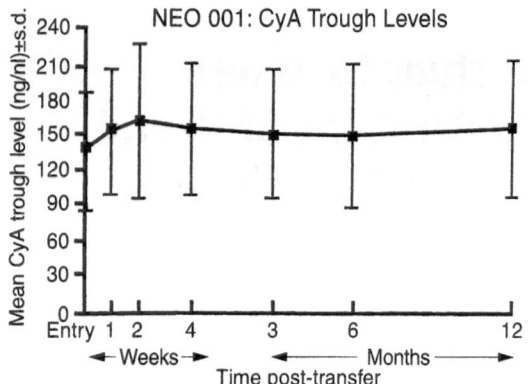

Fig. 1 Cyclosporin *(CyA)* trough levels in 75 maintained renal transplant patients following transfer from Sandimmun to Neoral

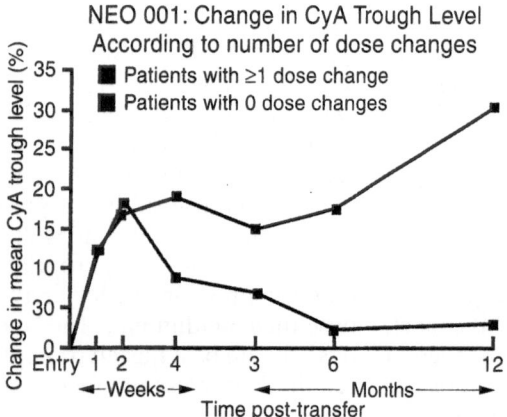

Fig. 2 Cyclosporin trough levels in 75 maintained renal transplant patients following transfer from Sandimmun to Neoral, stratified according to number of dose changes

Materials and methods

Subjects

Two hundred and fifty renal transplant recipients with a mean age of 49.4 years (range 17–80 years) and a median of 2.18 years post-transplant (range 0.3–10.9 years) were recruited at 22 centres. Seventy-seven patients were female, 170 were male. Two hundred and twelve patients (84.8 %) were primary transplants, 25 (10.0 %) were diabetic and 218 (87.2 %) were hypertensive. All patients were are least 6 months post-transplant and had experienced no episodes of rejection in the 3 months prior to entering the study.

Study design

The study was an open-label, single-arm study. Clinical and pharmacokinetic assessments were carried out at entry, 1, 2 and 4 weeks and at 3, 6 and 12 months. At the entry visit, all patients were transferred from Sandimmun to Neoral on a 1:1 dose conversion. Cyclosporin trough levels, dose, serum creatinine, blood pressure, use of antihypertensives, uric acid, presence of infection and adverse effects were recorded at each visit. Tolerability was assessed by the investigator and by the patient. Any change in dose and the reason for the dose change was also recorded.

Results

Data up to 12 months are now available for 75 of the patients enrolled in the study.

Cyclosporin trough levels

In this group of patients there was a slight trend to higher cyclosporin trough levels during the 12 months of the study, from 138.4 ng/ml at entry to 156.4 ng/ml at 12 months (Fig. 1). However, in those patients who had one or more dose changes, trough levels remained approximately unchanged, while those who did not receive a dose alteration showed a mean trough level increase of 30 %, accounting for the overall mean rise (Fig. 2).

Cyclosporin dose

The mean dose was reduced by 13 % over the study period, with 45 out of these 75 patients receiving one or more dose changes. There were 92 dose changes in total, of which 65 were decreases and 27 were increases. During the study period, the majority of dose changes (79 %) were made in response to trough cyclosporin levels.

Renal function

Creatinine levels showed a slight overall upward trend during the study period (151.5 µmol/l at entry to 169 µmol/l at 12 months), in line with the trend to an increase in trough cyclosporin levels resulting from the cohort of patients who did not receive a dose change (Fig. 3).

Adverse events and tolerability

Blood pressure was unchanged and there was no change in the use of antihypertensive medication. Uric acid levels were also unaltered 12 months after transfer to Neoral. Infections and adverse events were typical of those seen with Sandimmun therapy, with no unexpected events occurring.

Both the invesigators and patients reported 'very good' or 'good' tolerability in over 95 % of cases following transfer to Neoral.

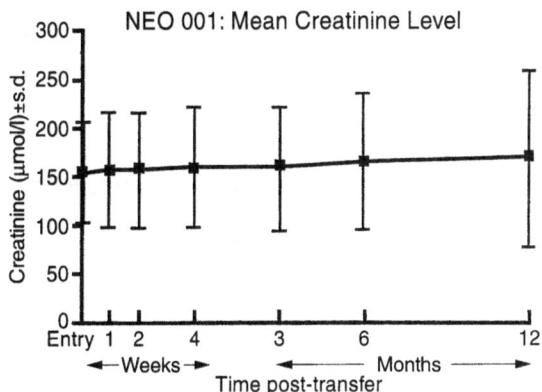

Fig.3 Serum creatinine levels in 75 maintained renal transplant patients following transfer from Sandimmun to Neoral

Status 3 months after transfer (full cohort)

Data up to 3 months post-transfer are now available from the full study cohort of 250 patients. Trough cyclosporin levels remained largely constant during the first 3 months of the study, from 161 ng/ml at entry to 155 ng/ml at 3 months (a change of 3.6 %). In patients who had a dose alteration following transfer to Neoral, mean trough levels fell from 182 ng/ml at entry to 162 ng/ml at 3 months. In the group who had no change in dose following transfer to Neoral, the trough level was 145 ng/ml at entry, rising marginally to 149 ng/ml after 3 months.

The mean creatinine level remained stable during the first 3 months of the study (146 µmol/l at entry compared to 149 µmol/l at 3 months) in this full cohort of 250 patients.

Discussion

These results support the findings of international double-blind trials in which renal transplant patients have been transferred from Sandimmun, the conventional formulation of cyclosporin, to Neoral. The transfer is safe and well-tolerated, with no significant change in the nature, incidence or severity of adverse effects.

Using Sandimmun, trough cyclosporin levels have provided only an imprecise estimate of total drug exposure. In patients receiving Neoral, however, it is clear that trough cyclosporin levels become a meaningful clinical measurement, and the result of this trial highlight that the dose of Neoral should therefore be adjusted promptly, where necessary, on the basis of trough cyclosporin measurements in order to maintain target blood levels.

Finally, these findings also confirm that Neoral can provide appropriate levels of immunosuppression at a lower mean dose than Sandimmun, offering the potential for considerable cost savings. In the clinical setting, a mean dose reduction of around 10 % could realistically be expected following transfer to Neoral. Since any new immunosuppressive agent must now be assessed in health economic terms as well as incremental clinical benefit, this fulfils an important criterion for transplant centres evaluating their current immunosuppressive protocols.

Acknowledgements The members of the UK Neoral Study Group are as follows: R. W. G. Johnson (Manchester Royal Infirmary), P. Sweny (Royal Free Hospital, London), J. D. Briggs (Western Infirmary), A. T. Raftery (Southern General Hospital, Sheffield), K. M. Rigg (Nottingham City Hospital), H. N. Riad (Royal Devon and Exeter Hospital, Exeter), P. Lear (Southmead Hospital, Bristol), H. Lee (St Mary's Hospital, Portsmouth), R. H. Moore (Cardiff Royal Infirmary), M. C. Jones (Ninewells Hospital, Dundee), G. Neild (Middlesex Hospital, London), A. J. Eisinger (St. Helier Hospital, Carshalton), J. Scoble (Dulwich Hospital, London), F. T. Lam (Walsgrave Hospital, Coventry), N. Richards (Queen Elizabeth Hospital, Birmingham), P. E. Gower (Charing Cross Hospital, London), R. J. Lechler (Hammersmith Hospital, London), M. J. Goggin (Kent and Canterbury Hospital, Canterbury), P. Veitch (Leicester General Hospital), J. C. Kingswood (Royal Sussex County Hospital, Brighton), M. Carmody (Beaumont Hospital, Dublin), R. Taylor (Royal Victoria Infirmary, Newcastle).

References

1. Kovarik JM, Mueller EA, Bree JB van, et al (1994) Reduced inter- and intraindividual variability in cyclosporin pharmacokinetics from a microemulsion formulation. J Pharm Sci 83: 444–446

2. Kovarik JM, Mueller EA, Bree JB van, et al (1994) Cyclosporine pharmacokinetics and variability from a microemulsion formulation – a multicenter investigation in kidney transplant patients. Transplantation 58: 658–663

3. Opelz G, for the Collaborative Transplant Study (1992) Collaborative transplant Study – 10-year report. Transplant Proc 24: 2342–2355

Transpl Int (1996) 9 [Suppl 1]: S314–S317
© Springer-Verlag 1996

A. J. Hoitsma
The IMM 125 Multicentre
Study Group

Comparison of Sandimmun with a new cyclosporin derivative (IMM 125) in renal transplant patients with stable renal function

A. J. Hoitsma (✉)
Division of Nephrology,
Sint Radboud Hospital,
Geert Grooteplein 8,
NL-6525 GA Nijmegen,
The Netherlands

Abstract A double-blind switch-over study was carried out on 70 renal transplant patients to assess the value of a new cyclosporin derivative, IMM 125. Preclinical in vitro and in vivo studies indicated that IMM 125 was as equally immunosuppressive as Sandimmun, but that its therapeutic index should be superior. The duration of the treatment was 24 weeks. The assumption that the dosage of IMM 125 could be 2.5 times lower than Sandimmun proved to be false; three patients suffered acute rejection episodes, probably as a consequence of the low dosage, and dosage adjustments had to be made for all patients receiving IMM 125 after only a few weeks. Although IMM 125 is an effective immunosuppressive agent, it does not appear to offer advantages over Sandimmun with regard to renal function. In addition, IMM 125 causes some disturbances in liver function.

Key words Cyclosporin IMM 125 · Immunosuppression

Introduction

With cyclosporin A, the initial and long-term survival rates in virtually all forms of transplantation have improved considerably [5]. In addition, its use is accompanied by a reduced rejection incidence and less morbidity [6, 7]. Nevertheless, the nephrotoxicity of this drug remains a major drawback, particularly in renal transplantation. When renal function deteriorates, it is often very hard to differentiate between an acute rejection and cyclosporin nephrotoxicity. Attempts to circumvent this side effect include the production of a new cyclosporin derivative with the same or stronger immunosuppressive potency, but without the nephrotoxic side effects. IMM 125 is such a derivative of the cyclosporin family with powerful immunosuppressive properties in vitro. IMM 125 is made from D-serine-8-cyclosporin followed by chemical modification [1]. It is neither cytostatic nor cytotoxic. In preclinical in vitro and in vivo studies it has been shown to be equally as immunosuppressive as Sandimmun [3, 4].

Based on biochemical and histological studies, IMM 125 has a toxicological profile qualitatively similar to Sandimmun. However, quantitative comparison suggests that the therapeutic index for IMM 125 should be superior to that of Sandimmun in clinical use [2]. In human volunteers, single doses of IMM 125 up to 800 mg were only followed by a transient increase in transaminases. The pharmacokinetics of IMM 125 have already been described [4].

In this study, IMM 125 is compared with Sandimmun in renal transplant patients with stable renal function to evaluate its immunosuppressive properties and side effects. Because in animals the toxicity of IMM 125 is lower than that of Sandimmun, reduction of side effects, especially an improvement in renal function, is expected after conversion from Sandimmun to IMM 125.

Patients and methods

In this double-blind switch-over study, patients either remained on Sandimmun or were switched to IMM 125, while the blood level of IMM 125 was kept the same as the blood level of Sandimmun before switching. Important end-points were side effects, especially renal dysfunction, the incidence of acute rejections and the frequency of graft loss in both groups.

Table 1 Reasons for discontinuation of the study

IMM 125 group ($n = 8$)
Acute rejection ($n = 3$)
Elevated liver enzymes ($n = 2$)
Poor compliance
Persistent increase in serum creatinine
Medication error (Sandimmun instead of IMM 125) causing creatinine increase
Sandimmun ($n = 3$)
Acute pancreatitis
Inclusion criteria violation ($n = 2$)

Included in this study were only adult recipients of a cadaveric renal allograft, who were 7–24 months after transplantation, and received a stable immunosuppressive regimen with Sandimmun and steroids for 2 months prior to entry. The Sandimmun dose should not be lower than 4 mg/kg per day and renal function had to be stable (serum creatinine between 150 µmol/l and 300 µmol/l, irrespective of gender) for 2 months prior to entry. Excluded from this study were patients with a third or subsequent renal transplantation, with diabetes, with proteinuria of more than 3 g/24 h, with a bilirubin level of more than 1.5 times the upper limit of normal, or with transaminases more than 2 times the upper limit of normal. Also excluded were patients taking any drugs potentiating nephrotoxicity of Sandimmun in the 2 weeks before entry or drugs interfering with Sandimmun pharmacokinetics in the 2 months before entry. Finally, treatment with ATG, OKT3 or azathioprine during 2 months prior to entry was also prohibited.

Patients were randomly assigned to either continuation of Sandimmun at the same maintenance dose or to switch-over to IMM 125. The starting number of capsules of IMM 125 was the same as the number of Sandimmun capsules taken the day before switching therapy. Dosages were taken in two separate and equal (if possible) doses, 12 h apart and, preferably, before meals. The duration of the treatment of 24 weeks. Sandimmun capsules contained 25 or 100 mg and IMM 125 capsules were of 10 or 40 mg according to the assumption (based on previous studies) that the bioavailability of IMM 125 capsules (versus Sandimmun capsules)

was 2.5 times higher. Dose adjustments based on whole blood trough levels were made in steps of 50 or 100 mg for Sandimmun and in equivalent doses for IMM 125, again equally divided between morning and evening. Blood levels were determined at one central place (Dr. Holt, London), and only the value of the blood level was passed to the centre.

Results and discussion

The study population consisted of 58 males and 12 females in seven centres. The mean age of the participants was 46.5 years (range 18–65 years). Thirty-four continued with Sandimmun and 36 were switched to IMM 125. Eleven patients prematurely discontinued the study medication for reasons shown in Table 1. None of the patients who were withdrawn from the study suffered from serious problems for a prolonged time. In three cases, IMM 125 medication was discontinued because of an acute rejection episode. These rejection episodes occurred between weeks 10 and 12 after the switch and were all reversible by treatment with i. v. steroids. Up to the time of rejection, the blood level of IMM 125 was consistently lower than the baseline Sandimmun level, despite dosage increments. After the initial three acute rejections in the IMM 125 group, probably caused by undertreatment, dosage adjustments in the case of low blood levels were more vigorously carried out (Table 2). Since the remaining 28 patients had no immunological problems one can state that, with trough levels in the therapeutic range, IMM 125 is an effective anti-rejection immunosuppressive agent. Adverse events are shown in Table 3. All except 11 adverse events were mild to moderate in severity according to predefined criteria. The 11 adverse events that were classified as severe were hypertension, acute pancreati-

Table 2 Percentage changes in creatinine, dose, blood level and alanine aminotransferase *(ALAT)* relative to baseline in both the IMM 125 and Sandimmun groups (means ± SD)

Period of study	Sandimmun				IMM 125			
	Creatinine (% diff)	Dose (% diff)	Blood level[a] (% diff)	ALAT (% diff)	Creatinine (% diff)	Dose (% diff)	Blood level[a] (% diff)	ALAT (% diff)
Baseline	0	0	0	0	0	0	0	0
Week 1	2 ± 12**	0 ± 0	8 ± 23	−4 ± 33**	−5 ± 11*,**	0 ± 0	7 ± 29	41 ± 74*,**
Week 2	2 ± 12**	−1 ± 6**	6 ± 30**	−10 ± 29**	−8 ± 9*,**	52 ± 47*,**	−59 ± 24*,**	79 ± 109*,**
Week 3	2 ± 11**	−3 ± 7**	17 ± 41*,**	−1 ± 26**	−8 ± 14*,**	62 ± 52*,**	−29 ± 41*,**	94 ± 137*,**
Week 4	2 ± 12**	−3 ± 10**	8 ± 32**	1 ± 39**	−7 ± 14*,**	71 ± 47*,**	−30 ± 39*,**	113 ± 140*,**
Week 6	2 ± 13**	−4 ± 10**	9 ± 40**	2 ± 40**	−7 ± 12*,**	81 ± 50*,**	−20 ± 40*,**	99 ± 140*,**
Week 8	2 ± 13	−3 ± 11**	2 ± 35**	5 ± 39**	−5 ± 10*	85 ± 50*,**	−19 ± 41*,**	92 ± 174*,**
Week 10	3 ± 13**	−3 ± 13**	8 ± 36**	3 ± 44**	−5 ± 12*,**	94 ± 58*,**	−19 ± 33*,**	158 ± 254*,**
Week 12	0 ± 11	−3 ± 13**	12 ± 51**	−2 ± 37**	−7 ± 14*	93 ± 54*,**	−4 ± 57**	178 ± 462*,**
Week 16	2 ± 10**	−3 ± 13**	10 ± 41	3 ± 37**	−9 ± 11*,**	94 ± 53*,**	−14 ± 33*	163 ± 269*,**
Week 20	1 ± 13**	−3 ± 13**	4 ± 37**	3 ± 36**	−6 ± 14*,**	102 ± 47*,**	−17 ± 31*,**	215 ± 350*,**
Week 24	1 ± 16	−5 ± 14**	3 ± 36**	4 ± 32**	−7 ± 15*	107 ± 41*,**	−18 ± 28*,**	191 ± 323*,**

* $P < 0.05$ versus baseline; ** $P < 0.05$ versus other group during same observation week
[a] Trough blood level of cyclosporin and IMM 125, respectively

Table 3 Adverse events

	IMM 125	Sand-immun
Total number of patients	36	34
Patients with adverse events	23	16
Total number of events	52	28
Gastrointestinal Dry mouth, gastritis, diarrhoea, retrosternal pain, acute pancreatitis, flatulence, increased liver enzymes, gingival hyperplasia, cholelithiasis, gastric reflux	11	5
Central nervous system Tremor, dizziness, tiredness, headache, burning feeling in hands, sleepiness, anorexia, paraesthesia, vision decrease	8	2
Locomotor Gout, backache, pain in thumb, chest plus shoulder pain, leg trauma, hyper-uricaemia, hydrops left knee, bone pain, pain right leg	10	3
Cardiovascular System Heart failure, flushing, hypotension, ankle oedema	5	10
Skin Acne rash, skin tenderness, hair loss, itch	5	
Renal Increase serum creatinine, rejection	4	1
General Weight gain, thirst, fever, fatigue, apathy, sensation of heat	5	5
Other Psychosis, paradontosis, anaemia, thyroid hypertrophy, hypercholesterolaemia	4	2

tis, diarrhoea, creatinine increase and psychosis in the Sandimmun group, and rejection (3×), anaemia, liver enzyme increase and gout in the IMM 125 group.

In the Sandimmun control group, serum creatinine values were stable over time, with fluctuations from visit to visit in the range of 0 % to 3 % versus baseline (Table 2). No significant changes could be detected. In the group switched from Sandimmun to IMM 125, serum creatinine dropped significantly by 5 % at week 1. Till week 24 the creatinine levels remained significantly lower at each visit as compared with baseline values. This is obviously caused by persistent lower blood levels, despite the fact that IMM 125 dosages were increased (Table 2). After 1 week of treatment with IMM 125, the levels were still unchanged, but thereafter blood levels decreased significantly, ranging from 59 % to 4 % in comparison with baseline values. In the Sandimmun control group the blood levels hardly changed and were significantly higher than the levels in the IMM 125-treated patients in the corresponding week.

Also, the dose in the Sandimmun control group remained the same during the investigation (decrease from 1 % to 5 %).

The assumption that the dosage of IMM 125 could be 2.5 times lower than the dosage of Sandimmun proved to be false. From the data of this trial one can conclude that the dosage of IMM 125 should be equal to that of Sandimmun to achieve similar trough levels. Due to this fact it is clear that the double blindness of this trial was hampered; after a few weeks the clinicians could guess what medication was given on the basis of the need for dose adjustments.

No substantial changes were observed with respect to alanine aminotransferase (ALAT), aspartate aminotransferase (ASAT) and alkaline phosphatase in the Sandimmun control group. In contrast, a rise in ALAT was readily detected after therapy was switched from Sandimmun to IMM 125 (Table 2). The rise in ALAT was detected as soon as the first visit after switching. On average, the increase was maximal at week 20 when the mean levels more than tripled the baseline value. Ten out of 26 patients had at that time point ALAT levels above normal. This may be explained by the progressive increase in the dose of IMM 125. The rise in ASAT was much milder, reaching 60 % at week 20. No signs of cholestasis were observed and the alkaline phosphatase level was unchanged, even in the patients who had the largest increase in ALAT. The liver intolerance constituted a new adverse event in comparison with Sandimmun. The rise in ALAT was dose-dependent, of quick onset (a few days), stable on a given dose of IMM 125, and reversible in a few days after therapy was stopped. Because of the liver intolerance, the ceiling dose of IMM 125 is currently limited to 350 mg/day. This means that IMM 125 can only be used as maintenance therapy, since the induction therapy after transplantation generally involves dosages above 350 mg/day.

With respect to blood pressure, no major changes were found after switch-over from Sandimmun to IMM 125 (data not shown).

In conclusion, one can state that IMM 125 is an effective immunosuppressive agent. As compared to Sandimmun, IMM 125 does not appear to offer important advantages with regard to renal function, while IMM 125 causes more liver function disturbances.

Acknowledgements Members the IMM 125 Multicentre Study Group are as follows: Dr. H. Wilczek, Prof. C. Groth, Huddinge sjukhus, Huddinge, Prof. Y. Vanrenterghem, Gasthuisberg, Leuven, Prof. W. Weimar, Dr. M. van Ierland-van Leeuwen, Dr. R. Zietse, University Hospital Rotterdam, Rotterdam, Dr. W. Diemont, Dr. L. Hilbrands, Dr. A. Hoitsma, University Hospital Nijmegen, Nijmegen, Dr. D. Albrechtsen, P. Fauchald, Rikshospitalet, Oslo, Prof. J. Salaman, Dr. R. Moore, Cardiff Royal Infirmary, Cardiff, Prof. R. Calne, Addenbrookes Hospital, Cambridge, Dr. Th. Beveridge, Dr. W. Collins, Dr. U. Gugerli, Sandoz, Basle.

This study was supported by Sandoz Pharma Ltd.

References

1. Baumann G, Andersen E, Quesniaux V, Eberle MK (1992) Cyclosporin and its analogue SDZ IMM 125 mediate very similar effects on T-cell activation – a comparative analysis in vitro. Transplant Proc 24 (Suppl 2): 43–48
2. Donatsch P, Mason J, Richardson BP, Ryffel B (1992) Toxicologic evaluation of the new cyclosporin derivative, SDZ IMM 125, in a comparative, subchronic toxicity study in rats. Transplant Proc 24 (Suppl 2): 39–42
3. Hiestand PC, Gräber M, Hurtenbach U, Herrmann P, Cammisuli S, Richardson BP, Eberle MK, Borel JF (1992) The new cyclosporin derivative, SDZ IMM 125: in vitro and in vivo pharmacologic effects. Transplant Proc 24 (Suppl 2): 31–38
4. Hiestand PC, Gräber M, Hurtenbach U, Herrmann P, Cammisuli S, Richardson BP, Eberle MK, Donatsch P, Ryffel B, Borel JF (1993) New cyclosporin derivative, SDZ IMM 125: in vitro and in vivo pharmacologic effects and toxicologic evaluation. Transplant Proc 25: 691–692
5. Kahan BD (1989) Cyclosporine. N Engl J Med 321: 1725–1738
6. The Canadian Multicentre Transplant Study Group (1986) A randomized clinical trial of cyclosporine in cadaveric renal transplantation: analysis at three years. N Engl J Med 314: 1219–1225
7. The European Multicentre Trial Group (1982) Cyclosporin A as a sole immunosuppressive agent in recipients of kidney allografts from cadaver donors. Lancet 2: 57–60

Transpl Int (1996) 9 [Suppl 1]: S318–S322
© Springer-Verlag 1996

Georg A. Böhmig
Thomas Wekerle
Marcus D. Säemann
Josef Kovarik
Gerhard J. Zlabinger

Induction of alloantigen-specific hyporesponsiveness in vitro by n-butyrate: antagonistic effect of cyclosporin A

G. A. Böhmig · M. D. Säemann ·
G. J. Zlabinger (✉)
Institute of Immunology,
University of Vienna, Borschkegasse 8 A,
A-1090 Vienna, Austria
Tel. +43 1 401 54/3 56;
Fax +43 1 408 66 70

T. Wekerle
Department of Transplant Surgery,
University of Vienna,
Währinger Gürtel 18–20,
A-1090 Vienna, Austria

J. Kovarik
Department of Internal Medicine,
University of Vienna,
Währinger Gürtel 18–20,
A-1090 Vienna, Austria

Abstract The short-chain fatty acid n-butyrate has recently been shown in vitro to specifically downregulate T cell reactivity to nominal antigen or to alloantigen, which possibly results from inhibition of cell cycle progression in early G_1 phase during antigen contact. In the present study, we investigated the effect of cyclosporin A (CyA) on the modulation of alloreactivity in human mixed lymphocyte culture (MLC) by n-butyrate. Whereas in primary culture, CyA additively enhanced inhibition of DNA synthesis by n-butyrate, the effect of this agent on secondary T cell reactivity was clearly antagonized by CyA. Thus, specific downregulation of proliferative responsiveness to restimulation with antigen from the original donor, observed in cultures pretreated with n-butyrate alone, was at least partially prevented by the addition of CyA to the primary culture. Our in vitro finding indicates that specific downregulation of T cell alloreactivity by n-butyrate might depend on a calcium-dependent T cell receptor (TCR)-mediated signal sensitive to the immunosuppressive action of CyA.

Key words n-Butyrate · Cyclosporin A · T cell · Alloantigen · Hyporesponsiveness

Introduction

n-Butyrate has been described as having multiple biological effects on various types of mammalian cells, such as modulation of gene expression, inhibition of proliferation, and induction of cellular differentiation [1]. This short-chain fatty acid, as well as related organic compounds, has also been reported to block proliferative responses of murine or human lymphocytes to mitogens [2–4], and to suppress the proliferation as well as generation of cytotoxic T cells in human primary and secondary MLC [5]. Furthermore, supplementation of drinking water with n-butyric acid resulted in modest but significant prolongation of skin allograft survival in mice [5]. Recently, Gilbert and Weigle [6] demonstrated in a human HGG-specific T cell clone that antigen contact in the presence of n-butyrate results in a state of antigen-specific unresponsiveness. Blockade of cell cycle progression in G_{1a} phase during antigen contact was proposed to be the mechanism underlying anergy induction in this model [6, 7]. We could further demonstrate that beyond inhibiting T cell proliferation in primary MLC, pretreatment of primary cultures with n-butyrate also resulted in a profound state of alloantigen-specific hyporesponsiveness as assessed in restimulation culture, suggesting a possible application of this agent for tolerance induction to allografts [8].

A series of data indicates that the immunosuppressive drug CyA might alter distinct forms of immunological tolerance [9]. Thus, CyA has been shown to prevent the induction of T cell anergy in vitro [10–12] as well as in vivo [13, 14]. Furthermore, this agent might interfere with the process of clonal deletion during thymic maturation [15–17]. On the other hand, however, CyA is well known to induce tolerance to allografts particularly in rodents [18]. In addition, this immunosuppressant has recently been shown to enhance peripheral T cell deletion [13, 14] and to induce alloantigen-specific anergy in vitro when combined with a monoclonal antibody against B7 [19].

The present study was designed to examine the impact of CyA on the modulation of alloreactivity by n-butyrate. Our observation that CyA enhances the inhibitory effect of n-butyrate on DNA synthesis in primary MLC, but antagonizes specific downregulation of T cell reactivity as assessed in secondary culture, suggests that the induction of specific hyporesponsiveness by n-butyrate critically depends on a calcium-dependent TCR-triggered signal that is sensitive to the immunosuppressive action of CyA.

Materials and methods

Primary MLC

Human peripheral blood mononuclear cells (PBMC) were isolated from heparinized peripheral blood by density gradient centrifugation on Ficoll-Hypaque (Pharmacia, Uppsala, Sweden) and resuspended in RPMI 1640 supplemented with 2 mM L-glutamine, antibiotics (100 U/ml penicillin and 100 µg/ml streptomycin), and 10 % fetal calf serum that had been inactivated at 56 °C for 30 min. For the primary culture, 4×10^4 PBMC from healthy volunteers were mixed with 4×10^4 irradiated (6000 rad) PBMC from unrelated donors in medium with or without n-butyrate (Sigma Chemical Co., St. Louis, Mo.) or CyA (a gift from Dr. Wiskott, Sandoz Ltd.). The cultures were set up in triplicate at 37 °C in a 5 % CO_2 atmosphere in round-bottomed 96-well plates. Proliferation was assessed on day 7 of culture. For measurement of DNA synthesis, the cultures were pulsed with 1 µCi [^{3}H]thymidine 16 h prior to harvesting. Incorporated radioactivity was measured by liquid scintillation spectrometry. Data are reported as mean cpm ± SD of triplicate cultures.

Secondary MLC

For secondary MLC, 1×10^6 PBMC were cocultured with an equal number of irradiated allogeneic PBMC in 75×12 mm tissue culture tubes in the presence or absence of the above-mentioned agents using culture conditions as described for primary MLC. After 7 days of culture, the cells were washed and incubated in fresh medium for another 7 days. Precultured cells (3×10^3) were then rechallenged with an equal number of freshly isolated irradiated autologous cells, of irradiated cells from the original donor or from unrelated third party donors, or with phytohemagglutinin (PHA) (1 µg/ml; Murex Diagnostics Limited, Dartford, UK). Secondary cultures were carried out in round-bottomed 96-well plates, and DNA synthesis was assessed on four consecutive days (days 3–6).

Flow Cytometry

For the determination of cell viability, cells were harvested at the day of restimulation, pelleted, and resuspended in PBS containing proidium iodide (PI) (0.1 µg/ml). After 15 min incubation at room temperature, the percentage of viable cells was assessed according to scatter characteristics and exclusion of PI using a FACScan (Becton Dickinson, Sunnyvale, Ca).

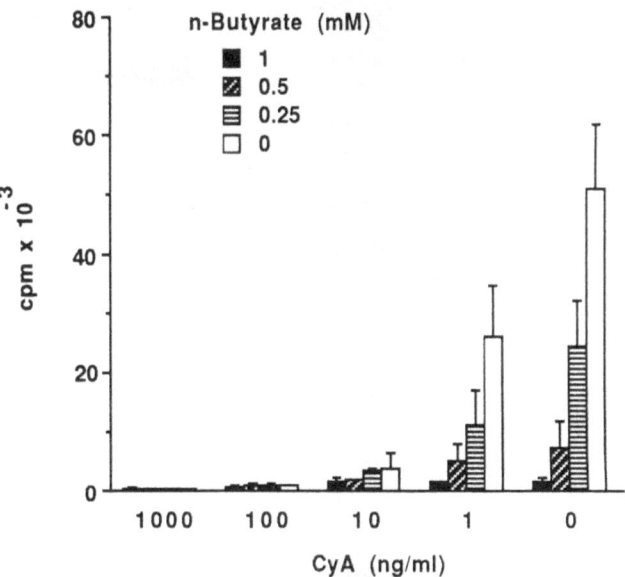

Fig. 1 Effect of CyA on inhibition of T cell alloreactivity in primary MLC by n-butyrate. DNA synthesis was assessed on day 7 of culture. Mean cpm ± SD of triplicate cultures are depicted. The experiment shown is a representative of two experiments each testing two different donor combinations

Results

Effect of CyA on inhibition of primary alloresponses by n-butyrate

In order to examine the effect of CyA on n-butyrate-mediated suppression of DNA synthesis in primary MLC, freshly isolated PBMC were mixed with irradiated allogeneic PBMC in medium containing n-butyrate at increasing concentrations in the presence or absence of CyA at various concentrations. As shown in Fig. 1, the n-butyrate dose dependently inhibited proliferation, with complete inhibition at 1 mM. CyA additively suppressed proliferative alloresponsiveness in n-butyrate-treated cultures.

Effect of CyA on specific downregulation of proliferative T cell alloreactivity by n-butyrate

To investigate the impact of CyA on the induction of alloantigen-specific hyporesponsiveness by n-butyrate, primary cultures were carried out in medium containing this agent at 1 mM in the presence or absence of CyA. CyA was added at 1 µg/ml, a concentration which in all experiments blocked primary alloresponses by more than 95 % (Table 1). In order to determine proliferative T cell responsiveness in restimulation culture, cells from primary cultures were washed on day 7 and incubated for another week in fresh medium until they were restim-

Table 1 Effect of CyA on the induction of alloantigen-specific hyporesponsiveness by n-butyrate. The results obtained in two different donor combinations *(A, B)* are depicted. Similar data were obtained in another two responder-stimulator combinations. Data are reported as mean cpm ± SD

Additions to primary MLC	Primary culture (day 7)	Percentage viability	Secondary culture (peak proliferation)			
			Autologous antigen	Specific antigen	Third party antigen	Phytohemagglutinin
A						
None	69 254 ± 11 326	46	3 177 ± 1 016	71 632 ± 7 035	30 712 ± 2 901	51 580 ± 3 072
n-Butyrate	1 100 ± 413	42	2 104 ± 1 077	10 690 ± 1 330	24 258 ± 4 952	56 412 ± 2 518
CyA	665 ± 207	45	1 016 ± 651	17 928 ± 1 296	22 781 ± 10 624	68 481 ± 5 844
CyA + n-butyrate	285 ± 147	44	3 710 ± 1 729	29 956 ± 5 371	47 535 ± 7 106	52 734 ± 3 650
B						
None	43 095 ± 8 695	42	1 575 ± 756	20 858 ± 5 194	13 673 ± 3 641	38 425 ± 3 370
n-Butyrate	1 975 ± 405	48	1 597 ± 386	12 041 ± 4 262	12 987 ± 4 181	67 952 ± 1 150
CyA	561 ± 214	51	967 ± 706	23 965 ± 4 241	14 204 ± 478	51 499 ± 655
CyA + n-butyrate	238 ± 39	51	2 589 ± 1 209	39 585 ± 1 649	10 910 ± 5 215	51 008 ± 7 213

ulated. To exclude non-specific toxic effects of the tested agents, the cells were harvested after this culture period and cell viability was assessed by PI staining. No significant reduction of cell viability was observed in cultures pretreated with n-butyrate, CyA, or with a combination of both substances (Table 1). Next, pretreated cells were rechallenged with freshly isolated irradiated autologous cells, irradiated cells from the original donor, from unrelated third party donors, or with PHA (1 µg/ml). In Table 1, the results obtained in two representative responder-stimulator combinations are shown. As previously reported [8], pretreatment of primary MLC with n-butyrate resulted in a marked reduction of proliferative reactivity to alloantigen from the original donor, whereas no such effect was observed regarding responsiveness to third party antigen or to mitogenic stimulation. Compared to cultures pretreated with n-butyrate alone, the addition of CyA to n-butyrate-treated primary cultures resulted in a marked, approximately three-fold, increase of alloresponsiveness to the same donor in secondary culture. In cultures pretreated with both CyA and n-butyrate, proliferative responses to the specific donor were clearly delayed (peaking on day 5 or 6) when compared to responses observed in control cultures or cultures pretreated with n-butyrate alone (peaking on day 3 or 4) and, thus, were characteristic of primary type alloresponses (not shown). Accordingly, as observed in three out of four donor combinations, in cultures pretreated with both CyA and n-butyrate, specific responses did not achieve levels observed in primed control cultures. Furthermore, in three donor combinations, the addition of CyA to primary MLC resulted in a significant decrease of reactivity to the specific donor, whereas reactivity to third party antigen or to PHA was not or only slightly reduced (see also Table 1). After pretreatment with both CyA and n-butyrate, responsiveness to the original donor was increased above levels observed in cultures pretreated with CyA alone.

Discussion

We have previously shown that beyond inhibition of primary alloresponses, the short-chain fatty acid n-butyrate induces a state of alloantigen-specific hyporesponsiveness, when added during primary contact with alloantigen [8]. In the present study, we analyzed the effect of the immunosuppressant CyA on n-butyrate-mediated inhibition of DNA synthesis in primary MLC and, further, on the induction of donor-specific hyporesponsiveness. Here, we describe that this agent enhances suppression of proliferation in primary MLC, but clearly antagonizes specific downregulation of T cell reactivity by n-butyrate. The latter finding suggests that specific downregulation of T cell alloreactivity might depend on an active TCR-triggered intracellular signal that is sensitive to the immunosuppressive action of CyA. Our finding that in most cases CyA did not restore specific T cell reactivity to levels observed in primed control cultures might be explained by prevention of T cell priming to alloantigen in cultures pretreated with both CyA and n-butyrate, as supported also by the time kinetics of proliferative responses to antigen from the original donor, which were delayed when compared to the secondary type response in untreated cultures.

CyA has been shown to inhibit a calcium-dependent TCR signal transduction pathway by blocking the activity of calcineurin, a calcium- and calmodulin-dependent protein phosphatase, which is responsible for the dephosphorylation and nuclear translocation of the cytoplasmic subunit of NF-AT (nuclear factor of activated T cells). As a consequence, the expression of numerous T cell activation genes, including genes encoding cytokines, is blocked [20].

Besides its immunosuppressive properties, CyA has been shown to alter distinct forms of immunological tolerance. It has also been reported that CyA prevents the induction of anergy in vitro [10–12] as well as in vivo

[13, 14], indicating an important role of TCR-triggered calcium-dependent signal transduction in the induction of functional T cell unresponsiveness. Recently, CyA has been shown to inhibit the induction of binding activity to the negative regulatory element A (NRE-A) of the IL-2 promotor following anergy induction in a human T cell clone [21]. These data are in line with the previously suggested model, that the induction of clonal anergy might result from the accumulation of a TCR-triggered negative regulator of IL-2 gene transcription, that is normally diluted out by proliferation [22, 23]. In addition, CyA has also been reported to interfere with other tolerance mechanisms, e. g., the blocking of intrathymic clonal deletion [15–17] or the inhibition of suppressor cell mechanisms [9].

In contrast to its reported prohibitive effects on various tolerance mechanisms, a short course of CyA has been reported to induce by itself a state of long-term tolerance to allografts in rats and in other species, which was attributed to the action of suppressor cells [18]. Furthermore, CyA has also been shown to increase peripheral deletion of reactive T cells induced by superantigens or anti-TCR monoclonal antibody in mice [13, 14]. Recently, Van Gool et al. [19] demonstrated that CyA synergizes with blockade of costimulation using a monoclonal antibody to B 7–1 in the induction of alloantigen-specific anergy in freshly isolated human T cells as assessed at the cytotoxic effector level. These authors suggested that, in this model, CyA might block additional calcium-dependent costimulatory signals and postulated that a calcium-independent limb of the TCR signaling pathway is required for anergy induction and remains unaffected by their treatment protocol [19].

Pretreatment of primary cultures with CyA alone sometimes led to a significant reduction of T cell responsiveness to the specific donor in secondary MLC, which appeared not to be a result of non-specific toxicity. This observation might fit in with a previous report demonstrating specific downregulation of alloantigen-specific T cell reactivity by CyA in murine MLC [24]. In addition, in human MLC, alloantigen-activated suppressor cells have been reported to be more resistant to CyA treatment than effector cells [25, 26]. Interestingly, the combined addition of both CyA and n-butyrate increased specific reactivity above levels observed in cultures pretreated with CyA or n-butyrate alone, suggesting that inversely n-butyrate might interfere with the modulation of T cell alloreactivity by CyA.

In conclusion, the observation that CyA antagonizes the induction of alloantigen-specific hyporesponsiveness by n-butyrate indicates that specific downregulation of T cell alloresponsiveness by n-butyrate critically depends on a calcium-dependent TCR-triggered signal that is sensitive to the immunosuppressive action of CyA. Our finding further supports previous results showing that immunosuppression by CyA might paradoxically interfere with distinct strategies of tolerance induction, which might be of importance in the introduction of new therapeutic strategies to induce tolerance to allografts.

Acknowledgements The authors wish to thank Gabriele Hölzl and Claus Wenhardt for excellent technical assistance. This study was supported by grant P10425 from the Fonds zur Förderung der wissenschaftlichen Forschung, Österreich.

References

1. Kruh J, Defer N, Tichonicky L (1995) Effects of butyrate on cell proliferation and gene expression. In: Cummings JH, Rombeau JL, Sakata T (eds) Physiological and clinical aspects of short-chain fatty acids. Cambridge University Press, Cambridge, pp 275–283
2. Kyner D, Zabos P, Christman J, Acs G (1976) Effect of sodium butyrate on lymphocyte activation. J Exp Med 144: 1674–1678
3. Novogrodsky A, Rubin AL, Stenzel KH (1980) A new class of inhibitors of lymphocyte mitogenesis: agents that induce erythroid differentiation in Friend leukemia cells. J Immunol 124: 1892–1897
4. Stenzel KH, Schwartz R, Rubin AL, Novogrodsky A (1980) Chemical inducers of differentiation in Friend leukemia cells inhibit lymphocyte mitogenesis. Nature 285: 106–108

5. Suthanthiran M, Rubin AL, Novogrodsky A, Stenzel KH (1982) Immunosuppressive properties of polar organic compounds that induce cellular differentiation in Friend erythroleukemia cells. Transplantation 33: 534–540
6. Gilbert KM, Weigle WO (1993) Th 1 cell anergy and blockade in G 1 a phase of the cell cycle. J Immunol 151: 1245–1254
7. Gilbert KM (1994) T cell clonal anergy. Chem Immunol 58: 92–116
8. Böhmig GA, Csmarits B, Cerwenka A, Alaei P, Kovarik J, Zlabinger GJ (1995) Induction of alloantigen-specific hyporesponsiveness in vitro by the short-chain fatty acid n-butyrate. Transplantation 59: 1500–1503
9. Prud'homme GJ, Vanier LE (1993) Cyclosporine, tolerance, and autoimmunity. Clin Immunol Immunopathol 66: 185–192

10. Jenkins MK, Ashwell JD, Schwartz RH (1988) Allogenic non-T spleen cells restore the responsiveness of normal T cell clones stimulated with antigen and chemically modified antigen-presenting cells. J Immunol 140: 3324–3330
11. Sloan-Lancaster J, Evavold BD, Allen PM (1993) Induction of T-cell anergy by altered T-cell-receptor ligand on live antigen-presenting cells. Nature 363: 156–159
12. Becker JC, Czerny C, Bröcker E-B (1994) Maintenance of clonal anergy by enogenously produced IL-10. Int Immunol 6: 1605–1612
13. Vanier LE, Prud'homme GJ (1992) Cyclosporin A markedly enhances superantigen-induced peripheral T cell deletion and inhibits anergy induction. J Exp Med 176: 37–46

14. Prud'homme GJ, Vanier LE, Bocarro DC, Ste-Croix H (1995) Effects of cyclosporin A, rapamycin, and FK520 on peripheral T-cell deletion and anergy. Cell Immunol 164: 47–56

15. Jenkins MK, Schwartz RH, Pardoll DM (1988) Effects of cyclosporine A on T cell development and clonal deletion. Science 241: 1655–1658

16. Gao E-K, Lo D, Cheney R, Kanagawa O, Sprent J (1988) Abnormal differentiation of thymocytes in mice treated with cyclosporin A. Nature 336: 176–179

17. Shi Y, Sahai BM, Green DR (1989) Cyclosporin A inhibits activation-induced cell death in T-cell hybridomas and thymocytes. Nature 339: 625–626

18. White DJG, Lim SML (1988) The induction of tolerance by cyclosporine. Transplantation 46: 118S–121S

19. Van Gool SW, de Boer M, Ceuppens JL (1994) The combination of anti-B7 monoclonal antibody and cyclosporin A induces alloantigen-specific anergy during a primary mixed lymphocyte reaction. J Exp Med 179: 715–720

20. Liu J (1993) FK 506 and cyclosporin, molecular probes for studying intracellular signal transduction. Immunol Today 14: 290–295

21. Becker JC, Brabletz T, Kirchner T, Conrad CT, Bröcker E-B, Reisfeld RA (1995) Negative transcriptional regulation in anergic T cells. Proc Natl Acad Sci USA 92: 2375–2378

22. DeSilva DR, Urdahl KB, Jenkins MK (1991) Clonal anergy is induced in vitro by T cell receptor occupancy in the absence of proliferation. J Immunol 147: 3261–3267

23. Jenkins MK (1992) The role of cell division in the induction of clonal anergy. Immunol Today 13: 69–73

24. Wang BS, Heacock EH, Collins KH, Hutchinson IF, Tilney NL, Mannick JA (1981) Suppressive effects of cyclosporin A on the induction of alloreactivity in vitro and in vivo. J Immunol 127: 89–93

25. Hess AD, Tutschka PJ (1980) Effect of cyclosporin A on human lymphocyte responses in vitro. I. CsA allows for the expression of alloantigen-activated suppressor cells while preferentially inhibiting the induction of cytolytic effector lymphocytes in MLR. J Immunol 124: 2601–2608

26. Mohagheghpour N, Benike CJ, Kansas G, Bieber C, Engleman EG (1983) Activation of antigen-specific suppressor T cells in the presence of cyclosporin requires interactions between T cells of inducer and suppressor lineage. J Clin Invest 72: 2092–2100

Transpl Int (1996) 9 [Suppl 1]: S 323–S 327
© Springer-Verlag 1996

B. Sido
G. Otto
R. Zimmermann
P. Müller
S. Meuer
T. J. Dengler

Prolonged allograft survival by the inhibition of costimulatory CD2 signals but not by modulation of CD48 (CD2 ligand) in the rat

B. Sido (✉) · G. Otto
Department of Surgery,
University of Heidelberg,
Im Neuenheimer Feld 110,
D-69120 Heidelberg, Germany

R. Zimmermann · T. J. Dengler
Department of Internal Medicine,
University of Heidelberg,
Heidelberg,
Germany

P. Müller · S. Meuer
Institute of Immunology,
University of Heidelberg,
Heidelberg,
Germany

Abstract The CD2 receptor is an important costimulatory molecule in T cell activation. Its ligand CD48 in rodents is supposed to be a homologue of human CD58, because of its similarities in structure and distribution. We evaluated the immunosuppressive activity of CD2/CD48-directed therapy in vitro and in vivo for the efficacy in prolonging rat heart allograft survival in a high responder transplant model. CD2-directed monoclonal antibody (mAb) therapy significantly prolonged median survival time to 45 days ($P < 0.001$). Suppression was mediated by down-modulation of CD2 below 20 % on lymph node cells without considerable cell depletion. In contrast, CD48 mAb could not prolong graft survival. Rejection occurred in the presence of complete CD48 modulation and, therefore, despite disruption of the CD2-CD48 interaction. CD48 mAb failed to inhibit lymphocyte activation via a mitogenic pair of CD2 mAbs and inhibited mixed lymphocyte reaction (MLR) only by an unspecific mechanism. In conclusion, our results suggest a negative regulatory signal transduction by inhibitory CD2 mAbs and argue against a pivotal role of mere disruption of the CD2-CD48 interaction in CD2-mediated immunosuppression.

Key words Transplantation · Graft survival · Antibody therapy · Costimulatory activation signals · Receptor-ligand binding

Introduction

Recently, it was shown in a rat heart transplant model that inhibition of costimulatory CD2 signals is highly immunosuppressive with induction of indefinite allograft survival [8]. CD2 is not only an important cell adhesion molecule that regulates cell to cell interaction and cell locomotion [5], but can also activate T lymphocytes via the "alternative pathway" [14]. The ligand of CD2 in humans is CD58 (LFA-3) that is expressed widely on haematopoietic and various non-haematopoietic cells including endothelial cells [5, 17]. So far, no equivalent of CD58 has been found in rodents. Kato et al. [9] have shown murine CD2 to bind CD48. van der Merwe et al. [12] has recently demonstrated a CD2-CD48 interaction in the rat by rosetting rat CD2 transfected COS-7

cells with soluble CD48-CD4-coated polystyrene Dynabeads. However, binding is of low affinity and can be completely blocked by a CD2 (OX34) and CD48 (OX45) mAb, respectively. CD48 is thought to be the CD58 homologue in rodents because of its similar distribution [2] and structural homology to the extracellular part of CD58 [10].

In the present study, we report on the in vivo and in vitro efficacy of a CD48 mAb (OX45) in the rat alone or in combination with an inhibitory CD2 mAb (OX34). Although a CD48 mAb has recently been used successfully in a murine transplant model [16] and CD48 is supposed to be the ligand of CD2 in the rat [13], we show that rat CD48 mAb does not produce any specific immunosuppression in vitro and in vivo. Based on the given results, we hypothesize that the in-

Table 1 Effect of CD2 and/or CD48 mAb therapy on rat cardiac allograft survival. The specified amount of mAb was i. v. injected into male Lew rats (220–250 g) that received a heterotopic cardiac transplant from DA rats

Monoclonal antibody (mAb)	Number	Total amount of mAb (mg)	Treatment (days)	Graft survival[a] (days)	Median graft survival time (days)
Control	16	–	–	6 (×4), 7 (×11), 8	7
OX34	6	2	0,1	35, 36, 36, 55, 71, 74	45.5
OX45	6	2	0,1	7, 7, 7, 7, 7, 7	7
OX45	6	6	0,1	7, 7, 7, 7, 7, 7	7
OX45	6	12	0–7	7, 7, 7, 7, 7, 7	7
OX34 + OX45	6	2	0,1	36, 42, 47, 49, 54, 65	48

[a] Complete rejection was defined as cessation of palpable heart beat and electrical activity in the ECG

hibitory CD2 mAb OX34 transduces a negative signal as compared to CD48 mAb and mere disruption of the CD2-CD48 interaction might not be the primary mechanism of CD2-mediated immunosuppression in the rat.

Materials and methods

Animals

Inbred rat strains blood group D-Agouti-RT1[a] (DA) and Lewis-RT1[1] (LEW) were obtained from Harlan CPB (Zeist, The Netherlands). Male rats were used, exclusively.

Heart Transplantation

We used a fully allogeneic high responder rat heart transplant model from DA (200–220 g) to LEW (220–250 g). Heterotopic intraabdominal heart transplantation was performed according to standard microsurgical techniques with an end-to-side anastomosis of the pulmonary artery to the vena cava and of the ascending aorta to the abdominal aorta. Total ischemic time was about 30 min. Rejection was defined as loss of palpable contraction and cessation of electrical activity in the ECG. For antibody therapy, a specified dose of CD2 (OX34) or CD48 (OX45) mAb was injected intravenously on two consecutive days starting immediately after transplantation.

Cells

For in vitro studies, cells were prepared and cultured from cervical and mesenteric lymph nodes (LNC) and the spleen by standard procedures [4].

Antibodies

Hybridoma cells for the following antibodies were obtained from European Collection of Animal Cell Cultures (Porton, England): OX1 (leucocyte common antigen), OX6 (MHC Class II), OX8 ($T_{c/s}$ and NK cells), OX12 (B cells), OX19 (CD5), OX21 (human C3b INA), OX34 (CD2), OX35 (T_h cells and macrophages), OX45 (CD48), OX54 (CD2), OX55 (CD2) and R73 ($\alpha\beta$TcR). Purified antibody was used for in vitro and in vivo experiments, unspecific mouse anti-human CD58 antibodies 1C7 (IgG1) and 1A10 (IgG2a) were used as controls.

Studies of lymphocyte proliferation in vitro

T cells were stimulated via the alternative pathway of CD2 by coincubation with a pair of mitogenic CD2 antibodies. 2.5×10^5 LEW-LNC and 5×10^5 syngeneic irradiated (30 Gy) spleen cells as a source of accessory cells were cultured together in the presence of a 1:1 mixture of OX54 and OX55 (20 µg/ml each final concentration) in a total volume of 200 µl/well in round-bottomed microtiter plates. 50 µl of [³H]thymidine (1 µCi, Amersham, Karlsruhe, Germany) were added for the last 18 h of a 72 h incubation period before harvesting the cells on an automatic harvester (Pharmacia, Freiburg, Germany). Thymidine uptake was measured with a β-counter (Pharmacia, Freiburg, Germany).

Inhibition of allogeneic stimulation of lymphocytes by CD2 and/or CD48 antibodies was tested in a primary mixed lymphocyte reaction (MLR). 1.75×10^5 responder LEW-LNC and 2.5×10^5 irradiated (30 Gy) stimulator DA-LNC were incubated with various concentrations of CD2 and/or CD48 antibodies for 2–6 days in round-bottomed microtiter plates at 37 °C in 7.5 % CO₂. [³H]Thymidine (1 µCi) was added for the last 18 h before harvesting the cells.

Flow cytometry analysis

5×10^5 LEW-LNC were incubated with 50 µl staining antibody (10 µg/ml) for 30 min at 4 °C and then washed twice with PBS. OX1 was used as a positive control, unspecific binding of OX21 as a negative control. After washing, the cells were labelled with a second-stage fluorescein-conjugated goat anti-mouse antibody (Southern Biotechnology Associates, USA) for 15 min at 4 °C, washed twice in PBS and fixed in 1 % formaldehyde. FACS analysis was performed on an EPICS flow cytometer (Hileah, Florida, USA).

Statistical analysis

Graft survival after heart transplantation in antibody-treated animals was compared with the untreated control group in a log-rank sum test. P values < 0.05 were regarded as significant.

Results

Graft survival

The CD2 mAb OX34 and the CD48 mAb OX45 were tested in vivo for their efficacy in prolonging allograft survival (Table 1). 1 mg OX34 administered on day 0 and 1 i. v. significantly prolonged median graft survival

Flow Cytometry

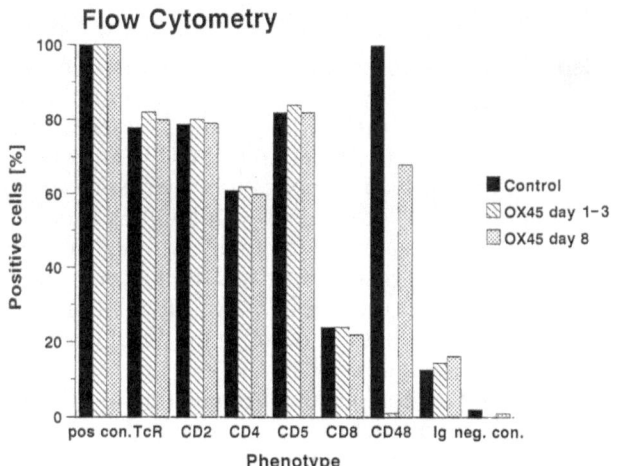

Fig. 1 Flow cytometry analysis of LNC on various days after treatment of non-transplanted LEW rats with i.v. injection 0f 3 mg OX45 on days 0 and 1. OX1 (leukocyte common antigen) was used as a positive control, OX21 (human C3b INA) as a negative control. OX45 specificly down-modulates CD48 without influencing other cell surface antigens

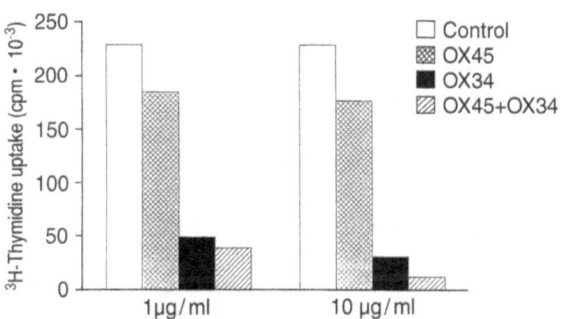

Fig. 2 CD2-mediated stimulation of 2.5×10^5 LEW-LNC by a 1:1 combination of mitogenic CD2 mAbs (OX54 + OX55; 20 μg/ml each final concentration) in the presence of 5×10^5 irradiated syngeneic spleen cells for 72 h. Results represent [³H]thymidine uptake during the last 18 h period

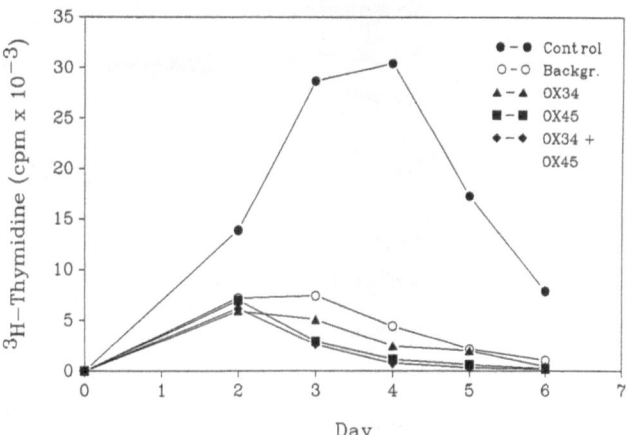

Fig. 3 Inhibition of MLR (LEW LNC vs. irradiated DA LNC) by 10 μg/ml OX34 and/or OX45 on day 2–6. Values represent [³H]thymidine uptake during the last 18 h of culture.

time (MST) to 45.5 days as compared with 7 days in untreated control animals ($P < 0.001$). This immunosuppression was dose dependent, but increasing the total amount of OX34 to 5 mg (1 mg on days 0, 1, 3, 5, 7) could not produce indefinite survival (data not shown).

As CD48 is supposed to be the major ligand for CD2 in rodents, we used OX45 in the same transplant model. OX45 failed to prolong allograft survival both at an equivalent dose of 2×1 mg (MST = 7 days) and at a dose three times higher of 2×3 mg (MST = 7 days) to compensate for the wide distribution of CD48 including endothelial cells and erythrocytes. Combination of 2×1 mg OX45 with 2×1 mg OX34 did not lead to an additive or supraadditive immunosuppressive effect in vivo compared to OX34 alone (MST = 48 days; P = n.s. vs OX34).

Phenotypic analysis

Dynamic phenotypic changes of surface antigens on LNC after intravenous injection of 1 mg mAb (CD2 or CD48 mAb) on days 0 and 1 in non-transplanted rats were investigated by flow cytometry analysis at various time-points after injection until the pretreatment phenotype was reestablished. OX34 led to a rapid and almost complete (> 80 %) down-modulation of CD2 from 76 % to 13 % positive cells, residual CD2 was antibody bound. CD2 reexpression started 5 weeks after injection and was completely restored after 72 days with 68 % positive cells and no receptor-bound OX34. Circulating OX34 mAb in the serum was present until day 72. A partial and only temporary T cell depleting effect, mainly of the CD4+ subset, was observed from day 14 to day 30 with a minimum of 20 % αβTcR+ cells (data not shown).

Application of 2×3 mg OX45 led to a complete down-modulation of CD48 within 1 day in the absence of any cell depletion, lasting for more than 3 days (Fig. 1). OX45 did not change expression of several other cell surface molecules, such as CD4, CD8 or TcR. Parallel to the removal of circulating mAb from serum, CD48 was partially, but functionally, reexpressed on 67 % of LNC after 8 days and fully reexpressed after 14 days. As the lack of effect of OX45 in prolonging allograft survival might be attributed to the fast biological clearance of the mAb from the circulation due to the wide distribution of CD48 along with early functional reexpression of CD48, we treated transplanted LEW rats daily from day 0–7 with a total of 12 m i.v. Even such a high-dose regimen with circulating mAb and persisting CD48 modulation for more than 8 days did not prolong allograft survival vs controls (MST = 7 days, P = n.s.).

CD2-mediated stimulation of LNC

LNC were stimulated via the CD2 receptor with a mitogenic combination of CD2 mAb (OX54 + OX55) in the presence of syngeneic irradiated spleen cells (Fig. 2). OX34 does not inhibit binding of both OX54 and OX55 [4]. While OX34 highly efficiently inhibited CD2-mediated stimulation, OX45 was not effective up to a final concentration of 100 µg/ml. Inhibition of CD2-induced proliferation by the combination of OX34 and OX45 did not differ from OX34 alone.

Allogeneic LNC stimulation in the MLR

Responder LNC were stimulated by irradiated stimulator LNC in the presence of different amounts of CD2 and/or CD48 mAb (Fig. 3). Peak proliferation was found to be on day 4 in the control MLR. The immunosuppressive effect of OX34 is fully established on days 3 and 4 with a biphasic dependence on mAb concentration. Interestingly, OX45 suppressed allogeneic LNC proliferation in this assay in a very similar manner, as seen with OX34 alone. Inhibition by OX45 is identical to the combination of OX34 and OX45.

As it is known that the inhibition of MLR by OX45 is dependent on the presence of macrophages [1], it was speculated that OX45 activates unspecific immunosuppressive activity of macrophages. We could demonstrate the non-specificity of OX45-mediated suppression of the MLR by preincubating the responder and stimulator LNC, respectively, with either OX34 or OX45 (10 µg/ml). After 24 h, cells were washed twice and stimulated in a 3 day MLR as described above. Inhibition of proliferation was exactly the same independent of whether the responder or the irradiated stimulator cells were pretreated with OX45. Inhibition was most prominent, when preincubated responder and preincubated stimulator cells were cultured together. On the contrary, the immunosuppressive effect of OX34 was exclusively restricted to pretreatment of responder cells with the CD2 mAb (data not shown).

Discussion

In the present study, we report on the in vivo efficacy of a treatment with anti-CD48 mAb OX45 after rat heart transplantation. Dynamic phenotypic changes of LNC after intravenous injection of 1 mg mAb (CD2 or CD48 mAb) on days 0 and 1 in non-transplanted rats were investigated by flow cytometry analysis on various days after injection until the pretreatment phenotype was reestablished. Even at very high doses, OX45 could not prolonged allograft survival vs untreated controls, when used alone, and had no additional immunosup-

pressive effect in conjunction with CD2 mAb, although it led to a dose-dependent down-modulation of CD48 without cell depletion. While the duration of allograft survival correlated with the long-lasting presence of circulating CD2 mAb in the serum and CD2 antigen modulation after antibody application, persisting down-modulation of CD48 for 7 days with the high-dose regimen of OX45 remained completely without an effect upon allograft survival. Thus, rejection occurs during ongoing OX45 therapy despite down-modulation of the ligand CD48, but does not occur in the absence of CD2 expression in the rat.

Qin et al. [16] could show prolongation of graft survival in a mouse model of non-vascularised heart transplantation. Equivalent doses of 100 µg of CD2 and CD48 mAb, respectively, were used, although CD48 has a much wider distribution comprising all haematopoietic and various non-haematopoietic cells including endothelium. While CD2 and CD48 mAb were immunosuppressive on their own, the authors demonstrated a synergistic effect with indefinite graft survival in mice treated concomitantly with CD2 and CD48 mAb. This synergistic action is in marked contrast to the findings presented in this study. These discrepant results might be explained by insufficient mAb binding affinity to rat CD48 to disrupt receptor-ligand interaction. This appears unlikely, however, as mAb binding is of much higher affinity compared with the weak CD2-CD48 interaction [13]. An alternative explanation is that there is another major functional ligand of CD2 in rats not as yet identified.

We investigated the immunosuppressive activity of OX34 and OX45, respectively, in different assays of lymphocyte activation in vitro. OX34 highly efficiently inhibited lymphocyte proliferation induced by a pair of mitogenic CD2 mAbs (OX54 + OX55), whereas OX45 failed to inhibit CD2-mediated T cell activation. The three CD2 mAbs bind to different epitopes of the CD2 molecule without cross-inhibition of binding [4]. Therefore, it might be speculated that OX34 actively transfers a negative regulatory signal via the CD2 receptor to neutralize OX54/55-mediated stimulation, provided that CD48 is the major functional ligand of CD2 in the rat. This suggestion is substantiated by the finding that mere lack of CD2 signal transduction in CD2 knock out mice does not mediate suppression [7, 11]. Transduction of negative regulatory signals by non-cross-linking CD2 mAbs has been suggested in earlier studies [3, 15, 18]. Alternatively, OX45 might be directed against an epitope of CD48, which is not involved in CD2 binding. van der Merwe et al. [13] could show, however, that COS-7 cells expressing surface CD2 specifically bind to a soluble form of CD48 (sCD48-CD4) coated on polystyrene Dynabeads and that this CD2-sCD48 interaction could be specifically blocked by OX34 as well as by OX45.

OX45 effectively suppressed lymphocyte proliferation in the allogeneic MLR, but by an unspecific mechanism as shown by preincubation experiments. This finding is in accordance with data by Arvieux et al. [1], who proposed that inhibition by OX45 is mediated via activation of non-specific suppression by accessory cells that are thought to be macrophages. The authors showed that OX45 failed to inhibit T cell activation in the presence of dendritic cells, but not when spleen cells or macrophages were used as stimulators.

In summary, CD48 is thought to be the equivalent of human CD58 in rodents because of its similar distribution and structure. Both OX34 and OX45 are known to inhibit specifically CD2-CD48 binding in vitro. As we could show, the use of CD48 mAb OX45 in vitro and in an experimental animal transplant model failed to show any specific immunosuppressive activity as opposed to the CD2 mAb OX34, indicating that negative regulatory signaling may be involved in CD2-mediated suppression rather than mere disruption of the CD2-CD48 interaction. Alternatively, an as yet unidentified ligand other than CD48 might be of major importance in binding to the CD2 receptor in the rat in vivo and in vitro.

References

1. Arvieux J, Jefferies WA, Paterson DJ, Williams AF, Green JR (1986) Monoclonal antibodies against a rat leukocyte antigen block antigen-induced T-cell responses via an effect on accessory cells. Immunol 58: 337–342
2. Arvieux J, Willis AC, Williams AF (1986) MRC OX-45 antigen: a leukocyte/endothelium rat membrane glycoprotein of 45 000 molecular weight. Mol Immunol 23: 983–990
3. Chavin KD, Qin L, Lin J, Woodward J, Baliga P, Kato K, Yagita H, Bromberg JS (1994) Anti-CD48 (murine CD2 ligand) mAbs suppress cell-mediated imunity in vivo. Int Immunol 6: 701–709
4. Clark SJ, Law DA, Paterson DJ, Puklavec M, Williams AF (1988) Activation of rat lymphocytes by anti-CD2 monoclonal antibodies. J Exp Med 167: 1861–1872
5. Dustin ML, Springer TA (1991) Role of lymphocyte adhesion receptors in transient interactions and cell locomotion. Ann Rev Immunol 9: 27–66
6. Dustin ML, Selvyraj P, Mattaliano RJ, Springer TA (1987) Anchoring mechanisms for LFA-3 cell adhesion glycoprotein at membrane surface. Nature 329: 846–848
7. Evans CF, Rall GF, Killeen N, Littmann D, Oldstone MBA (1993) CD2-deficient mice generate virus-specificcytotoxic T lymphocytes upon infection with lymphocytic choriomeningitis virus. J Immunol 151: 6259–6264
8. Hirahara H, Tsuchida M, Watanabe T, Haga M, Matsumoto Y, Abo T, Eguchi S (1995) Long-term survival of cardiac allografts in rats treated before and after surgery with monoclonal antibody to CD2. Transplant 59: 85–90
9. Kato K, Koyanaga M, Okada H, Takanashi T, Wong Y, Williams AF, Okumura K, Yagita H (1992) CD48 is a counter-receptor for mouse CD2 and is involved in T cell activation. J Exp Med 176: 1241–1249
10. Killeen N, Moessner R, Arvieux J, Willis A, Williams AF (1988) The MRC OX-45 antigen of rat leukocytes and endothelium is a subset of the immunoglobulin superfamily with CD2, LFA-3 and carcinoembryonic antigens. EMBO J 7: 3087–3091
11. Killeen M, Stuart SG, Littman DR (1992) Development and function of T cells in mice with a disrupted CD2 gene. EMBO J 11: 4329–4336
12. Merwe A van der, Brown PA, Davis MH, Barclay SJ (1993) Affinity and kinetic analysis of the interaction of the cell adhesion molecules rat CD2 and CD48. EMBO J 12: 4945–4954
13. Merwe A van der, McPherson DC, Brown MH, Barclay AN, Cyster JG, Williams AF, Davis SJ (1993) The NH$_2$-terminal domain of rat CD2 binds rat CD48 with a low affinity and binding does not require glycosilation of CD2. Eur J Immunol 23: 1373–1377
14. Meuer SC, Hussey RE, Fabbi M, Fox D, Acuto O, Fitzgerald KA, Hodgdon JC, Protentis JP, Schlossman SF, Reinherz EL (1984) An alternative pathway of T-cell activation: a functional role for the 50 kd T11 sheep erythrocyte receptor protein. Cell 36: 897–906
15. Ohno H, Nakamura T, Yagita H, Okumura K, Taniguchi M, Saito T (1991) Induction of negative signal through CD2 during antigen-specific T cell activation. J Immunol 147: 2100–2106
16. Qin L, Chavin K, Lin J, Yagita H, Bromberg JS (1994) Anti-CD2 receptor and anti-CD2 ligand (CD48) antibodies synergize to prolong allograft survival. J Exp Med 179: 341–346
17. Selvaraj P, Plunkett ML, Dustin M, Sanders ME, Shaw S, Springer TA (1987) The lymphocyte glycoprotein CD2 binds the cell surface ligand LFA-3. Nature 326: 400–403
18. Yokoyama A, Suzuki H, Kamitani T, Yagita H, Okumura K, Yano S (1991) Characterization of inhibitory effect of an anti-murine CD2 monoclonal antibody on the proliferation of T cell clones. Immunol Lett 28: 219–225

Transpl Int (1996) 9 [Suppl 1]: S 328–S 330
© Springer-Verlag 1996

Yuan Lin
Michel Vandeputte
Mark Waer

A short-term combination therapy with cyclosporine and rapamycin or leflunomide induces long-term heart allograft survival in a strongly immunogenic strain combination in rats

Y. Lin · M. Vandeputte · M. Waer (✉)
Division of Nephrology and Laboratory for
Experimental Transplantation,
University of Leuven, O & N, Herestraat 49,
B-3000 Leuven, Belgium

Abstract Synergism between cyclosporine (CsA) and rapamycin (RAPA) or leflunomide (LF) was studied in a strongly immunogenic cardiac allograft model in rats. In the absence of immunosuppression, PVG recipients rejected WKAH heart grafts after a mean survival time (MST) of 5.2 ± 1.1 days. A dose of 7.5 mg/kg per day CsA did not prolong graft survival (MST 5.6 ± 1.2 days). CsA given at 10 mg/kg per day for 30 days extended MST of the grafts to 48 ± 7 days. A short course of combination therapy consisting of adding a non-therapeutic dose of RAPA or a subtherapeutic dose of LF to a 1-month course of CsA resulted in permanent graft survival. These data suggest that RAPA and LF synergize with CsA enabling not only the lowering of the dose of CsA, but also inducing transplantation tolerance.

Key words Allograft · Tolerance · Cyclosporine · Rapamycin · Leflunomide

Introduction

Efficient T lymphocyte activation requires two signals. Signal 1 is provided by an interaction between the T cell receptor (TCR) and antigens in association with self-MHC molecules (TCR-antigen pathway). Signal 2 results from an interaction between non-MHC molecules and their ligands. As a costimulatory signal, signal 2 determines whether T lymphocytes undergo mitosis, apoptosis or anergy. It is well recognized that the CD 28–B 7 interaction is one of the most important in signal 2 transduction. Cyclosporine (CsA) and FK 506 suppress T lymphocyte activation mainly by blocking the TCR-antigen pathway [1]. In contrast, rapamycin (RAPA) can also block the CD 28–B 7 pathway [2]. Leftunomide (LF), an isoxazol derivative which recently raised a lot of interest as a potential immunosuppressant, is also believed to be able to block the CD 28–B 7 pathway [3].

In various rat strain combinations, transplantation tolerance can be readily induced using CsA or RAPA monotherapy [4]. However, we found that in a strongly immunogenic strain combinations, induction of the tolerance using only one drug appeared to be more difficult. Hence, we investigated the potential of drugs blocking signal 2, such as RAPA and LF, to synergize with CsA which blocks signal 1 in this highly immunogenic model.

Materials and methods

T lymphocyte proliferation in vitro

The mixed lymphocyte reaction (MLR) as well as the proliferation assay of purified T cells through the CD 3 and CD 28 pathways were performed on human peripheral blood mononuclear cells (PBMC) using the methods described elsewhere [3].

Animals

Inbred male PVG rats (RT1^c), weighing 200–250 g were used as recipients. Inbred WKAH rats (RT1^k), weighing 100–150 g were used as donors.

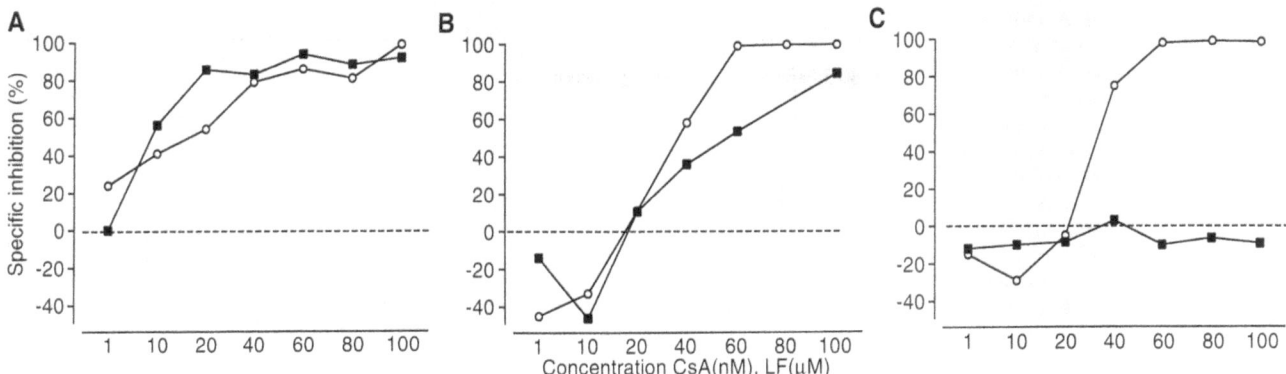

Fig. 1 A–C Effect of CsA and LF on human T cell proliferation in vitro. **A** T cell proliferation in MLR. **B** Purified T cell proliferation by stimulation with OKT 3 + PMA. **C** Purified T cell proliferation by stimulation with anti-CD 28 + PMA. (■ Inhibition mediated by CsA, ○ inhibition mediated by LF)

Heterotopic heart transplantation

Heterotopic heart transplantation was performed by implanting the heart grafts into the neck of recipients using methods described previously [5]. The function of grafts was monitored by daily inspection and palpation. Rejection was determined by the cessation of the graft beating and confirmed by histology.

Immunosuppressive therapy

LF (HWA 486) and RAPA were freshly suspended in 1% carboxymethylcellulose and given by gavage and i.p., respectively. CsA was diluted in olive oil and given by gavage.

Results

Effect of CsA and LF in different T cell stimulation pathways

CsA and LF both inhibited T cell proliferation in a dose-dependent manner in the MLR (Fig. 1 A, B), as well as through the CD 3 (OKT 3) stimulation pathway (Fig. 1 C). In contrast, the CD 28 pathway was only inhibited by LF. These results are similar to those previously published for RAPA and confirmed what has been reported for LF (Fig. 1 C) [3].

Effect of CsA, RAPA and LF on graft survival

Graft survival is shown in Fig. 2. Untreated PVG rats rejected WKAH heart allografts after a mean survival time (MST) of 5.2 ± 1.1 days. CsA at 7.5 mg/kg per day and RAPA at 2.5 mg/kg per day did not affect graft survival (MST 5.6 ± 2 and 4.2 ± 1 days, respectively) (Fig. 2 A). CsA and LF both given at 10 mg/kg per day for 30 days prolonged graft survival to 48 ± 7 and 32 ± 7.4 days, respectively (Fig. 2 B). Combination of RAPA (2.5 mg/kg per day, day 0–15) with CsA (7.5 mg/

kg per day, day 0–30) (Fig. 2 A) or combination of LF (10 mg/kg per day, day 0–30) with CsA (10 mg/kg per day, from day 0–30) (Fig. 2 B) resulted in indefinite graft survival.

Discussion

Looking for new immunosuppressants which can provide additive or synergistic effects on CsA remains an option for reducing the side effects of CsA and so achieving better immunosuppression. As T cell activation is now generally believed to be dependent on two activation pathways and as CsA and FK 506 only suppress the first one (delivered by the TCR), much interest exists in drugs that can suppress the second pathway (delivered by the B 7–CD 28 interaction). RAPA and LF clearly seem to belong to the latter class of the drugs as was shown previously [2, 3], and this is also confirmed in the present study.

Here we show that in a strongly immunogenic heart allograft model in rats, synergism between the two types of drugs is also observed in vivo. The immune mechanisms involved are not precisely known as yet, but they seem to be different from what was previously found in a weaker immunogenic rat combination also using the RAPA + CsA combination therapy [6]. Indeed, in contrast to the latter study, we found no arguments for the presence of suppressor cells, nor for the existence of circulating blocking antibodies. It, therefore, seems that a combination therapy of immunosuppressants blocking signal 1 and signal 2 of T cell activation, respectively, may lead to long-term graft survival without maintenance therapy based on different immune mechanisms. The mechanism responsible for the long-term graft survival in our study is at present being further investigated.

Acknowledgements This work was supported by grants from the "National fund for scientific research-NFWO" and of the "ONDERZOEKSRAAD" from the University of Leuven.

Fig. 2 A Effect of CsA and RAPA given alone or in combination on graft survival; no treatment (○) CsA 7.5 mg/kg per day (■), RAPA 2.5 mg/kg per day (□), combination of CsA (day 0–30) and RAPA (day 0–15) (▲). **B** Effect of CsA and LF given alone or in combination on graft survival; no treatment (○), CsA 10 mg/kg per day, day 0–30 (■), LF 10 mg/kg per day, day 0–30 (□), combination of CsA (day 0–30) and LF (day 0–30) (▲)

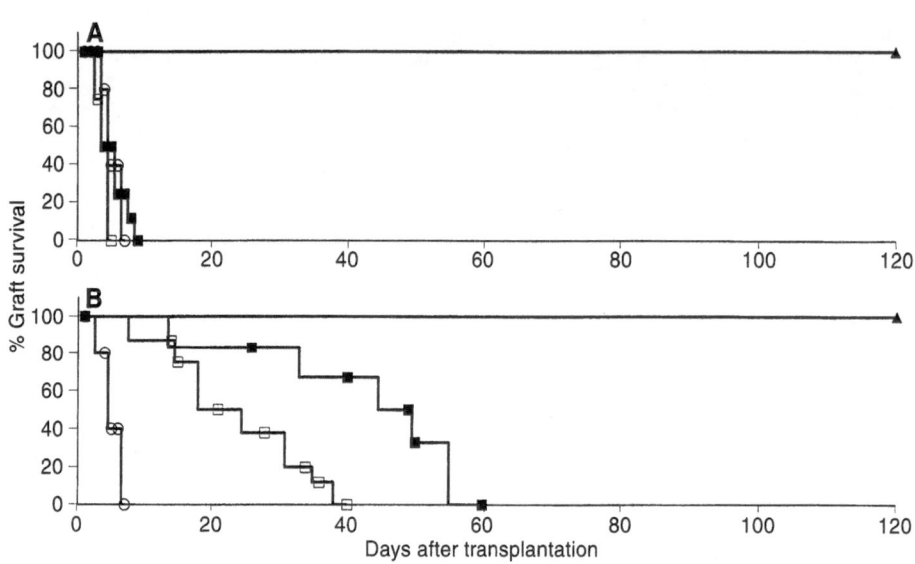

References

1. Tocci MJ, Matkovich DA, Kwok KA, Dumont F, Lin S, et al (1989) The immuno-suppressant FK 506 selectively inhibits expression of early T cell activation genes. J Immunol 143: 718
2. Luo H, Chen H, Daloze P, St-Louis G, Wu J (1993) Anti-CD 28 antibody- and IL-4-induced human T cell proliferation is sensitive to Rapamycin. Clin Exp Immunol 94: 371
3. Chong ASF, Gebel H, Finnegan A, Petraitis EE, Jiang XL, Sankary HN, Foster P, Williams JM (1993) Leflunomide, a novel immunomodulatory agent: in vitro analyses of the mechanism of immunosuppression. Transplant Proc 25: 747
4. Chen HF, Luo HY, Daloze P, Xu DS, Wu JP (1994) Rapamycin-induced long-term allograft survival depends on persistence of alloantigen. J Immunol 152: 3107
5. Lin Y, Sobis H, Vanderputte M, Waer M (1994) Long-term xenograft survival and suppression of xenoantibody formation in the hamster-to-rat heart transplant model using a combination therapy of Leflunomide and Cyclosporine. Transplant Proc 26: 3202
6. Ferraresso M, Ghobrial R, Stepkowski SM, Kahan B (1993) The mechanism of unresponsiveness to allografts induced by Rapamycin/Cyclosporine treatment in rats. Transplantation 55: 888

Transpl Int (1996) 9 [Suppl 1]: S331–S333
© Springer-Verlag 1996

E. Antoniou
A. DeRoover
Y. Nishimura
A. J. Howie
P. McMaster
M. D'Silva

Effect of RS61443 in combination with leflunomide or FK506 on rat heart allograft survival

E. Antoniou · A. DeRoover · Y. Nishimura ·
M. D'Silva (✉)
Transplantation Microsurgery Laboratory,
The Liver Research Laboratories,
Clinical Research Block,
Queen Elizabeth Hospital and
Medical Center, Edgbaston,
Birmingham B15 2TH, UK
Fax + 44 121 627 24 97

A. J. Howie
Department of Pathology,
University of Birmingham, Edgbaston,
Birmingham B15 2TH, UK

P. McMaster
The Liver and Hepatobiliary Unit,
Queen Elizabeth Hospital and
Medical Center, Birmingham, UK

Abstract Mycophenolate Mofetil (RS61443) is a potent inhibitor of de novo purine synthesis and lymphocyte proliferation. It is known to prevent ongoing rejection and even reverse established rejection, alone and in combination with, cyclosporin. We investigated whether RS61443 in combination with leflunomide (Lef) or FK506 (FK) could prolong allograft survival in a rat heart model, since combination therapy might help to overcome drug toxicity. Abdominal heart grafting was performed from DA to LEW rats (250 g) and RS61443, 10 mg/kg or 30 mg/kg monotherapy or combination treatment (RS 10 mg/kg with Lef 5 mg/kg or FK 0.5 mg/kg) was begun orally at transplantation and continued daily until the ninth posttransplant (post-Tx) day. Ventricular motion was graded daily and rejection was defined as lack of contractions, confirmed by histology. Results were analysed using non-parametric tests. A two-tail P value < 0.05 was considered significant. RS at 10 mg/kg was ineffective and all grafts were rejected under immunosuppression between 5 and 6 post-Tx day, whereas RS at 30 mg/kg was immunosuppressive for as long as it was given. The combinations of RS at 10 mg/kg with either Lef at 5 mg/kg or FK at 0.5 mg/kg were immunosuppressive in the majority of cases, for as long as they were given. However, the combination of RS at 10 mg/kg with FK at 0.5 mg/kg was attendant with graft vein anastomosis rupture (3/5). The combination of RS with Lef was clinically therapeutic for as long as it was given; grafts were rejected 3–4 days after withdrawing immunosuppression. The combination of RS with FK resulted in over-immunosuppression, leading to graft vein anastomosis non-healing and rupture within 5 days of grafting; histology demonstrated evidence of bacterial infection with complete destruction of the vein wall. These data suggest that the combination of RS with Lef or FK in subtherapeutic doses might be a potentially promising strategy for combination therapy in solid organ transplantation.

Key words Immunosuppression · Rejection · Combination therapy · RS61443 · Heterotopic heart transplantation

Introduction

Mycophenolate Mofetil (RS61443) is a semisynthetic prodrug of mycophenolic acid (MPA), which selectively, non-competitevely and reversibly inhibits the de novo pathway for the purine synthesis required for T and B cells proliferative responses to antigens and mitogens [5]. This drug has been found to have antifungal, antiviral and antibacterial properties, and it has also been tested clinically in the treatment of psoriasis [6]. RS61443

Table 1 Heart allograft survival under monotherapy or combination therapy immunosuppression (*RS* RS61443, *Lef* leflunomide, *FK* FK506)

Group	Treatment (days 0–9 post-transplantation)	Survival (days), median (range)	P	Comments	Graft histology
1 (*n* = 6)	–	5 (4–5)		–	Severe AR 5/5
2 (*n* = 4)	RS 10 mg/kg	5.5 (5–6)	0.14	–	Severe AR 4/4
3 (*n* = 5)	RS 30 mg/kg	13 (13–14)	0.009	–	Severe AR 5/5
4 (*n* = 5)	RS 10 mg/kg + Lef 5 mg/kg	13 (13–14)	0.009	–	Severe AR 5/5
5 (*n* = 5)	RS 10 mg/kg + FK 0.5 mg/kg	17.5 (14–21)[a]	0.05	3/5 vein anastomosis rupture	Severe AR 2/5

[a] Excluding grafts with ruptured vein anastomoses

has shown efficacy in several models of organ transplantation, preventing ongoing rejection and even reversing established rejection, alone and in combination with, cyclosporin [3, 4].

We investigated whether RS61443 (RS) in combination with leflunomide (Lef) or FK506 (FK) could prolong allograft survival in a rat heart model, since combination therapy might help to overcome drug toxicity.

Materials and methods

Heterotopic intraabdominal heart transplantation was performed, according to a previously reported technique [1], using adult male DA(RT1^a) as donors and Lewis-RT1^1 (LEW) rats as recipients, weighing 200–250 g. The subjects were commercially obtained from Charles River, UK and cared for humanely during the course of the study, according to prevailing Home Office Guidelines in the UK. RS and Lef were suspended in 1 % carboxymethyl cellulose (CMC). FK was dissolved in normal saline.

RS monotherapy or combination therapy was administered orally daily for 10 days, starting the day of grafting until the ninth posttransplant day. Ventricular motion was graded daily and rejection was defined as lack of contractions, confirmed by histology. Recipients with rejected grafts or adverse clinical signs were euthanised and tissues analysed histologically. Results are expressed as median survival days and analysed using non-parametric tests. A two-tail *P* value < 0.05 was considered significant.

Results

Table 1 shows the results of this study using a fully major histocompatibility complex (MHC) incompatible strain combination (DA to LEW), in which freshly harvested DA hearts were transplanted intraabdominally to LEW recipients. In the control group, graft rejection was complete between 4 and 5 days postoperatively. The median survival time was 5 days. RS at 10 mg/kg was ineffective and all grafts were rejected under immunosuppression between 5 and 6 days posttransplantation, whereas RS at 30 mg/kg was found to be immunosuppressive for as long as it was given, prolonging graft survival for a period of 4–5 days after termination of immunosuppres-

sion. The median survival time in the first group (RS 10 mg/kg) was 5.5 days, not significantly different from controls. In the second group (RS 30 mg/kg) the median survival time was 13 days (range 13–14 days), significantly different from controls.

The combinations of RS at 10 mg/kg with either Lef at 5 mg/kg or FK at 0.5 mg/kg were immunosuppressive in the majority of cases, for as long as they were given. However, the combination of RS at 10 mg/kg with FK at 0.5 mg/kg led to graft vein anastomosis rupture (3/5). The median survival time in the first combination (RS + Lef) was the same as the RS at 30 mg/kg group. Apart from the rats with the ruptured vein anastomoses in the second combination group (RS + FK), the grafts of the remainder rats achieved a prolonged survival of 14–21 days (median survival time 17.5 days), significantly different from controls.

Discussion

In this study, we have used RS monotherapy (10 and 30 mg/kg) and RS in combination with Lef or FK in an effort to prolong heterotopic heart allograft survival in the rat. RS at 10 mg/kg was found to be subtherapeutic, all grafts rejecting under treatment, whereas 30-mg/kg dose prolonged allograft survival 8 days beyond DA × LEW controls. Moreover, combination therapy of RS at 10 mg/kg with Lef at 5 mg/kg was clinically therapeutic for as long as it was given; grafts were rejected 3–4 days after withdrawing immunosuppression. On the other hand, the combination of RS at 10 mg/kg with FK at 0.5 mg/kg resulted in over-immunosuppression, leading to graft pulmonary vein anastomotic non-healing and rupture within 5 days of grafting. Histology demonstrated evidence of bacterial infection with complete destruction of the vein wall. However, 2/5 grafts survived an additional 14 and 21 days after discontinuing treatment. Previous studies [2] have demonstrated that long-term heart allograft survival was achieved with RS at 20 mg/kg per day and brequinar at 3 or 6 mg/kg, 3 times per week. Our data, however, suggest that the combination of RS with Lef or FK in subtherapeutic doses may be a potentially promising strategy for combination therapy in solid organ transplantation.

Acknowledgement E.A. is a recipient of a scholarship of The Scholarships State Foundation of Greece.

References

1. D'Silva M, Candinas D, Achilleos O, et al (1995) Transplantation 60: 1–8
2. Kawamura T, Hullett DA, Suzuki Y, et al (1993) Transplantation 55: 691–695
3. Knechtle SJ, Wang J, Burlingham WJ, et al (1992) Transplantation 53: 699–701
4. Laskow DA, Deierhoi MH, Hudson SL, et al (1994) Transplantation 57: 640–643
5. Morris ER, Hoyt EG, Murphy MP, et al (1990) Transplant Proc 22: 1659–1662
6. Platz KP, Sollinger HW, Hullett DA, et al (1991) Transplantation 51: 27–31

Immunobiology

Transpl Int (1996) 9 [Suppl 1]: S 337–S 339
© Springer-Verlag 1996

Rat MHC class I peptides are immunogenic

N. Zavazava
F. Fandrich
K. A. Y. Ott
A. Freese
K. Turnewitsch

N. Zavazava (✉) · F. Fandrich ·
K. A. Y. Ott · A. Freese · K. Turnewitsch
Institute of Immunologie and Klinik
für Allgemeine Chirurgie und
Thoraxchirurgie, University of Kiel,
Brunswikerstr. 4, D-24105 Kiel, Germany
Tel.: +49-431-597-33 46/47
Fax: +49-431-597-33 35

Acknowledgements: This work was supported partially by a grant of the Sandoz Therapeutische Stiftung; Nürnberg and partially by the VW-Stiftung, Wolfsburg.

Abstract We postulated that indirect recognition of MHC-derived peptides might modulate the alloresponse to donor antigen. In this study, we looked at the potential of two class I peptides derived from the α1 and α2 regions of the DA RT1A^a molecule. Lew responder rats were immunized by varying concentrations of two 25mer peptides covering residues 56–81 and 96–120. The injections were under the footpad and were repeated on day 14. The thickness of the footpads was measured to control delayed-type hypersensitivity (DTH). The animals were sacrificed on day 16 and the splenocytes were tested in mixed lymphocyte culture as responders against DA stimulator cells and CAP third-party splenocytes. In addition, the phenotype of the cells was measured using flow cytometry with antibodies against CD4, CD8, CD5, MHC class II, CD25, CD14 and CD19. Peptide 96–120 induced strong sensitization of the Lew recipient animals at concentrations of 200–500 μg ($n = 4$). The stimulation index was 2–3 times higher than that of untreated animals. Peptide 56–81 failed to induce sensitization at the concentrations used, but surprisingly induced a concentration-dependent immunosuppression that was highest at 400 μg ($n = 4$). In proliferation experiments responder Lew rats proliferated only to peptide 56–81 in vitro.

Introduction

Indirect presentation of alloantigen can have beneficial or detrimental effects on graft outcome. It has become well established that antigen-presenting cells of recipient origin pick up soluble donor antigen, process it and induce anti-donor reactivity [6]. The antigen-presenting cells present antigen to T cells that are either CD4 or CD8 and to B cells that produce antibodies against the graft. Since the structure of the HLA-A2 molecule was published [1] it has become much easier to better define the polymorphic regions of human and murine MHC class I molecules, and also those of class II. Peptides derived from these regions have been shown to sensitize and induce accelerated rejection [3].

Class II derived 25mers have been shown to induce tolerance after intrathymic injection [5]. Nisco et al. [4] have shown prolonged survival induced by a human class I peptide in rats and mice. Up to now there have been no systematic studies on rat class I peptides to investigate their efficacy in prolonging graft survival. In the current study, we looked at the potential of two DA-derived class I peptides to induce sensitization and unresponsiveness in Lew responder rats.

Materials and methods

Peptides

Peptides of the DA RT1A^a strain were synthesized using the Fmoc technique. Peptides were analysed by reversed phase high-pressure liquid chromatography (HPLC) and mass spectrometry. In these experiments peptides with the sequences 56–81 and 96–120 were used. Sequences were confirmed by mass spectrometry. The amino acid sequences of the two peptides were as follows:

56–81: NH2-Gly-Pro-glu-Tyr-Trp-Glu-Gln-Gln-Thr-Arg-Ile-Ala-
Lys-Glu-Trp-Glu-Gln-Ile-Tyr-Arg-Val-Asp-Leu-Arg-Thr-COOH
96–120: NH2-Gln-Glu-Met-Tyr-Gly-Cys-Asp-Val-Gly-Ser-Asp-
Gly-Ser-Leu-Leu-Arg-Gly-Tyr-Arg-Gln-Asp-Ala-Tyr-Asp-Gly-C-
OOH

Immunization

Lew rats were immunized under the footpads with various peptide
concentrations: 200, 300, 400 and 500 µg/animal. In preliminary
studies, we had been able to show that 100 µg of either peptide
was ineffective, so that the concentrations used in the current studies were higher. The immunizations were repeated on day 14. On
day 16 the thickness of the footpads was measured to detect any
delayed-type hypersensitivity (DTH), and the animals were subsequently sacrificed. Splenocytes were used for both mixed lymphocyte reactions and phenotyping studies. Four animals were immunized for each concentration.

Mixed lymphocyte reaction and proliferation assays

Irradiated DA stimulator cells (10 Gy) were added to 2×10^5 Lew
responder splenocytes at 1:1 and 1:2 cell ratios in RPMI supplemented with 10 % foetal calf serum (Gibco, UK) and 1 % rat normal serum. In addition, untreated Lew rats were used as controls.
As third-party stimulator cells the rat strain CAP was used. The
cells were incubated for 4 days and pulsed with H^3-thymidine for
18 h before harvesting. In the proliferation assays, the responder
cells were co-cultivated with peptide concentrations of 100, 50, 25
and 12.5 µg/ml, pulsed after 4 days and harvested after another
18 h.

Phenotyping

OX12, Ox41 and antibodies against CD4, CD8, CD5, CD25 and
MHC class II molecules were used to study the phenotype of the
Lew cells by flow cytometry. Antibodies were purchased from Serotec, Germany. Antibodies were diluted 1:100 and incubated
with 5×10^5 splenocytes for 30 min at 4 °C. Cells were washed three
times and further incubated with a fluorescein-conjugated goat
anti-mouse serum for another 30 min. The cells were subsequently
washed and cell fluorescence measured by flow cytometry.

Results

Rats received two injections of the DA peptides on
days 0 and 14. The peptides were not supplemented
with adjuvant in order to be able to study the effect of
peptides alone as one would expect in a transplantation
set-up. On day 16, the rats were sacrificed and the splenocytes were used in mixed lymphocyte cultures. The
splenocytes were responders both to irradiated DA
stimulator cells and third-party CAP splenocytes. Peptide 56–81 (RT1) induced a concentration-dependent
immunosuppression as can be seen on Fig. 1. The lowest
response was measured at 400 µg/rat. This result was rather unexpected. Interestingly third-party stimulator
cells, CAP, failed to abolish this suppression, suggesting
that the effect was not allospecific.

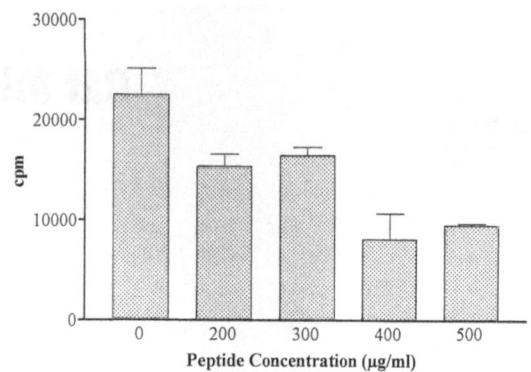

Fig. 1 Lew responder rats treated with peptide RT1 showed a concentration-dependent suppression of the mixed lymphocyte reaction to DA stimulator cells. The lowest response was measured in
the animals treated with 400 mg

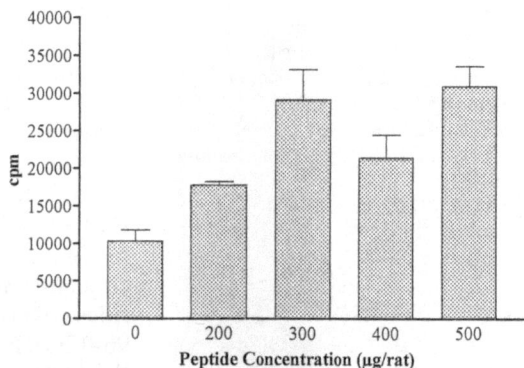

Fig. 2 Lew responder rats were treated by peptide RT4. A significant enhancement of the response was measured in all animals
that had received the peptide. This result shows that the peptide
sensitized and that this region is apparently a relevant region of
the native DA class I molecule

The second sequence studied, 96–120 (RT4), had contrary effects. A concentration-dependent augmentation
of the alloresponse was observed in the mixed lymphocyte response (Fig. 2). This result suggested that this peptide represented a region of the class I molecule that is
immunogeneic in vivo and, thus, sensitizes. To study the
mode of peptide recognition, we performed proliferation
studies in which the splenocytes of the immunized animals were used as responders to peptides added in culture. Only peptide RT1 was clearly presented and led to
T-cell proliferation, as shown in Fig. 3. RT4 and a control
human peptide 19 (HLA-A3: 56–69) failed to induce proliferation. Further, antigen-presenting cells were enriched by adherence and pulsed by these peptides be-
fore-hand. The cells were subsequently irradiated and
then used as stimulator cells. Only antigen-presenting
cells pulsed with RT1 could induce T-cell proliferation
(data not shown). This experiment showed that recognition was through the indirect presentation. On phenotyping, animals treated with either RT1 or with RT4 did not

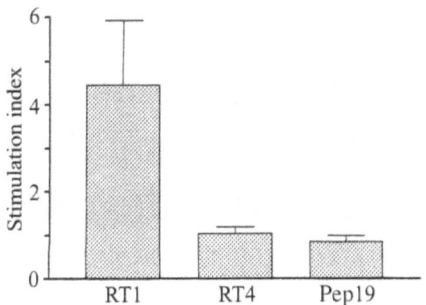

Fig. 3 Indirect recognition of RT1. Splenocytes of responder Lew rats previously treated by 200 µg of each peptide were cultivated in 50 µg of each of these for 4 days. After pulsing for 18 h, the cells were harvested. The highest proliferation was measured in the splenocytes of the rat treated by RT1. RT4 and the control human peptide 19 were not presented. RT1 appears to contain anchor residues for the Lew MHC class II molecule

show any significant differences to control untreated animals for all cell markers studied.

DTH has been clearly shown to be one of the mechanisms by which allografts are damaged and subsequently rejected during rejection episodes. We immunized rats by subcutaneous injection of 400 µg (RT1) or 200 µg (RT4) peptide and the thickness of the footpads was measured after reimmunization 14 days later. None of these peptides was able to induce DTH. However, when the peptides were supplemented with Freud's complete adjuvant, peptide RT1 strongly induced foot thickness and inflammation. When both peptides were mixed and used for immunization, DTH was as severe as that observed by injecting RT1 alone (data not shown).

Discussion

Although the two peptides described here have been described by others [3], few in vitro studies have been performed. Our data showed two different reaction patterns. RT1 was well presented in vitro, as shown by the proliferation assays. We assume that the peptide was presented by class II molecules of the Lew antigen-presenting cells, since enrichment of the class II expressing antigen-presenting cells resulted in augmentation of the immune response. Surprisingly, however, after in vivo treatment of Lew responder animals, RT1 decreased the T-cell response. Two possibilities are likely explanations for this phenomenon. First, it is quite likely that since this peptide is presented, there could be induction of T-cell suppressor cells or regulatory Th2 cells that downregulate the immune response [7]. Second, a much easier hypothesis could be that the peptide binds to some cell receptor required for T-cell proliferation and thus blocks cell response. This effect was not allospecific since response to third-party CAP stimulator cells was also reduced. Nisco et al. [4] and Cuturi et al. [2] have described a human decamer B7 peptide that induces prolongation of graft survival. Although our peptide RT1 is a 25mer, the B7 decamer and this peptide share the same residues at seven positions. It remains unclear whether we are describing a similar phenomenon or not.

The second peptide, RT4, sensitized recipient animals so that they reacted strongly in the mixed lymphocyte reaction. This peptide remained ineffective in proliferation assays, suggesting that it may require further processing in vivo before presentation. It was also interesting to observe that this peptide did not induce DTH, unlike RT1. In preliminary transplantation studies, recipient Lew responder rats were pre-treated with either peptide and received DA allogeneic cardiac allografts. The grafts were rejected in the normal fashion in both groups. This indicated that without further immunosuppression, the in vitro effects observed were not sufficient either to induce accelerated rejection or prolong survival. These studies are being continued with low levels of cyclosporin A.

References

1. Bjorkmann PJ, Saper MA, Samranoi B, et al (1987) Structure of the human class I histocompatibility antigen HLA-A2. Nature 329: 506–512
2. Cuturi M, Josien R, Douillard P, et al (1995) Prolongation of allogeneic heart graft survival in rats by administration of a peptide (a.a. 75–84) from the α helix of the first domain of HLA-B7 01. Transplantation 59: 661–669
3. Fangmann J, Dalchau R, Fabre JW (1992) Rejection of skin allografts by indirect allorecognition of donor class I major histocompatibility complex peptides. J Exp Med 175: 1521–1529
4. Nisco S, Vriens P, Hoyt G, et al (1994) Induction of allograft tolerance in rats by an HLA class I derived peptide and cyclosporine A. J Immunol 152: 3786–3792
5. Sayegh MH, Perico N, Imberti O, et al (1993) Thymic recognition of class II major histocompatibility complex allopeptide induces donor-specific unresponsiveness to renal allograft. Transplantation 56: 461–465
6. Siciu-Foca N, Ho E, King DW, et al (1991) Soluble HLA and anti-idiotypic antibodies in transplantation: modulation of anti-HLA antibodies by soluble HLA antigens from the raft and anti-idiotypic antibodies in renal and cardiac allograft recipients. Transplant Proc 23: 295–296
7. Shoskes D, Wood K (1994) Indirect presentation of MHC antigens in transplantation. Immunol Today 15: 32–38

Transpl Int (1996) 9 [Suppl 1]: S 340–S 344
© Springer-Verlag 1996

F. L. Li
G. Grauls
M. Yin
C. A. Bruggeman

Correlation between the intensity of cytomegalovirus infection and the amount of perivasculitis in aortic allografts

F. L. Li · G. Grauls · M. Yin
Department of Medical Microbiology,
University Hospital Maastricht, University
of Limburg, NL-6202 AZ Maastricht,
The Netherlands

C. A. Bruggeman (✉)
Department of Medical Microbiology,
University of Limburg, P. O. Box 5800,
NL-6202 AZ Maastricht, The Netherlands
Tel. +31 433876644; Fax +31 433876643

Abstract We previously demonstrated that cytomegalovirus (CMV) infection enhanced perivascular inflammation in rat aortic allografts. In this study, we investigated the relationship between the CMV infection load and the magnitude of perivasculitis (chronic rejection) in aortic transplants. Rats received orthotopic abdominal aortic grafts, different degrees of total body irradiation (TBI) for immunosuppression and CMV inoculation. The spleens of the rats receiving 5 Gy of TBI contained more infectious virus and viral antigens than those of rats receiving 3 Gy of TBI or no TBI. Although the number of inflammatory cells infiltrating the perivascular area was decreased after TBI, CMV infection resulted in increased perivasculitis in rats that received 5 Gy of TBI as compared to non-infected animals. This virus-induced effect was characterized predominantly by an increased T-cell infiltration, including CD4 and CD8 T-cells. It is concluded that an enhanced systemic CMV infection during severe immunosuppressive therapy can accelerate the development of chronic rejection, which seems to be mediated mainly by T-cells.

Key words Chronic rejection · Transplant-associated · arteriosclerosis (TAA) · Cytomegalovirus (CMV) infection · Perivasculitis · Immunosuppression

Introduction

Transplant-associated arteriosclerosis (TAA) or chronic rejection is the major cause of diminished long-term survival of transplanted organs [13]. In cardiac allograft recipients the incidence of TAA is nearly 50 % at 5 years posttransplantation [7]. The most common pathological features of TAA are persistent perivascular inflammation (perivasculitis) and intimal thickening in arteries (arteriosclerotic changes) of grafts [9].

The factors responsible for initiation and progression of TAA are not completely understood. Among others, TAA may be induced or accelerated by virus infections, such as cytomegalovirus (CMV) infection [11]. There is strong clinical evidence to show that CMV infections play a role in the pathogenesis of cardiac allograft arteriosclerosis [12]. CMV nucleic acids have been identified in the coronary arteries of heart allografts with severe accelerated arteriosclerosis [10, 18].

Previous work in our laboratory showed that immunosuppression enhanced the replication of CMV in the host leading to massive viral infection in almost all the organs [14] and that treatment with antiCMV therapy reduced the development of intimal thickening in the vascular wall of allografts [5]. However, it has not been elucidated whether the systemic CMV infection load, dependent on the degree of immunosuppression, influences the extent of transplant perivasculitis. For this purpose we used the rat aorta transplantation (Tx) as a specific model to investigate the effects of enhanced viral infection on the perivascular inflammatory response.

Table 1 Summary of experimental groups

Group	Transplantation	Number of rats	TBI[a]	RCMV[b] infection	Day of sacrifice
1	Syngeneic	5	No	+	7
2	Syngeneic	5	No	−	7
3	Allogeneic	5	No	+	7
4	Allogeneic	5	No	−	7
5	Allogeneic	4	3Gy	+	7
6	Allogeneic	4	3Gy	−	7
7	Allogeneic	3	5Gy	+	7
8	Allogeneic	4	5Gy	−	7
9	Syngeneic	5	No	+	28
10	Syngeneic	5	No	−	28
11	Allogeneic	5	No	+	28
12	Allogeneic	5	No	−	28
13	Allogeneic	3	3Gy	+	28
14	Allogeneic	3	3Gy	−	28
15	Allogeneic	6	5Gy	+	28
16	Allogeneic	5	5Gy	−	28
17	Allogeneic	4	5Gy	iRCMV	28

[a] Total body irradiation (TBI) was performed on day 1 after transplantation
[b] RCMV inoculation was performed intraperitoneally at 6 h after TBI

Materials and methods

Animals and aorta transplantation

Male inbred Brown Norway (BN/M; RT_{1n}) and Lewis (LEW/N; RT_{11}) rats, weighing 250–300 g, were used as donors and recipients. In the donor operation, a segment of the abdominal aorta (1.8–2 cm) between the left renal artery and the bifurcation was removed with all side branches ligated after intravenous administration of heparin (50 IU). The grafts were transplanted orthotopically into recipients by the end-to-end anastomosis technique. Total ischemic times varied from 25 to 35 min, during which the grafts were kept cold with 4 °C PBS.

Experimental design

The aortic grafts from BN/M rats were transplanted into LEW/N recipients (allogeneic) or into BN/M recipients (syngeneic). After Tx, the animals were randomly divided into several groups (Table 1). A total body irradiation (TBI) of 3 or 5 Gy was used as immunosuppression therapy. The rats of the RCMV-infected group were inoculated intraperitoneally with 10^5 plaque forming units of rat CMV (RCMV, Maastricht strain [1]). The animals used as controls received either inactivated RCMV (iRCMV), which was derived from the same virus pool and inactivated by UV irradiation, or no virus at all. The recipients were sacrificed either on day 7 or day 28 after Tx. Tissue samples of the grafts and other organs were removed and divided into several pieces, which were processed either for frozen and paraffin sections, or for plaque assay.

Virus detection

Immunocytochemical techniques [14] were used for the detection of rat CMV antigens in grafts using RCMV monoclonal antibodies [4]. For the detection of general viral infection, the salivary glands, spleen and liver were placed aseptically into culture medium at sacrifice. These organs were homogenized in a tissue grinder and suspended in MEM with 2 % FCS. Quantification of infectious virus was done by means of plaque assay [1, 2]. For this, ten-fold dilutions of 10 % homogenates (wt/vol) were inoculated on a confluent rat embryonal fibroblast monolayer. After an incubation period of 7 days, the number of plaques was monitored microscopically after fixation and methylene blue staining.

Histological and immunohistochemical staining of grafts

A segment of the graft fixed in 3.7 % buffered formalin was embedded in paraffin, and examined histologically after sectioning and staining with haematoxylin and eosin. The aortas from non-transplanted rats were used as normal controls.

Four-micron-thick cross-sections of grafts were stained with three-layer (paraffin sections) or two-layer (frozen sections) indirect immunoperoxidase technique using monoclonal antibodies: W3/13 (Sera-lab, Crawley Down, UK), a mouse monoclonal antibody to rat pan T-cells; ED-1 (kindly supplied by Dr. Dijkstra, Department of Immunology, Free University, Amsterdam, The Netherlands), a mouse monoclonal antibody to rat monocytes/macrophages (mo/mΦ); Ox-8 (Sera-lab, Crawley Down, UK), a mouse IgG_1 monoclonal antibody to rat CD8 T-cells; and W3/25 (Sera-lab, Crawley Down, UK), a mouse IgG_1 monoclonal antibody to rat CD4 T-cells.

Quantification of the extent of perivasculitis

The total number of nuclei (TNN) and positively stained cells for W3/13 (T-cells), ED-1 (mo/mΦ) and Ox-8 (CD8 T-cells) in aortic adventitia was quantified in the cross-sectioned grafts and expressed as point score units (PSU), i.e. the mean number of points falling over given anatomical areas using straight, cross-sectional lines, and a 100 mm² square eye piece micrometre under a magnification of 400 ×. Under this magnification, a total area of 400 mm² was counted. The positively stained cells for W3/25 were scored from 0 to 5 (0, no staining; 1, very weak; 2, weak; 3, moderate; 4, intense; 5, very intense specific staining). Data are expressed as mean ± SEM. The number of positive cells or TNN in different groups were statistically compared with the aid of the non-parametric Mann-Whitney U-test. P values < 0.05 were regarded as statistically significant.

Results

RCMV infection

Two out of four RCMV-inoculated rats that received 3 Gy of TBI (3 Gy-TBI) and five out of six rats that received 5 Gy of TBI (5 Gy-TBI) harboured infectious RCMV in their spleens at 7 days after Tx. Viral culture from the salivary glands and liver was negative. On day 28, only the salivary glands harboured infectious RCMV, while no infectious virus was found in the liver and spleen of both syngeneic and allogeneic recipients that received 3 or 5 Gy-TBI. In iRCMV-inoculated control rats, no virus was cultured from any organs.

Sporadic RCMV-antigen-harbouring cells in the adventitia were detected in the allografts at 7 and 28 days

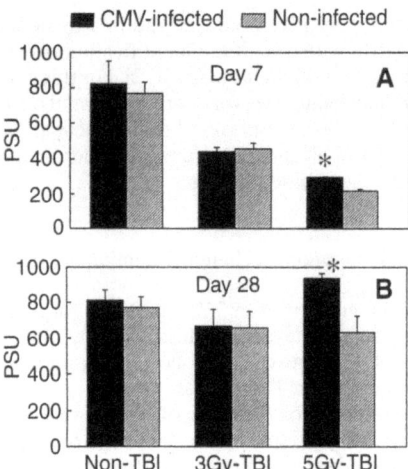

Fig. 1A, B Total number of nuclei in the adventitia of aortic allografts at **A** 7 and **B** 28 days after transplantation. Data are expressed as mean ± SEM/PSU. (* $P < 0.05$ when compared with the non-infected group)

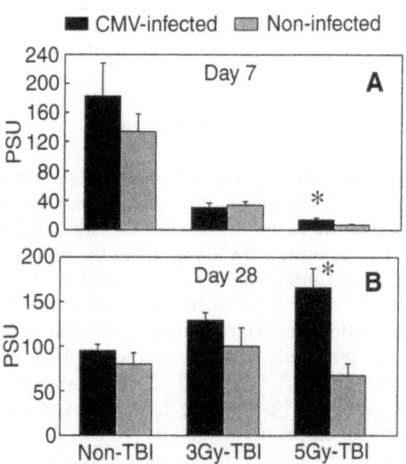

Fig. 2A, B The number of total T-cells in the adventitia of aortic allografts at **A** 7 and **B** 28 days after transplantation. Data are expressed as mean ± SEM/PSU. (* $P < 0.05$ when compared with the non-infected group)

after Tx. There was a tendency that slightly more RCMV-reactive cells were present in recipients with TBI than without TBI. No viral antigens were detectable in isografts and allografts of iRCMV-inoculated rats irrespective of TBI.

Magnitude of perivasculitis

Without the application of TBI, the TNN in the allografts of the RCMV-infected group did not differ from that in the non-infected group at 7 days after Tx (Fig. 1A). The TNN was decreased in rats that received 3 Gy-TBI as compared to that of non-TBI rats

($P < 0.05$). Nevertheless, after 3 Gy-TBI no significant difference in TNN was observed between the RCMV-infected and non-infected rats. In animals that received 5 Gy-TBI, the TNN was further decreased as compared to animals that received 3 Gy-TBI ($P < 0.05$). However, after 5 Gy-TBI, a significant difference in the TNN was observed between the RCMV-infected and non-infected groups ($P < 0.05$). At 28 days after Tx in the animals that received either non-TBI or 3 Gy-TBI, no significant difference in TNN could be found between the RCMV-infected and non-infected rats (Fig. 1B). However, in the rats that received 5 Gy-TBI the TNN in the RCMV-infected group was significantly higher than in the non-infected group ($P < 0.05$). Moreover, after RCMV infection, the TNN was higher in the animals that received 5 Gy-TBI than in those that received 3 Gy-TBI ($P < 0.05$). Meanwhile, the TNN in the rats that received iRCMV did not differ from that in the non-infected rats, but was significantly less than in the RCMV-infected rats that received 5 Gy-TBI ($P < 0.05$).

The number of infiltrating T-cells in the allografts is shown in Fig. 2. At 7 days after Tx (Fig. 2A), the number of infiltrating T-cells decreased significantly with an increase in the degree of TBI from non-TBI to 3 Gy-TBI and 5 Gy-TBI, respectively ($P < 0.05$). Nevertheless, no significant difference in the number of T-cells could be found between the RCMV-infected group and the non-infected group that received either no TBI or 3 Gy-TBI. In contrast, after 5 Gy-TBI, there was a significant increase in the number of T-cells in the RCMV-infected group as compared to the non-infected group ($P < 0.05$). At 28 days after Tx (Fig. 2B), there was no significant difference in T-cell infiltration between the RCMV-infected and non-infected rats that received either no TBI or 3 Gy-TBI. However, when the animals received 5 Gy-TBI, the number of T-cells in the RCMV-infected group was more than twice that in the non-infected group ($P < 0.05$). Moreover, the number of T-cells in animals that received RCMV infection and 5 Gy-TBI was higher than that in rats that received RCMV infection without TBI and in animals that received iRCMV inoculation and 5 Gy-TBI ($P < 0.05$). The latter group was comparable to the non-infected animals with 5 Gy-TBI (PSU of 65 ± 21 and 67 ± 13, respectively).

In the allografts of animals that received RCMV infection and 5 Gy-TBI, the number of CD4 T-cells was higher than in the non-infected animals that received 5 Gy-TBI at 28 days after Tx only ($P < 0.05$, Fig. 3A). The number of CD8 T-cells, however, was significantly higher in the RCMV-infected group as compared to the non-infected group both at 7 and 28 days after Tx ($P < 0.05$, Fig. 3B).

Although with TBI the number of mo/mΦ in the allograft was decreased on day 7, no significant difference could be found between the RCMV-infected and the non-infected rats (Fig. 4A). Likewise, at 28 days after

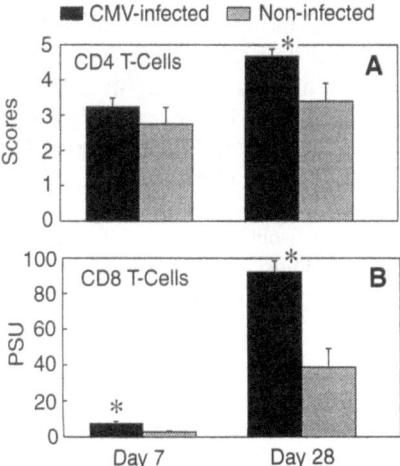

Fig. 3 A, B The number of CD4 and CD8 T-cells in the adventitia of aortic allografts in animals that received 5 Gy-TBI at 7 and 28 days after transplantation. Data are expressed as mean ± SEM/PSU or Scores. (* $P < 0.05$ when compared with the non-infected group)

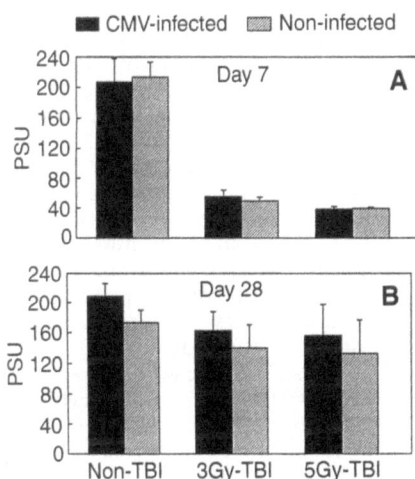

Fig. 4 A, B The number of monocytes/macrophages in the adventitia of aortic allografts at **A** day 7 and **B** day 28 after transplantation. Data are expressed as mean ± SEM/PSU. No statistical difference is found between the RCMV-infected and non-infected groups

Tx, no effect of TBI and RCMV infection on the number of mo/mⱷ (Fig. 4 B) was observed.

In the adventitia of non-transplanted normal aortas, almost no infiltrating cells (T-cells or mo/mⱷ) were found, only some fibroblasts were present. In syngeneic grafts (with or without RCMV infection), the TNN at 7 and 28 days after Tx was comparable with the normal aorta (data not shown). Sporadic, specifically stained T-cells and mo/mⱷ in the adventitia were observed.

Discussion

The present study demonstrates the effect of acute generalized RCMV infection on allograft perivasculitis in immunosuppressed recipients. Although previous work in rats and data obtained from human material suggested that CMV infection leads to an enhanced perivascular inflammation in the transplanted organs, this report describes, for the first time, the relationship between the active replication of the virus in the host and the enhanced perivasculitis in the allografts. The fact that the perivasculitis was not affected by the inoculation of iRCMV, as seen in our study, indicates that replication of the virus in the host is necessary for the increased inflammatory response in the allografts. In line with previous work in our laboratory [14], this study also demonstrates that increased TBI enhances RCMV replication in the host, resulting in massive RCMV infection in almost all the organs of the animals after 5 Gy-TBI.

It is noticeable that CMV infection enhances the perivascular inflammatory response in allografts but not in isografts. This result suggests that the virus-induced perivasculitis is not the result of direct interactions of the virus with vessel wall cells, but the result of interactions between the virus and the immune cells, such as the allospecific T-lymphocytes. Although the cellular and molecular factors leading to TAA are largely unknown and the mechanism of the effect of CMV infection on TAA remains unclear, there is some evidence that immune inflammatory cells and the factors they produce are important for the process [3]. In the vessel wall of immunocompetent (non-TBI) and immunocompromised (TBI) rats, almost no viral antigen and infectious virus were detectable, while the internal organs, such as the spleen, contained infectious virus and viral antigens during the acute infection period (the first week postinfection).

The spleen is known as an important lymphoid organ in the immune system and in the course of viral infection [2, 14]. In the immunosuppressed host, replicating virus is detectable in large amounts in this organ [14]. Studies in mice have shown that CMV infection can lead to polyclonal T-cell activation and upregulation of allospecific cytotoxic T-cells [15, 19]. In addition, it has been shown that CMV infection enhances the graft versus host reaction in mice [6]. The activated T-cells and the mediators they produce, such as IL-2, TNF [8], may contribute to the process of allograft rejection. Thus, it might be speculated that the CMV-associated effect is an immune-mediated process rather than direct viral damage [3]. In support of the above hypothesis, we did find that mainly T-cells, including both CD4 and CD8 T-cells, were involved in the perivasculitis.

Besides the effect of CMV infection on the T-cell response, the interaction of CMV with endothelial cells (EC) could also be of importance for the development of chronic rejection. In an in vitro study, Waldman [17] has demonstrated that CMV-infected EC provide a powerful stimulus for the activation of T-cells derived from CMV-seropositive donors, and that T-cells thus activated release IFN-γ sufficient to induce the expression of HLA-DR on the surrounding uninfected EC [16]. In addition, cytokines elaborated by CMV-activated T-cells are capable of enhancing endothelial HLA class I and ICAM-1 expression [17]. Therefore once CMV infects EC, several molecular inflammatory cascades may be triggered, and continue in the absence of the virus.

In conclusion, our results indicate that enhanced general RCMV infection has a detrimental effect on development of TAA of aortic allografts in highly immunocompromised recipients. This CMV-associated process, which appears to be T-cell mediated, is accelerated by an increased immunosuppressive regimen.

Acknowledgements The authors would like to thank Erik Beuken for the technical assistance and Frans S. Stals for critically reading the manuscript.

References

1. Bruggeman CA, Meijer H, Dormans PHJ, Debie WMH, Grauls GELM, Boven CPA van (1982) Isolation of a cytomegalovirus-like agent from wild rats. Arch Virol 73: 231–241
2. Bruggeman CA, Meijer H, Bosman F, Boven CPA van (1985) Biology of rat cytomegalovirus infection. Intervirology 24: 1–9
3. Bruggeman CA, Li FL, Stals FS (1995) Pathogenicity: Animal models. Scand J Infect (in press)
4. Bruning JH, Debie WHM, Dormans PHJ, Meijer H, Bruggeman CA (1987) The development and characterisation of monoclonal antibodies against rat cytomegalovirus induced antigens. Arch Virol 94: 55–70
5. Bruning JH, Persoons M, Lemström K, Stals FS, De Clercq E, Bruggeman CA (1994) Enhancement of transplantation-associated atherosclerosis by CMV, which can be prevented by antiviral therapy in the form of HPMPC. Transpl Int 7 [Suppl]: S365–S370
6. Cray C, Levy RB (1989) The ability of murine cytometalovirus and class I major histocompatibility complex-disparate parental cells to induce alterations characteristic of severe graft-versus-host reactions. Transplantation 48: 1057–1063
7. Gao SZ, Alderman EL, Schroeder JS, Siverman JF, Hunt SA (1988) Accelerated coronary vascular disease in the heart transplant patient: coronary arteriographic findings. J Am Coll Cardiol 12: 334–340
8. Geist LJ, Hunninghake GW (1994) Cytomegalovirus as a trans-activator of cellular genes. Semin Virol 5: 415–420
9. Häyry P (1994) Chronic allograft rejection: An update: Clin Transplant 8: 160–161
10. Hruban RT, Wu TC, Beschorner WE, Cameron DE, Ambinder RF, Baumgartner WA, Hutchins GM, Reitz BA (1990) Cytomegalovirus nucleic acids in allografted hearts. Hum Pathol 21: 981–983
11. Kendall TJ, Wilson JE, Radio SJ, Kandolf R, Gulizia JM, Winters GL, Costanzo-Nordin MR, Malcom GT, Thieszen SL, Miller LW, McManus BM (1992) Cytomegalovirus and other herpes viruses: do they have a role in the development of accelerated coronary arterial disease in human heart allografts? J Heart Lung Transplant 11: 14–20
12. McDonald K, Rector TS, Braunlin EA, Kubo SH, Olivari MT (1989) Association of coronary artery disease in cardiac transplant recipients with cytomegalovirus infection. Am J Cardiac 64: 359–362
13. Paul LC, Fellström B (1992) Chronic vascular rejection of the treatment options emerged? Transplantation 53: 1169–1179
14. Stals FS, Bosman F, Boven CPA van, Bruggeman CA (1990) An animal model for therapeutic intervention studies of CMV infection in the immunocompromised host. Arch Virol 114: 91–107
15. Via CS, Shanley JD, Shearer GM (1990) Synergistic effect of murine cytomegalovirus on the induction of acute graft-vs-host disease involving MHC Class I differences only. Analysis of in vitro T cell function. J Immunol 145: 3283–3289
16. Waldman WJ, Knight DA (1995) Cytokines-mediated induction of endothelial MHC and adhesion molecule expression by cytomegalovirus-activated T cells (abstract). International symposium on the etiology and pathobiology of transplant vascular sclerosis, March 1–5, Bermuda
17. Waldman WJ, Adams PW, Orosz CG, Sedmak DD (1992) T lymphocyte activation by cytomegalovirus-infected, allogeneic cultured human endothelial cells. Transplantation 54: 887–896
18. Wu TC, Hruban RH, Ambinder RF, Pizzorno M, Cameron DE, Baumgartner WA, Reitz BA, Haywaed GS, Hutchins GM (1992) Demonstration of cytomegalovirus nucleic acids in the coronary arteries of transplanted heart. Am J Pathol 140: 739–747
19. Yang H, Dundon PL, Nahill SR, Welsh RM (1989) Virus-induced polyclonal cytotoxic T lymphocytes stimulation. J Immunol 142: 1710–1718

Transpl Int (1996) 9 [Suppl 1]: S345–S347
© Springer-Verlag 1996

N. M. van Besouw
L. M. B. Vaessen
C. J. Knoop
A. H. M. M. Balk
B. Mochtar
F. H. J. Claas
W. Weimar

Evidence that cyclosporin A prevents clinical cardiac allograft rejection by blocking both direct and indirect antigen presentation pathways

N. M. van Besouw (✉) · L. M. B. Vaessen ·
C. J. Knoop · W. Weimar
Department of Internal Medicine I, Room
Bd299, University Hospital Rotterdam-
Dijkzigt, Dr Molewaterplein 40,
NL-3015 GD Rotterdam, The Netherlands
Tel. + 31-10-4 63 54 20
Fax + 31-10-4 63 54 30

A. H. M. M. Balk · B. Mochtar
Thorax Center, University Hospital
Rotterdam-Dijkzigt, Rotterdam, The
Netherlands

F. H. J. Claas
Department of Immunohematology and
Bloodbank, University Hospital Leiden,
Leiden, The Netherlands

Abstract Monitoring for the responses to alloantigens presented either by the direct or the indirect presentation pathway have been reported to be of clinical value after kidney transplantation. Amongst others, the level of these responses may be dependent on the immunosuppressive treatment. We studied both presentation routes in peripheral blood mononuclear cells (PBMC) of cardiac transplant patients, who experienced episodes of rejection, and related them to the *in vivo* cyclosporin A (CsA) levels in plasma. PBMC of the recipients were stimulated with irradiated donor cells to determine the direct presentation pathway. As a method for the activation of the immune response via the indirect pathway, PBMC were stimulated with tetanus toxoid. Both immune responses increased when CsA levels inadvertently decreased to inadequate concentrations and histological rejection was diagnosed. After clinical heart transplantation, CsA may prevent rejection by blocking both the direct and the indirect antigen presentation pathway.

Key words Clinical transplantation · Presentation pathways · Cyclosporin A · Rejection

Introduction

Both direct and indirect presentation pathways for alloantigens have been reported to be involved in rejection after kidney transplantation [5, 6]. Recently, it was suggested that the indirect pathway is more sensitive to immunosuppression than the direct route of alloantigen presentation [1, 3–5]. The latter presentation pathway involves direct activation of the recipient T-cells by donor antigen-presenting cells (APC). For the indirect alloantigen presentation pathway, allogeneic major histocompatibility complex (MHC) molecules are processed into peptides and presented on recipient APC by MHC molecules of the recipient. This pathway is similar to the one by which nominal antigens, such as tetanus toxoid (TET), are presented.

In order to test whether the use of the different presentation pathways is dependent on the immunosuppressive load [1, 3–5], we monitored both routes in PBMC of human cardiac transplant recipients and related them to the *in vivo* cyclosporin A (CsA) levels measured in plasma and to acute rejection. PBMC from transplant recipients were stimulated by spleen cells derived from the donor to measure the direct alloantigen presentation route in a mixed lymphocyte culture (MLC). Recently, we have shown that in MLC, complete removal of donor APC from the stimulator population is not a suitable tool for determining indirect presentation of donor antigens [1]. Therefore, we measured the indirect presentation route by stimulating PBMC with the nominal antigen, TET.

Materials and methods

PBMC sampling

We selected blood samples from three cardiac transplant recipients, who had experienced one or more periods of rejection during

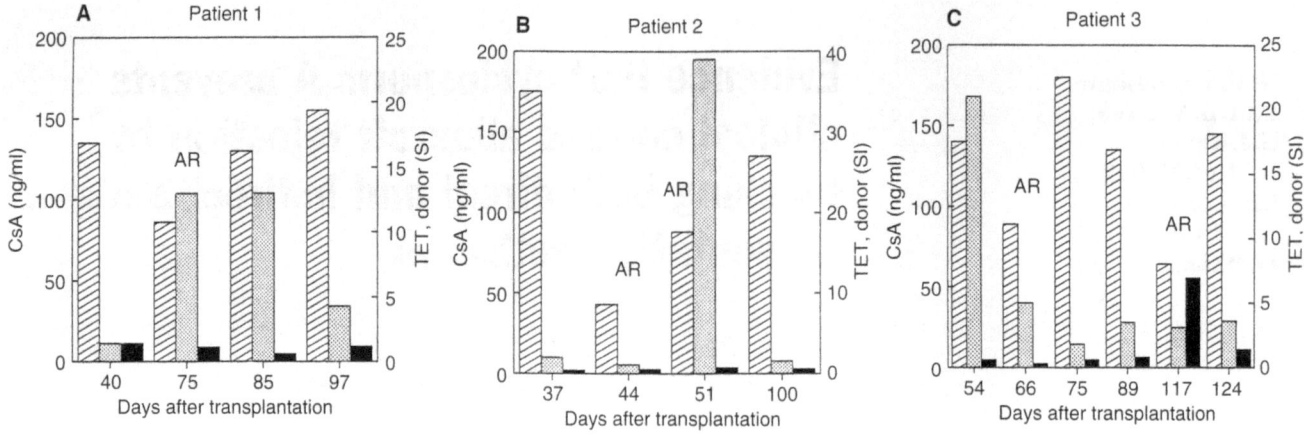

Fig. 1 Relationship of acute rejection *(AR)* and cyclosporin A *(CsA)* levels in plasma (▨) with the proliferative capacity of peripheral blood mononuclear cells to directly presented donor antigens (☐) and indirectly presented antigens tetanus toxoid *(TET)* (■)

the first 4 months after heart transplantation when CsA levels were inadvertently decreased to inadequate concentrations. Rejection was diagnosed histologically in endomyocardial biopsies (ISHLT grade 3 or more) [2].

PBMC were isolated from heparinised blood by density gradient centrifugation using Ficoll-Isopaque ($\delta = 1\,077$). Spleen cells were obtained by mechanical dissociation of small pieces of spleen derived from the organ donor as previously described [1].

Proliferation tests

For MLC and TET stimulation, 100 µl of a PBMC suspension of 5×10^5 cells/ml in culture medium (RPMI 1640-DM supplemented with 4 mM L-glutamine, 100 IU/ml penicillin and 10 % heat-inactivated human AB serum) was added to 5×10^4 irradiated (60 Gy) donor spleen cells (direct pathway); TET at 7.5 If/ml (RIVM, Bilthoven, The Netherlands) final concentration (indirect pathway); phytohaemagglutinin M (PHA, 1 : 100 final dilution) to control the viability of the cells; and culture medium. After 6 days of incubation at 37° in a humified atmosphere of 5 % CO_2 in air, cell proliferation was measured by the incorporation of [^{3}H]thymidine (0.5 µCi/well) added during the last 8 h of culture. The mean counts per minute (cpm) were determined and expressed as the stimulation index (SI). The SI is the ratio of the cpm obtained in the presence of antigen to the cpm obtained in the absence of antigen.

CsA levels

CsA trough levels were measured in plasma from the same blood samples as described above using a radioimmunoassay with [^{125}I]labelled CsA and CsA-specific monoclonal antibodies (Cyclo-Trac SP; Incstar, Stillwater, Minn., USA). CsA plasma levels were maintained at therapeutic concentrations of 100–150 ng/ml after transplantation. Levels below 100 ng/ml were considered inadequate.

Results

Patient 1 (Fig. 1 A) experienced a rejection episode on day 75 after transplantation. On this day, a decrease in the level of CsA was found, while at the same time the response to the direct donor antigen presentation pathway increased. In contrast to the situation 1 day before transplantation (SI = 11), the indirect pathway became and remained undetectable (SI < 2) after transplantation. After anti-rejection therapy with steroids and increasing the dose of CsA, the response to the direct presentation route slowly decreased when the CsA levels normalised.

Patient 2 (Fig. 1 B) had two successive biopsies with histological signs of acute rejection on day 44 and day 51 after transplantation, when the CsA plasma levels proved to be inadequate. After treatment with steroids and adjusting the CsA dose on day 44, only a small increase in the CsA plasma level was detected on day 51, while the PBMC strongly responded to the directly but not to the indirectly presented antigens. A second anti-rejection therapy with rabbit anti-thymocyte globulin and a higher dose of CsA proved to be necessary. Thereafter, the CsA concentrations in plasma reached normal levels, the direct pathway became undetectable and no further histological signs of rejection were found.

Patient 3 (Fig. 1 C) experienced the first rejection period 66 days after transplantation during a drop in CsA concentration in plasma, while 12 days before a high reactivity of PBMC to the directly presented donor antigens had been found. After anti-rejection treatment with steroids and increasing the CsA dose, the response to the direct pathway decreased. On day 117 after transplantation a second rejection episode was observed, accompanied by a combination of another fall in the CsA level in plasma and an increment of the response to the indirectly presented antigens. After anti-rejection therapy consisting of steroids and increasing the dose of CsA, the CsA levels normalised and reduction of the response of PBMC to the indirect pathway was found.

Discussion

In the present study, we analysed four rejection episodes occurring at a time when the CsA trough levels were inadequate. During only one of these episodes the indirect antigen presentation pathway was functional (SI > 2) (Fig. 1 C), while during the other three rejection periods (Fig. 1) only the direct pathway was found to be intact. This finding is consistent with data described by Muluk et al. [5], who showed that the indirect presentation pathway is more susceptible to CsA therapy than the direct pathway. In agreement with these results, Clerici et al. [3] demonstrated that *in vitro* exposure of CsA to stimulated PBMC suppressed the indirect presentation pathway more strongly than the direct presentation pathway. Also Gallon et al. [4] confirmed that CsA inhibits proliferation of *in vivo*-primed T-cells to indirectly presented MHC peptides. In addition, recently, we have shown that a TET response (indirect pathway) was more frequently found before (75 %) compared to the first year after (13 %) clinical heart transplantation [1].

Others suggested that only the indirect presentation pathway correlates with acute rejection, independently of the direct pathway [3, 5]. In contrast, from our data we conclude that acute rejection after clinical cardiac transplantation in the presence of inadequate CsA levels may be accompanied by an increment in the responses of PBMC both to directly presented donor antigens or indirectly presented antigens. Therefore we conclude that after clinical heart transplantation CsA may prevent rejection by blocking both the direct and indirect presentation routes.

Acknowledgements We thank C. R. Daane, C. C. Baan, W. M. Mol and C. J. Hesse for technical assistance. This work was supported by grant 92.094 from the Netherlands Heart Foundation.

References

1. Besouw NM van, Vaessen LMB, Daane CR, Jutte NHPM, Balk AHMM, Claas FHJ, Weimar W (1996) Peripheral monitoring of direct and indirect presentation pathways in clinical heart transplant recipients. Transplantation (in press)
2. Billingham ME, Cary NRB, Hammond ME, Kemnitz J, Marboe C, McCallister HA, Snovar DC, Winters GL, Zerbe A (1990) A working formulation for the standardization of nomenclature in the diagnosis of heart and lung rejection: Heart Rejection Study Group. J Heart Lung Transplant 9: 587–593
3. Clerici M, Shearer GM (1990) Differential sensitivity of human T helper cell pathways by in vitro exposure to cyclosporin A. J Immunol 144: 2480–2485
4. Gallon L, Watschinger B, Murphy B, Akalin E, Sayegh MH, Carpenter CB (1995) The indirect pathway of allorecognition. The occurrence of self-restricted T cell recognition of allo-MHC peptides early in acute renal allograft rejection and its inhibition by conventional immunosuppression. Transplantation 59: 612–616
5. Muluk SC, Clerici M, Via CS, Weir MR, Kimmel PL, Shearer GM (1991) Correlation of in vitro CD4$^+$ T helper cell function with clinical graft status in immunosuppressed kidney transplant recipients. Transplantation 52: 284–291
6. Schulick RD, Weir MB, Miller MW, Cohen DJ, Bermas BL, Shearer GM (1993) Longitudinal study of in vitro CD4$^+$ T helper cell function in recently transplanted renal allograft patients undergoing tapering of their immunosuppressive drugs. Transplantation 56: 590–596

Transpl Int (1996) 9 [Suppl 1]: S 348–S 351
© Springer-Verlag 1996

Liver sinusoidal lymphocytes: their immune functions

Sergiusz Durowicz
Danuta Sadowska-Ryffa
Ewa Cybulska
Urszula Wojewódzka
Waldemar L. Olszewski

S. Durowicz (✉) · D. Sadowska-Ryffa ·
E. Cybulska · U. Wojewódzka ·
W. L. Olszewski
Department of Surgical Research and
Transplantology, Medical Research Center,
Polish Academy of Sciences,
02-004 Warsaw, 5 Chalubinskiego, Poland
Tel./Fax +48 22 621 49 23

Abstract Recent studies strongly suggest that the liver plays an important immunoregulatory role. Evidence of its role in general immune responsiveness originates from observation that, in recipients of liver grafts, the survival of other allografts is significantly prolonged. The question arises as to which blood lymphocyte subsets, most likely to be responsible for this phenomenon, marginate in liver sinusoids. To study this problem, a liver ex vivo perfusion model was designed for rats. In situ W/WAG livers were washed clear of sinusoidal marginating cells prior to and after 1 h perfusion with syngeneic blood. The number of blood cells retained in liver sinusoids, their phenotypes, the responsiveness to mitogen (PHA, 90 μg/ml) and cytotoxicity against YAC-1 tumour cells were examined. Our studies showed that rat liver retains in the sinusoids a population of blood cells, enriched in NK, CD8$^+$ and MHC class II$^+$ cells, displaying a high cytotoxic activity and low responsiveness to mitogen stimulation, with a capacity of about 10^6 cells/g of tissue.

Key words Liver transplantation · Sinusoidal lymphocytes · Tolerance

Introduction

Recent studies from our and other laboratories strongly suggest that the liver plays an important immunoregulatory role in general and local immunity [2, 4, 6, 7, 9, 10, 12–16, 21, 22]. Evidence of its role in general immune responsiveness originates from the observation that in liver recipients who do not receive any immunosuppressive treatment, the survival of heart, skin and kidney allografts is significantly prolonged [1, 2, 6, 14]. Moreover, there are numerous examples of survival of liver grafts in man after the withdrawal of immunosuppressive treatment [1, 19, 21]. These data suggest that the role of the liver is not limited to elimination and inactivation of damaged cells and digestive and bacterial antigens, but also encompasses the immune responsiveness to non-self antigens. The main cell mediators in these reactions are lymphocytes. It appears that the local immune function of the liver is associated with a specific population of lymphocytes, most probably of blood origin, which are transiently retained in the liver [10]. These cells, marginating in hepatic sinusoids, appear to be responsible for the destruction of malignant cells reaching the liver via the bloodstream [3, 9, 22]. The question arises as to which blood lymphocyte subsets marginate in liver sinusoids. Since the in vivo studies on trapping of lymphocytes in liver sinusoids are difficult because of other functioning lymphatic organs (mainly the spleen) actively halting circulating lymphocytes, we decided to carry out studies on an extracorporeal liver perfusion model. The study was devoted to the investigation of the process of halting circulating blood lymphocytes in the liver sinusoids and the characterization of the phenotypes of these cells.

Materials and methods

Animals

Wistar (W/Wag) (RT1u) rats with body weights of 200–250 g were used.

Liver perfusion

The rat liver perfusion system consisted of a peristaltic pump, an oxygenator with 0.1 m² gas exchange surface, and a heat exchanger (Fig. 1). The temperature of 37 °C was maintained in the perfusion circuit by means of a water thermostat. The rats were heparinized and exsanguinated. Their livers were washed out cells through the portal vein with 40 ml of PBS and the collected wash-out cells isolated by centrifugation at 1600 rpm for 35 min on a Lymphoprep gradient (Nyegaard, Oslo, Norway) and collected for further studies. Subsequently, in situ perfusion of the liver was carried out for 1 h with syngeneic blood diluted 1 : 2 with PBS. After completion of perfusion, the liver vasculature was again washed out as described above and the collected cells were isolated.

Parameters measured

The following parameters were measured:
1. The number of blood cells washed out from the liver sinusoids
2. Phenotypical characteristics of cells using monoclonal antibodies. For immunohistochemical staining, the indirect alkaline phosphatase anti-alkaline phosphatase (APAAP) technique was applied. Cytospines fixed in acetone were incubated in normal rabbit serum (NRS), followed by the application of primary mouse MoAbs: W3/13 (CD3) – pan T cells, W3/25 (CD4) – helper/inducer cells, OX6 – MHC class II antigens bearing cells, OX8 (CD8) – suppressor/cytotoxic cells, OX19 (CD5) – T cells, 3.2.3 – NK cells (Serotec, UK). The secondary and tertiary antibodies consisted of rabbit-anti-mouse immunoglobulins and APAAP complex. All incubations were carried out at room temperature for 30 min, followed by a wash in two changes of TBS for 10 min. The reaction product was developed by incubation with chromogenic alkaline phosphatase substrate for 15 min. Then 400 cells were counted with light microscope.
3. Responsiveness of washed out cells to mitogen (PHA, 90 μg/ml, Wellcome, HA15). Microcultures containing 1×10^5/well cells suspended in medium RPMI 1640 + 15 % FCS were cultured with phytohemaglutinin (final mitogen concentration 10 μg/ml and 2 μg/ml) for 72 h. Proliferation was then measured with an 18-h pulse of [³H]thymidine and expressed as the number of counts per minute (cpm).
4. Cytotoxicity of washed out cells against YAC-1 tumour cells. Target cells (3×10^6) were labelled for 60 min at 37 °C using 100 μCi of sodium chromate (Amersham, UK) and resuspended in RPMI 1640 + 10 ml FCS to a concentration of 2.5×10^4/ml of lymphocytes. They were added to round-bottomed small culture tubes together with 0.2 ml of YAC-1 cells to make the effector-target ratio 20 : 1, 10 : 1 and 5 : 1. All tests were done in triplicate and incubated for 4 h at 37 °C in an atmosphere of 5 % CO_2 in air. After incubation, the tubes were centrifuged and 0.2 ml samples of supernatant were transferred to the other tubes and both aliquots counted on a gamma counter. The data were expressed as the percentage of ^{51}Cr release for each sample.

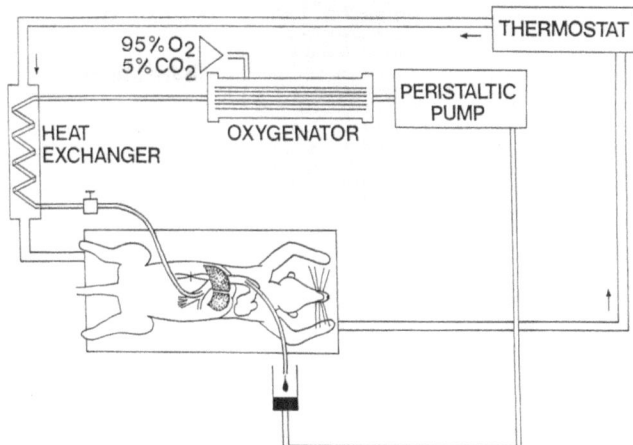

Fig. 1 The in situ ex vivo rat liver perfusion system

Table 1 Phenotypes of cells retrieved from liver sinusoids (median) ($n = 6$). Perfusion of liver with syngeneic blood in an extracorporeal circuit brought about reaccumulation in the sinusoids of similar populations of lymphocytes as had been found prior to perfusion. Both, pre- and postperfusion populations differed from blood populations (* ss vs blood)

MoAb	Prior to perfusion	After perfusion	Blood
W3/13	48.0	49.0	68.0
W3/25	36.6*	35.2*	49.7
OX6	32.0*	25.5*	21.7
OX8	33.0*	26.5*	24.5
OX19	28.0*	25.6*	58.2
3.2.3	25.3*	22.5*	10.0

Results

Number of blood cells retained in liver sinusoids

The number of cells retrieved from liver sinusoids before perfusion was $1.08 \pm 0.3 \times 10^6$/g of liver tissue and after perfusion it was $0.96 \pm 0.2 \times 10^6$/g of liver tissue.

Phenotypical characteristics of cells retained in liver sinusoids

The results of phenotypical characteristics of cells washed out from liver sinusoids and perfusing blood are presented in Table 1. Monoclonal antibody analysis showed a prevalence in the wash-out population before perfusion, as compared to the perfusing blood, of OX8⁺ suppressor/cytotoxic (33 % vs 24.5 %, respectively), OX6⁺ class II antigen⁺ (32 % vs 21.7 %) and 3.2.3⁺ NK cells (25.3 vs 10 %), whereas it contained fewer W3/25⁺ helper/inducer (36.6 % vs 49.7 %) and OX19⁺ T cells (28 % vs 58.2 %). Cells isolated from wash-out fluid af-

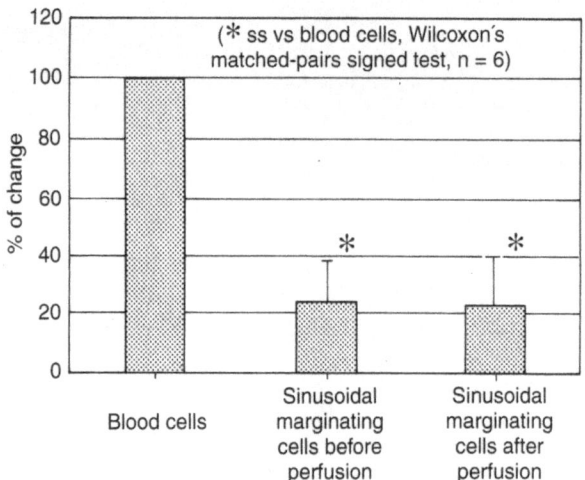

Fig. 2 The pre- and postperfusion responsiveness to mitogen (PHA, 90 μg/ml) of the liver sinusoidal wash-out cells compared to perfusing blood cells

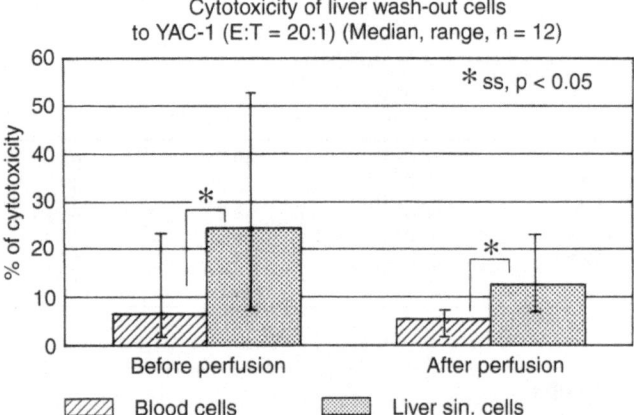

Fig. 3 The pre- and postperfusion level of cytotoxicity against YAC-1 of the liver sinusoidal wash-out cells and perfusing blood cells

ter perfusion displayed the same characteristics as the population washed out before perfusion.

Responsiveness to PHA

The responsiveness of lymphocytes to PHA in the wash-out fluid before perfusion was significantly lower (mean 76.4%) than of the perfusing blood lymphocytes and, similarly, the responsiveness of wash-out fluid after perfusion cells was also diminished (mean 77.2%) (Fig. 2).

Cytotoxicity against YAC-1 tumour cells

The cytotoxicity against YAC-1 (E : T = 20 : 1) cells of the wash-out fluid cells before perfusion was 24.49% (median values). It differed significantly from the cytotoxicity of cells in the perfusing blood, where it was 6.52%. Cytotoxicity of postperfusion wash-out cells was 12.58% and, again, it differed significantly compared to the cytotoxicity of cells in perfusing blood, where it was 5.43% (Fig. 3).

Discussion

These studies provided the following information: (a) a liver perfused ex vivo with syngeneic blood retained its in vivo function of marginating mononuclear cells in sinusoidal blood, at a concentration of approximately 1 million cells/g of tissue, (b) perfusion of a liver with syngeneic blood brought about the reacummulation in the sinusoids of a similar population of lymphocytes as found prior to perfusion, and (c) the blood mononuclear cells retained in the liver sinusoids after perfusion showed the same low responsiveness to PHA, and a high level of cytotoxicity to YAC-1 tumour cells as the preperfusion population.

The trapping of cells with NK and suppressor/cytotoxic characteristics in an ex vivo perfused liver, demonstrated in these experiments, points to the capacity of the liver to select certain cell population from sinusoidal blood. It has been shown in the in vivo studies that certain populations of blood lymphocytes have a predilection to accumulate temporarily in the liver [10, 11, 12, 18]. However, the mechanism of this process remains unclear. Circulating lymphocytes that arrive at the liver must adhere to the endothelial cells in order either to extravasate or to carry out their in situ tasks in the sinusoids. The adhesion molecules are present both on mononuclear and endothelial cells. These proteins fall into two main groups: (a) adhesion proteins which are constitutionally expressed by all normal microvascular endothelial cells, such as ICAM-2 (CD102, intracellular adhesion molecule-2), and (b) inducible proteins, absent from normal endothelial cells but upregulated by inflammatory cytokines, such as ICAM-1 (CD-54, intracellular adhesion molecule-1), VCAM-1 (CD106, vascular cell adhesion molecule-1), and E-selectin (CD62E) [8, 20]. Significant differences between sinusoidal endothelial cells and microvascular endothelial cells were only observed for ICAM-1. In contrast to most microvascular endothelial cells in the body, sinusoidal endothelial cells display a constitutionally high expression of ICAM-1 [17]. Like the other capillary endothelial cells, sinusoidal endothelial cells express ICAM-2, but do not display detectable levels of VCAM-1 and E-selectin. However, VCAM-1 and E-selectin can be upregulated on sinusoidal endothelial cells in inflammatory conditions. Adhering lymphocytes possess on their surface ligands to the endothelial cell adhesion molecules as LFA-1 (CD18/CD11a, lymphocyte function antigen), VLA 4 (CD 49d, very late antigen 4) and CD44 [3, 17].

Which of these molecules participate in the process of margination of NK and other sinusoidal populations in the rat liver remains the subject of our investigations. Recent results of our studies suggest that LFA-1/ICAMs and VLA-4/VCAM-1 are the main pathways of the lymphocyte-endothelial adhesion process in liver sinusoids [5]. These interactions could be further modulated and potentiated by the presence of other cell surface molecules. Cells from liver sinusoids strongly express LFA-2 (CD2), for which the specific ligand LFA-3 (CD58) is constitutionally present on sinusoidal endothelial cells. The action of these molecules may represent an additional factor in the adhesion of lymphocytes to endothelial and Kupffer cells in the sinusoidal lumen.

Taken together, perfused rat liver selectively retains in the sinusoids a specific population of blood cells, enriched in NK, CD8$^+$ and MHC class II$^+$ cells, displaying a high cytotoxic activity and low responsiveness to mitogen stimulation.

References

1. Calne R, Davies H (1994) Organ graft tolerance: the liver effect. Lancet 343: 67
2. Dahmen U, Qian S, Rao AS, et al (1994) Split tolerance induced by orthotopic liver transplantation in mice. Transplantation 58: 1
3. Garcia-Barcina M, Winnock M, Bidaurrazaga I, et al (1994) Detection of cell-adhesion molecules on human liver associated-lymphocytes. Immunol 82: 95
4. Garcia-Barcina M, Bedin C, Hemon C, et al (1995) Action of liver metastatic cells on lymphokine-activated killer activity of human liver-associated lymphocytes. In: Wisse E, Knook DL, Wake K (eds) Cells of the hepatic sinusoid. 5: 96
5. Garcia-Barcina M, Łukomska B, Gawron W, et al (1995) Expression of cell adhesion molecules on liver-associated lymphocytes and their ligands on sinusoidal lining cells in patients with benign and malignant liver disease. Am J Pathol 146: 1406
6. Gonwa TA, Nery JR, Husberg BS, et al (1988) Simultaneous liver and renal transplantation in man. Transplantation 46: 690
7. Howell CD, Yoder T, Claman N, Vierling JM (1989) Hepatic homing of mononuclear inflammatory cells isolated during murine chronic graft-vs-host disease. J Immunol 143: 476
8. Imhof BA, Dunon D (1994) Leucocyte migration and adhesion. Adv Immunol 58: 345
9. Łukomska B, Olszewski WL, Ryffa T, et al (1989) Liver sinusoidal blood containing natural killer-like cells. Scand J Immunol 29: 239
10. Łukomska B, Pieńkowska B, Andrzejewski W, et al (1991) Liver sinusoidal cytotoxic cells are recruited from blood and divide locally. J Hepatol 12: 332
11. Meusen E, Garrell MD, Brandon MR (1988) Presence of a distinct CD8+ and CD5− leucocyte subpopulation in the sheep liver. Immunology 64: 615
12. Pabst R, Binns R (1989) Heterogeneity of lymphocyte homing physiology: several mechanisms operate in the control of migration to lymphoid and non-lymphoid organs in vivo. Immunol Rev 108: 83
13. Pabst R, Nowara E (1982) Organ distribution and fate of newly formed splenic lymphocytes in the pig. Anat Record 202: 85
14. Rasmussen A, Davies HS, Jamieson NV, et al (1993) Combined transplantation of liver and kidney from the same donor protects the kidney from rejection and improves kidney graft survival (abstract). Sixth congress of the European society for organ transplantation, Rodos, Greece
15. Reynolds CW, Denn III AC, Barlozzari T, et al (1984) Natural killer activity in the rat. IV. Distribution of LGL following intravenous and intraperitoneal transfer. Cell Immunol 86: 371
16. Rolstad B, Herberman RB, Reynolds CW (1984) Natural killer cell activity in the rat. V. The circulation patterns and tissue localization of peripheral blood LGL. J Immunol 136: 2800
17. Scoazec J-Y, Feldman G (1994) The cell adhesion molecules of hepatic sinusoidal endothelial cells. J Hepatol 20: 296
18. Smith ME, Ford WL (1983) The recirculating lymphocyte pool of the rat: a systematic description of the migratory behaviour of recirculating lymphocytes. Immunol 49: 83
19. Starzl TE, Demetris AJ, Trucco M, et al (1992) Systemic chimerysm in human female recipients of male livers. Lancet 340: 876
20. Steinhoff G, Behrend M, Wonigeit K (1990) Expression of adhesion molecules on lymphocytes/monocytes and hepatocytes in human liver grafts. Hum Immunol 28: 123
21. Tzakis AG, Reyes J, Zeevi A, et al (1994) Early tolerance in pediatric liver allograft recipients. J Pediatr Surg 29: 754
22. Wisse E, Vanderkerken K, Crabbe E, et al (1995) The role of pit cells in the defense against tumor cells. In: Wisse E, Knook DL, Wake K (eds) Cells of the hepatic sinusoid. 5: 90

Transpl Int (1996) 9 [Suppl 1]: S 352–S 355
© Springer-Verlag 1996

Determination of HLA-B7 T-cell epitopes

A. Freese
N. Zavazava

A. Freese (✉) · N. Zavazava
Institute of Immunology,
University of Kiel,
Brunswiker Strasse 4, D-24105 Kiel,
Germany
Tel. + 49 (0)431/5 97 33 64;
Fax + 49 (0)431/5 97 33 35

Abstract A series of peptides derived from the α1 and α2 regions of the HLA-B7 and HLA-A2 molecules was synthesized with an automatic peptide synthesizer using the FMOC (9-fluorenylmethoxycarbonyl) technique. Peptides were analyzed and purified by reversed-phase high pressure liquid chromatography (HPLC). Peptide purity was > 96 %. The effect of B7 peptides on mixed lymphocyte cultures was tested in vivo. The alloresponse in the cultures with B7 peptides was strongly enhanced. The peptides that were most effective inhibited cytotoxic T-lymphocyte (CTL) cytolysis. The data show that the peptides are immunogenic and that they are recognised by both the direct and indirect pathways. Further, the mechanism of peptide recognition was studied. We coupled peptide B7 (residues 62–70 in HLA-B7) and peptide A2 (residues 62–70 in HLA-B2) covalently to fluorescein isothiocyanate (FITC). B7-specific CTLs were incubated with these peptides at 37 °C for 90 min and cell fluorescence measured by flow cytometry. The B7 peptide was bound by 60 % of the CTLs whereas the A2 peptide, as a negative control, bound only 10 %. The molecular size of the ligands to which the peptides bind are being characterized by immunoprecipitation.

Key words HLA-B7 · HLA-A2 · T-lymphocytes · Synthetic peptides · T-cell recognition

Introduction

Acute rejection of transplanted allogeneic organs is strongly dependent on T-cell activity against foreign human lymphocyte antigen (HLA) molecules. There are three possible explanations for the alloresponse. In one model, T-cell recognition requires the foreign HLA molecule together with a presented self peptide. Another model states that foreign HLA molecules are presented by antigen-presenting cells as processed peptides together with self HLA class I molecules on the cell surface. In the third model, the intact allogeneic HLA molecule is recognized independently of bound peptide [1]. The results of our inhibition assays showed that purified class I molecules [9] and papain-digested class I molecules [3] inhibit alloreactive cytotoxic T-lymphocytes (CTLs) specifically and so support the model of direct HLA recognition. CTLs show marked specificity for HLA class I molecules. These studies were continued using HLA-derived synthetic peptides. The major objective of the current studies is to perform CTL epitope mapping to determine those regions of the HLA molecule that are responsible for T-cell recognition. Defined overlapping peptides of the polymorphic region of the HLA-A2 and HLA-B7 molecules were utilized. Assuming that the differences between HLA specificities are anchored in this polymorphic region, the mismatched residues should be responsible for specific allo-recognition. To investigate the ligand bound on T-cells, peptides were coupled to a fluorescein isothiocyanate (FITC) molecule and tested in binding assays with allospecific T-cells. Furthermore, we investigated which regions of the HLA molecule are preferentially presented. For this reason we incubated HLA-B7-derived peptides with naive HLA-B7-negative peripheral blood lymphocytes.

Materials and methods

Peptide synthesis

We synthesized peptides derived from the polymorphic regions of the HLA-A2 and HLA-B7 molecule. The HLA-B7-derived peptides 10 (91-105: GSHTLQSMYGCDVGP), 11 (62-70: RNTQIY-KAQ), 12 (106–120: DGRLLRGHDQYAYDG), and the HLA-A2-derived peptides 4 (75–89: RVDLGTLRGYYNQSE) and 21 (62–70: GETRKVKAH) were synthesized by the standard FMOC (9-fluorenylmethoxycarbonyl) technique with an automatic peptide synthesizer (Millipore, USA). Peptide chains are generally assembled from the carboxyl-terminus to the amino-terminus. The first amino acid is covalently attached to an insoluble polystyrene support (PEG-PS). The remaining amino acids are added serially in cycles consisting of deblocking steps (i.e., removal of the alpha-amino-protecting FMOC group), dimethylformamide (DMF, Millipore, USA) washes, and binding of the next amino acid. The deblocking step is monitored by measuring the release of the UV-absorbing FMOC group.

Following synthesis, the product is cleaved from the resin and all side chain-protecting groups are removed. For this reaction we used a solution containing trifluoroaceticacid (Millipore, USA), phenol (Riedel-de Haen, Germany), and triisopropylsilane (Aldrich, UK). Cleavage was completed after 8 h. The peptide was finally precipitated and washed 3 times in cooled ether (Merck, Germany).

The peptide was analyzed and purified using reversed phase (Pep-S, C_2C_{18}, Pharmacia high pressure liquid chromatography (HPLC).

Generation of CTL lines

Peripheral blood lymphocytes (PBLs) were isolated from HLA-typed B7-negative volunteers. An HLA-B7-specific cell line, HN.B7, was generated by coculturing PBLs (HLA-A26,28, –B60,–C3, –DR3,6) with irradiated (50 Gy) stimulator Epstein-Barr virus (EBV)-transformed B cells, prostaglandin F (HLA-A3, –B7) at a 10 : 1 ratio in RPMI 1640 medium (Gibco, USA) supplemented with 15 % heat inactivated human AB serum, 125 µg/ml penicillin, and 250 µg/ml streptomycin. T-cells were restimulated every 10 days with stimulator cells. At the third and subsequent restimulations, interleukin-2 was added at a concentration of 30 U/ml. After the second restimulation, CTLs were used in functional assays.

Stimulation of PBLs with allogeneic peptides

PBLs were isolated from HLA-typed B7-negative volunteers. These PBLs were stimulated at day 0 with 10 µg/ml of a mixture of HLA-B7-derived peptides (peptides 10, 11, and 12). After 10 days, the cells were restimulated with autologous PBL blasts at a 10 : 1 ratio [6]. The blasts were preincubated with a 100-µg/ml peptide mixture for 90 min at 37 °C. After irradiation (25 Gy) the blasts together with the peptide mixture were added to the cells. At 5–6 days after the first restimulation, cells were tested in functional assays.

Proliferation assay

Primed PBLs were cocultivated with 100 µg/ml of the HLA-B7-derived peptides 10, 11, and 12. After 5 days the cells were pulsed with [^{3}H]thymidine and harvested after 16 h. The uptake was measured in a β-counter.

FITC coupling of synthetic peptides

We modified the method described by Kropshofer et al [4] by coupling peptides before cleavage. Peptides attached to the solid support were dissolved in 50 mM borate buffer and mixed with FITC in a molar ratio of 1 : 3. The solution was shaken gently for 6 h. The peptides were washed 3 times with borate buffer and then cleaved. The purity of the coupled peptides was analyzed by reversed-phase HPLC.

Binding assays with FITC-coupled peptide

An HLA-B7-specific cell line was incubated with 500 µg/ml of the HLA-B7-derived peptide 11 (residues 62–70) and the HLA-A2-derived peptide 21 (residues 62–70) as a negative control. We incubated the cells at 37 °C for 90 min. Subsequently, the cells were washed 3 times with phosphate-buffered saline (PBS) and the fluorescence intensity was measured in a FACScan.

Results

The efficiency of amino acid coupling was reflected in the HPLC profiles. After synthesis, the peptide was purified by means of preparative HPLC. A purity of more than 96 % was achieved. These highly purified peptides were used in the assays to study the regions of the HLA molecule responsible for T-cell recognition.

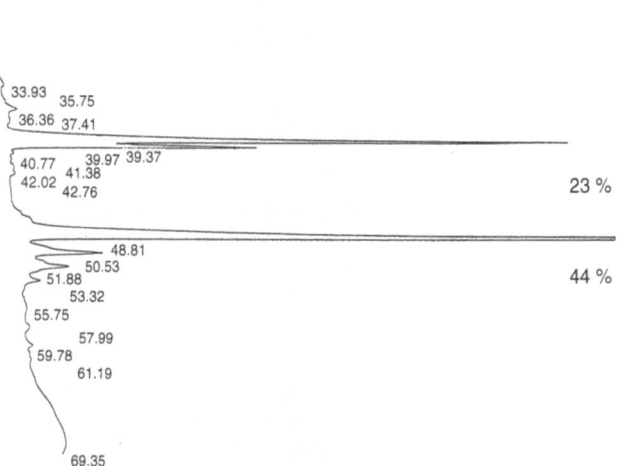

Fig. 1 The high pressure liquid chromatography (HPLC) profile of fluorescein isothiocyanate (FITC) coupled peptide 11 at 214 nm. The first peak, marked 23 %, represents the uncoupled peptide and that marked 44 % the FITC coupled peptide. This was the highest yield obtained

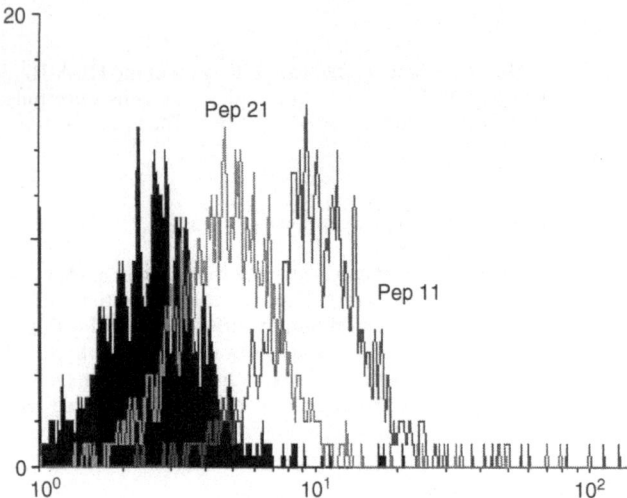

Fig. 2 Results of a binding assay with FITC-coupled peptides. The HLA-B7-derived peptide 11 *(Pep 11)* shows a greater affinity to the HLA-B7 cell line, HNB7, than does the HLA-B2-derived peptide 21 *(Pep 21)*. This result suggest that the binding is stable

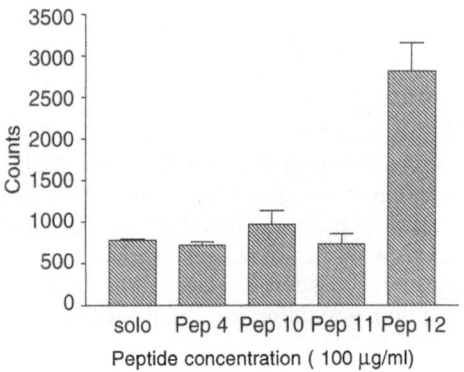

Fig. 3 Presentation of peptide 12. B7-negative peripheral blood lymphocytes (A2,−B51,60,−C3,−DR8,12) were cultured in 10 µg/ml peptides 4, 10, 11, and 12 for 10 days. Five days after restimulation, cells were cultivated in 100 µg/ml of each peptide. Cells were pulsed after 5 days and harvested. Peptide 12 *(Pep 12)* induced enhanced proliferation

The interaction of highly purified FITC-coupled peptides of the polymorphic region of the HLA molecule with allospecific cell lines was investigated in order to obtain information on the intensity, specificity, and duration of the binding of allopeptides to specific T-cells. FITC-coupling of the HLA-B7-derived peptide 11 (62–70), which was positive in several inhibition assays, was performed. The first coupling experiments were moderately successful. After numerous coupling experiments with slight modifications in the reaction time and in the molar ratio of peptide to FITC, the maximum yield of FITC-coupled peptide was raised to 44 % (Fig. 1). With this method established, it was possible to couple any peptide of interest. To have a perfect negative control

for our binding experiments we synthesized an HLA-A2 peptide of the same region as peptide 11, peptide 21 (A2: 62–70). This peptide was also FITC-coupled with a similar yield.

We tested the binding specificty of allopeptides to HLA-specific T-cells. For this reason, an HLA-B7-specific cell line was incubated with 500 µg/ml of the FITC-coupled peptide 11 and the HLA-A2-derived peptide 21 as a negative control. The result obtained is shown in Fig. 2. Peptide 11 showed a greater binding affinity to the B7-specific cell line than did the negative control, peptide 21. Many different cell lines were tested. The binding intensity to peptide 11 ranged from 15 % to 90 %.

Additionally, we investigated the capability of HLA-B7-derived peptides to induce a proliferative response to PBLs. The naive PBLs were coincubated with 100 µg/ml of the B7-derived peptides 10 (91–105), 11 (62–70), and 12 (106–120). Peptide 10 caused low cell proliferation, whereas peptide 12 doubled the response (not shown). Peptide 4 is an A2 (75–89) negative control peptide. To test if the naive PBLs could be primed with peptides they were cocultivated with a 10-µg/ml peptide mixture of peptides 10, 11, and 12 for 10 days. Five days after restimulation, cells were tested in a proliferation assay with the various peptides. As shown in Fig. 3, peptide 10 slightly increased cell proliferation, whereas peptide 12 was strongly presented. In other experiments, peptide presentation was shown to be mediated by antigen-presenting cells (data not shown).

Discussion

We previously showed that purified native HLA class I molecules are capable of specifically inhibiting allogeneic cytotoxic T-lymphocytes in vitro. Continuing these studies, we established the production of synthetic peptides. The inhibition assays using synthetic peptides confirm our previous data [3, 9]. Similarly to the whole purified HLA molecule, tested peptides of the polymorphic region of the HLA molecule are able to inhibit cytotoxic T-cell reactivity specifically. These results also confirm findings by others [2, 5]. The HLA-B7-specific CTL epitopes were located at positions 62–70 and 91–105. A simple explanation for this specific inhibition of the CTLs is that the peptides bind directly to the T-cell receptor (TCR). The blocked receptor can, thus, no longer come into contact with the foreign HLA molecule of the target cell, hence no cytolysis occurs. The nature of this binding is still, however, not clear. To further investigate the interaction between the allospecific peptide and the T-cells, we coupled the peptides to FITC. Our results showed that peptide binding to the membrane ligand is much stronger than expected. In studies done with soluble TCR heterodimers, the binding of class II major histocompatibility complex (MHC) molecules was reported to have a very fast off rate, with a $t_{1/2} \approx 12$ s [5]. Additionally, Seth et al. [7] reported that it was impossible to detect a class II-peptide-TCR complex in a native polyacrylamide gel because of the low affinity of these interactions. However, further characterization of this phenomenon is required. In light of these arguments, it is not clear whether our peptides directly interact with the TCR or some other cell-surface ligand. Since the interaction is allospecific, there is strong evidence for the involvement of the TCR.

The proliferation studies showed that one synthetic peptide was presented and led to T-cell proliferation. This observation is important for organ transplantation. As reported by others [8], donor soluble HLAs or their fragments could be picked up by recipient antigen-presenting cells and either lead to augmentation of the alloresponse or to T-cells that might down-regulate proliferation. These studies are helpful in elucidating alloreactivity and identification of relevant T-cell epitopes.

References

1. Benoist C, Mathis D (1991) Demystification of the alloresponse. Curr Biol 1: 143–144
2. Clayberger C, Parham P, Rothbard J, Ludwig DS, Schoolnik GK, Krensky AM (1987) HLA-A2 peptides can regulate cytolysis by human allogeneic T lymphocytes. Nature 330: 763
3. Hausmann R, Zavazava N, Steinmann J, Müller-Ruchholtz W (1993) Interaction of papain-digested HLA class I molecules with human alloreactive cytotoxic T lymphocytes (CTL). Clin Exp Immunol 91: 183–188
4. Kropshofer H, Max H, Kalbacher H (1993) Evidence for cobinding of self- and allopeptides to human class II major histocompatibility antigen DR1 by energy transfer. Proc Natl Acad Sci USA 90: 403–407
5. Matsui K, Boniface JJ, Steffner P, Reay PA, Davis MM (1994) Kinetics of T-cell receptor binding to peptide/I-E^{k}complexes: correlation of the dissociation rate with T-cell responsiveness. Proc Natl Acad Sci USA 9: 112862–112866
6. Schmidt C, Burrows SR, Moss DJ, Sculley TB, Misko IS (1991) Oligopeptide induction of a secondary cytotoxic T-cell response to Epstein-Barr virus in vitro. Scand J Immunol 33: 411
7. Seth A, Stern LJ, Ottenhoff THM, Engel I, Owen MJ, Lamb JR, Klausner R, Wiley DC (1994) Binary and ternary complexes between T-cell receptor, class II MHC and superantigen in vitro. Nature 369: 324
8. Siciu-Foca N, Ho E, King DW, et al (1991) Soluble HLA and anti-idiotypic antibodies in transplantation: modulation of anti-HLA antibodies by soluble HLA antigens from the graft and anti-idiotypic antibodies in renal and cardiac allograft recipients. Transplant Proc 23: 295–296
9. Zavazava N, Hausmann R, Müller-Ruchholtz W (1991) Inhibition of anti-HLA-B7 alloreactive CTL by affinity-purified soluble HLA. Transplantation 51: 838–842

Transpl Int (1996) 9 [Suppl 1]: S 356–S 363
© Springer-Verlag 1996

S. K. Hemmatpour
P. R. Evans
S. McQuilkin
D. A. Sage
W. M. Howell

HLA class I A and B typing in the clinical laboratory using DNA-based techniques

S. K. Hemmatpour (✉) · P. R. Evans ·
S. McQuilkin · D. A. Sage · W. M. Howell
Wessex Histocompatibility Service,
Tenovus Laboratory,
Southampton University Hospitals,
Southampton, SO16 6YD, UK
Tel. +44 1703 796638;
Fax +44 1703 701416

Abstract The potential for clinical HLA class I A and B typing utilizing the polymerase chain reaction combined with sequence-specific oligonucleotide probes (PCR-SSOP) was investigated. Two hundred and ten clinical samples for the HLA-B locus and 100 clinical samples for the HLA-A locus were typed by DNA-based methods and serology. For the HLA-B locus an improved SSOP typing system was developed which involved using HLA-B specific 5′ primers and two 3′ primers, in separate reactions. Using a panel of 30 digoxigenin-labelled SSOPs, HLA-B types were assigned for all 210 individuals with an improvement in resolution over previously described DNA-based systems and confirming serologically assigned types in all cases except one. In addition, using a single primer pair and a panel of 16 SSOPs, 100 samples were successfully HLA-A typed by PCR-SSOP resolving ambiguous serological types, including HLA-A19 subtypes and A2 homozygosity. In 25 samples, the assigned types were also confirmed by the amplification refractory mutation system (ARMS-PCR). These results indicate that non-urgent clinical HLA-A and -B typing may be performed by PCR-SSOP with a resolution at least equal to that of serology.

Key words Polymerase chain reaction · HLA-A · HLA-B · PCR-SSOP · Clinical transplantation

Introduction

The influence of patient-donor HLA matching on allograft survival in renal and bone marrow transplantation is well documented. This has been demonstrated by the highly successful survival rate of kidneys transplanted between either living related individuals or HLA identical siblings, 90 % of which have a graft survival in excess of 5 years. Martin and Dyer [12] and Opelz [18] have emphasized that a favourable HLA-DR and HLA-B match is the optimal requirement for a successful transplant. It is also known that the outcome of bone marrow transplantation critically depends on the degree of HLA matching, for example, one case has been reported in which T-cell mediated allograft rejection correlated with a single amino acid difference in an HLA-B allele (specifically HLA-B44) [5]. A further report by Steinle et al. [19] also suggested that single, naturally occurring, sequence variations in the HLA-B35 group of alleles influence allorecognition and could be of importance in clinical transplant matching. It is essential, therefore, that any HLA class I tissue typing method is ultimately capable of determining all allelic subtypes that may be of clinical importance and which may give rise to a rejection response.

Until recently, all routine HLA typing has been performed by serology, using the microlymphocytotoxicity test. However, the introduction of DNA-based testing for HLA class II typing has revealed that serological HLA-DR typing has error rates of up to 25 % [16]. The serological 'errors' incurred are mainly due to the limited availability of specific alloantisera and poor viability or low yield of lymphocytes isolated from the sample to be typed. These limitations do not apply to DNA-based typing techniques. Thus, these methods can confirm homozygosity and identify additional genetic variation not detectable by serology. More recently, the availability of DNA sequence data for the HLA class I alleles has permitted the development of a number of PCR based typing methods for the HLA-A, -B and -C loci using the polymerase chain reaction [10, 17, 24], a technically more demanding task for class I than class II loci. Therefore, it is now possible to use DNA-based typing methods to investigate the accuracy of clinical HLA class I serological typing and from this, to develop more precise DNA-based methods for routine use.

The HLA class I A, B and C genes each consist of seven exons, of which exons II, III and IV code for the three external domains ($\alpha 1$, $\alpha 2$ and $\alpha 3$). The $\alpha 1$ and $\alpha 2$ domains are the most polymorphic, forming the peptide binding groove of the molecule which contains several hypervariable regions. These domains are encoded by exons II and III of the gene in question [11]. Identification of sequence polymorphism in these exons should form the basis of any DNA-based PCR typing system for the HLA class I loci.

The aim of this study, therefore, was to develop an appropriate system for clinical HLA-A and -B PCR typing of homozygous and heterozygous individuals, using panels of sequence-specific oligonucleotide probes (SSOPs) of a manageable size. For the HLA-B locus, the specific aim was to extend a recently developed DNA-based typing system [24], which was based only on exon II sequences. In order to further distinguish most clinically relevant specificities, this system was expanded into a more comprehensive form by extending the region amplified into exon III and by using a further 7 SSOPs specific for two hypervariable regions in this exon. In addition, typing of the HLA-A locus was performed using a protocol based on the method devised by Oh et al. [17] but with careful selection of the SSOPs used, reducing their number from 28 to 16. Further confirmation of certain assigned HLA-A types was achieved by supplementary use of a multiplex PCR amplification refractory mutation system (ARMS-PCR) [2, 21]. The development of these typing systems allowed a retrospective assessment of the accuracy of serological typing for the HLA-A and HLA-B loci and lead to the establishment of a manageable system for clinical HLA-A and -B PCR-SSOP typing.

Materials and methods

Cell lines

Initially, DNA from 36 B-lymphoblastoid cell lines [14, 22, 23], covering the majority of the WHO designated HLA-A and -B serological specificities, were used as control material. These cell lines were selected to give both positive and negative reactivities with all probes tested.

Patients and donors

One hundred and seventy renal donors and recipients (including 66 donor-recipient pairs transplanted between January 1992 and October 1993) were selected for inclusion in this study along with 40 bone marrow transplant-related samples (12 patients and 28 donors). All samples were HLA-B typed by a modified PCR-SSOP method. A further 100 samples (randomly selected bone marrow and renal, patients and donors) were HLA-A typed by PCR-SSOP, with 26 of these typed by both PCR-SSOP and ARMS-PCR. All 310 of these individuals were previously HLA-A and -B typed by serology using the standard microlymphocytotoxicity test [20].

DNA preparation

Genomic DNA was prepared from 1 ml of peripheral blood or 0.5 ml of frozen lymphocytes using a phenol/chloroform miniprep method [1] or by using a salting-out technique [15]. In both of the above methods the DNA was dissolved in 30 µl sterile double-distilled water.

HLA-B PCR primers and DNA amplification

Two HLA-B locus specific 5'-sided primers, CG4 (5'-GAC GAC ACC CAG TTC GTG A-3') and CG5 (5'-GAC GAC ACG CTG TTC GTG A-3'), designed by Yoshida et al. [24], and derived from nucleotides 84–102 in exon II were employed, amplifying all HLA-B alleles except B54. The two 3'-sided primers, D1 (5'-GCC GCG GTC CAG GAG CT-3') and D1X (5'-GCG GCG GTC CAG GAG CG-3'), were based on nucleotides 120–136 in exon III and amplify all alleles, regardless of a nucleotide mismatch at position 134 in exon III, generating a 560 bp PCR product. Each DNA sample was amplified using an equal mix of the 5' primers and either the D1 or D1X 3' primer in separate reactions to increase the resolution of HLA-B allele assignment over the original system described by Yoshida et al. [24].

Genomic DNA (1 µg) was amplified in a 50 µl reaction mix [67 mM TRIS-HCl pH 8.0, 16.6 mM ammonium sulphate, 6.7 µM EDTA, 0.017 % BSA, 2 mM $MgCl_2$, 200 µM of each deoxynucleotide (dATP, dCTP, dGTP and dTTP), 0.2 µM of each primer and 1 unit of Taq polymerase (Amplitaq, Perkin-Elmer Cetus, CA)]. The reaction mix was overlaid with mineral oil and amplified in a thermal cycler (Omnigene, Hybaid, Limited, Middlesex, UK) according to the following protocol: 5 cycles of 1 min denaturation at 95°C, 1 min annealing at 65°C and 2 min extension at 72°C, followed by 25 cycles of 1 min denaturation at 95°C, 1 min annealing at 55°C and 2 min extension at 72°C. Successful PCR amplifications were determined by agarose gel electrophoresis.

Table 1 Oligonucleotide probe sequences for exon II and III of the HLA-B gene

Hypervariable region/exon	Probe name	Sequence (5'–3')	Corresponding nucleotide number
A/exon II	01	GAG GAA GGA GCC GCG GGC	128–145
	02	GAG GAC GGA GCC CCG GGC	128–145
	07	GAG GAT GGC GCC CCG GGC	128–145
	09	GAG TCC GAG AGA GGA GCC	122–139
B/exon II	03	ACA CGG AAC ATG AAG GCC	189–206
	04	ACA CAG ATC TCC AAG ACC	189–206
	24	GGG AGA CAC AGA TCT CCA	184–201
	25	GGA ACA CAC AGA TCT CCA	184–201
	05	ACA CAG ATC TTC AAG ACC	189–206
	08	ACA CAG ATC TGC AAG ACC	189–206
	10	GAT CTA CAA GGC CCA GGC	195–212
	11	GAA GTA CAA GCG CCA GGC	195–212
	12	ATC TGC AAG GCC AAG GCA	195–212
C/exon II	13	ACT GAC CGA GAG AGC CTG	216–233
	14	GAC TTA CCG AGA GAA CCT	215–232
	15	GAC TGA CCG AGA GAA CCT	215–232
	16	TTA CCG AGA GGA CCT GCG	218–235
	17	ACT TAC CGA GAG AGC CTG	216–233
	18	ACT GAC CGA GTG AGC CTG	216–233
D/exon II	20	AGC GGA GCG CGG TGC GCA	232–249
	21	CGG AAC CTG CGC GGC TAC	234–251
	22	CGG ACC CTG CTC CGC TAC	234–251
	23	CGG ATC GCG CTC CGC TAC	234–251
E/exon III	E1	CTC ACA CTT GGC AGA CGA	4–21
	E2	CAG AGC ATG TAC GGC TGC	15–32
	E3	CTG CGA CCT GGG GCC CGA	29–46
	E4	CTC ACA CTT GGC AGA GGA	4–21
	E5	CCA GTG GAT GTA TGG CTG	14–31
F/exon III	F1	CTC CGC GGG CAT GAC CAG	57–74
	F2	GGC ATA ACC AGT TAG CCT	64–81

HLA-A PCR primers and DNA amplification

PCR primers (5'-GAC GCC GCG AGC CAG AGG AT-3' and 5'-TGC AGC GTC TCC TTC CCG TT-3') and amplification protocols based on those of Oh et al. [17], amplified a 671 bp PCR product, spanning exons II and III.

Genomic DNA (0.5 µg) was amplified in a 50 µl reaction mix [10 mM TRIS-HCl pH 8.3, 50 mM potassium chloride, 0.01 % gelatin, 1.5 mM MgCl$_2$, 200 µM of each deoxynucleotide (dATP, dCTP, dGTP and dTTP), 0.2 µM of each primer and 1 unit of Taq polymerase]. The reaction mix was overlaid with mineral oil and amplified in a thermal cycler according to the following protocol: 5 min denaturation at 95 °C followed by 30 cycles of 1 min denaturation at 96 °C, 50 s annealing at 60 °C and 1.5 min extension at 72 °C. Successful amplifications were determined by agarose gel electrophoresis.

Sequence-specific oligonucleotide probes (SSOPs)

Initially, 23 SSOPs described by Yoshida et al. [24], designed to detect variations in sequences in four hypervariable regions in exon II of the HLA-B gene, were utilized. To expand the system into a more comprehensive form a further 7 probes (Table 1) were designed and used to detect sequence variations in two hypervariable regions of exon III of the HLA-B gene.

Originally, Oh et al. [17] described 28 SSOPs which were designed to detect sequences in the hypervariable regions of exons II

and III of the HLA-A gene. However, in this study a simplified panel of 16 SSOPs (Table 2) was selected to provide a PCR-SSOP typing system with a resolution equivalent to that of serology.

The HLA-A and HLA-B oligoprobes were 15 and 18 bases in length, respectively. This allowed the use of tetramethylammonium chloride (TEMACl)-based buffers in single temperature hybridization and wash steps. All of the probes were also 3'-end labelled with digoxigenin-11-2',3'-dideoxyuridine 5'-triphosphate (DIG-11-ddUTP; Boehringer Mannheim, Mannheim, Germany) using the enzyme terminal deoxynucleotidyl transferase (TdT; Boehringer Mannheim, Germany) according to the manufacturers instructions.

Dot-blot hybridization and signal detection

Successfully amplified DNA was spotted onto a series of replicate, positively charged, nylon-based membranes (Boehringer Mannheim, Germany) and then soaked in denaturation solution (0.5 M NaOH, 1.5 M NaCl) for 5 min followed by a neutralizing solution (0.5 M TRIS-HCl pH 7.2, 1.5 M NaCl, 1 mM EDTA) for 1 min. The DNA was then immobilised by UV irradiation on a transilluminator for 1.5 min.

The membranes were prehybridized for 50 min, at either 52 °C for HLA-B or 46 °C for HLA-A, in 5 ml of hybridization buffer (3 M TEMACl, 50 mM TRIS-HCl pH 8.0, 2 mM EDTA and 0.1 % SDS). Subsequently, 10 pmol of the labelled SSOPs were hybridized with the membranes for 75 min at either 52 °C for HLA-B

Table 2 Oligonucleotide probe sequences for exon II and III of the HLA-A gene

Probe name	Exon II/III	Sequence (5'–3')	Corresponding amino acid position
56R	II	GAG AGG CCT GAG TAT	55–59
62LQ	II	TGG GAC CTG CAG ACA	60–64
62G	II	GAC GGG GAG ACA CGG	61–65
62RN	II	GAC CGG AAC ACA CGG	61–65
62EG	II	GAG GAG ACA GGG AAA	62–66
73I	II	TCA CAG ATT GAC CGA	71–75
77S	II	GAG AGC CTG CGG ATC	76–80
114EH	III	TAT GAA CAG CAC GCC	113–117
131R	III	CGC TCT TGG ACC GCG	131–135
142TK	III	ACC ACC AAG CAC AAG	142–146
149T	III	TGG GAG ACG GCC CAT	147–151
150V	III	GAG GCG GTC CAT GCG	148–152
151R	III	GCG GCC CGT GTG GCG	149–153
156Q	III	GAG CAG CAG AGA GCC	154–158
161D	III	CTG GAT GGC ACG TGC	160–164
163R	III	GAG GGC CGG TGC GTG	161–165

or 46 °C for HLA-A. The prehybridization and hybridization stages were performed in a hybridization incubator (Hybaid Maxi Hybridization Oven, Hybaid Limited, Middlesex, UK). The membranes were then subjected to the following stringency washes: two 5 min washes in $2 \times$ SSPE pH 7.4 (0.3 M NaCl, 0.02 M NaH$_2$. PO$_4$·H$_2$O, 2 mM EDTA) and 0.1 % SDS at room temperature with constant agitation; and two 10 min washes in TEMACl wash (3 M TEMACl, 50 mM TRIS-HCl pH 8.0, 2 mM EDTA, 0.1 % SDS) at either 58 °C (exon II probes) or 62 °C (exon III probes) for HLA-B and at 50 °C for HLA-A.

The hybridized SSOPs were subjected to immunodetection of digoxigenin label using anti-DIG-AP fab fragments conjugated to alkaline phosphatase (Boehringer Mannheim, Germany) and Lumigen-PPD (Boehringer Mannheim, Germany). The resulting chemiluminescent reaction was visualized by autoradiography and the allelic type assigned by probe reactivity (HLA-B Table 3; HLA-A Table 4).

HLA-A ARMS-PCR typing

The ARMS-PCR system (Cellmark Diagnostics, Cheshire, UK) used in this study for confirmation of certain assigned HLA-A types, utilized five separate multiplex PCR reactions. In brief, DNA samples were amplified by ARMS-PCR and the products detected by gel electrophoresis. The HLA-A type was then assigned after interpreting the resulting band patterns. Each reaction detects between 2 and 6 HLA-A locus specificities, with 20 different specificities being able to be detected in total [2, 21].

Results

HLA-B typing

All samples (36 control cell lines and 210 clinical samples) were successfully amplified by one or both of the two PCR reactions employed. All alleles with sequences complementary to the primers amplified. In addition, the 5'-sided primers amplified 15 alleles (0801, 1401/2, 3801, 3901/13/2/3, 5401, 5501/2, 5601/2, 1503, 7901) re-

gardless of either a G/G primer/template mismatch at position 92 or an A/A mismatch at position 94 of exon II. A further allele (1801) also amplified successfully despite a C/A mismatch at position 88 of exon II. Similarly, the 3'-sided primers amplified all alleles including 8 alleles (2702/3/5/5w, 4101, 4701, 0801, 4201) with either a C/C or a G/G mismatch at position 134 of exon III.

The SSOP dot-blot hybridization patterns obtained usually had low backgrounds and a strong signal intensity. Twenty-three of the thirty SSOPs were highly specific and showed a strong hybridization signal intensity. Probe 13, although showing variable hybridization reactions with respect to the amount of non-specific hybridization, was still useful in assigning HLA-B alleles. Six probes (25, 8, 15, 16, 18 and F1) were of little use in assigning alleles because of the high degree of non-specific hybridization that occurred under the conditions used.

The types obtained for all 36 B-lymphoblastoid control cell lines agreed with published serological assignments except for the cell line FLE. This cell line is reported as a B63(15) in the literature [8], however, by PCR-SSOP typing it was found to be B*5701/2.

Of the 210 individuals typed, 17 were confirmed to be homozygotes and the remaining 193 were confirmed to be heterozygotes. Initially, the use of the two 3' primers in separate reactions partially resolved some of the four ambiguous groups of alleles described by Yoshida et al. [24]. Subsequently, the use of seven extra oligoprobes improved the resolution further, as summarised in Table 5. Two ambiguous heterozygote combinations were also found to be resolved by using the probes based on sequences in exon III of the HLA-B locus (B44, B15 or B45/B50, B13 resolved as B44, B15 and B44, B1503/B4802/B7901 resolved as B44, B1503). Finally, one discrepancy between the molecular and serology types was found. This sample was typed by serology as B35, B70 and by PCR-SSOP as B35, B45/B50.

Table 3 HLA-B oligoprobe reactivities

Allele	0000 1279	0022001111 3445580123	11111 45678	2222 0123	EEEEE 12345	FF 12
D1 amplifications						
4701	+ − − −	− + + − − − − − − −	− − + − −	− − + −	− − − − −	− −
4401	+ − − −	− + + − − − − − − −	+ − − − −	− − − −	− − − − −	− −
4402/3	+ − − −	− + + − − − − − − −	+ − − − −	+ − − −	− − − − −	− −
4501	+ − − −	− + + − − − − − − −	− − − + −	− + − −	− − + + −	− −
4901	+ − − −	− + + − − − − − − −	+ − − − −	− − − +	− − + + −	− −
5001	+ − − −	− + + − − − − − − −	− − − + −	− + − −	− − + + −	− −
1801	− + − −	− + − + − − − − − −	− − − + −	− + − −	− − − − −	+ −
3701	− + − −	− + + − − − − − − −	− − + − −	− − + −	− − − − −	− −
3501/3	− + − −	− − − − + − − − − −	− − − + −	− + − −	− − + − −	+ −
3502/4/6	− + − −	− − − − + − − − − −	− − − + −	− + − −	− − + − −	− −
3505	− + − −	− − − − + − − − − −	− − − + −	− + − −	− + + − −	+ −
5301	− + − −	− − − − + − − − − −	+ − − − −	− − − +	− − + − −	+ −
5101/2/3	− + − −	− − − − + − − − − −	+ − − − −	− − − +	+ − − − −	− −
5104	− + − −	− − − − + − − − − −	+ − − − −	− − − +	− − − − −	− −
5201/12	− + − −	− + + − − − − − − −	+ − − − −	− − − +	+ − − − −	− −
7801	− + − −	− − − − + − − − − +	− − − − −	− + − −	+ − − − −	− −
5801	− + − −	+ − − − − − − − − −	+ − − − −	− − − +	− − + − −	+ −
1301	− − + −	− + + − − − − − − −	+ − − − −	+ − − −	− − − − −	− +
1302	− − + −	− + + − − − − − − −	+ − − − −	+ − − −	+ − − − −	− +
1501	− − + −	− + + − − − − − − −	− − − + −	− + − −	− − − − −	+ −
1502	− − + −	− + − + − − − − − −	− − − + −	− + − −	− − − − −	− −
1504	− − + −	− + + − − − − − − −	− − − + −	− + − −	+ − − − −	+ −
4601	− − + −	− − − − − − − + − −	− − − − +	− + − −	− − − − −	+ −
5701	− − + −	+ − − − − − − − − −	+ − − − −	− − − +	− − − − −	+ −
5702	− − + −	+ − − − − − − − − −	+ − − − −	− − − +	− − − − −	− −
2702	− − − +	− − − − − + − − + −	− + − − −	− − − +	− − − − −	− −
2703/5/54	− − − +	− − − − − + − − + −	− − − − −	− − + −	− − − − −	− −
1401/2	− − − +	− − − − − + − − − +	− − − − −	− + − −	− − − − +	− −
3801	− − − +	− − − − − + − − − −	+ − − − −	− − − +	− − − − −	− −
3901/13	− − − +	− − − − − + − − − +	− − − − −	− + − −	− − − − −	− −
3902	− − − +	− + + − − − − − − +	− − − − −	− + − −	− − − − −	− −
3903	− − − +	− − − − − + − − − +	− − − − −	− + − −	− + − − −	− −
4802	− − − +	− + + − − − − − − −	− − − + −	− + − −	− − + − −	+ −
5501/2	− − − +	− − − − − − + − − +	− − − − −	− + − −	+ − − − −	− +
5601	− − − +	− − − − − − + − − +	− − − − −	− + − −	+ − − − −	− +
5602	− − − +	− − − − − − + − − +	− − − − −	− + − −	− − − − −	− +
1503	− − − +	− + + − − − − − − −	− − − + −	− + − −	− − − − −	+ −
7901	− − − +	− − − − − + − − − −	− − − + −	− + − −	− − − − −	+ −
D1X amplifications						
4001/4	+ − − −	− + + − − − − − − −	− − − + −	− + − −	− − − − −	− −
4002/5	+ − − −	− + + − − − − − − −	− − − + −	− + − −	− + − − −	− −
4003	+ − − −	− + + − − − − − − −	− − − + −	− + − −	− + − − −	+ −
4101	+ − − −	− + + − − − − − − −	− − − + −	− + − −	− − − + −	− −
2707	− − − +	− − − − − + − − + −	− − − − −	− − + −	− + − − −	− −
0701	− − − +	− − − − − − + − − +	− − − − −	− + − −	− − − − −	+ −
0702/3	− − − +	− − − − − − + − − +	− − − − −	− + − −	− + − − −	+ −
0801	− − − +	− − − − + − − − − +	− − − − −	− + − −	− + − − −	− −
4201	− − − +	− − − − − − + − − +	− − − − −	− + − −	− + − − −	− −
4801	− − − +	− + + − − − − − − −	− − − + −	− + − −	− + − − −	− −

HLA-A typing

All samples (36 control cell lines and 100 clinical samples) were successfully amplified despite an A/C mismatch in exon II at position 127 (0202/5) and 130 (0101, 3601) in the 5′ primer. The PCR products were dotted onto nylon membranes and hybridized with 16 SSOPs derived from hypervariable regions of exons II and III of the HLA-A locus. The hybridization patterns with all 16 SSOPs showed low backgrounds and a strong signal intensity.

All 36 B-lymphoblastoid cell lines were successfully typed and results agreed with those obtained by serology. All 100 clinical samples were also successfully

S 361

Table 4 HLA-A oligoprobe reactivities

Allele	56 R	62 LQ	62 G	62 RN	62 EG	73 I	77 S	114 EH	131 R	142 TK	149 T	150 V	151 R	156 Q	161 D	163 R
31011/2	+	–	–	–	–	+	–	–	+	–	–	–	+	–	–	–
3001/2	+	–	–	–	–	–	–	+	+	–	–	–	–	–	–	–
4301	–	+	–	–	–	–	–	–	+	–	+	–	–	–	–	+
2901/2	–	+	–	–	–	–	–	–	+	–	–	–	+	–	–	–
0201–10	–	–	+	–	–	–	–	–	+	+	–	–	–	–	–	–
0211	–	–	+	–	–	+	–	–	+	+	–	–	–	–	–	–
0212	–	–	+	–	–	–	–	–	+	+	–	–	–	+	–	–
6801/2	–	–	–	+	–	–	–	–	+	+	–	–	–	–	–	–
6901	–	–	–	+	–	–	–	–	+	+	–	–	–	–	–	–
2501	–	–	–	+	–	–	+	–	+	–	+	–	–	–	–	+
2601	–	–	–	+	–	–	–	–	+	–	+	–	–	–	–	+
3401/2	–	–	–	+	–	–	–	–	+	–	+	–	–	–	–	–
6601	–	–	–	+	–	–	–	–	+	–	+	–	–	–	–	+
6602	–	–	–	+	–	–	–	–	+	–	+	–	–	–	–	–
3301	–	–	–	+	–	+	–	–	+	–	–	–	+	–	–	–
2301	–	–	–	–	+	–	–	–	+	–	–	–	+	–	–	–
2401–3	–	–	–	–	+	–	–	–	+	–	–	–	–	+	–	–
3201	–	–	–	–	–	–	+	–	+	–	–	–	+	–	–	–
7401	–	–	–	–	–	–	–	–	+	–	–	–	+	–	–	–
0101	–	–	–	–	–	–	–	–	+	–	–	+	–	–	–	+
0301	–	–	–	–	–	–	–	–	+	–	–	–	–	–	+	–
0302	–	–	–	–	–	–	–	–	+	–	–	–	–	+	+	–
1101/2	–	–	–	–	–	–	–	–	+	–	–	–	–	+	–	+
3601	–	–	–	–	–	–	–	–	+	–	–	+	–	–	–	–

Table 5 Summary of resolved ambiguous allele groups

Allele group	Initial resolution using separate 3′ primers		Final resolution using seven extra oligoprobes	Number of cases
	Primer	Resolution		
'B7' (B7,42,55,56)	D1	B55,B56	No resolution possible	7
	D1X	B7,B42	B*07	69
			B*42	0
'B51' (B51,53)	D1	B51,B53	B*51	12
			B*53	0
'B14' (B14,39)	D1	B14,B39	B*14	9
			B*39	4
'B40' (B40,41,45,50)	D1	B45,B50	No resolution possible	2
	D1X	B40,B41	B*4001/4	11
			B*4002/3/5	8
			B*41	0

typed by PCR-SSOP, including 15 samples that could not be unambiguously typed by serology. Of these 15 samples, 5 were subtyped for the A*19 allele (1 × A*30, 3 × A*32, 1 × A*33), 1 was A*10 subtyped (A*26) and 3 had their A*03 status confirmed. In addition, 5 samples were also confirmed to be A*02 homozygotes and 1 was confirmed to be an A*02, A*28 heterozygote.

Further typing was performed on 26 of the 100 samples using ARMS-PCR. There was shown to be complete agreement between serology, PCR-SSOP and ARMS-PCR in 23 of these samples. However, 3 samples were found to be incorrectly typed by serology when comparing the results with PCR-SSOP and ARMS-PCR. These 3 samples were serologically typed as either A2, A2 or A2, A28 (2 cases) or A2, A29 (1 case), but were all confirmed to be A*02 homozygotes by PCR-SSOP and ARMS-PCR.

Discussion

Molecular typing of the HLA system has, until recently, been restricted to the class II region (HLA-DR, -DQ, -DP) because of the complexity and dispersed nature of the polymorphism of the class I loci [7]. In addition, homologous sequences shared between different class I loci, including pseudogenes, can lead to coamplification of these sequences, making locus-specific PCR or probing difficult. However, it has been previously reported that the HLA-B 5′ primers used in this study are unlikely to coamplify any pseudogenes [24]. The HLA-A primers, though, are known to coamplify three alleles of the HLA-H pseudogene [17], although the products obtained do not interfere with the typing results.

This study has improved upon the resolution reported in an earlier study by Yoshida et al. [24] for HLA-B typing, by using different 3′ primers (D1 and D1X) and extra oligoprobes derived from exon III of the HLA-B locus. In this original study, 22 unambiguous specificities could be identified, along with four unresolvable 'allele groups' (see Table 5). Initially, using the two 3′ primers in separate reaction mixes enabled certain of these 'allele groups' to be split up (Table 5); for example, the 'B7' group was subdivided into two groups, B55, B56 and B7, B42. The resolution was further improved by using seven extra oligoprobes; for example, the subgroup B7, B42 could be resolved into the alleles B*0701, B*0702/3 and B*4201. A parallel study [13] has also reported some improvements upon Yoshida et al.'s original HLA-B PCR-SSOP system. However, this parallel study used various amounts of probe and a range of stringency wash temperatures, resulting in a less manageable system than described in the present study which uses 10 pmol of probe throughout and only two stringency wash temperatures (58 °C and 62 °C). In addition, this latter study also reported a problem in differentiating between the alleles B*4201 and B*6701, and similarly B*1503 and B*4801. However, in the system described here we can distinguish between these alleles by using the 3′ primers in separate PCR reactions, thus improving the resolution of typing.

The number of HLA-B oligoprobes used in this study could also be slimmed down to 24 probes as 6 were found to be of little use in assigning alleles. The resolution of typing achieved by this system is comparable to serology utilizing 24 of the 30 oligoprobes tested, but can also be expanded into a higher resolution typing system. Such a high resolution typing system has been reported by Fernandez-Vina and colleagues [4] using different primers (for group-specific amplification) and many more probes. However, the number of group-specific PCR reactions (nine in total) in association with the number of probes required for typing (in excess of 40) gives rise to a system that is unwieldy for use in routine laboratory work. The system described here is more amenable for use in a clinical tissue typing laboratory and achieves a resolution at least equivalent to that of good serology.

However, there are a number of shortcomings. For example, it has been shown that the 5′ primers used in this study do not amplify HLA-B54 because of a nucleotide mismatch at the 3′-end of the primers. This could be overcome by using primers described by Cereb et al. [3] which are derived from locus-specific sequences in the noncoding introns flanking exons II and III. However, initial data published under the auspices of the 12th International Histocompatibility Workshop indicate that the 3′ HLA-B primers used in two separate PCR reactions in this study achieve a higher level of resolution compared with the intron primers used in a single reaction [9]. A possible solution (although not investigated here) may be achieved by combining the 5′ primer described by Cereb et al. [3] with the 3′ primers (D1 and D1X) in separate reactions, as used in this study.

Finally, in considering the application of the improved HLA-B PCR-SSOP typing system, developed in this study, the B-lymphoblastoid cell line FLE was found to type as a B*5701/2 with the oligoprobes used in this study, but had been previously reported as B63 in the literature [8]. The sequence data published by Hildebrand and colleagues [6] has designated B63 as B*1517 and, on comparison with previously published HLA class I nucleotide sequences, shows that this allele shares sequence motifs with B*5701/2 accounting for the identical oligoprobe reaction pattern and ambiguous typing using the current panel of probes. In addition, the discrepancy found between serology and PCR-SSOP in one sample remains to be resolved, but it is unlikely to be due to a failure of the PCR-SSOP typing system.

Generally, the HLA-A PCR-SSOP typing system described in this study is a simplified version of one described by Oh et al. [17]. Originally 28 SSOPs were used to type the HLA-A locus but this was reduced to 16 SSOPs for the purpose of this study. The results show that this modified version of the typing system can achieve a comparable level of resolution to that achievable by good serology. The use of the ARMS-PCR system on a small series of samples verified the PCR-SSOP results and also showed that the molecular methods could discriminate between alleles that can be difficult to assign by serology.

The application of improved PCR-SSOP methods for HLA-A and HLA-B as applied in this study shows it is possible to routinely type these loci in the laboratory with a resolution at least equal to that of serology. In addition, the PCR-SSOP typing methods can be used to supplement serological typing of 'problem' HLA-A and -B specificities, e.g. subtypes of A19. Both methods are an improvement over previously published systems offering a higher level of resolution without using a high number of probes for the B locus and a streamlined typing system, without significant loss of resolution, for the HLA-A locus.

Acknowledgements Thanks are due to Dr. M. Browning (University of Leicester) and Dr. P. Krausa (Institute of Molecular Medicine, Oxford) for making available HLA-B primer sequences and to Dr. J. Bidwell, Dr. N. Wood (University of Bristol), Dr. K. Poulton (University of Manchester) and Mrs. F. Williams (Northern Ireland Tissue Typing Laboratory) for probe design and synthesis under the auspices of a working group of the British Society for Histocompatibility and Immunogenetics. Financial support from the South and West Regional Health Authority and Hybaid Limited is gratefully acknowledged.

References

1. Bidwell JL, Jarrold EA (1986) HLA-DR allogenotyping using exon-specific cDNA probes and application of rapid mini-gel methods. Mol Immunol 23: 1111–1116

2. Bodmer JG, Petronzelli F, Browning M, Krausa P (1995) Pilot study on an ARMS-PCR class I DNA typing method. Eur J Immunogen 22: 25

3. Cereb N, Maye P, Lee S, Kong Y, Yang SY (1995) Locus-specific amplification of HLA class I genes from genomic DNA: locus-specific sequences in the first and third introns of HLA-A, -B, and -C alleles. Tissue Antigens 45: 1–11

4. Fernandez-Viña M, Lazaro AM, Sun Y, Miller S, Forero L, Stastny P (1995) Population diversity of B-locus alleles observed by high-resolution DNA typing. Tissue Antigens 45: 153–168

5. Fleischhauer K, Kernan NA, O'Reilly RJ, Dupont B, Yang SY (1990) Bone marrow allograft rejection by T lymphocytes recognizing a single amino acid difference in HLA-B44. N Engl J Med 323: 1818–1822

6. Hildebrand WH, Domena JD, Shen SY, Lau M, Terasaki PI, Bunce M, Marsh SGE, Guttridge MG, Bias WB, Parham P (1994) HLA-B15: A widespread and diverse family of HLA-B alleles. Tissue Antigens 43: 209–218

7. Huetz F, Mariotti M, Lucotte G (1987) Taq I restriction polymorphism of HLA Class-I genes, and hybridization with HLA-A and HLA-B specific probes. Expl Clin Immunogen 4: 1–7

8. Jaraquemada D, Reinsmoen NL, Ollier W, Okoye R, Bach FH, Festenstein H (1984) First level testing of HLA-DR4-associated new HLA-D specificities: Dw13(DB3), Dw14(LD40), Dw15(DYT), and DKT2. In: Albert ED, Baur MP, Mayr WR (eds) Histocompatibility Testing 1984. Springer, Heidelberg, pp 270–274

9. Kennedy L, Poulton K (1995) BSHI class I SSOP pilot study: full report. 12th W Express 4: 23–29

10. Levine JE, Yang SY (1994) SSOP typing of the 10th International Histocompatibility Workshop reference cell lines for HLA-C alleles. Tissue Antigens 44: 174–183

11. Lund T, Festenstein H (1991) HLA and disease. In: Brostoff J, Scadding GK, Male D, Roitt IM (eds) Clinical immunology. Gower Medical Publishing, London, pp 2.1–2.10

12. Martin S, Dyer PA (1993) The case for matching MHC genes in human organ transplantation. Nature Genetics 5: 210–213

13. Middleton D, Williams F, Cullen C, Mallon E (1995) Modification of a HLA-B PCR-SSOP typing system leading to improved allele determination. Tissue Antigens 45: 232–236

14. Milford EL, Kennedy LJ, Yang SY, Dupont B, Lalouel J-M, Yunis EJ (1989) Serologic characterization of the reference panel of B-lymphoblastoid cell lines for factors of the HLA system. In: Dupont B (ed) Immunobiology of HLA, vol I, Histocompatibility Testing 1987. Springer, New York, pp 19–38

15. Miller SA, Dykes DD, Polesky HF (1988) A simple salting-out procedure for extracting DNA from human nucleated cells. Nucleic Acids Res 16: 1215

16. Mytileneos J, Scherer S, Opelz G (1990) Comparison of RFLP-DR beta and serological HLA-DR typing in 1500 individuals. Transplantation 50: 870–873

17. Oh S, Fleischhauer K, Yang SY (1993) Isoelectric focussing subtypes of HLA-A can be defined by oligonucleotide typing. Tissue Antigens 41: 135–142

18. Opelz G, Wujciak T, Mytilineos J, Scherer S (1993) Revisting HLA matching for kidney transplantation. Transplant Proc 25: 173–175

19. Steinle A, Reinhardt C, Nößner E, Uchanska-Ziegler B, Ziegler A, Schendel DJ (1993) Microheterogeneity in HLA-B35 alleles influences peptide-dependent allorecognition by cytotoxic T cells but not binding of a peptide-restricted monoclonal antibody. Hum Immunol 38: 261–269

20. Terasaki PI, Bernoco D, Pane MS, Ozturk G, Iwaki Y (1978) Microdroplet testing for HLA-A, -B, -C and -D antigens. Am J Clin Pathol 69: 103–120

21. Weston SL, Jack D, Robertson NH, Ferrie RM, O'Keefe C, Buckel A, Little S (1995) Development of a multiplex ARMS method for HLA A-locus DNA typing. Eur J Immunogen 22: 25

22. Yang SY (1989) Assignment of HLA-A and HLA-B antigens for the reference panel of B-lymphoblastoid cell lines determined by one-dimensional isoelectric focusing (1D-IEF) gel electrophoresis. In: Dupont B (ed) Immunobiology of HLA, vol I, Histocompatibility Testing 1987. Springer, New York, pp 43–44

23. Yang SY, Milford E, Hammerling U, Dupont B (1989) Description of the reference panel of B-lymphoblastoid cell lines for factors of the HLA system: The B-cell line panel designed for the Tenth International Histocompatibility Workshop. In: Dupont B (ed) Immunobiology of HLA, vol I, Histocompatibility Testing 1987. Springer, New York, pp 11–19

24. Yoshida M, Kimura A, Numaro F, Sasazuki T (1992) Polymerase-chain-reaction-based analysis of polymorphism in the HLA-B gene. Hum Immunol 34: 257–266

Transpl Int (1996) 9 [Suppl 1]: S 364–S 367
© Springer-Verlag 1996

D. Talbot
M. White
B. K. Shenton
A. Bell
D. Manas
G. Proud
R. M. R. Taylor

Flow cytometric crossmatching in renal transplantation – outcome after five years

D. Talbot (✉) · M. White · B. K. Shenton ·
A. Bell · D. Manas · G. Proud ·
R. M. R. Taylor
Renal Transplant Unit, Royal Victoria
Infirmary, Newcastle-upon-Tyne NE1 4LP,
UK

Abstract The association of a positive flow cytometric crossmatch between recipient IgG directed against donor T lymphocytes and poor outcome is well described in renal transplantation. Until now, no long-term follow-up on such patients has been available. A total of 117 renal transplant patients were followed up for a period of 5 years. Of these, 21 were known to have donor T cell-directed IgG and 5 had B lymphocyte-directed IgG. Both groups of patients with these antibodies had a significantly poorer outcome at 5 years than did the group of patients without IgG ($P < 0.0001$ Handel Maenzel test). Patients with antibody detected preoperatively were tested again, either at the time of graft failure or at 5 years posttrans-plantation. The sera were tested against stored donor cells and the intensity of surface IgG compared with the preoperative levels. In those recipients who lost their grafts, the levels increased in 60 % of cases but those that retained their grafts also had an increase in levels of donor-directed antibody in 50 % of cases. The changing levels of antibody therefore appeared to have little relevance to outcome. However, when IgG isotypes were considered, for those who experienced graft failure and also had a γ_3 isotype, a rise in IgG was demonstrated in all cases. Conversely, successful grafts with γ_3 had a decline in levels between preoperative and 5-year samples in three of the four cases (p not significant).

Introduction

The association of a positive flow cytometric crossmatch between recipient IgG directed against donor T lymphocytes and poor outcome is well described in renal transplantation. Most series to date demonstrate the outcome up to 1 year [1, 5, 6, 7, 8] after transplantation but no long-term data exist regarding graft survival after 5 years from transplantation.

Materials and methods

Patient group

A total of 117 renal transplants was studied retrospectively. The transplants were performed between August 1985 and April 1988 during the time when the flow cytometric crossmatch was under investigation. At this time although the results of the flow cytometric crossmatch were known by the research team, this knowledge was not shared with the clinicians involved.

The transplants were from cadaveric donors and the recipients were receiving their first graft in 81.4 % of cases, the remainder being regrafts. There was a mean of 1.53 A/B locus match and 0.83 DR match between donor and recipient human lymphocyte antigen (HLA). At that time there was a policy of not transplanting across a warm or cold, historic or current cytotoxic T cell crossmatch, immaterial of B crossmatch or panel reactivity. The mean current panel reactivity was 7.1 % for the whole group with a

S365

Fig. 1 Renal graft survival with and without preoperative donor-directed IgG as detected by flow cytometry

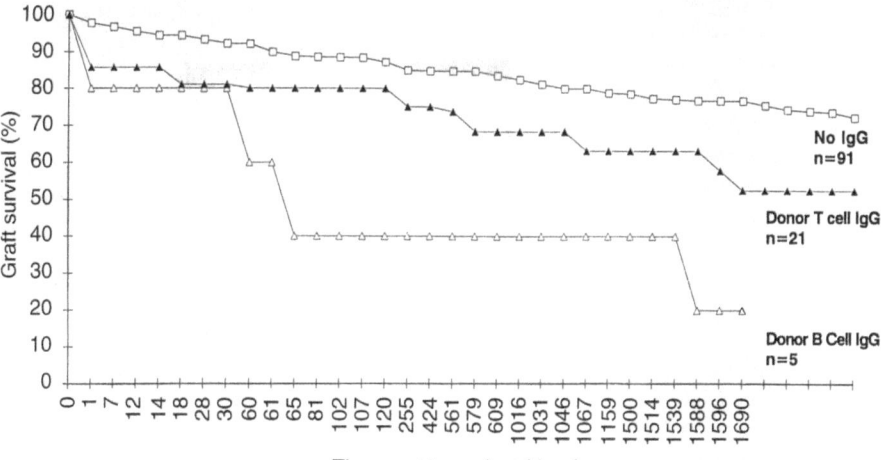

mean peak of 21.6 %. Cyclosporin was used as the base-line immunosuppression in 94 % of cases.

The flow cytometric crossmatch

This was performed as described previously [9] using donor splenocytes and current recipient sera. Six sera from healthy volunteers were used as controls. Anti-CD3 and anti-CD20 (Becton Dickinson) were used to label T and B cells, respectively, and anti-human IgG Fc (Sigma) was used to label the test or control sera. The cell/sera combinations after incubation and washings were exposed to the labelling antibodies. After further incubation and washing, the cells were analysed in a FACS 420 using Consort 30 software (Becton Dickinson).

Second serum analysis

Serum samples were obtained, when available, from the Tissue Typing laboratories where they were stored after routine periodic panel reactivity testing. When a graft failed, the nearest serum sample was obtained prior to the failure. Otherwise, the second sample of serum was obtained approximately 5 years after transplantation. The second sample was tested against the appropriate donor cells which had been stored in liquid nitrogen since the time of transplantation. In this way, 18 combinations were retested for the second sera out of the original 26 transplants known to have lymphocyte-directed IgG, as detected by flow cytometry.

With small numbers of cells viable after thawing the samples 5 or more years after transplantation, it was not possible to discriminate between B or T lymphocytes and therefore data analysis was performed on ungated samples. The 530-nm fluorescence (proportional to surface IgG) was determined for test and control sera and expressed as a ratio. The ratios determined for preoperative and 5-year samples were obtained with the flow cytometer aligned in the same way using fluorescent marker beads (Becton Dickinson).

IgG isotype detection

This has been previously described [10]. Briefly, donor splenocytes were incubated with the control or test sera. After incubation and washing, the cells were incubated with mouse anti-human γ_1, γ_2, γ_3 or γ_4 monoclonal antibodies (Serotec). The cells after washing

were incubated with goat anti-mouse antibody conjugated with fluorescein isothiocyanate (Becton Dickinson). After further washing, the cells were incubated with a non-specific mouse serum to saturate spare binding sites. Finally, after more washing, the cells were incubated with anti-CD3 or anti-CD20 conjugated with phycoerythrin depending on the known affinity of the recipient sera. The cells were then analysed in the flow cytometer. The 530-nm fluorescence (fluorescein) of the 575-nm positively fluorescent cells (phycoerythrin) was compared between the recipient/donor combinations and the control/donor combinations.

Results

The outcome of the total group of 117 recipients is illustrated in Fig. 1. The total graft survival at 5 years was 59 %. There were 13 deaths with functioning grafts; if these are considered lost to follow-up, the proportion of patients with functioning grafts rises to 66.3 %. When the patients are subdivided into those without antibodies detectable preoperatively, the 5-year graft survival is 72.5 % (58/80 with 11 deaths). Those recipients with T-directed IgG as detected by flow cytometry preoperatively ($n = 21$), had a 5-year graft survival of 52.6 % (with 2 deaths). All these patients had no cytotoxic antibodies detectable by standard means and the grafts lost were for biopsy-proven rejection in 90 % of cases. When recipients with B-directed IgG are considered ($n = 5$), the 5-year graft survival is considerably less at 20 %. Both these survival curves are significantly worse than the zero antibody group, as assessed by the Handel Maenzel test ($P < 0.0001$).

Obviously, there were still some recipients with donor-directed IgG as detected by flow cytometry preoperatively who had no problem with rejection and did quite well (11 surviving at 5 years). These patients were no different regarding risk factors of tissue match (1.6 versus 1.4 match for A/B loci, 0.6 versus 0.6 match for DR, fail versus success, respectively), ischaemic times

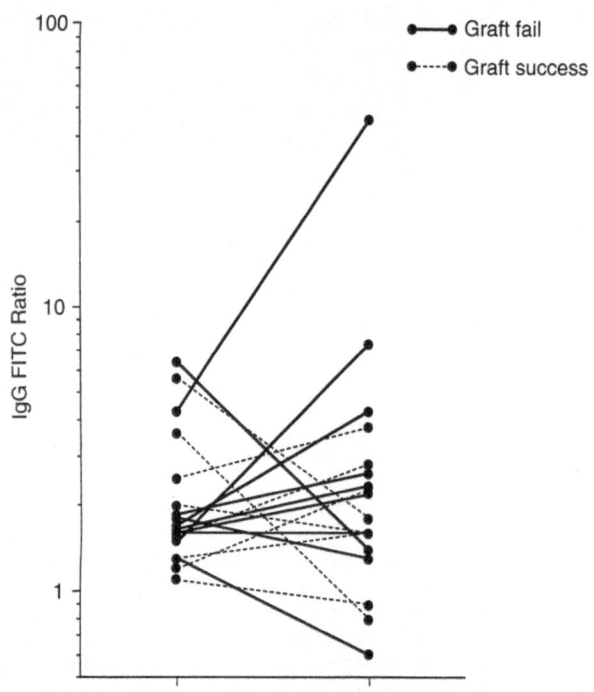

Fig. 2 Recipient/control sera ratio of IgG fluorescein isothiocyanate *(FITC)* before and after renal transplantation

(cold: 1174 versus 1156 min, warm: 34 versus 31 min, fail versus success, respectively) and regraft (42 % versus 36 %, fail versus success, respectively). This led us to retest the recipients at 5 years for the presence of donor-directed IgG. Figure 2 illustrates the changing antibody ratios with time (test/control). On first inspection of the figure it appears that the group that failed generally has an increasing level of antibody, as would be expected. However, this did not occur in all cases (60 %). Considering the converse, where grafts were retained, one would expect a decline in levels of antibody but the findings actually showed a rise in 50 % of cases. There were insufficient samples to retest for IgG isotypes to clarify the situation in the second sample but isotype

testing had been performed in a number (16) of cases preoperatively. The results are summarised in Table 1. In eight cases, γ_3 only was identified and in these cases a subsequent rise always indicated failure (100 %) whereas a decline indicated that the graft would be retained in most cases (75 %). Statistical significance was not achieved but this was probably due to insufficient numbers ($P = 0.07$, Fishers exact test).

Discussion

The survival curves illustrated in Fig. 1, whilst showing a worse outcome with T- or B-directed IgG, suggest that the biggest impact for T-directed IgG occurs early. The curves then are largely parallel, suggesting that control has been achieved at a cost. This is obviously not the situation for the B-positive group where the lines diverge. Admittedly, the numbers of B-positive combinations were small ($n = 5$) but they confirm the finding of others where outcome was noted to be worse [2–4].

Why outcome should vary in the flow cytometric crossmatch combinations led us to to test other factors such as regraft, mismatch and ischaemic times, but no differences could be established between those that functioned and those that failed. Retesting for donor-directed antibody at 5 years was interesting in so far as this also did not reflect outcome. This would suggest that late rejection bears no relationship to antibody changes and that cellular events are the important factors.

However, IgG isotypes were apparently of some help, with rising IgG and γ_3 in preoperative samples indicating failure and falling levels indicating salvage. However, graft failure could still be seen in recipients with $\gamma_{1,2}$ and γ_4 isotypes, again suggesting that cellular events were of more importance.

Further conclusions could possibly have been drawn if the target of the antibodies was established. Unfortunately, there was insufficient donor material to establish anti-class I or II activity.

Table 1 Outcome after renal transplantation in flow cytometric positive combinations with known donor lymphocyte-directed IgG. The ratio of fluorescence to control is shown for preoperative samples and for sera collected prior to graft loss or at 5 years posttransplantation

Recipient	IgG target	γ Isotype	Test/control fluorescence (pretransplant sera)	Test/control fluorescence (5 years post-transplant sera)	Outcome
Jo	T	γ_3	4.3	45.8	Fail
Si	T	γ_3	1.5	7.4	Fail
Go	T	γ_3	5.6	1.8	OK
Ho	T	γ_3	1.1	0.9	OK
Sn	T	γ_3	1.6	2.2	Fail
Cr	T	γ_3	1.3	1.6	OK
Wh	T	γ_{2+3}	1.2	2.3	OK
Mc	B	γ_3	1.6	1.6	Fail
Sw	T	γ_2	2.5	3.8	OK
Da	B	γ_2	1.7	4.4	Fail
Ri	T	γ_3	3.6	0.9	OK

In summary, this study serves to confirm the original concept that a positive preoperative flow cytometric crossmatch for IgG to T lymphocytes carries a poorer prognosis for outcome. The principal effect is seen early, with the survival curves subsequently paralleling those of the zero antibody group. For B-directed IgG, the results appear to be even worse and this is now currently under evaluation in our centre.

Acknowledgements This work was supported by the Northern Counties Kidney Research Fund.

References

1. Evans PR, Lane AC, Lambert CM, et al (1992) Lack of correlation between IgG T-lymphocyte flow cytometric crossmatches with primary renal allograft outcome. Transpl Int [Suppl] 5: 609–612
2. Farley TJ, Shanahan TC, Bartholomew WR (1989) Resolution of the B cell positive crossmatch by a modified flow cytometric procedure. Transplantation 48: 535–537
3. Garovoy MR, Colombe BW, Melzer J, et al (1985) Flow cytometry crossmatching for donor specific transfusion recipients and cadaveric transplantation. Transplant Proc 17: 693–695
4. Lazda VA (1994) Identification of patients at risk for inferior renal allograft outcome by a strongly positive B cell flow cytometry crossmatch. Transplantation 57: 964–969
5. Mahoney RJ, Ault K, Given SR, et al (1990) The flow cytometric crossmatch and early transplant loss. Transplantation 49: 527–534
6. Talbot D (1993) The flow cytometric crossmatch in perspective. Transpl Immunol 1: 155–162
7. Talbot D, Givan AL, Shenton BK, et al (1989) The relevance of a more sensitive crossmatch to renal transplantation. Transplantation 47: 552–555
8. Talbot D, Givan AL, Shenton BK, et al (1990) The prospective value of the preoperative flow cytometric crossmatch in renal transplantation. Transplantation 49: 809–810
9. Talbot D, Givan AL, Shenton BK, et al (1988) Rapid detection of low levels of donor specific IgG by flow cytometry with single and dual colour fluorescence in renal transplantation. J Immunol Methods 112: 279–283
10. Talbot D, Givan AL, Shenton BK, et al (1988) The nature of donor specific IgG isotypes identified by flow cytometry in the preoperative crossmatch. Transplant Proc 20: 84–85

Transpl Int (1996) 9 [Suppl 1]: S368–S371
© Springer-Verlag 1996

D. C. Wahoff*
B. E. Papalois
L. A. Nelson
J. P. Leone
J. A. Everett
D. E. R. Sutherland

Allograft tolerance by intrathymic donor splenocyte transfer: an age-dependent, species-specific phenomenon?

D. C. Wahoff · B. E. Papalois · L. A. Nelson ·
J. P. Leone · J. A. Everett ·
D. E. R. Sutherland
Department of Surgery,
University of Minnesota, Minneapolis,
Minnesota, USA

D. E. R. Sutherland (✉)
Box 280 UMHC,
420 Delaware St. S. E.,
Minneapolis, MN 55455, USA
Ph + 1-612-625-7600
FAX + 1-612-625-8496

Abstract Protocols that allow allograft survival without immunosuppression remain the ultimate goal in transplantation. Intrathymic injection of donor splenocytes into a transiently immunosuppressed recipient has induced tolerance to a variety of subsequently transplanted allografts in rats. The purpose of this study was to determine if recipient age is critical to intrathymic tolerance in light of age-dependent thymic changes, and if this protocol can be extended to an outbred, large animal model. Prepubertal and postpubertal Wistar-Furth rats underwent intrathymic injection of splenocytes from Lewis rats and antilymphocyte serum (ALS) intraperitoneally. On day 21, a heterotopic Lewis heart was transplanted, with graft survival evaluated by cardiac palpation. Graft tolerance (> 100 days) occurred in four out of five (80 %) of the prepubertal rats compared to two out of six (33 %) postpubertal rats. Tolerance was not demonstrated in rats receiving intrathymic injection of buffer only. In puppies, groups 1 and 2 underwent splenectomy with intrathymic injec-

tion of *allo* splenocytes. Control puppies (group 3) received intrathymic *auto* splenocytes. Groups 1 and 3 were given antilymphocyte gamma globulin (ALG) on days 7 to 0 with respect to the intrathymic injection. Group 2 did not receive ALG, but instead received cyclosporin A (CSA) on days 0–2. On day 21, all puppies underwent bilateral nephrectomy and single renal transplantation. No additional immunosuppression was given. Tolerance (creatinine < 7 mg/dl for 100 days) was not obtained by any dog in all three groups. There was no difference in graft survival between control and experimental dogs, with the longest surviving graft seen in a control dog (26 days). Our results suggest that thymic change during maturation may alter the ability to induce tolerance by intrathymic injection of donor cells in rats, and that the protocol is not easily adapted to large animals.

Key words Transplant tolerance · Intrathymic injection · Rodent · Canine

* Recipient of an American College of Surgeons research scholarship

Introduction

Permanent acceptance of an allograft without long-term nonspecific immunosuppressant medications is the goal of transplantation research. The concept of induction of transplantation tolerance was pioneered in the 1950's by Medawar [1]; since then many protocols have successfully induced donor-specific unresponsiveness in selected inbred rodent donor-recipient strain combinations [4–8]. In other reports, cyclosporin (CSA), a common immunosuppressive agent, has been used as an adjunct to tolerance induction [2, 3]. It is thought that the mechanism of action of CSA is that it interferes with secondary signals involved in cellular immunological interactions. Unfortunately, many of the experimental protocols described in rodents have either not been successful or have not been completely tested in outbred, large animal models [2–8].

One of the most recent and novel schemes to induce allograft tolerance in mice and rats as described by Posselt et al., involves injection of donor antigen or tissue into the thymus of a recipient transiently immunosuppressed with an antilymphocyte antibody prior to transplantation [6]. Previously published reports on variations of the Posselt protocol have used prepubertal rodents [4]. However, the thymus undergoes spontaneous involution at puberty in humans, possibly restricting the time period in which the thymus must be exposed to donor antigen. This possibility must be investigated prior to using the Posselt protocol in human beings. The purpose of this study was threefold: (1) to determine if allograft (heart) tolerance by intrathymic injection is equally successful in pre- and postpubertal rats, (2) to translate the protocol to prepubertal outbred dogs in a renal allograft model, and (3) to determine if the use of CSA rather than antilymphocyte antibody in the protocol could promote unresponsiveness in conjunction with intrathymic injection of donor cells.

Materials and methods

Rodent experiment

Animals

Prepubertal (< 6 weeks, 100 to 150 g) and postpubertal (> 8 months, > 400 g) Wistar-Furth (RT1, WF) rats were used as recipients. Prepubertal Lewis (RT1, LEW) rats were the donor animals for the splenocytes and heart allografts.

Preparation of donor splenocytes

Donor LEW splenocytes were obtained by dispersion of the pulp through a 100-μm plastic screen followed by erythrocyte lysis with Tris-NH$_4$Cl (0.83 %) at 37 °C. The splenocytes were then washed three times with Hank's balanced salt solution (HBSS, Celox, Hopkins, Minn.) and stored at 4 °C until injection.

Intrathymic injection and immunosuppression

The thymus of the LEW recipients was exposed through a partial median sternotomy and either a total of 3×10^7 splenocytes or HBSS was injected into both lobes with a 30-guage needle. After intrathymic injection, a single 1-ml dose of rabbit anti-rat antilymphocyte serum (ALS, Accurate Chemical Corp, Westbury, N.Y.) was injected intraperitoneally.

Heterotopic cardiac transplantion

Twenty-one days after intrathymic injection, heterotopic abdominal cardiac allografts were performed by the technique developed by Ono and Lindsey [5]. Graft survival was determined by daily palpation. A palpable heartbeat indicated graft function; cessation of a heartbeat along with histologic rejection defined graft failure. Tolerance was defined as graft survival > 100 days

Canine experiment

Animals

Outbred puppies (< 3 months old and weighing 5–10 kg) were used as both the recipients and donors.

Intrathymic injection and immunosuppression

On day 0, all puppies underwent splenectomy and intrathymic injection of 2×10^9 donor allo- or autosplenocytes. Splenocytes were isolated by straining through a 100-μm screen after tissue was minced and gently crushed at 37 °C in Tris-NH$_4$Cl (0.83 %) buffer. In groups 1 and 3, antilymphocyte gamma globulin IV (ALG; 40 mg/kg per day) was administered intravenously from day – 7 to day 0 (with respect to the day on which the splenocyte injection was performed). Group 2 puppies received oral CSA (20 mg/kg per day) for 3 days from day 0 to day 2 following splenocyte transplantation. This group did not receive ALG, and CSA was not given following kidney transplantation. Instead of allosplenocytes, the control puppies (group 3) received an intrathymic injection of autologous splenocytes following splenectomy.

Renal transplantation

Twenty-one days after splenocyte injection, the puppies underwent bilateral nephrectomies followed by single kidney allotransplantations from the previous splenocyte donors for groups 1 and 2, except for the control group puppies (group 3) who received an injection of their own splenocytes. Surgically, the renal artery was anastamosed end-to-end to the external iliac artery and the renal vein was anastomosed to the external iliac vein in an end-to-side fashion. The ureteral-bladder anastomosis was done by pulling the ureter into the bladder through a puncture on its underside and then fixed in place with a simple suture. No postoperative immunosuppression was given, and rejection was monitored by measuring urine creatinine levels daily. Graft failure was defined by a creatinine level > 7 mg/dl and was histologically confirmed to be rejection. Tolerance was defined as graft survival > 100 days.

Statistics

The Mann-Whitney *U*-test was used for comparison of independent samples with nonuniform sampling distributions to determine the probability that differences between graft survivals were due to chance alone. Fisher's exact test for comparison of two proportions in independent samples was used to compare differences in tolerance between treatment groups.

Animal care

For the animal experiments, the *Principles of laboratory animal care* (NIH publication No. 86-23, revised 1985) were followed, as well as the regulations required by the USDA Animal Welfare Act and the University of Minnesota animal care committee.

Results

Rodents (Table 1)

In the prepubertal rodents four out of five (80%) animals were tolerant (grafts functioned > 100 days), while in the postpubertal group two out of six (33%) animals achieved tolerance (Fisher's exact $P = 0.24$). Prepubertal ($n = 2$) and postpubertal ($n = 4$) WF rats that received buffer only intrathymically plus ALS did not become tolerant (mean graft survival 14 ± 2 days). No animals died due to intrathymic injection of splenocytes, intraperitoneal injection of ALS, or technical complications of the cardiac transplant.

Canine (Table 2)

Tolerance was not achieved in the large animal model (Table 2). In the experimental group that received allosplenocytes intrathymically, ten out of ten grafts failed before 26 days; the longest duration of function was seen in the three controls who received an intrathymic injection of autosplenocytes. The addition of a short course of CSA following allosplenocyte injection did not prolong renal allograft survival. No animals died due to intrathymic injection of splenocytes, nor did ALG or CSA therapy result in death. Three allografts failed due to technical failure (i.e., urine leak or thrombosis), and the dogs were not included in analysis.

Discussion

Many investigators have shown that donor-specific tolerance can be induced in rodents after intrathymic injection of donor alloantigen followed by subsequent transplant of various allografts [4–7]. In humans the thymus undergoes spontaneous postpubertal involution. Therefore, thymic change may alter the effect of induced tolerance by donor intrathymic transfer in animals. In our study, tolerance was more frequent in prepubertal rats after intrathymic injection of allosplenocytes and ALS therapy. However, further studies using larger numbers of rats are needed to determine if the differences are statistically significant.

When a similar protocol of intrathymic injection of alloantigen and ALS for donor-specific tolerance was transferred to large animals, puppies were chosen as the experimental model based on the improved results in the prepubertal rats. With our protocol, puppies receiving intrathymic allosplenocytes and ALS prior to renal allograft transplantation failed to demonstrate graft survival consistent with tolerance as defined in this study. The substitution of CSA as an adjunct to intrathymic injection of splenocytes was also unsuccessful in prolonging graft survival. Thus, a protocol designed to inhibit antigen recognition and sensitization via secondary signals at the time of antigen presentation did not alter time to graft rejection in this model.

Failure to replicate long-term survival by intrathymic transplant in the dog model implies that this phenomenon may be species specific. Thus, tolerance by intrathymic donor splenocyte injection, like many other tolerance schemes, may be unique to young, inbred rodents. Variations in lymphocyte depletion, intrathymic tissue type and dose, timing of the allograft placement, and the duration and dose of adjunct therapies (i.e., total lymphoid irradiation, immunosuppressive drugs, ultraviolet irradiation of donor tissue, etc.) need to be studied further if allograft unresponsiveness is to be obtained in higher mammals.

Table 1 Lewis cardiac allograft survival in prepubertal (Pre) and postpubertal (Post) Wistar-Furth (WF) rats after receiving Lewis splenocytes intrathymically (IT) and antilymphocyte serum (ALS)

Group	n	Treatment	Graft survival time		Tolerance[b] (%)
			days[a]	median	
Pre	5	IT Lew SC + ALS	15, > 100 × 4	100	4/5 (80)
Post	6	IT Lew SC + ALS	9, 9, 10, 53, > 100 × 2	37.5	2/6 (33)

[a] Mann-Whitney $P = 0.14$
[b] Fisher's Exact – $P = 0.24$

Table 2 Renal allograft survival in prepubertal dogs after intrathymic (IT) injection of auto- or allosplenocytes with antilymphocyte gamma globulin (ALG) or cyclosporin (CSA) immunosuppression (*SC* splenocytes)

Group	Treatment	n	Graft survival time		Tolerance (%)
			days[a]	median	
1	T allo SC + ALG	10	3, 5, 6 × 3, 7, 8, 15 × 2, 25	6.5	0/10 (0)
2	IT allo SC + CSA	5	7, 7, 8, 8, 11	8.0	0/5 (0)
3	IT auto SC + ALG	3	7, 7, 26	7.0	0/3 (0)

[a] Mann-Whitney 1 vs 2 $P = 0.46$; 1 vs 3 P 0.31; 2 vs 3 $P = 0.88$

References

1. Billingham R, Brent L, Medawar P (1956) Actively acquired tolerance of foreign cells. Nature 172: 603–605
2. Calne RY, Watson CJE, Brons IGM, Makisalo H, Metcalfe SM, Sriwatana-wongsa V, Davies HS (1994) Tolerance of porcine renal allografts induced by donor spleen cells and seven days' treatment with cyclosporine. Transplantation 57: 1433–1435
3. Hartner WC, Markees TG, De Fazio SR, Shaffer D, Van der Werf WJ, Gilchrist B, Yatko C, Monaco AP, Gozzo JJ (1995) Effect of early administration of donor bone marrow cells on renal allograft survival in dogs treated with antilymphocyte serum and cyclosporine. Transplantation 59: 131–155
4. Nakafusa Y, Goss JA, Mohanakumar T, Flye MW (1993) Induction of donor-specific tolerance to cardiac but not skin or renal allografts by intrathymic injection of splenocyte alloantigen. Transplantation 55: 877–882
5. Ono K, Lindsey ES (1969) Improved technique of heart transplantation in rats. J Thorac Cardiovasc Surg 57: 225
6. Posselt AM, Barker CF, Thomaszewski JE, Markmann JF, Choti MA, Naji A (1990) Induction of donor-specific unresponsiveness by intrathymic islet transplantation. Science 249: 1293
7. Remuzzi G, Rossini M, Imberti O, Perico N (1991) Kidney graft survival in rats without immunosuppressants after intrathymic glomerular transplantation. Lancet 337: 750–752
8. Vriens PW, Nisco SJ, Hoyt EG, Lyu S-C, Pierre P, Reitz BA, Clayberger C (1994) Tissue-specific differences in the establishment of tolerance: tolerogenic effects of lung allografts in rats. Transplantation 57: 1795–1798

Transpl Int (1996) 9 [Suppl 1]: S 372–S 378
© Springer-Verlag 1996

Basil E. Papalois
David C. Wahoff
Tor C. Aasheim
Robert J. Griffin
Jose Jessurun
Sue M. Clemmings
Jane M. Field
John P. Leone
David E. R. Sutherland

Total lymphoid irradiation, without intrathymic injection of donor cells, induces indefinite acceptance of heart but not islet or skin allografts in rats

B. E. Papalois · D. C. Wahoff · T. C. Aasheim
S. M. Clemmings · J. M. Fields · J. P. Leone ·
D. E. R. Sutherland (✉)
Department of Surgery, Box 280, UMHC,
420 Delaware Street, S. E.,
Minneapolis, MN 55455, USA
Tel. +1 612 625 7600;
Fax +1 612 625 8496

R. J. Griffin
Department of Therapeutic Radiology,
University of Minnesota, Minneapolis,
Minnesota, USA

J. Jessurun
Laboratory of Medicine and Pathology,
University of Minnesota, Minneapolis,
Minnesota, USA

Abstract Allograft tolerance occurs in rodents given a dose of anti-lymphocyte serum (ALS) and intrathymic injection (ITI) of donor splenocytes (SC) 1–3 weeks prior to transplant (TX). The purpose of our study was to test total lymphoid irradiation (TLI) as an alternative to ALS in ITI tolerance induction to heart, islet, and skin allografts. Prepubertal Wistar Furth rats were recipients. ITI of donor (Lewis) SC was done at the end of the TLI course. Rats received either a heterotopic heart, a skin graft, or 2300 islets (diabetic recipients) intraportally from Lewis donors. TLI (without ITI) in a dose of 200 rads/day for 5 consecutive days, followed by TX in 3 weeks resulted in indefinite acceptance of heart (but not islet or skin) grafts in 60 % of the recipients. These data indicate that TLI by a dose schedule of 200 rads/day for 5 days should be tested for clinical relevance in large animal recipients of immediately vascularized grafts.

Key words Transplantation · Tolerance · Thymus · Irradiation · Rodents

Introduction

Systemic immunosuppression for organ transplantation often results in drug-specific toxicity and long-term immunosuppression is a major cause of morbidity and mortality [5]. These complications could be avoided if it were possible to achieve a state of donor-specific unresponsiveness without subsequent immunosuppression [2], and tolerance is the ultimate goal of transplantation.

It is known that thymocytes originate from bone marrow multipotential hematopoietic stem cells and mature in the thymus into antigen-reactive T-lymphocytes before migrating to the peripheral lymphoid organs [4]. A variety of protocols has been able to achieve donor-specific unresponsiveness to organ allografts in rodents [2]. One approach developed recently has involved depletion of mature T-cells followed by intrathymic exposure to alloantigen [3] or donor hematopoietic cells [7]. With such a protocol the recipient theoretically "relearns" self in the context of the new alloantigen, but this theory does not explain why the unresponsiveness may be organ-specific (e. g., heart accepted, skin or kidney rejected) [6]. In rodents, most protocols that used intrathymic injection (ITI) gave a single dose of anti-lymphocyte serum (ALS) at the time when donor cells were inoculated, 3 weeks prior to transplantation [3, 6, 7]. Whether it is important to use an anti-T-cell agent in ITI protocols, or whether a transient generalized immunosuppressant would work as well, has not been determined. The purpose of our study was to determine whether total lymphoid irradiation (TLI) can be used as an alternative to ALS in combination with ITI to induce tolerance to heart, islet or skin allografts in rats. A further rationale to test TLI results from the fact that anti-T-cell agents are not readily available for large animal recipients in which the intrathymic approach would ideally be tested in a preclinical model.

Materials and methods

Animals

For all experiments, the "Principles of laboratory animal care" (NIH publication 86-23, revised 1985) and the regulations of the University of Minnesota Animal Care Committee were followed. Lewis (LEW, RT1') adult male rats were donors and Wistar Furth (WF, RT1^u) prepubertal (age < 6 weeks) male rats were recipients. Brown Norway (BN, RT1^n) adult male rats were used as third party for the in vitro studies.

TLI

WF rats were anesthetized with an i.m. injection of 60 mg/kg of ketamine and the skull, lungs, part of the pelvis, the hind limbs, and the tail were covered with lead shields. In some goups the thymus was also shielded (TS). A Phillips Rt-250 kV orthovoltage X-ray machine was used, and the dose rate was 139.9 rad/min. The rats received either 200 rad/day (a single or five consecutive doses) or 1000 rad/day in a single dose. Total lymphocyte count (LC) was monitored before the administration of TLI, after completion of TLI and before the transplant.

ITI

Donor LEW rats underwent splenectomy under ether anesthesia. The splenocytes were obtained by mincing and then passing the spleen through a 60-μm brass screen, and then lysing the erythrocytes with TRIS-NH$_4$Cl (0.83 %) at 37 °C. The remaining splenocytes were washed 3 times with Hank's balanced solution. After completion of TLI, WF rats were anesthetized with ether, the thymus was exposed through a partial median sternotomy, and a total of 30×10^6 LEW splenocytes were injected into the thymus (approximately 15×10^6 splenocytes in each lobe).

Heart transplantation

Donor (LEW) and recipient (WF) rats were anesthetized with an i.m. injection of 60 mg/kg of ketamine and an i.p. injection of 30 mg/kg of sodium pentobarbital. Heterotopic abdominal heart transplantation was performed using the modified technique of Ono and Lindsey [9]. Graft survival was assessed by daily transabdominal palpation. Rejection was defined by cessation of heart beat and confirmed by histological (hematoxylin and eosin staining) evaluation.

Islet transplantation

WF rats were made diabetic (blood glucose > 400 mg/dl for 2 consecutive days) by a single injection in the tail vein of 55 mg/kg of streptozotocin. Two LEW donors were sacrificed, their pancreata were harvested, and the islets were isolated and purified by a technique which has been previously described [11]. A total of 2300 islet, were transplanted into the portal vein of WF diabetic recipients. Graft survival was assessed by daily blood glucose count and rejection was defined as 2 consecutive days of blood glucose 0062 200 mg/dl. In addition, in order to test islet viability, diabetic LEW rats were transplanted intraportally with 2000 isogenic islets.

Skin transplantation

Donor LEW rats were sacrificed and abdominal skin grafts were harvested using the method of Billingham [1]. The skin grafts were then transplanted (sutured to the dorsal thorax after creating an integument deficit) to WF recipients which were under ether anesthesia. Graft survival was assessed by daily inspection and rejection was defined as graft necrosis and sloughing (> 90 %).

Mixed lymphocyte culture (MLC)

Responder splenocytes were harvested from transplanted WF rats. The spleens were dispersed into a single-cell suspension and washed 3 times in Dubecco's modified Eagle medium (DMEM) supplemented with sodium pyruvate, HEPES, 2-mercaptoethanol, L-glutamine, L-arginine, L-aspaginine, folic acid, penicillin, streptomycin, and 1 % heat-inactivated normal rat serum (HI-NRS, complete C-DMEM). Responder cells (2.5×10^5) were cultured in C-DMEM, 1 % HI-NRS with irradiated stimulator splenocytes (1×10^6 LEW, BN, or autologous splenocytes) in quadruplet 200-ul cultures, pulsed with ^{3}H-thymidine on days 3–7, and then harvested for scintillation counting. Proliferation was assayed by ^{3}H-thymidine incorporation.

Thymus histology

Four prepubertal naive WF rats were sacrificed and the thymus was harvested. The thymus was also harvested from prepubertal WF rats that were sacrificed after receiving 1×200 rad, 1×1000 rad and 5×200 rad (four animals in each group). The samples were stained with hematoxylin and eosin and the cortex/medulla ratio was assessed for the thymic lobules.

Statistical analysis

The Student's t-test was used to compare means. The chi-square test and, when applicable, the Fisher's exact test were used to compare categorical variables. Graft survival rates between groups were compared using the Wilcoxon test. For all statistical tests, a P value of < 0.05 was considered significant.

Experimental design

The heart allograft model is the one for which many previous ITI protocols have achieved good results [3, 6, 7] and in our study was used to assess the most successful TLI/ITI protocol: for each irradiation dose schedule recipients were transplanted either immediately after completion of TLI, or 3 weeks after completion of TLI with or without ITI. The protocols by which the highest rate of graft function > 100 days was achieved were then applied again to the heart allograft model, but with the thymus of the recipients shielded during TLI in order to further explore its role in induction of donor-specific unresponsiveness. In addition, for the same groups of animals with the highest rate of graft function > 100 days, the recipients received a skin transplant at 150 days in order to test their unresponsiveness to different grafts, and MLC studies were conducted (for animals with hearts functioning for at least 150 days) to test in vitro donor-specific unresponsiveness of those recipients. Finally, the protocols that gave the best results in the heart allograft model were tested for ability to prolong islet and skin allograft survival.

Table 1 Heart allograft survival. $P \leq 0.001$ for II versus I, III and V, $P \leq 0.005$ for III versus I, and V, $P \leq 0.04$ for IV versus I and V, $P \leq 0.02$ for IV versus I, III and V, $P \leq 0.02$ for IX versus I, III, IV, and V, $P \leq 0.04$ for X versus I, III, IV, V, VII, VIII, XII, and XIII, $P \leq 0.03$ for XI versus I, II, III, IV, V, VII, and VIII, $P = 0.02$ for XIII versus V. (*ITI* Intrathymic injection, *TS* thymus shielding, *TLI* total lymphoid irradiation)

Group	n	Treatment	Transplant	Graft survival (days)	Median
I	4	None		8, 9, 9, 10	9
II	7	ITI	In 3 weeks[a]	14, 16, 27, 31, 53, 55, 130	31
III	6	1×200 rad	Immediately[b]	11, 11, 12, 14, 17, 22	13
IV	6	1×200 rad	In 3 weeks	9, 9, 12, 15, 23, 62	13.5
V	5	1×200 rad + ITI	In 3 weeks	5, 5, 8, 8, 11	8
VI	5	1×1000 rad	Immediately	15, 22, 30, 174, 192	30
VII	6	1×1000 rad	In 3 weeks	4, 6, 19, 22, 79, 88	21
VIII	6	1×1000 rad + ITI	In 3 weeks	4, 10, 13, 38, 39, 99	25.5
IX	7	5×200 rad	Immediately	23, 27, 30, 37, 57, 65, 348[c]	37
X	10	5×200 rad	In 3 weeks	15, 16, 20, 65, 108, 184, 195, 198[d], 221[d], 269[d]	> 100
XI	11	5×200 rad + ITI	In 3 weeks	6, 35, 38, 81, 84, 118, 137, 145, 214[d], 241[d], 353[d]	> 100
XII	6	5×200 rad + TS	In 3 weeks	4, 9, 24, 29, 41, 45	26.5
XIII	6	5×200 rad + TS + ITI	In 3 weeks	7, 12, 23, 24, 42, 100	23.5

[a] Transplant immediately after comletion of ITI, TLI, or TLI + ITI
[b] Transplant in 3 weeks after completion of ITI, TLI, or TLI + ITI
[c] Sacrificed with a functioning graft because of old age
[d] Sacrificed with a functioning graft for the in vitro studies

Results

TLI was effective in decreasing peripheral blood LC, particularly when 200 rad was given in five consecutive doses. The mean ($\pm$ SD) reduction of the total LC (cells/mm^3) was 7000 ± 1900 for 1×200 rad (the LC for all rats after TLI was between 39 % and 48 % of the LC before TLI), 7600 ± 1400 for 1×1000 rad (the LC for all rats after TLI was between 37 % and 40 % of the LC before TLI), and 17266 ± 2100 for 5×200 rad (the LC for all rats after TLI was between 0 and 17 % of the LC before TLI), ($P = 0.01$ for the mean $\pm$ SD reduction of the LC for 5×200 rad versus 1×200 rad and 1×1000 rad). The total LC reverted to normal range 3 weeks after completion of TLI and regardless of the TLI dose and the induction or not of ITI. There were no apparent side effects after completion of TLI with either the 1×200 rad or 5×200 rad dose schedule. All the rats that received 1×1000 rad developed mild diarrhea and weight loss after completion of TLI.

The results for the heart transplants are presented in Table 1. One protocol (group X, 5×200 rad, transplantation in 3 weeks after TLI) was effective in prolonging median heart allograft survival > 100 days without ITI, and heart allograft survival was > 100 days in 60 % of the recipients in that group. All the other TLI protocols (group III, 1×200 rad, transplant immediately after TLI; group IV, 1×200 rad, transplant 3 weeks after TLI; group VI, 1×1000 rad, transplant immediately after TLI; group VII, 1×1000 rad, transplant 3 weeks after TLI; and group IX, 5×200 rad, transplant immediately after TLI) were less effective in prolonging heart allograft survival (median graft survival was 13 days in group III, 13.5 days in group IV, 30 days in group VI, 21 days in group VII, and 37 days in group IX). How-

ever, in two (40 %) recipients in group VI and in one recipient (14.3 %) in group IX, graft survival was prolonged > 100 days ($P = 0.6$ for X versus VI and $P = 0.1$ for X versus IX).

ITI injection by itself (group II) significantly prolonged heart allograft survival (median 31 days) compared to controls but only one recipient (14.3 %) had graft function > 100 days ($P = 0.5$ for II versus VI, $P > 0.9$ for II versus IX, and $P = 0.1$ for II versus X). An additive or synergistic effect of ITI with TLI could not be demonstrated when ITI was combined with TLI protocols that were partially effective (group V, 1×200 rad + ITI, transplantation 3 weeks after TLI + ITI; group VIII, 1×1000 rad + ITI, transplantation 3 weeks after TLI + ITI). When ITI was combined with the most effective TLI protocol (group XI, 5×200 rad + ITI, transplantation 3 weeks after TLI + ITI), the median graft survival was > 100 days and prolongation of graft survival > 100 days occurred in 54 % of the recipients ($P = 0.1$ for XI versus II, $P > 0.9$ for XI versus VI, $P = 0.1$ for XI versus IX, and $P > 0.9$ for XI versus X).

The importance of thymus irradiation was demonstrated when the protocols of groups X and XI were modified by TS during TLI. Median graft survival was only 26.5 days in group XII (5×200 rad + TS, transplantation 3 weeks after TLI) and 23.5 days in group XIII (5×200 rad + TS + ITI, transplantation 3 weeks after TLI + ITI) with no grafts functioning > 100 days in both groups. The skin grafts that were transplanted to the animals in groups X and XI with hearts functioning > 150 days were rejected at 7–15 days while the hearts continued to beat.

In the in vitro studies (Fig. 1), the mean $\pm$ SD (mean for four different counts for each animal and for three

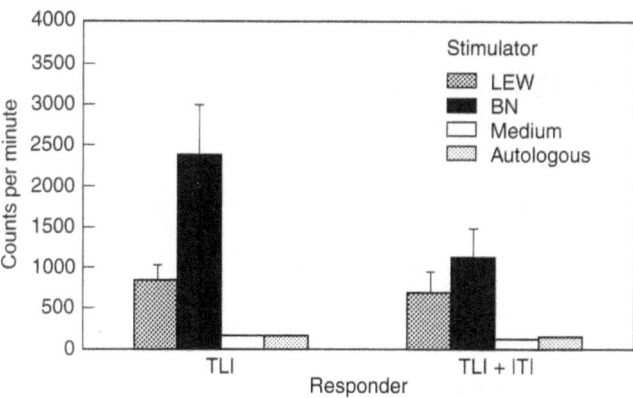

Fig. 1 Effect of total lymphocyte irradiation *(TLI)* and intrathymic injection *(ITI)* on mixed lymphocyte culture. Responder splenocytes were harvested from three Wistar Furth rat (WF) recipients in group X (5×200 rad, transplantation 3 weeks after TLI) and three WF recipients in group XI (5×200 rad + ITI, transplantation 3 weeks after TLI + ITI) with heart allografts functioning > 150 days. Responder cells (2.5×10^5) were cultured with irradiated stimulator splenocytes [1×10^6 Lewis *(LEW)*, Brown Norway *(BN)*, or autologous splenocytes]. Proliferation was assayed by ^{3}H-thymidine incorporation. When comparing the mean ± SD counts per min (proliferation on day 5) for different stimulators in group X, the *P* values were: 0.08 for LEW versus BN cells, 0.03 for LEW versus autologous cells or medium, 0.02 for BN versus autologous cells and medium, and 0.4 for autologous cells versus medium. For the same comparison in group XI, the *P* values were: 0.4 for LEW versus BN cells, 0.1 for LEW versus autologous cells or medium, 0.6 for BN versus autologous cells, 0.052 for BN cells versus medium, and 0.4 for autologous cells versus medium. There was no difference between groups X and XI when comparing response to LEW ($P = 0.7$), BN ($P = 0.2$), autologous stimulator cells ($P = 0.6$), and medium ($P = 0.09$)

different animals in each group) counts per min (proliferation on day 5) in group X (5×200 rad, transplantation in 3 weeks after TLI) was not different when comparing response to LEW (allo-specific) versus BN (third party) stimulator cells ($P = 0.08$), or when comparing response to autologous stimulator cells versus medium ($P = 0.4$). There was a significant difference when response to LEW stimulator cells was compared to autologous cells or medium ($P = 0.03$ in both cases), and when response to BN stimulator cells was compared to autologous cells or medium ($P = 0.02$ in both cases). In group XI (5×200 rad + ITI, transplantation in 3 weeks after TLI + ITI), there was no significant difference when comparing response to LEW versus BN stimulator cells ($P = 0.4$), or when response to autologous cells was compared to medium ($P = 0.4$). In group XI (in contrast to group X) there was no significant difference when response to LEW stimulator cells was compared to autologous cells or medium ($P = 0.1$ in both cases), or when response to BN stimulator cells was compared to autologous cells ($P = 0.6$) or medium ($P = 0.052$). There was no difference between groups X and XI when comparing response to LEW ($P = 0.7$), BN

($P = 0.2$), autologous stimulator cells ($P = 0.6$) and medium ($P = 0.09$).

The histological findings of the heart allografts after cessation of beating (Fig. 2) revealed either rejection with massive lymphocyte infiltration, or necrosis with trophic calcification. Both ot those types of histological findings were present in all groups and no difference in the incidence of one type versus the other was observed in a specific group. Of note, heart allografts functioning > 150 days from animals that were sacrificed for the in vitro studies also had some histological evidence of either lymphocyte infiltration or necrosis.

The results for islet and skin allograft survival are presented in Tables 2 and 3, respectively. The diabetic LEW rats, which were transplanted with isogenic islets in order to test islet viability, were normoglycemic on the first posttransplant day and remain normoglycemic > 100 days. When the two most effective protocols in prolonging heart allograft survival (5×200 rad ± ITI, transplantation 3 weeks after TLI ± ITI) were applied to islet and skin allograft recipients, there was no prolongation of survival of either islet or skin allografts.

The cortex/medulla ratio (Fig. 3) in the lobules of normal rats was 1:1. The cortex/medulla ratio was decreased to 1:1.5 in the animals that received 1×200 rad, 1:2 in the animals that received 1×1000 rad, and 1:1.5 in the animals that received 5×200 rad.

Discussion

Different TLI protocols gave different results in the heart allograft model. A total dose of 1000 rad fractionated in five consecutive doses of 200 rad/day and followed by transplantation in 3 weeks was the most effective TLI protocol in depleting the lymphocytes (without any apparent side effects) and it was also the most successful in prolonging graft survival even without ITI. However, recipients treated with 5×200 rad ± ITI (transplantation in 3 weeks after TLI ± ITI) with hearts functioning > 100 days, rejected the skin grafts that were transplanted to them at 150 days while the hearts continued to beat. That indicates that they were not tolerant to the donor and that their allo-responsiveness was reduced only to heart allografts. However, the results of histology for heart grafts of the animals that were sacrificed for in vitro studies (while their heart grafts continued to beat) demonstrated some evidence of lymphocyte infiltration or myocardial necrosis. These histological data indicate that the recipients were rather hyporesponsive than unresponsive to heart allografts, since those allografts were sensitive to rejection-effective mechanisms.

ITI by itself did not have a synergistic effect in vivo with either the less effective TLI protocols or with the most successful TLI protocol of 5×200 rad followed by

Fig. 2 The histological findings of the heart allografts after cessation of beating revealed either rejection with massive lymphocyte infiltration *(left)*, or necrosis *(right)* with trophic calcification. Both of these types of histological findings were present in all groups and no difference in the incidence of one type versus the other was observed in a specific group

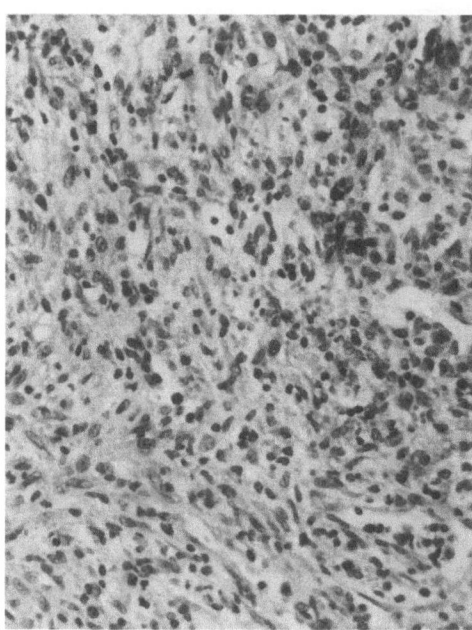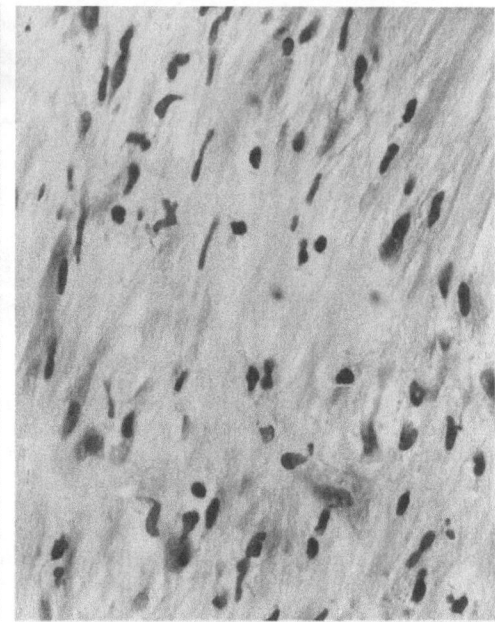

Table 2 Islet allograft survival. $P = 0.2$ for I versus II and III

Group	n	Treatment	Transplant	Graft survival (days)	Median
I	4	None		0, 0, 1, 3	1
II	12	5 × 200 rad	In 3 weeks[a]	0, 0, 0, 0, 0, 0, 0, 1, 1, 4, 5, 6	0
III	13	5 × 200 rad + ITI	In 3 weeks	0, 0, 0, 0, 0, 0, 0, 1, 1, 1, 1, 1, 3	0

[a] Transplant in 3 weeks after completion of TLI or TLI + ITI

Table 3 Skin allograft survival. $P = 0.5$ for I versus II and III

Group	n	Treatment	Transplant	Graft survival (days)	Median
I	3	None		13, 15, 15	15
II	11	5 × 200 rad	In 3 weeks[a]	9, 10, 10, 13, 14, 15, 15, 15, 16, 17, 19	15
III	9	5 × 200 rad + ITI	In 3 weeks	11, 11, 13, 15, 17, 17, 17, 20, 21	17

[a] Transplant in 3 weeks after completion of TLI or TLI + ITI

transplantation in 3 weeks. This demonstrates a difference with the protocols that used ALS + ITI for inducing donor-specific unresponsiveness where ITI had a significant additional effect to the use of ALS only, and indicates that TLI (by the protocols used) is not a substitute for ALS. However, the 5 × 200 rad protocol (followed by transplantation in 3 weeks) can replace both ALS and ITI in inducing indefinite acceptance of heart allografts in rats. Nevertheless, there is some evidence in our in vitro data that recipients treated with ITI and TLI (5 × 200 rad, transplantation in 3 weeks after TLI + ITI) had lower responsiveness to donor and third party stimulator cells compared to recipients that were treated only with TLI. These data indicate that pretransplant treatment with ITI could possibly have had a positive effect in prolonging heart allograft survival in the long run–that is if the recipients had not been sacrificed

for in vitro studies. However, since only three animals were used in each group for the in vitro experiments, further in vitro studies are necessary to verify these results.

The 5 × 200 rad TLI protocol (without ITI) was more effective when transplantation was performed 3 weeks after completion of TLI (when the total LC had reverted to normal range) than immediately after completion of TLI (total LC reduced between 0 and 17 % of the LC before TLI). This might indicate that what is really important for prolonging heart allograft survival by using TLI is not the generalized immunosuppressive effect of TLI but the correct timing between lymphocyte depletion and transplantation. The presence of the heart allograft could be considered as donor-specific antigen presentation to the recipient (having the role that ITI is supposed to have in making the recipient relearn self)

Fig. 3 The cortex *(C)*/medulla *(M)* ratio in the lobules of the thymus of normal rats was 1:1 *(left)*. The cortex/medulla ratio after TLI was decreased to 1:1.5 in the animals that received 1 × 200 rad, 1:2 in the animals that received 1 × 1000 rad *(right)*, and 1:1.5 in the animals that received 5 × 200 rad

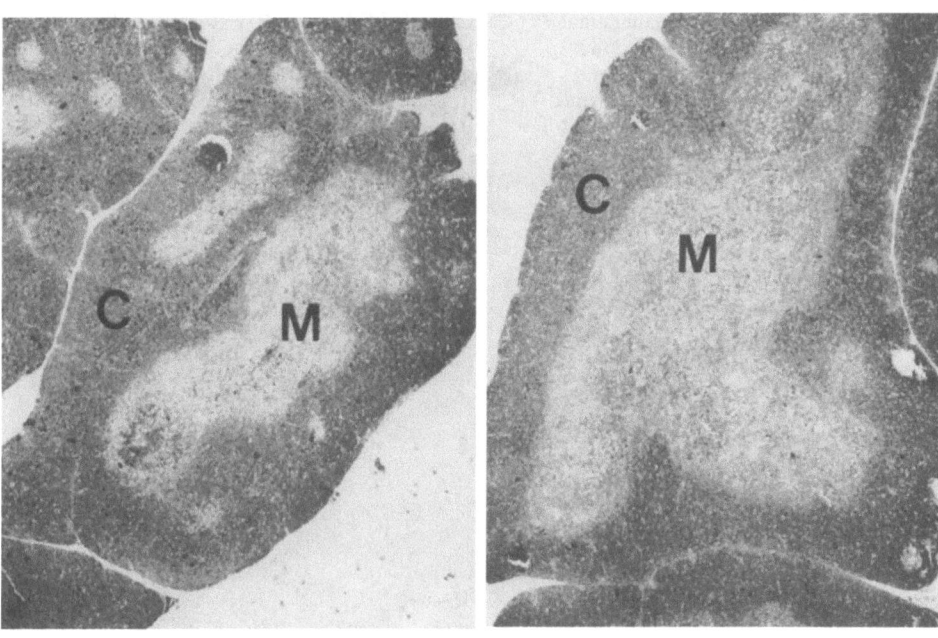

and 3 weeks post-TLI might be the optimum time for the new immature T-cells to "meet" the donor antigens in the peripheral blood and become hyporesponsive to them. This hypothesis is in accordance with similar observations for development of donor-specific unresponsiveness by using peritransplant immunosuppression and i. v. injection of donor cells [8].

The 5 × 200 rad protocol (with or without ITI, followed by transplantation in 3 weeks) was effective only when the thymus was exposed to irradiation, indicating that depeletion of the T-cells that exist in the thymus (and have already learned what is self and non-self) is probably important for inducing donor-specific hyporesponsiveness.

TLI altered the histology of the thymus, decreasing the cortex/medulla ratio from 1:1 before to 1:1.5 after 1 × or 5 × 200 rad and 1:2 after 1 × 1000 rad. The histological picture after TLI resembled that of an old, nonfunctioning thymus [10] and further supports the hypothesis that donor-specific hyporesponsiveness develops in the periphery, and the heart allograft by itself serves for donor-specific antigen presentation to the re-

cipient. However, the in vitro results that suggest donor and third party hyporesponsiveness in recipients treated with TLI + ITI versus TLI alone is consistent with at least partial function of the thymus after TLI.

The fact that prolongation of islet or skin allograft survival was not achieved by using the two most effective protocols in prolonging heart allograft survival (5 × 200 rad ± ITI, transplantation in 3 weeks after TLI ± ITI) indicates that the effect of TLI ± ITI in inducing donor-specific hyporesponsiveness is organ-specific, as is the effect of the use of ALS in combination with ITI [6]. These results also indicate a difference between immediately (heart) and later (islets, skin) vascularized grafts.

In conclusion, TLI in a dose schedule of 200 rad/day for 5 consecutive days followed by transplantation in 3 weeks was effective (even without ITI) in inducing indefinite acceptance of heart but not islet or skin allografts in rats. Thus, TLI by this scheme should be tested for prolonging survival of immediately vascularized grafts in a preclinical large animal model.

References

1. Billingham RE (1961) Free skin grafts in mammals. In: Billingham RE, Silver WK, (eds) Transplantation of tissues and cells. Wistar Institute, Philadelphia
2. Charlton B, Auchincloss H, Fathman CG (1994) Mechanisms of transplantation tolerance. Annu Rev Immunol 12: 707–734
3. Goss JA, Nakafusa Y, Sam Y, Flye MW (1993) Intrathymic injection of donor alloantigens induces specific tolerance to cardiac allografts. Transplantation 56: 166–173
4. Miller JFAP, Marshall A, White R (1962) The immunological significance of the thymus. Adv Immunol 2: 111–116
5. Monaco AP (1991) Future trends in transplantation in the 1990s: prospects for the induction of clinical tolerance. Transplant Proc 23: 67–71

6. Nakafusa Y, Goss JA, Mohanakumar T, Flye MW (1993) Induction of donor-specific tolerance to cardiac but not skin or renal allografts by intrathymic injection of splenocyte alloantigen. Transplantation 55: 877–882

7. Odorico JS, Barker CF, Posselt AM, Naji A (1992) Induction of donor-specific tolerance to rat cardiac allografts by intrathymic inoculation of bone marrow. Surgery 112: 370–377

8. Oluwole SF, Fawwaz RA, Reemtsma K, Hardy MA (1988) Permanent rat cardiac allograft survival by ultraviolet B-irradiated donor lymphocytes and peritransplant cyclosporine. Surgery 104: 231–238

9. Ono K, Lindsey ES (1969) Improved technique of heart transplantation in rats. J Thorac Cardiovasc Surg 57:225–230

10. Roitt I, Brostoff J, Male D (1993) Immunology, 3rd edn. Mosby, London

11. Xenos ES, Stevens RB, Sutherland DER, Lokeh A, Ansite JD, Casanova D, Gores PF, Platt JL (1994) The role of nitric oxide in IL-1b-mediated dysfunction of rodent islets of Langerhans. Transplantation 57: 1208–1212

Transpl Int (1996) 9 [Suppl 1]: S379–S381
© Springer-Verlag 1996

IMMUNOBIOLOGY

R. L. Marquet
R. W. F. de Bruin
J. N. M. IJzermans

Induction of specific inhibition of alloreactivity in beagle dogs by intrathymic injection of donor splenocytes

R. L. Marquet (✉) · R. W. F. de Bruin ·
J. N. M. IJzermans
Laboratory for Experimental Surgery,
Erasmus University, P. O. Box 1738,
NL-3000 DR, Rotterdam,
The Netherlands
Fax +31 10-4 36 91 40

Abstract The aim of this study was to investigate whether intrathymic injection (ITI) of donor splenocytes in dogs might lead to specific immunomodulation as assessed by mixed lymphocyte culture (MLC) tests. Two groups of five beagles each were used. Group 1 contained animals that were 2 years old, group 2 consisted of animals that were 6 months old. One animal was splenectomized per experimental group and 1×10^9 splenocytes were injected into the thymic lobes or thymic remnant of the four remaining dogs. On the day of ITI the dogs were treated subcutaneously with a single dose of 2 ml/kg anti-lymphocyte serum (ALS). In group 1 the thymus of all dogs was found to be atrophic. ITI in this group did not result in a decreased immunoreactivity but rather in an enhanced immune response. In group 2 the thymus was still clearly present and ITI was easy to perform. ITI induced a significant reduction of specific MLC reactivity at 1 week after treatment. The effect was transient and not significantly further diminished at week 2. These results indicate that ITI is a technically feasible procedure in a preclinical animal model. It may induce temporary sensitization as well as immunosuppression, possibly depending on the age of the recipient.

Key words Intrathymic · Unresponsiveness · Dogs

Introduction

Posselt et al. [1, 2] were the first to show in rats that intrathymic injection (ITI) of pancreatic islets could lead to induction of specific unresponsiveness. Extension of this original finding by many groups in various rat and mouse models revealed also that ITI of lymphocytes or purified alloantigens, combined with a brief course of immunosuppression, was able to evoke donor-specific unresponsiveness of subsequent allo- and xenografts [3–8]. The question remained whether this new way of inducing unresponsiveness was just a typical rodent phenomenon or also would hold for preclinical animal models and even might be extrapolated to man. Recently, it was claimed by Une et al. [9] that ITI of islets in NIH minipigs, in conjunction with a short course of anti-lymphocyte serum (ALS), did induce donor-specific inhibition of cell-mediated cytotoxicity shortly after inoculation. In some cases, this reactivity even became undetectable after 1 month. In contrast, Merhav et al. [10] failed to produce prolonged survival of cardiac or renal allografts in mongrel dogs by donor-specific ITI of splenocytes and transient immunosuppression. The aim of the present study was to further investigate this issue in a well-defined preclinical animal model. Beagle dogs of different ages were used to study the feasibility of ITI. The capacity to induce unresponsiveness by ITI of spleen cells was monitored by performing mixed lymphocyte culture (MLC) tests.

Materials and methods

Animals

Two groups of male and female beagle dogs (Harlan, Zeist, The Netherlands), each containing five animals, were used. Group 1 consisted of adult dogs, which were about 2 years old, group 2 consisted of young dogs, which were 6 months old.

DLA matching and MLC monitoring

Tissue typing for class I and II antigens of the dog MHC (DLA) was achieved by serology and MLC tests, as described previously [11]. For both groups of experimental animals, only dogs were selected that were unrelated and DLA-incompatible. MLC tests for monitoring of immune reactivity were performed in a similar manner as for DLA class II typing [12]. The results were expressed as stimulation index (SI). To control for inter-assay variations during time, changes in donor-specific MLC reactivity after ITI were assessed by using normalized SIs. Therefore, a ratio was calculated by dividing the experimental SI by the mean SI of controls, being the results of mutual MLCs between the four ITI dogs. The SI ratio (SIR) is given as a percentage.

Antilymphocyte serum

Goat anti-dog lymphocyte serum (ALS) was produced by immunizing a goat 3 times subcutaneously (s.c.) with beagle mesenteric lymph node cells. The serum was collected 1 week after the last immunization. The lymphocytotoxic titer of the product was 1:126.

Experimental design

The beagle in each group of five dogs showing the highest stimulatory capacity in MLC against the four other dogs was selected to undergo splenectomy. Spleen lymphocytes were prepared in RPMI by standard methods and divided into four aliquots, each containing about 1×10^9 cells. The cells were cryopreserved in dimethyl sulfoxide (DMSO) employing programmed, stepwise freezing, and stored at $-196\,°C$ until used for ITI. ITI of splenocytes in the four remaining dogs of the group was performed under general anesthesia. Via a lateral incision in the neck, access was gained to the thymic region, after which the thymus (young animals) or its atrophic remnant (adult animals) was exposed. Biopsies were taken to ensure that the appropriate region was explored. The spleen cells were then injected into the two lobes of the thymus or into the thymic remnant, in a volume of 0.5 ml per lobe. After ITI, a single injection of ALS was given s.c. at a dose of 2 ml/kg body weight. The number of peripheral blood leukocytes was determined regularly and MLCs were performed at weekly intervals to monitor specific alterations in immune reactivity. The criteria for a significant change in immune reactivity were twofold: (1) specific SIs in a given assay had to be significantly different from control SIs; and (2) SIRs had to be significantly different from the baseline SIR.

Results

Feasibility of ITI

In all four adult dogs of group 1, the thymus was found to be atrophic. Histology revealed that small thymic remnants were still present. Injection of spleen cells into the atrophied tissue was feasible but leakage could not be prevented. In the young animals of group 2, the two thymic lobes were easily identified and injection of

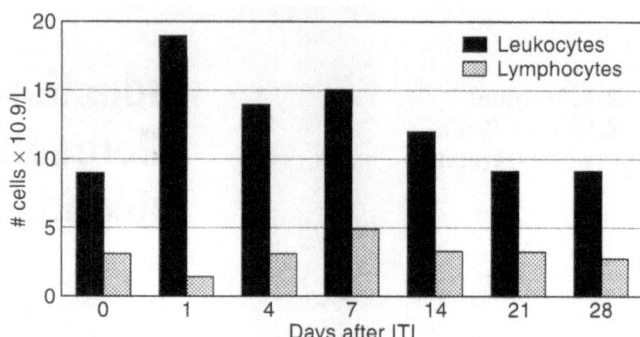

Fig. 1 Mean number of peripheral blood leukocytes and lymphocytes ($\times 10^9$/l) after a single subcutaneous injection of 2 ml/kg goat anti-dog lymphocyte serum ($n = 4$). The number of leukocytes is significantly increased on days 1, 4, and 7; the number of lymphocytes is significantly decreased on day 1. (*ITI* Intrathymic injection)

cells in a volume of 0.5 ml/lobe was easy to perform. Leakage of cells into surrounding tissue did not seem to occur.

Effect of ALS on lymphocytes

Total leukocyte and differential lymphocyte countings were performed in the four dogs of group 1. The results are given in Fig. 1. The number of leukocytes was elevated significantly during the first week after ITI, possibly due to the surgical procedure or to ALS-induced leukocytosis. ALS produced a transient lymphopenia (less than 50% of normal) on day 1 after ITI, after which the number of lymphocytes normalized again rapidly.

Immune reactivity after ITI

The results are depicted in Fig. 2. In group 1, monitoring of MLC reactivity was only performed once, at 1 week after ITI. Surprisingly, it was found that the mean SIR of the four dogs against the spleen cell donor was not diminished but, rather, had increased from $179 \pm 82\%$ to $700 \pm 538\%$ (Wilcoxon: $P = 0.05$). The results in group 2 were quite different. One week after ITI the mean SIR had dropped from $260 \pm 86\%$ to $50 \pm 39\%$ ($P = 0.02$); 1 week later the mean SIR was $68 \pm 28\%$ (not significant); at 4 weeks the mean SIR was normalized to $103 \pm 19\%$.

Discussion

Three major conclusions can be drawn from the current experiments: (1) ITI in dogs is a feasible procedure with no morbidity; (2) ITI in adult dogs with an atro-

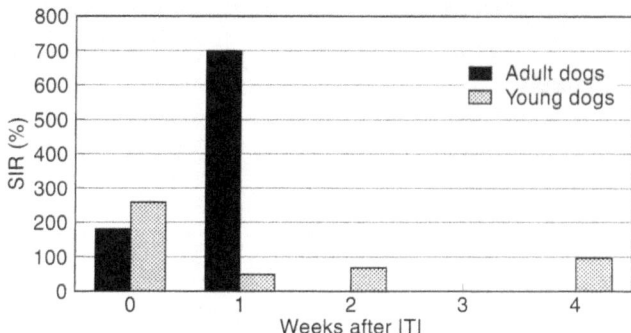

Fig. 2 Changes in specific immune reactivity as assessed by mixed lymphocyte culture (MLC) reactivity after intrathymic injection *(ITI)* of donor spleen cells into the thymus of four adult dogs (group 1) and four young dogs (group 2). MLC reactivity was calculated as the stimulation index (SI), which was normalized to a ratio *(SIR* in %) by dividing the mean donor-specific SI per group by the mean SI of controls. One week after ITI the mean SIR of group 1 was significantly increased ($P = 0.05$), whereas the mean SIR of group 2 was significantly decreased ($P = 0.02$)

phied thymus may lead to specific immunization; and (3) ITI in young dogs with an intact thymus leads to a transient form of specific immunosuppression. The latter result implies that ITI-induced unresponsiveness in not just a rodent phenomenon but also applies to a preclinical model. Although less striking, our results are in

agreement with those of Une et al. [9] obtained in minipigs. Following ITI of islets, these authors found a profound and durable suppression of MLC reactivity, whereas we observed a moderate and transient suppression. A major reason for this difference in efficacy of ITI may have been the quality or dose of the ALS used. The goat anti-dog ALS employed by us may have been of moderate quality, evidenced by the finding that it only induced a short-term reduction in the number of peripheral blood lymphocytes. On the other hand, the fact that we did find a significant degree of specific unresponsiveness may cast doubt on the dogma that depletion of peripheral lymphocytes at the time of ITI is essential in larger animals; it may even be counterproductive. We recently observed in a specific rat model that ITI of spleen cells, in combination with a single dose of ALS, did not lead to prolonged acceptance but to accelerated rejection of heart allografts [13]. The current findings in adult dogs that ITI may lead to sensitization are very reminiscent of these observations.

It is obvious that the reduced MLC reactivity observed in our young dog model is only a remote parameter for the ultimate aim of ITI: prolonged graft survival. In this respect, the first transplantation results obtained by Merhav et al. [10] in dogs are very sobering. They indicate that the clinical road to tolerance may, as ever, not be as easy as the rodent's.

References

1. Posselt AM, Barker CF, Tomaszewski JE, Markmann JF, Choti MA, Naji A (1990) Induction of donor-specific unresponsiveness by intrathymic islet transplantation. Science 249: 1293–1295
2. Posselt AM, Naji A, Roark JH, Markmann JF, Barker CF (1991) Intrathymic islet transplantation in the spontaneously diabetic BB rat. Ann Surg 214: 363–373
3. Remuzzi G, Rossini M, Imberti O, Perico N (1991) Kidney graft survival in rats without immunosuppression after intrathymic glomerular transplantation. Lancet 337: 750
4. Goss J, Nakafusa Y, Flye W (1992) Intrathymic injection of donor alloantigens induces donor-specific vascularized allograft tolerance without immunosuppression. Ann Surg 216: 409–416
5. Ohzako H, Monaco AP (1992) Induction of specific unresponsiveness (tolerance) to skin allografts by intrathymic donor-specific splenocyte injection in antilymphocyte serum-treated mice. Transplantation 54: 1090–1095

6. Sheffield CD, Hadley GA, Dirden BM, Bartlett ST (1994) Prolonged cardiac xenograft survival is induced by intrathymic splenocyte injection. J Surg Res 57: 55–59
7. Mayo GL, Posselt AM, Campos L, Noorchashm N, Barker CF, Naji A (1994) Intrathymic transplantation promotes survival of islet xenografts (rat to mouse). Transplant Proc 26: 758
8. Zeng Y, Bluestone JA, Ildstad ST, Torres MA, Montag AG, Thistlewaite RJ (1994) Long-term functional xenograft tolerance after intrathymic islet transplantation (rat to mouse). Transplant Proc 25: 438–439
9. Une S, Kenmochi T, Miyamoto M, Nakagawa Y, Benhamou PY, Sangkharat A, Mulle Y (1994) Induction of donor-specific unresponsiveness in NIH minipigs following intrathymic islet transplantation. Transplant Proc 27: 142–144

10. Merhav H, Ye Y, Niekrasz M, Luo Y, Kobayashi T, Kosanke S, Baker J, Smith D, Cooper DKC (1995) Failure of intrathymic inoculation of donor-specific splenocytes to prolong cardiac or renal allograft survival in dogs. Transpl Immunol 3: 39–44
11. Bull RW, Vriesendorp HM, Cech R, Grosse-Wilde H, Bijma AM, Ladiges WL, Krumbacher K, Doxiadis I, Ejima H, Templeton J, Albert ED, Storb R, Deeg HJ (1987) Joint report on the third international workshop on canine immunogenetics II. Analysis of the serological typing of cells. Transplantation 43: 154–158
12. Bijnen AB, Dekkers-Bijma AM, Vriesendorp HJ, Westbroek DL (1979) The value of the mixed lymphocyte reaction in dogs as a genetic assay. Immunogenetics 8: 287–291
13. Bruin RWF de, Rossum TJ van, Scheringa M, Bonthuis F, IJzermans JNM, Marquet RL (1995) Intrathymic injection of alloantigen may lead to hyperacute rejection as well as prolonged graft survival of heart allografts in the rat. Transplantation 60: 1061–1063

Xenotransplantation

Transpl Int (1996) 9 [Suppl 1]: S385–S387
© Springer-Verlag 1996

A. Pascher
Ch. Poehlein
M. Storck
D. Abendroth
J. Mueller-Hoecker
W. Koenig
V. K. Young
D. J. G. White
C. Hammer

Expression of human decay accelerating factor (hDAF) in transgenic pigs regulates complement activation during ex vivo liver perfusion – immunopathological findings

A. Pascher · Ch. Poehlein · C. Hammer (✉)
Institute for Surgical Research,
Klinikum Grosshadern, LMU Munich,
Marchioninistrasse 15, D-81366 Munich,
Germany

M. Storck · D. Abendroth
Department of Surgery II,
University of Ulm, Germany

J. Mueller-Hoecker
Institute for Pathology,
Klinikum Grosshadern, LMU Munich,
Germany

V. K. Young
Department of Cardiothoracic Surgery,
Papworth Hospital, Cambridge, UK

W. Koenig · D. J. G. White
Department of Surgery,
University of Cambridge, UK

Abstract Ex vivo perfusions of human decay accelerating factor-expressing transgenic ($n = 3$), and nontransgenic ($n = 6$) porcine livers with human blood revealed a higher degree of organ damage in nontransgenic pig livers. Transgenic livers were protected from immunohistologically detectable complement deposition, despite corresponding IgM and IgG deposits in both groups. Complement activation and consumption of C3 and C4 turned out to be lower in transgenic pig livers. In contrast to livers of normal landrace pigs, livers from genetically manipulated pigs showed no morphological alterations after perfusion.

Key words Decay accelerating factor · Transgenic pig · Ex vivo perfusion · Immunohistology · Complement

Introduction

Extracorporeal liver perfusion for elimination of toxic metabolic products causing hepatic encephalopathy after fulminant hepatic failure has regained importance in the last few years. Due to progress in immunosuppression and, for example, antibody depletion techniques, some obstacles for its clinical use could be cleared. The current case reports [4, 6] about discordant heterotopical hepatic transplantation and extracorporeal perfusion, however, show that there are still severe problems ahead, influencing the viability of the perfused organ and the clinical outcome of patients as well. Xenogeneic ex vivo perfusion of isolated pig livers is closely related to the idea of therapeutic extracorporeal perfusion, providing the possibility of simulating benefits and, even more important, risks of extracorporeal liver perfusion prior to clinical application. A new aspect is the use of genetically manipulated porcine livers expressing the membrane-bound human decay accelerating factor (hDAF) [5, 9, 11]. The purpose of this study was to compare the degree of complement activation during perfusion of transgenic, hDAF-expressing and nontransgenic pig livers, as well as to examine differences in the deposition of complement components on their endothelial cells.

Materials and methods

After hypothermic perfusion via the portal vein and the hepatic artery with 4 °C University of Wisconsin (UW) solution, three transgenic pigs were hepatectomised in deep anaesthesia within a multiorgan explantation. Cold storage and preparation time were 90 min in total. The median liver weight (LW) was 535 ± 42 g. Livers of six nontransgenic pigs (LW = 689 ± 29 g) were treated equally and served as the control group. The livers were wrapped in a waterproof plastic bag and suspended in a waterfilled perfusion chamber. Heparinised human blood (10 IU/ml) of two donors with identical blood group (BG 0, A or B) and Rh factor was diluted to a haematocrit of 30 % for perfusion. The volume of diluted blood amounted to approximately 1500 ml. After the first passage through the liver, a blood volume which corresponded to about 1 ml/g organ weight was removed from the circuit, to avoid a wash- in of UW solution, potassium, etc. into the circuit. Perfusion was carried out for 3 h. During perfusion, pressure, temperature, pH and oxygenation were controlled, and blood samples taken at several time points. Tissue specimens taken before and after perfusion were prepared for routine staining, detection of neutrophils and platelets, immunohistology and fine-structural analysis. An indirect immunoperoxidase technique was used for immunohistology. An avidin-biotin complex (ABC) kit (Dianova-Immunotech, Hamburg, Germany) was combined with an avidin-biotin blocking kit (Vector Laboratories, Calif., USA) and aminoethylcarbazole (AEC, Sigma-Aldrich, Deisenhofen, Germany) as chromophore. The antibodies chosen for detailed analysis of complement and preformed natural antibody deposition included monoclonal mouse anti-human antibodies against C3c, C3d, C4c, C4d, SC5b-9 neoantigen (MAC), factor P (Quidel, San Diego, Calif., USA), IgM and IgG (Dako, Hamburg, Germany). Sections from at least ten corresponding loci of each organ were stained for these antigens. In addition, biochemical parameters such as electrolytes, transaminases and other enzymes, as well as bile flow, increase of organ weight and vascular resistance, indicating liver cell damage and functional restrictions of the organs, were determined (data not shown). CH50 and AP50, as well as serum levels of C3 and C4 as markers for complement activation and consumption were analyzed.

Results

In the control group (n = 6), organs were positive for all complement factors in six to nine sections of, in average, 14 treated sections per single factor and organ (43–65 %). Livers of transgenic pigs (n = 3) were C3d-, C4c- and MAC-negative. C3c staining occurred in one single case. C4d and properdin were detectable though less extensive than in nontransgenic livers. The main effects concentrated on branches of the interlobular arteries. Venous staining occurred less often and, in this case, affected portal venous vessels. In both, control and transgenic livers, there was no complement and antibody deposition on hepatocytes, sinusoidal lining cells, central veins, epithelia of bile tracts and on hepatic veins. Hence, the immunoreactive product was predominantly detectable on endothelial cells and, to a minor degree, on the myothel and perithel of arteries. No difference occurred in the deposition of the preformed natural antibodies (PNAB), IgM and IgG, between transgenic and nontransgenic organs. Concerning morphological alterations, predominantly midzonal, but sometimes also pericentral areas of necrosis were present in nontransgenic livers, accompanied by hyperaemia, sometimes even haemorrhagia, whereas specimens from transgenic livers showed no signs of necrosis. Correspondingly, the fine structural analysis of transgenic liv-

ers revealed no alterations of morphology. In both groups, however, disseminated infiltration and sequestration of granulocytes appeared in the sinusoids, accompanied by leucocyte casts in vessels. Furthermore, there was evidence of thrombocyte aggregation in sinusoids of livers in each group. Moreover, thrombosis, especially in portal venous vessels, occurred in transgenic and nontransgenic pig livers. Biochemical analysis of the blood samples supported the histological results. In particular, transaminases, glutamate dehydrogenase and potassium reached higher levels in control livers (data not shown). Plasma levels of C3 and C4 showed a decrease during perfusion of both transgenic and nontransgenic livers. In human DAF-expressing livers, a steady state was reached at about 85 ± 5 % (C3) and 84 ± 2 % (C4) of original values after 60 min. In normal pig livers, no steady state was reached and levels decreased to 60–70 %. CH50 and AP50 determination by total haemolytic complement assay confirmed a higher degree of complement activation in the control livers. Classical and alternative pathways of the complement cascade were activated similarly in the control group.

Discussion

The results of ex vivo liver perfusions of hDAF-expressing organs evidenced the effectiveness of this strategy to overcome the activation of the human complement cascade following the binding of human preformed natural anti-pig antibodies to the porcine liver endothelium [3]. Though it was reported previously that the targets of these antibodies, gal α(1,3)gal epitopes, were more or less omnipresent in pig livers [7], binding of IgG and IgM as well as complement factors concentrated on arterial and, less distinctly, on portal venous vessels in nontransgenic livers. Despite the corresponding antibody deposition in transgenic livers, only trace deposits of C4d and properdin could be observed in transgenic livers. The plasma complement levels concurrently remained higher during perfusion of transgenic livers. Morphological changes in the nontransgenic livers and the lack of alterations in transgenic organs confirmed a higher extent of organ damage. These findings suggest that genetic manipulation of domestic pigs in the sense of expressing human complement regulatory proteins [1] is an advance towards the reliable clinical application of pig liver perfusion either for transient therapeutic purposes till the original liver has regenerated or as a bridge to allotransplantation [2]. In combination with an improved perfusion protocol, including optimal circulation in the portal venous low pressure system by floating suspension and pneumosynchronous pressure changes [8, 10], a prolonged viability and function of the livers can be reached, reducing the need for organs during one perfusion procedure.

References

1. Baldwin WM III, Pruitt SK, Brauer RB, et al (1995) Complement in organ transplantation – contributions to inflammation, injury and rejection. Transplantation 59: 797–808
2. Burdick JF, Fair JH (1994) Xenoperfusion: the pig liver as a bridge. Xeno 2: 3–5
3. Carrington CA, Richards AC, Cozzi E, et al (1995) Expression of human DAF and MCP on pig endothelial cells protects from human complement. Transplant Proc 27: 321–323
4. Chari RS, Collins BH, Magee JC, et al (1994) Treatment of hepatic failure with ex vivo pig liver perfusion followed by liver transplantation. N Engl J Med 331: 234–237
5. Cozzi E, Langford GA, Wright L, et al (1995) Comparative analysis of human DAF expression in the tissues of transgenic pigs and man. Transplant Proc 27: 319–320
6. Makowka L, Cramer DV, Hoffman A, et al (1995) The use of a pig liver xenograft for temporary support of a patient with fulminant hepatic failure. Transplantation 59: 1654–1659
7. McKenzie IFC, Koulmanda M, Mandel T, et al (1995) Comparative studies of the major xenoantigen galα(1,3)gal in pigs and mice. Transplant Proc 27: 247–248
8. Neuhaus P, Blumhardt G (1993) Extracorporeal liver perfusion: applications of an improved model for experimental studies of the liver. Int J Artif Organs 16: 729–739
9. Rosengard AM, Cary NRB, Langford GA, et al (1995) Tissue expression of human complement inhibitor, decay accelerating factor, in transgenic pigs – a potential approach for preventing xenograft rejection. Transplantation 59: 1325–1333
10. Schön MR, Lemmens HP, Neuhaus P, et al (1994) Improved xenogeneic extracorporeal liver perfusion. Transplant Proc 26: 1293–1297
11. Yannoutsos N, Langford GA, Cozzi E et al (1995) Production of pigs transgenic for human regulators of complement activation. Transplant Proc 27: 324–325

Transpl Int (1996) 9 [Suppl 1]: S388–S391
© Springer-Verlag 1996

H. Terajima
Y. Shirakata
T. Yagi
S. Mashima
H. Shinohara
S. Satoh
Y. Arima
T. Gomi
T. Hirose
I. Ikai
T. Morimoto
T. Inamoto
Y. Yamaoka

Long-duration xenogeneic extracorporeal pig liver perfusion with human blood

H. Terajima (✉) · Y. Shirakata · T. Yagi ·
S. Mashima · H. Shinohara · S. Satoh ·
Y. Arima · T. Gomi · T. Hirose · I. Ikai ·
T. Morimoto · T. Inamoto · Y. Yamaoka
Second Department of Surgery,
Faculty of Medicine,
Kyoto University 54 Kawara-cho,
Shogoin, Sakyo-ku, Kyoto,
606-01 Japan
Fax +81 75 752 45 19

Abstract Hepatic xenografts can tolerate hyperacute rejection owing to their lower susceptibility to humorally mediated injury. We investigated the possibility of long-duration xenoperfusion without immunologically controlling natural antibodies or complements. Pig livers were perfused for 9 h with human blood (Group 1) or pig blood (Group 2). Physiological conditioning and administration of prostaglandin E_1 and insulin was characteristic of our system. The portal vein and hepatic artery pressure and bile production did not significantly differ between the two groups. Despite a gradual decrease throughout the perfusion, overall oxygen consumption was significantly higher in Group 1. Liver enzymes were released at higher levels in Group 1. Histological examination revealed intact hepatic architecture in Group 2, while in Group 1 interlobular morphology was severely damaged by endothelial disruption, although hepatic sinusoidal architecture was preserved. It is concluded that, despite biochemically and histologically confirmed tissue injury, graft viability was well-maintained in xenoperfusion even without immunological manipulations.

Key words Xenoperfusion · Liver · Hyperacute rejection · Prostaglandin E_1

Introduction

In the 1960s and 1970s, extracorporeal liver perfusion (ECLP) to support failed liver functions was extensively studied [1, 5] but this procedure was abandoned for a while because of poor outcome and the advent of orthotopic liver transplantation. The current shortage of donors has shed new light on the concept of ECLP as a bridge to liver transplantation and as a diagnostic technique to assess whether patients with untreatable fulminant hepatic failure will recover from neurological dysfunction by transplantation. Porcine livers, though discordant, are considered to be the most suitable graft in terms of size, disease transmission, domestication, and anatomical similarities. However, unlike concordant xenografts, they are inevitably injured by xenogeneic hyperacute rejection mediated by preformed xenoreactive natural antibodies and complements. It is crucial to suppress this xenoreactive immune response for successful discordant xenotransplantation. Immunological manipulations for the control of hyperacute rejection may not necessarily be required in short-term xenogeneic ECLP, however, as long as the graft can function long enough to assist failed liver functions, since the liver is less susceptible to humorally mediated injury than the kidney and the heart. In this study, we explored the possibility of long-duration xenoperfusion without immunological manipulations.

Materials and methods

Ten Large White pigs from 16 to 21 kg were used as graft donors. At the procurement, the liver was completely freed from the surrounding tissues through incising the diaphragm circularly around the suprahepatic inferior vena cava (IVC), and flushed out through

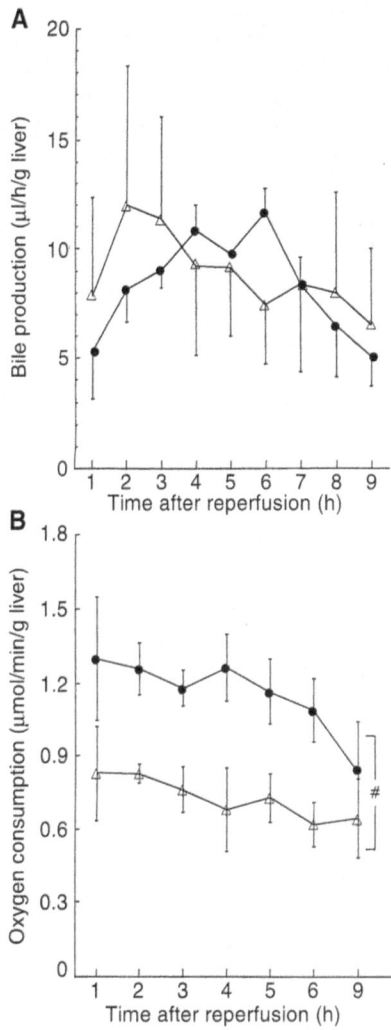

Fig.1 A Bile production was not significantly different between Groups 1 (●) and 2 (△). **B** Oxygen consumption of Group 1 (●) was significantly higher than that of Group 2 (△) (# P <0.001)

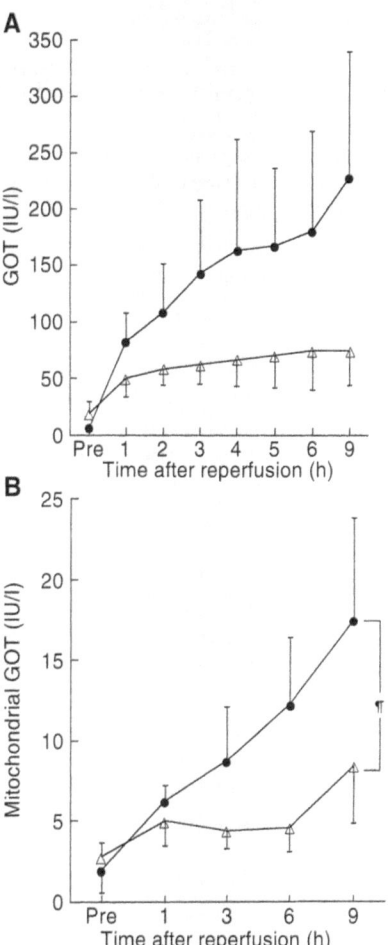

Fig.2 A, B The changes in the release of liver enzymes in Groups 1 (●) and 2 (△). **A** Glutamate oxaloacetate transferase *(GOT)* release continuously increased and tended to be higher in Group 1, but not significantly so. **B** Mitochondrial GOT was significantly higher in Group 1 ($P < 0.05$)

the portal vein (PV) and the hepatic artery (HA) with 1.5 l of cold lactated Ringer's solution containing heparin. The liver was perfused via PV and HA by separate roller pumps. Total hepatic blood flow was kept constant at 1 ml/min per g liver and HA flow was adjusted to approximately 25 % of PV flow. The blood outflow was allowed through infrahepatic IVC by a hydrostatic pressure gradient of 15–20 cm H_2O. The perfusate consisted of fresh human blood or pig blood diluted with lactated Ringer's solution containing low molecular dextran, with a subsequent hematocrit value of 25–30 %. Two membrane oxygenators with heat exchanging function (Menox AL-2000, Kurare, Okayama, Japan) were used to provide a partial oxygen pressure (pO_2) of between 45 and 60 mm Hg for PV and a pO_2 of between 100 and 150 mm Hg for HA, similar to physiological levels. The liver was immersed in a 37 °C heating chamber to prevent the compression of portal vessels by the liver mass, and the temperature of the perfusate was maintained between 35.8 °C and 37.5 °C. Prostaglandin E_1 (PGE$_1$), supplied by Ono (Japan), and regular insulin (Humalin R, Shionogi, Tokyo, Japan) were administered continuously via PV at the rate of 25 mg/h and 1 IU/h, respectively.

In Group 1, pig livers were perfused with human blood ($n = 5$), and in Group 2, perfused with pig blood ($n = 5$). The livers were perfused for 9 h.

Graft viability and hepatocellular injury were verified by PV and HA pressures, bile production and oxygen consumption, and by the release of glutamate oxaloacetate transferase (GOT) and mitochondrial GOT (mGOT). For histological examination, liver tissues were stained with hematoxylin and eosin and analyzed by light microscopy.

Values are expressed as means ± SD. The statistical analysis was performed by two-way repeated-measure analysis of variance (ANOVA). A P-value of less than 0.05 was considered to be statistically significant.

In this animal experiment, the "Principles of laboratory animal care" (NIH publication 86-23, 1985) was followed.

Results

Cold ischemic time could be considerably shortened by our manipulation of organ procurement in both groups (24.3 ± 3.3 min in Group 1 and 23.8 ± 4.7 min in Group 2). The fluctuations of PV and HA pressures did not significantly differ between the two groups. They did not exceed 20 cm H_2O and 180 mm Hg, respectively, even in Group 2. No significant differences in bile production were found (Fig. 1 A). Oxygen consumption was significantly higher in Group 1 ($P < 0.001$, Fig. 1 B), but it tended to gradually decrease in both groups. Regardless of this fluctuation, oxygen consumption remained at a high level even at the end of perfusion (0.83 ± 0.21 µmol/ml per min in Group 1 and 0.64 ± 0.16 µmol/ml per min in Group 2). The release of GOT and mGOT continuously increased and tended to be higher in Group 1, and significant differences were found in mGOT ($P < 0.05$, Fig. 2).

Histological examination revealed that during the early phase of the perfusion, mild sinusoidal dilatation and neutrophil infiltration were observed in both groups. Thereafter, no marked hepatocellular damage was evident in Group 2, while in Group 1 severe periportal edema and extensive interlobular hemorrhage developed in addition to extravasation of fibrinous exudate. In spite of interlobular morphological deterioration, the hepatic sinusoidal architecture was comparatively preserved without massive hepatocellular necrosis.

Discussion

Xenogeneic hyperacute rejection causes endothelial disruption and loss of anticoagulant properties, thus leading to increased vascular permeability, interstitial hemorrhage, intravascular thrombosis, and rapid destruction of the graft [2]. Because of this, the xenoperfused kidney or heart would usually cease to function within minutes when unmanipulated, but the liver is specifically less susceptible to humorally mediated rejection and there is evidence that discordant hepatic xenografts may tolerate hyperacute rejection [8]. This may be related to the liver's ability to neutralize and inactivate cytotoxic antibodies by the release of soluble

MHC antigens and by Kupffer cell absorption, and to the unique double blood supply of the hepatic sinusoid, which confers protective effects from ischemic damage [3, 4]. The comparatively intact architecture of the hepatic sinusoid in xenoperfused livers in this study represents this peculiar characteristic. Considering this resistance of the liver to humorally mediated injury, xenogeneic ECLP without any immunological treatment seems to be possible for a limited period.

For successful, longer-duration xenoperfusion without immunological manipulation, three problems need to be settled: deterioration of the graft viability during procurement and preservation; damage to the graft induced by ischemia reperfusion injury and extracorporeal perfusion; extracorporeal perfusion conditions far from the physiological environment, leading to inhomogeneous perfusion and hypoxia of the graft. Cold ischemic time and ischemia reperfusion injury were reduced as much as possible by reconsidering the procurement procedure. Intraportal administration of insulin can exert a beneficial influence on hepatic mitochondrial energy metabolism and has the potential to enhance the ATP-generating systems in the hepatic mitochondria [9], and PGE_1 not only ameliorates hepatic microcirculatory disturbances by vasodilatation and by inhibiting platelet aggregation [6] but also has direct cytoprotective effects on hepatocytes through stabilization of membrane microviscosity [7]. These cytoprotective properties were considered to bring about stable graft viability even in xenoperfusion. It is very difficult to create completely physiological conditions in extracorporeal circumstances, but by modifying the placement of the liver graft and regulating pO_2, and by simplified pressure gradient drainage of outflow blood, homogeneous perfusion was provided in our system.

It is concluded that, despite biochemically and histologically confirmed tissue injury, graft viability was well-maintained in xenoperfusion even without immunological manipulations. Artificial liver support devices could play an increasing role in the success of liver transplantation but no artificial livers which can completely take over all metabolic functions are in experimental or clinical use. Our newly designed ECLP could be a useful tool to provide a sufficient, stable, supporting environment for a restricted duration of less than 9 h.

References

1. Abouna GM, Fischer LM, Porter KA, Andres G (1973) Experience in the treatment of hepatic failure by intermittent liver hemoperfusions. Surg Gynecol Obstet 137: 741–752

2. Bach FH, Robson SC, Ferran C, Winkler H, Millan MT, Stuhlmeier KM, Vanhove B, Blakely ML, Van Der Werf WJ, Hofer E, De Martin R, Hancock WW (1994) Endothelial cell activation and thromboregulation during xenograft rejection. Immunol Rev 141: 5–29

3. Colletti LM, Johnson KJ, Kunkel BG, Merion RM (1994) Mechanisms of hyperacute rejection in porcine liver transplantation. Antibody-mediated endothelial injury. Transplantation 57: 1357–1363

4. Collins BH, Chari RS, Magee JC, Harland RC, Lindman BJ, Logan JS, Bollinger RR, Meyers WC, Platt JL (1994) Mechanisms of injury in porcine livers perfused with blood of patients with fulminant hepatic failure. Transplantation 58: 1162–1171

5. Eisman B, Liem DS, Raffucci F (1965) Heterologous liver perfusion in treatment of hepatic failure. Ann Surg 162: 329–345

6. Helling TS, Hacker KA, Kragel PJ, Eisenstein CL (1994) Evidence for cytoprotection by prostaglandin E_1 with normothermic hepatic ischemia. J Surg Res 56: 309–313

7. Masaki N, Ohta Y, Shirataki H, Ogata I, Hayashi S, Yamada S, Hirata K, Nagoshi S, Mochida S, Tomiya T, Ohno A, Ohta Y, Fujiwara K (1992) Hepatocyte membrane stabilization by prostaglandins E_1 and E_2: favorable effects on rat liver injury. Gastroenterology 102: 572–576

8. Merion RM, Colletti LM (1990) Hyperacute rejection in porcine liver transplantation. Transplantation 49: 861–868

9. Mori K, Ozawa K, Kiuchi T, Takada Y, Yamaguchi T, Sadamoto T, Shimahara Y, Kobayashi N, Yamaoka Y, Kumada K (1991) Insulinopenia as a risk factor in hepatectomy and its resolution by intraportal insulin administration. Ann Surg 162: 43–49

Transpl Int (1996) 9 [Suppl 1]: S 392–S 396
© Springer-Verlag 1996

Ch. Pöhlein
A. Pascher
M. Storck
V. K. Young
W. König
D. Abendroth
M. Wick
J. Thiery
D. J. G. White
C. Hammer

The function of transgenic human DAF-expressing porcine livers during hemoperfusion with human blood

Ch. Pöhlein (✉) · A. Pascher · C. Hammer
Institute for Surgical Research,
Grosshadern,
Ludwig-Maximilians-University,
Marchioninistrasse 15,
D-81366 Munich, Germany

M. Storck · D. Abendroth
Department of Surgery II,
University of Ulm, Germany

V. K. Young · W. König · D. J. G. White
Department of Surgery and Pathology,
University of Cambridge, UK

M. Wick · J. Thiery
Department of Clinical Chemistry,
Grosshadern,
Ludwig-Maximilians-University,
Munich, Germany

Abstract Extracorporal pig liver perfusion could bridge the deadly problem of acute human liver failure. However, preformed natural antibodies and complement activation (CA) are the predominant mechanisms of hyperacute xenogeneic rejection. The blockade of both pathways of CA in the xenograft, using transgenic livers expressing human decay accelerating factor on the endothelial surface results in prolonged graft survival and lower release of mediators.

Key words Hyperacute xenogeneic rejection · Transgenic pig · Liver · Human DAF · Complement · Preformed natural antibodies

Introduction

In the search for a temporary substitute for a non-functioning liver during hepatic coma, animal organs such as pig livers were connected to the patients' circulation [4]. These xenografts were rejected hyperacutely without major effect. New means have been found recently to improve this situation. Beside the absorption of multireactive preformed natural antibodies (PNAb) by plasmaphereses or apheresis, the breeding of transgenic pigs expressing human complement regulatory proteins such as decay accelerating factor (DAF) on the endothelial cell surface is the most advanced technique [8]. The combination of these methods seems to be able to prolong the survival time (SVT) of extracorporeal livers due to inhibition or reduction of antibody binding, complement activation, cell adherence and, finally, cytokine release.

Applying these means it seems to be possible to substitute metabolic liver failures after intoxication for a clinically relevant time [1, 2, 6]. In case the patient's own liver recovers, allogeneic transplantation could be avoided. We constructed and tested, therefore, an extracorporeal hepatic perfusion device, which allows investigation of the function of porcine livers when perfused with native, heparinized human blood undergoing hyperacute rejection (HXR). This system allows monitoring of the immediate reaction of the xenogeneic human blood elements when contacting the endothelium or the sinusoidal cells of the porcine liver [7].

Materials and methods

Three transgenic pigs (TP) (body weight 16.3 ± 1.5 kg) and six ordinary landrace pigs (NP) (body weight 25.0 ± 1.6 kg) were heparinized and underwent hepatectomy. The livers (TP: 535 ± 42 g; NP: 689 ± 29 g) were washed clear by infusion of 2000 ml of UW solution at 4 °C via catheters in the portal vein and hepatic artery. After a cold ischemia time of 92 ± 8 min the livers were perfused

Table 1 Data presented (mean ± SEM) of the transgenic human decay accelerating factor (DAF)-expressing pig livers ($n = 3$) perfused with human blood. (*Rah* Vascular resistance of the hepatic artery, *Rvp* vascular resistance of the portal vein, *WBC* white blood cells, *GLDH* glutamate dehydrogenase, *AST* aspartate aminotransferase, *ALT* alanine aminotransferase, *LDH* lactate dehydrogenase, *CK* creatinine kinase, *Hggt* hemagglutination, *TNFα* tumor necrosis factor α, *IL-6* interleukin-6, *IFNγ* interferon-γ)

Parameter measured	Perfusate sampling time (min)								
	0	EF	5	15	30	60	90	120	180
Rah (mm Hg/ml per min)	0.76 ± 0.23	0.66 ± 0.22	0.87 ± 0.57	0.87 ± 0.57	0.80 ± 0.47	0.43 ± 0.03	0.44 ± 0.01	0.41 ± 0.02	0.40 ± 0.01
Rvp (mm Hg/ml per min)	0.09 ± 0.01	0.09 ± 0.01	0.09 ± 0.01	0.10 ± 0.01	0.10 ± 0.01	0.11 ± 0.01	0.13 ± 0.02	0.13 ± 0.01	0.13 ± 0.01
WBC (1000/µl)	3.23 ± 0.09	2.70 ± 0.61	1.07 ± 0.15	1.37 ± 0.27	1.30 ± 0.26	1.27 ± 0.29	1.33 ± 0.32	1.33 ± 0.32	1.23 ± 0.17
GLDH (U/l)	0.27 ± 0.13	8.87 ± 3.25	3.77 ± 1.31	4.47 ± 1.54	5.57 ± 1.28	6.07+2.02	6.87 ± 1.56	8.53 ± 2.27	9.20 ± 2.88
AST (U/l)	4 ± 1	198 ± 131	71 ± 43	83 ± 41	92 ± 42	103 ± 48	118 ± 52	139 ± 56	168 ± 60
ALT (U/l)	4 ± 1	12 ± 5	6 ± 2	7 ± 2	8 ± 2	8 ± 2	10 ± 3	10 ± 3	11 ± 3
LDH (U/l)	62 ± 4	487 ± 279	208 ± 97	242 ± 84	293 ± 89	335 ± 113	396 ± 124	489 ± 136	651 ± 158
CK (U/l)	18 ± 3	94 ± 24	58 ± 27	101 ± 32	135 ± 38	178 ± 62	232 ± 79	276 ± 96	342 ± 119
Hggt (%)	100.0 ± 0	4.67 ± 3.94	1.53 ± 0.90	1.53 ± 0.90	0 ± 0	0 ± 0	0 ± 0	0 ± 0	0 ± 0
CH50 (%)	100.0 ± 0	–	–	–	–	81.5 ± 2.4	–	81.5 ± 1.0	77.7 ± 4.5
AP50 (%)	100.0 ± 0	–	–	–	–	85.7 ± 5.9	–	83.4 ± 5.3	81.2 ± 10.4
C4 (%)	100.0 ± 0	–	–	–	–	84.1 ± 2.5	–	83.5 ± 2.7	86.8 ± 3.1
C3 (%)	100.0 ± 0	–	–	–	–	85.2 ± 5.1	–	85.1 ± 3.9	86.1 ± 4.9
TNFα (pg/ml)	1.0 ± 0.3	4.7 ± 4.2	2.0 ± 1.2	3.7 ± 2.7	39.3 ± 15.4	266.7 ± 114.4	496.0 ± 98.8	666.0 ± 140.0	1003.0 ± 115.9
IL-6 (pg/ml)	0 ± 0	0 ± 0	0 ± 0	0 ± 0	0 ± 0	1.0 ± 0.5	8.0 ± 2.9	39.0 ± 19.7	275.3 ± 50.2
IFNγ (pg/ml)	0 ± 0	48.0 ± 36.2	28.3 ± 14.7	38.3 ± 19.2	43.7 ± 30.0	71.0 ± 34.4	92.0 ± 41.5	117.0 ± 23.5	114.0 ± 19.9
6kPGF1α (pg/ml)	22 ± 3	1230 ± 400	625 ± 80	1087 ± 317	974 ± 321	1120 ± 161	2815 ± 182	3995 ± 848	5118 ± 743

Principle of Perfusion

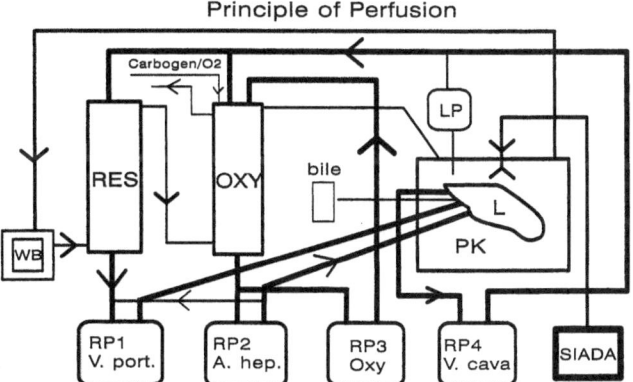

Fig. 1 Scheme of the pig liver perfusion model. (*WB* Warm water bath at 38 °C, *RES* heated blood reservoir, *OXY* heated oxygenator, *RP1–4* roller pumps for the portal vein, hepatic artery, oxygenator, and vena cava, respectively, *LP* Lenz pump to recirculate extrahepatic bleeding, *L* liver packed in a bag, *PK* perfusion chamber filled with 38 °C NaCl solution, *SIADA* simulation of the intraabdominal pressure amplitude)

with heparinized blood in which the pH was adjusted to 7.4 and the temperature to 37 °C. Fresh human blood (1.6 l) from three donors of identical blood groups was diluted to a hematocrit of 30 % with a multielectrolyte solution. The blood was oxygenized and applied under a flow rate of 1.0 ml/g per min (25–30 % over the hepatic artery and 70–75 % over the portal vein). Steady pressure was controlled electronically. The livers were mounted in a plastic bag which was fitted into a transparent perfusion chamber. Around the plastic bag, phosphate-buffered saline (PBS) of 38 °C was circulating. The liver was placed in physiological saline in a vertical position in the air-fed chamber. This fixation allowed changes during the respiratory cycle to be mimicked (Fig. 1).

The metabolic capacity of the xenoperfused liver was determined measuring bile production and oxygen consumption (artery-vein oxygen difference). Perfusate was sampled at times 0, EF, 5, 15, 30, 45, 90, 120, and 180 min. In order to monitor the mechanisms of HXR, liver weights (g), liver-specific enzymes (U/l), electrolyte (mmol/l), white blood cells and platelets (1000 cells/µl), and vascular resistance (as a quotient of perfusion pressure to flow) of the hepatic artery and of the portal vein (mm Hg/min per ml) were determined. Human tumor necrosis factor α (TNFα), interleukin-6 (IL-6), and interferon-γ (IFNγ) (pg/ml) were detected by enzyme-linked immunosorbent assays, the prostaglandin I$_2$ metabolite, 6kPGF1α (pg/ml), by radioimmunoassay. The quantity of PNAb was titrated in a hemagglutination assay using pig red blood cells [5]. Complement consumption was

Table 2 Data (mean ± SEM) from ordinary pig livers ($n = 6$) hemoperfused with human blood. For abbreviations, see Table 1

Parameter measured	Perfusate sampling time (min)								
	0	EF	5	15	30	60	90	120	180
Rah (mm Hg/ml per min)	1.17 ± 0.12	1.16 ± 0.12	1.17 ± 0.09	1.24 ± 0.10	1.22 ± 0.09	1.25 ± 0.10	1.29 ± 0.08	1.33 ± 0.08	1.32 ± 0.07
Rvp (mm Hg/ml per min)	0.06 ± 0.01	0.05 ± 0.01	0.05 ± 0.01	0.06 ± 0.01	0.06 ± 0.01	0.07 ± 0.01	0.07 ± 0.01	0.07 ± 0.01	0.07 ± 0.01
WBC (1000/μl)	4.88 ± 0.16	6.95 ± 0.94	2.90 ± 0.43	2.15 ± 0.29	2.13 ± 0.18	2.08 ± 0.62	2.87 ± 0.49	3.22 ± 1.10	3.78 ± 1.76
GLDH (U/l)	2 ± 1	6 ± 2	7 ± 3	8 ± 2	8 ± 4	9 ± 3	10 ± 3	10 ± 3	12 ± 4
AST (U/l)	7 ± 1	256 ± 104	148 ± 44	194 ± 56	215 ± 51	241 ± 54	311 ± 80	353 ± 93	591 ± 157
ALT (U/l)	5 ± 1	14 ± 4	11 ± 2	13 ± 3	14 ± 2	15 ± 3	18 ± 4	20 ± 5	29 ± 8
LDH (U/l)	144 ± 9	541 ± 230	406 ± 121	473 ± 110	609 ± 152	682 ± 146	782 ± 144	850 ± 139	1218 ± 260
CK (U/l)	26 ± 4	79 ± 23	143 ± 40	228 ± 62	273 ± 67	340 ± 81	427 ± 136	434 ± 118	512 ± 130
Hggt (%)	100.0 ± 0	1.05 ± 0.43	0.30 ± 0.15	0.40 ± 0.18	0.17 ± 0.13	0 ± 0	0 ± 0	0 ± 0	0 ± 0
CH50 (%)	100.0 ± 0	–	–	–	–	66.4 ± 4.0	–	63.1 ± 8.5	57 ± 7.3
AP50 (%)	100.0 ± 0	–	–	–	–	67.9 ± 10.5	–	61.3 ± 7.5	60.1 ± 6.5
C4 (%)	100.0 ± 0	–	–	–	–	71.2 ± 7.8	–	60.6 ± 14.4	59.0 ± 13.9
C3 (%)	100.0 ± 0	–	–	–	–	78.3 ± 2.3	–	79.2 ± 9.4	71.1 ± 8.03
TNFα (pg/ml)	8.8 ± 5.9	65.3 ± 11.5	38.3 ± 13.8	58.7 ± 15.4	178.0 ± 31.6	419.8 ± 65.1	561.8 ± 73.0	861.2 ± 126.3	1103.2 ± 179.4
IL-6 (pg/ml)	2.0 ± 1.0	1.0 ± 0.5	1.8 ± 0.7	2.0 ± 0.7	2.3 ± 0.6	11.7 ± 1.6	46.8 ± 5.8	146.8 ± 20.0	370.0 ± 58.8
IFNγ (pg/ml)	2.5 ± 2.5	4.5 ± 4.5	6.0 ± 3.9	14.7 ± 11.6	19.5 ± 14.3	45.8 ± 16.7	72.2 ± 13.6	137.2 ± 17.4	146.8 ± 25.1
6kPGF1α (pg/ml)	0 ± 0	303 ± 62	359 ± 21	364 ± 52	435 ± 69	1042 ± 152	1403 ± 122	1499 ± 163	1720 ± 198

measured using the CH50 (%) and AP50 (%) tests. C4 and C3 (mg/l) were directly determined in the plasma aliquots. At completion of the perfusion, tissue sections were snap-frozen for histological and immunohistological examination.

PNAb of IgM and IgG types and the complement components of the classical and alternative complement pathways were stained using the appropriate secondary detecting antibodies.

Results

All data were tested by the Wilcoxon test in each group and by variance analysis and LS means test between groups ($P < 0.05$). Because $n = 3$ in the TP group, statistical tests did not reach significant levels, but the trend was positive. Data can be compared in Tables 1–3.

Physical characteristics

In the NP group, the mean liver weight increased by 14.1 % in contrast to only 9 % in the TP group. Bile flow (expressed in ml/h) increased by 28.6 % during reperfusion but did not change in the TP group. Resistance values showed marked differences between the hepatic artery and the portal vein, with a very high initial resistance in the portal vein. Resistance in the he-

patic artery showed no particular pattern. All values were found to be lower in the TP than in the NP group. A traumatic leukocyte depletion, directly after starting reperfusion, was found to be identical in both groups.

Biochemical characteristics

A significant difference existed in plasma levels of creatinine kinase (CK), lactate dehydrogenase (LDH), aspartate aminotransferase (AST), [glutamate oxaloacetate transferase (GOT)], alanine aminotransferase (ALT) [glutamate phosphotransferase (GPT)], and glutamate dehydrogenase (GLDH) immediately after reperfusion and at the end of the experiment between the two groups. The perfusing system only had no impact on biochemical results or white blood cell counts and cytokines, nor did the titers of PNAb or the amount of complement change.

Immunological parameters

Both the TP and NP groups showed a rapid decrease of white blood cells and thrombocytes after circulating

Table 3 Data (mean ± SEM) of the controls (human blood circulating the system without a graft; $n = 5$). For abbreviations, see Table 1

Parameter measured	Perfusate sampling time (min)							
	0	5	15	30	60	90	120	180
WBC (1000/µl)	4.28 ± 0.48	4.04 ± 0.48	3.78 ± 0.36	3.76 ± 0.37	3.20 ± 0.28	3.34 ± 0.47	3.40 ± 0.42	3.27 ± 0.30
GLDH (U/l)	0.62 ± 0.23	0.48 ± 0.16	0.46 ± 0.07	0.58 ± 0.17	0.62 ± 0.16	0.80 ± 0.20	0.84 ± 0.20	0.72 ± 0.24
AST (U/l)	5 ± 1	5 ± 1	5 ± 1	5 ± 1	5 ± 1	5 ± 1	6 ± 1	6 ± 1
ALT (U/l)	3 ± 1	3 ± 1	3 ± 1	3 ± 1	3 ± 1	3 ± 1	3 ± 1	4 ± 1
LDH (U/l)	122 ± 15	119 ± 10	127 ± 10	141 ± 13	155 ± 20	180 ± 29	191 ± 35	230 ± 45
CK (U/l)	25 ± 7	25 ± 7	26 ± 8	26 ± 8	25 ± 7	25 ± 7	25 ± 7	25 ± 7
Hggt (%)	100.0 ± 0	100.0 ± 0	100.0 ± 0	100.0 ± 0	100.0 ± 0	100.0 ± 0	100.0 ± 0	100.0 ± 0
CH50 (%)	100.0 ± 0	–	–	–	99.4 ± 0.6	–	96.8 ± 2.4	98.0 ± 2.0
AP50 (%)	100.0 ± 0	–	–	–	96.1 ± 3.9	–	99.4 ± 0.6	100.0 ± 0
C4 (%)	100.0 ± 0	–	–	–	98.8 ± 1.2	–	100.0 ± 0	100.0 ± 0
C3 (%)	100.0 ± 0	–	–	–	100.0 ± 0	–	100.0 ± 0	96.3 ± 3.7
TNFα (pg/ml)	14.4 ± 11.8	9.8 ± 7.9	10.0 ± 8.1	12.0 ± 8.7	200.8 ± 87.4	642.6 ± 324.2	957.8 ± 324.2	1318.0 ± 289.8
IL-6 (pg/ml)	4.0 ± 1.4	2.2 ± 0.4	2.6 ± 0.9	3.8 ± 0.7	6.8 ± 3.6	72.6 ± 41.3	312.4 ± 93.4	519.8 ± 65.4
IFNγ (pg/ml)	2.0 ± 1.1	25.2 ± 13.3	23.4 ± 10.6	21.6 ± 9.1	27.4 ± 12.5	38.2 ± 20.3	23.4 ± 8.9	31.6 ± 12.7
6kPGF1α (pg/ml)	30 ± 28	36 ± 32	36 ± 25	7 ± 3	7 ± 3	6 ± 2	16 ± 8	46 ± 21

the xenograft. PNAb were depleted rapidly from the circulating blood in both groups.

Marked differences were found in complement consumption. In the NP group, the CH50 and AP50 tests revealed a 70 % decrease but this was only 20 % in the transgenic group. In plasma, C4 and C3 showed no decrease in the peripheral blood of the TP group but a significant reduction in the NP group. This was reflected by immunohistology showing no staining for C4/d/d and C3/c/d in the NP group but marked staining in the NP group.

Levels of the proinflammatory cytokines, TNFα, IL-6, and IFNγ, increased significantly during the first 60 min of reperfusion without noticeable differences, however, between the two groups. Values of 6kPGF1α were found to increase significantly during hemoperfusion of livers of both groups with a much higher release in the TP group.

Discussion

Until recently the temporary xenogeneic hemoperfusion of porcine livers was one of the only clinical applications of discordant xenografts. New developments in many directions, especially in producing transgenic pigs, could further improve the beneficial results achieved.

Our reperfusion system allows a careful management of the organ in applying physiological conditions. The specially prepared tubing system and oxygenator but,

even more, the modification of the transgenic pigs, [3, 9] improved the perfusion parameters significantly. Dramatic differences were seen in the release of specific enzymes, prostaglandins, and cytokines. This might be due to the significantly lower consumption of complement and its activation on the endothelial cells surfaces, as shown by immunohistology.

The expression of human DAF on endothelial cells seems to reduce the early endothelial cell stimulation by preventing the extreme hemorrhage and edema seen in normal livers. The significantly reduced complement activation by these complement regulator proteins also prevents endothelial cell activation, as shown by the low release of cytokines and high release of prostaglandins. In the event that the observed increase of resistance can be inhibited by DAF antagonists and antibody aphereses, this temporary approach could be the first clinically relevant application of a discordant xenograft.

References

1. Abouna GM, et al (1972) Br Med J 1: 23
2. Burdick JF, et al (1994) Xenotransplantation 2: 3
3. Carrington CA, et al (1995) Transplant Proc 27: 321
4. Fox IJ, et al (1993) Am J Gastroenterol 88: 1876
5. Hammer C (1987) Transplant Proc 19: 4443
6. Makowka L, et al (1993) Xenotransplantation 1: 27
7. Pöhlein Ch, et al (1994) Transplant Int 7 (Suppl 1): 643
8. Rosengard AM, et al (1995) Transplant Proc 27: 326
9. White DJG (1994) Xenotransplantation 2: 1

Ethics

Transpl Int (1996) 9 [Suppl 1]: S 399–S 402
© Springer-Verlag 1996

ETHICS

L. B. Hilbrands
A. J. Hoitsma
R. A. P. Koene

Costs of drugs used after renal transplantation

L. B. Hilbrands (✉) · A. J. Hoitsma ·
R. A. P. Koene
Department of Medicine, Division of
Nephrology, University Hospital
Nijmegen,
PO Box 9101, NL-6500 HB Nijmegen,
The Netherlands
Tel. +31 24 361 47 61; Fax +31 24 354 00 22

Abstract There are no detailed data on the relative contributions to overall health care costs of the various drugs that are commonly used in renal transplant patients. We performed a cost analysis in 122 patients, using the medical records and our hospital administration service as data sources, for all health care-related costs during the first year after renal transplantation. During the first 3 months all patients were on cyclosporine (CsA) and prednisone. Subsequently, they were randomly allocated to CsA monotherapy or to conversion from CsA to azathioprine. Cost of drugs comprised about 25 % of total health care expenses. In CsA-treated patients, the following costs per patient per year were calculated: CsA, DFL 9929 (1 DFL is about US $ 0.60; 67.5 % of total drug costs); antilymphocyte agents, DFL 2613 (17.8 %); other immunosuppressive drugs, DFL 455 (3.1 %); antimicrobial agents, DFL 687 (4.7 %); antihypertensive drugs, DFL 467 (3.2 %); remaining drugs, DFL 554 (3.8 %). Conversion from CsA to azathioprine resulted in a decrease in mean drug costs for the remainder of the first posttransplant year of DFL 4597 ($P < 0.01$). Although the incidence of acute rejections tended to be higher after steroid withdrawal than after conversion (39 % versus 26 %, not significant), the costs of anti-rejection therapy, hospitalization, and laboratory services did not differ. We conclude that CsA is the main determinant of overall drug costs. When compared to CsA monotherapy, conversion from CsA to azathioprine at 3 months after transplantation may result in subsequent cost savings of about DFL 5000 per patient per year without a higher incidence of rejection or graft loss.

Key words Renal transplantation · Cost analysis · Cyclosporine · Immunosuppressive drugs

Introduction

Costs of drugs, especially cyclosporine (CsA) and antilymphocyte agents, considerably add to overall expenses of health care in renal allograft recipients. Detailed data on the relative contribution of various drugs to health care expenditure in this population are not available. We performed a cost-effectiveness analysis in renal transplant patients who participated in a prospective randomized trial comparing CSA monotherapy with the combination of azathioprine and prednisone from 3 months after transplantation. The data that were gathered for this analysis during the first year after transplantation allowed us to answer the following questions:

1. How do the costs of drugs compare to the costs of other items (e.g., hospital admission days, laboratory services)?
2. What is the relative contribution of various classes of drugs to total drug costs?

3. How do different immunosuppressive regimens affect costs of drugs and of other items?

Patients and methods

Patient population and treatment protocol

Our study population comprised 127 recipients (age between 18 and 65 years) of a first or second cadaveric renal allograft, with a functioning graft at 3 months after transplantation. None of the patients had received induction therapy with antilymphocyte agents. CsA was given in an oral dose of 12 mg/kg per day during the first month. This was gradually reduced to about 4 mg/kg per day at 3 months after transplantation. The prednisone dose was 25 mg/day during the first month and 20 mg/day during the second and third months after transplantation. At 3 months after transplantation, patients were allocated to withdrawal of steroids, resulting in CsA monotherapy, or to replacement of CsA by azathioprine. In the CsA group, CsA was continued in the same dosage with adjustments to reach trough blood levels between 100 and 200 ng/ml (monoclonal antibody assay). The daily prednisone dosage was reduced by 5 mg every 2 weeks, resulting in CsA monotherapy after 6 weeks. In patients allocated to azathioprine-prednisone therapy, CsA was replaced without overlap by azathioprine at a dosage of 3 mg/kg. Their prednisone dosage was temporarily increased from 20 to 25 mg/day and reduced by 5 mg every 2 weeks until a maintenance dose of 10 mg/day was reached. Antimicrobial prophylactic therapy was not applied, but all patients received an H_2-receptor antagonist during the first 3 to 4 months after transplantation as prophylaxis against peptic ulcers.

During the first 3 months after transplantation, acute rejection episodes were treated with methylprednisolone (1 g/day i.v. on 3 consecutive days) or antithymocyte globulin (ATG, RIVM Bilthoven, The Netherlands; 200 mg/day i.v. on alternate days for 10 days). An oral course of high-dose prednisone (initial dosage 200 mg/day tapering to 25 mg/day in 12 days) was given after failure of one or both of these treatments. From 3 months after transplantation (i.e., after randomization), acute rejections were primarily treated with ATG in all cases. High-dose prednisone courses were given in case of failure of ATG, bone marrow suppression, or previous treatment with ATG for rejection. Occasionally, acute rejections were treated with monoclonal anti-CD3 antibodies.

Cost analysis

Health care costs were calculated for the first year after transplantation. Costs of kidney-acquisition and indirect costs for society, e.g., costs related to disablement, were not considered. Otherwise, no restrictions were made in the services that were included, regardless of the probability of a relationship between a particular service or activity on the one hand and the renal transplantation on the other hand. The medical records were used as data source for the amounts of all kinds of drugs that were used during hospital stays (except drugs used in the operating room) as well as on an outpatient basis. Similarly, number of admission days, number of visits to the outpatient clinic, and number of CsA blood level measurements were counted from the medical records. The clinical laboratory and blood transfusion service supplied quantitative information on their services for the patients concerned. Our hospital financial administration service provided data on activities regarding to following items: operating room and anesthesia, diagnostic radiology, nuclear medicine, endoscopy, pathology, and physiotherapy. Prices current during 1993 or 1994, and expressed in Dutch guilders (1 DFL is about U.S. $ 0.60), were used to calculate costs.

Table 1 Health care costs per patient during the first year after transplantation in patients who were allocated treatment with cyclosporine monotherapy *(CsA)* or a combination of azathioprine and prednisone *(Aza-Pred)*. Costs are expressed in Dutch guilders (means ± SD)

Item	Treatment period (months)	CsA	Aza-Pred
Drugs	1–3	5641 ± 2598	5829 ± 2677
	4–12	9064 ± 4713	4280 ± 4062*
	Entire year	14706 ± 5361	10109 ± 4680*
Hospitalization	1–3	8311 ± 4692	8036 ± 4351
	4–12	10520 ± 30609	5579 ± 8925
	Entire year	18831 ± 31444	13615 ± 10159
Visits to outpatient clinic	1–3	816 ± 189	852 ± 185
	4–12	1554 ± 597	1499 ± 449
	Entire year	2370 ± 625	2351 ± 502
CsA level measurements	1–3	965 ± 365	1020 ± 387
	4–12	1009 ± 459	173 ± 347*
	Entire year	1975 ± 675	1194 ± 495*
Renal replacement therapy	1–3	551 ± 1316	374 ± 881
	4–12	109 ± 788	35 ± 273
	Entire year	660 ± 1497	409 ± 908
Laboratory services (excluding CsA level measurements)		9453 ± 7352	8516 ± 3207
Other diagnostic and therapeutic activities		4944 ± 3882	4335 ± 4425
Blood products		545 ± 1168	355 ± 571
Total costs		53484 ± 44828	40882 ± 18895**

* $P < 0.001$, ** $P < 0.05$ for differences between both groups

Prices of the medication that was used were obtained from the hospital pharmacy. The direct costs of hospital days and visits to the outpatient clinic were estimated on the basis of personnel costs and material expenses (excluding medication and blood products) and amounted to about DFL 300 and DFL 75, respectively. For the intensive care unit, costs were estimated at DFL 2000 per day. The costs of other services were assessed in an analogous way and in case reliable estimations were not attainable (as for laboratory services), charges were used as a proxy for costs.

Statistical analysis

Although a number of patients switched from one treatment to another (e.g., because of CsA nephrotoxicity), all data were analyzed on an intention-to-treat basis. Calculations were performed with the SAS system (SAS Institute, Cary, North Carolina, USA). Data are given as means with SD. Comparisons of numerical data were performed with Wilcoxon's rank sum test. Proportions were compared with chi-square analysis using continuity correction. A P value smaller than 0.05 was considered statistically significant.

Results

Two patients who died, two patients with graft loss, and one patient for whom insufficient data were available, were excluded from the analysis (death and graft loss were evenly distributed among both groups). Of the re-

Table 2 Costs of various classes of drugs that were used during the first year after transplantation by patients who were allocated treatment with cyclosporine monotherapy *(CsA)* or a combination of azathioprine and prednisone *(Aza-Pred)* from 3 months after transplantation. Added costs for all patients in each group are expressed in Dutch guilders

Drug	Treatment period (months)	CsA ($n = 61$)		Aza-Pred ($n = 61$)	
		Absolute	Percentage of total	Absolute	Percentage of total
Cyclosporine	1–3	238083		249920	
	4–12	367597		48694	
	Entire year	605680	67.5	297985	48.3
Azathioprine	1–3	1453		1168	
	4–12	19842		63719	
	Entire year	21296	2.4	64888	10.5
Prednisone	1–3	2078		2083	
	4–12	2583		3087	
	Entire year	4662	0.5	5170	0.8
Antilymphocyte agents	1–3	73716		75425	
	4–12	85720		82421	
	Entire year	159436	17.8	157847	25.6
Steroids for rejection	1–3	1028		1307	
	4–12	741		380	
	Entire year	1770	0.2	1687	0.3
Antihypertensive drugs	1–3	5251		4386	
	4–12	23251		17966	
	Entire year	28502	3.2	22353	3.6
Antimicrobial agents	1–3	13323		14683	
	4–12	28574		29907	
	Entire year	41898	4.7	44591	7.2
Other drugs	1–3	9164		7191	
	4–12	24616		14908	
	Entire year	33780	3.8	22099	3.6
Total	1–3	344104		355540	
	4–12	552932		261088	
	Entire year	897037	100	616629	100

maining 122 patients, the mean age was 43 ± 13 years, 64 % were male, and 83 % had a first transplant. Each treatment group consisted of 61 patients. The number of patients with one or more acute rejection episodes during the first 3 months after transplantation did not differ between the groups (CsA: 25 %, azathioprine-prednisone: 26 %). From the time of randomization until the end of the first posttransplant year, the incidence of at least one rejection was 39 % in the CsA group and 26 % in the azathioprine-prednisone group (not significant).

Table 1 shows the costs of drugs and of several other items for all patients, and for both treatment groups separately. When available, separate data are given for months 1–3 and months 4–12 after transplantation. Costs of drugs comprised about 25 % of all expenses to health care during the first year after transplantation in these patients. As expected, in 62 patients who experienced one or more rejection episodes during the first year after transplantation, total costs per patient were significantly higher than in 60 patients without a rejection (DFL 56717 ± 39406 versus 37333 ± 26250; $P < 0.001$). When patients with any acute rejection episode after transplantation were excluded from calculations, total costs were DFL 43582 ± 34398 in the CsA

group ($n = 28$) and DFL 31865 ± 14654 in the azathioprine-prednisone group ($n = 32$) ($P < 0.05$).

In Table 2, costs of different classes of drugs are summarized. In the CsA group, whole-year costs of CsA made up 68 % of all drug costs, as compared to 48 % in the azathioprine-prednisone group. When only the period after randomization was included in the calculations (months 4–12), these figures were 67 % and 19 %, respectively. Antilymphocyte agents formed the next most expensive drug category. The costs of drugs other than immunosuppressive agents amounted to only 10–15 % of total drug costs during the first year after transplantation.

The lower total costs in the azathioprine-prednisone group (Table 1), in part, resulted from significantly lower drug costs and less expenditure on measurements of CsA levels. During the 9 months after randomization, the costs of base-line immunosuppressive therapy (CsA, prednisone, and azathioprine) differed significantly between groups, despite the inclusion of patients who changed from one treatment group to the other at some time (CsA, DFL 6394 ± 274; azathioprine-prednisone, DFL 1893 ± 192; $P < 0.001$). From the data obtained during the last 3 months of the first posttransplant year, we estimate that conversion from CsA to azathioprine might result in subsequent savings of about DFL 4700 per year.

Discussion

Drugs substantially contribute to the costs of renal transplantation. In our population of renal transplant patients, drugs accounted for about 25 % of the financial expenses to health care during the first year after transplantation. Together with a decrease in the number of hospital admission days, the relative contribution of drugs to total costs can be expected to be even larger during subsequent years. CsA is the main determinant of overall drug costs, since costs of CsA amounted to nearly 70 % of all drug costs in CsA-treated patients.

We recognize that these figures cannot be generalized to all renal transplant patients. First, a number of the criteria included (only first and second transplants, age between 18 and 65 years) may have caused some selection bias. Second, only the data of patients who were alive with a functioning graft at 1 year after transplantation were analyzed. Some of the patients with severe or multiple complications, ultimately leading to death or graft loss, may generate unusually high or low costs on certain items. In addition, it has to be mentioned that for several entries in our calculations, hospital charges were used as a proxy for costs. In some instances these charges can at best be used as a rough estimate of how the costs of comparable activities (e. g., different laboratory services) relate to each other. Nevertheless, we believe that our data provide valuable information, which is currently scarce, on the relative contribution of various drugs and other services to the costs of renal transplantation.

The use of CsA has substantially increased graft survival rates after renal transplantation [2, 3]. This improvement in graft survival appears to result mainly from a decrease in the number of rejection episodes during the first months after transplantation. From an economic point of view, switching from CsA to azathioprine at some time after transplantation seems an attractive treatment strategy. In our hands, azathioprine-prednisone from 3 months after transplantation appeared to be a more cost-effective treatment than CsA monotherapy. The tendency to a higher frequency of rejections in the CsA group could not sufficiently explain the higher costs in this group, since the difference in costs remained present after exclusion of patients with one or more rejection episodes from both groups. Previous studies have demonstrated the cost-effectiveness of CsA-containing immunosuppressive regimens [1, 6]. However, in these studies, control patients did not receive CsA at all, whereas in the current study all patients were treated with CsA during the first 3 months after transplantation. This initial treatment with CsA protected our patients from the high risk of rejection and associated costs of hospital readmissions during the early phase after transplantation. Indeed, the finding of lower costs associated with the use of CsA in the study of Showstack et al. [6] was confined to the direct posttransplantation hospitalization period, while total charges did not differ from those in the control group during the follow-up period.

Our data do not allow a comparison of the cost-effectiveness of conversion from CsA to azathioprine versus continued treatment with CsA and prednisone. Given the impression that a number of rejections in our CsA group were related to the withdrawal of steroids, continued treatment with both CsA and prednisone will most likely result in a rejection incidence that is lower than that observed after conversion from CsA to azathioprine [5]. In that case, the reduced frequency of rejections may compensate for the higher costs of base-line immunosuppressive therapy. Nevertheless, recent reports of similar graft survival rates after conversion from CsA to azathioprine as compared to continued treatment with CsA and prednisone [4, 5], support a deliberate use of a conversion regimen, which may save about DFL 5000 per patient per year.

Acknowledgements Supported by a research grant from Sandoz, Basle, Switzerland.

References

1. Canafax DM, Gruber SA, Chan GL, Miles CJ, Matas AJ, Najarian JS, Cipolle RJ (1990) The pharmacoeconomics of renal transplantation: increased drug costs with decreased hospitalization costs. Pharmacotherapy 10: 205–210
2. European Multicentre Trial Group (1983) Cyclosporin in cadaveric renal transplantation: one year follow-up of a multicentre trial. Lancet 2: 986–989
3. Hall BM, Tiller DJ, Hardie I, Mahony J, Mathew T, Thatcher G, Miach P, Thomson N, Sheil AG (1988) Comparison of three immunosuppressive regimens in cadaver renal transplantation: long-term cyclosporine, short-term cyclosporine followed by azathioprine and prednisolone, and azathioprine and prednisolone without cyclosporine. N Engl J Med 318: 1499–1507
4. Hollander AAMJ, Saase JLCM van, Kootte AM, Dorp WT van, Bockel HJ van, Es LA van, Woude FJ van der (1995) Beneficial effects of conversion from cyclosporin to azathioprine after kidney transplantation. Lancet 345: 610–614
5. Kasiske BL, Heim-Duthoy K, Ma JZ (1993) Elective cyclosporine withdrawal after renal transplantation. A meta-analysis. J Am Med Assoc 269: 395–400
6. Showstack J, Katz P, Amend W, Salvatierra O (1990) The association of cyclosporine with the 1-year costs of cadaver-donor kidney transplants. J Am Med Assoc 264: 1818–1823

Transpl Int (1996) 9 [Suppl 1]: S403–S406
© Springer-Verlag 1996

ETHICS

L. Berardinelli
M. Raiteri
B. Costantino

Ethical aspects of using "marginal" kidneys for transplant

L. Berardinelli · M. Raiteri · B. Costantino
Kidney Transplant Unit, Policlinico
University Hospital, Via Francesco Sforza
35, I-20122 Milan, Italy
Tel. +39 2 55 03 56 53; Fax +39 2 55 18 56 02

L. Berardinelli (✉)
Kidney Transplant Unit,
Policlinico University
Hospital, Via F. Sforza 35,
I-20122 Milan, Italy

Abstract The continuing demand for transplantable organs leads to ongoing debates about organ procurement, even with arguments in favour of xenotransplantation as a valid alternative. This article examines the management of kidneys with major anatomical anomalies, almost one-quarter of those available for transplantation in our experience: the decision-making is considered from a scientific and an ethical standpoint. Surgical techniques include primary revascularization (PR) and/or bench-top reconstructions (BR). The results, examined for 1311 normal grafts (Group I) and 362 grafts presenting major anatomical anomalies (Group II), all transplanted for the first time, showed almost the same rates of failures due to surgical causes in these two groups. No operative mortality was associated with any of the vascular techniques, BR being easier and safer than PR. Graft survival at 1 year is the same for Group I and Group II (85 % versus 84 %, respectively). An ethical allocation system ought to take into account the experience of the transplant surgeon for maximizing outcome and minimizing cost and risk for transplantation.

Key words Marginal kidneys · Renal anomalies · Surgical complications · Kidney transplantation · Microsurgery in kidney transplantation

Introduction

The success of kidney transplantation (KT) has increased the need for transplantable organs: over 2000 dialysis patients die each year in the United States on the waiting list for a kidney [7]. The discrepancy between request and offer continues to grow, making it imperative to transplant all functioning organs, including kidneys with abnormal anatomy, which constitute in some series up to 28 % of the total available [6]. On the other hand, graft quality is important for transplant outcome and must be taken into account in kidney sharing.

The purpose of the present study is to examine our experience with anomalous kidneys that are generally considered to be at higher risk for surgical complications [1, 5, 6] and delayed graft function [5], evaluating the question of transplanting so-called marginal kidneys from an ethical standpoint.

Patients and methods

From May 1969 to July 1995, 1760 renal transplants were performed at our Institution, the majority (89.2 %) from cadaver donors (CD). Eighty-five patients received a second transplant and two of them a third transplant (Table 1). From the outset, we have adopted a wide policy of kidney procurement and graft exchange.

Where donor nephrectomy is done by our team and the abnormality is unilateral, the normal kidney is generally sent away and the anomalous one transplanted at our center. A total of 385 anomalous kidneys, with major anatomical abnormalities or repaired renal arteries, has been transplanted, coming from either CD (375) or living donors (LD) (10). In 115 of these grafts, 123 extracorporeal bench reconstructions (95 arterial and 28 venous) had to be performed before transplantation. The earliest microvascular

Table 1 Kidney transplants performed at the Policlinico University Hospital of Milan (May 1969–July 1995). Fourteen simultaneous multivisceral transplants were performed between 1986 and 1995

Transplants at different time periods	Number	Live donors	Retransplants
1969–1973	132	4	2
1974–1978	257	21	10
1979–1983	360	28	15
1984–1988	501	43	46
1989–1995	490	93	14
1969–July 1995	1760	189	87

Table 2 Causes of variations from the standard technique in vascular anastomoses (1760 renal transplantations). (In 115 transplantations with vascular anomalies of the grafts, 123 extracorporeal reconstructions (95 arterial and 28 venous) were performed before transplantation. Two of the en-bloc transplants were of horseshoe kidneys

	Artery	Vein
Vascular anomalies of the graft	371	120
Arterial sclerosis of the recipient	301	–
Vascular anomalies of the recipient	6	5
Discrepancy of vascular size	41	19
En-bloc transplant	14	14
Ligature of thin vessels	55	144

bench reconstructions were successfully made on grafts from LD found to have at nephrectomy supernumerary vessels, which had not been visualized by preoperative arteriography. Later on, our Institution, as the most experienced center of KT in Italy, took on the role of collecting anomalous cadaver kidneys that would otherwise have been discarded from other transplant centers.

The lack of hypoperfused areas and the absence of severe atherosclerotic disease were the criteria requested for repairing the organs whose vessels had been damaged at nephrectomy. In only 55 cases could a simple ligation of thin arterial vessels less than 1 mm in diameter be made, as hilar branches or small capsular arteries of the upper pole, supplying areas smaller than 2 cm in diameter (Table 2). Multiple arteries supplying the lower pole are always revascularized to avoid ureteral necrosis and fistula or stenosis.

A total of 1673 grafts coming from CD or LD and transplanted for the first time are considered for the present study:

1. Group 1: 1311 normal kidneys [776 treated with cyclosporine (CsA) and 535 with conventional therapy].
2. Group II: 362 kidneys with major anatomical anomalies (194 under CsA and 168 under conventional therapy). Group II comprises 348 kidneys having an abnormal vascular supply (two arteries in 303 cases, three arteries in 40 cases and four arteries in 5 cases; not included are grafts in which thin supernumerary arteries were ligated); 12 organs presenting a complete ureteral duplication (treated by two separate ureterocistoneostomies with an antireflux technique); 2 indivisible horseshoe kidneys [transplanted en-bloc into two recipients using different techniques (Fig. 1)].

A variety of surgical techniques has been employed to solve the problem of multiple arterial supply, using primary revascularization (PR) in 265 cases and/or 95 arterial bench-top reconstructions (BR). End-to-side anastomosis of an aortic patch bearing the multiple vessels, separate end-to-side anastomoses of multiple renal ar-

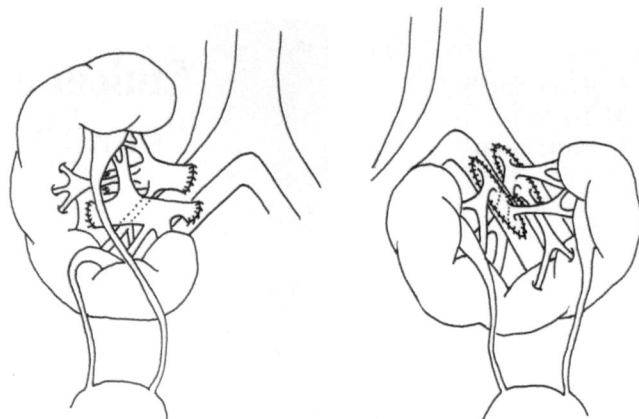

Fig. 1 Two different techniques for en-bloc transplantation of indivisible horseshoe kidneys

teries, removed without a patch, end-to-end anastomoses of multiple renal arteries to the bifurcation of the hypogastric artery, and end-to-end anastomosis of a lower polar artery to the recipient epigastric artery are some of the techniques employed for primary revascularization.

BR techniques have been adopted for transplanting 95 grafts (Fig. 2) with repair of a damaged accessory artery at the aortic patch junction (6 cases), anastomosis of multiple arteries end-to-side to the main renal artery (67 cases), end-to-end anastomosis of the supernumerary artery after having cut off the damaged segment (3 cases), where necessary by interposing an inverted homologous vein graft to extend the length of the artery (6 cases), a vena cava patch (6 cases) or an aortic patch (2 cases), both derived from the actual CD, were employed for an end-to-side anastomosis of accessory artery or arteries. Where a donor patch was unavailable, a homologous saphenous vein patch acquired from a stripping was adopted to anastomose one or more accessory arteries (5 cases).

Our vascular shield [2], used as an intraluminal stent, prevents the inferior wall being entrapped. This simple device allowed the microsurgical repairing of damaged vessels, even in infant necrokidneys: in the World Transplant Records 1994 reported by P. Terasaki we are the first center successfully to transplant the youngest (and smallest) CD renal allografts reconstructed at the bench [9].

Group I and Group II, similar in demographic variables and clinical profiles such as sex, age, original disease, source of organs, HLA matching, prior transfusions, sensitization, mean warm/cold ischemia time and preservation, are separately evaluated on the basis of the immunosuppressive treatments by actuarial graft survival according to Kaplan-Meier curves and compared by means of the log-rank test. No patients were excluded from the analysis.

Results

There was no operative mortality associated with any of these vascular techniques. In Group I, overall failures related to a surgical cause were 45 (3.4%), while in Group II, 15 kidneys were lost through surgical complications (5.6%); the difference is not significant. Moreover, the majority (80%) of these complications belong to the initial stages of our study. Infact, in the 95 BR

Fig. 2 Some bench-top techniques employed for transplanting kidneys with multiple or damaged arteries

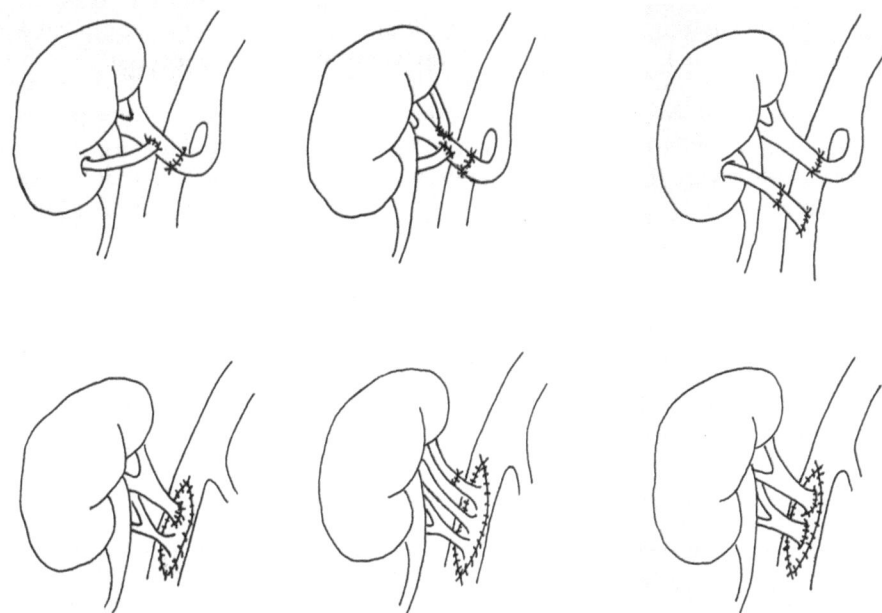

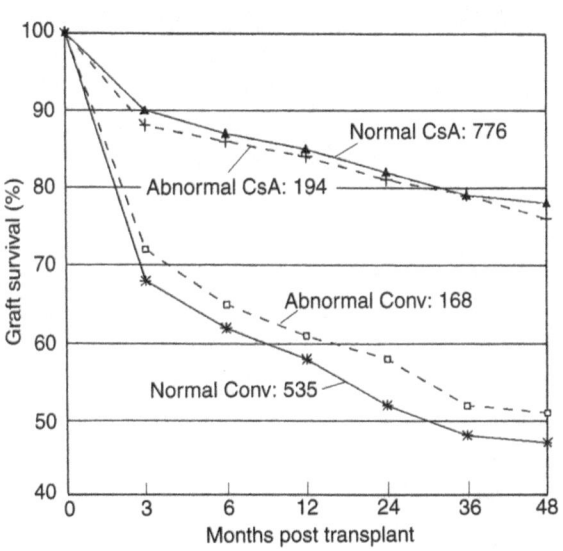

Fig. 3 Actuarial first graft survival of normal and abnormal kidneys on the basis of the immunosuppressive treatment. (*CsA* Cyclosporine)

The two indivisible horseshoe kidneys had a postoperative course free of complications and immediate diuresis in both cases. The function remained good for 25 and 61 months, when the grafts were lost due to non-compliance and rejection, respectively [9].

The presence of renal anomalies did not influence the primary function of 194 patients under CsA, transplanted with an anomalous graft, in comparison with those receiving a normal one (88.9 %, versus 90.1 %).

The results of graft survival are significantly better under CsA therapy [3] in comparison with historical series of transplants under conventional immunosuppression (Fig. 3); moreover, actuarial graft survival of 776 normal grafts, transplanted for the first time and treated with CsA, evidenced the same success rate as the 194 "marginal" kidneys under CsA, at all time intervals (85 % versus 84 % at 1 year, and 78 % versus 76.8 % at 4 years).

Lastly, vascular supply does not appear to influence function, as measured by creatinine clearance at the first postoperative year, as we have previously noted [8].

grafts belonging to Group II, only one kidney had to be removed due to a surgical complication, which was a result of spontaneous parenchymal rupture. Of the 12 patients receiving organs with a double ureter, two have been treated by conventional therapy and ten were submitted to CsA therapy; none had any surgical problem; two patients lost their graft at 1 and 53 months respectively due to irreversible rejection; one patient died 37 months after transplantation in a road accident; the other nine patients have a well-functioning kidney from 3 to 152 months after transplant (57.3 ± 52.9 months).

Discussion

Our results indicate that anomalous kidneys must not be considered as high-risk grafts, contrary to the experience of others, who report an increase of 22.9 % in vascular complications after transplantation of kidneys with multiple arteries [1]. Some of the contradictory results of studies analyzing surgical complications of anomalous kidneys may be explained by different management and different experience in microsurgical techniques. The current allocation system ought to take into account the anatomical anomalies of the kidney, and the experience of the transplant surgeon who is responsible for the decision to transplant a kidney. In order to reduce organ shortage and maximize outcome of transplantation, anomalous kidneys ought to be collected in those centers with the most experience, where a critical evaluation is mandatory. The anomalous kidney becomes a "marginal" graft only for those operators having poor experience.

Routine use of extracorporeal reconstruction allows a liberalization of the eligibility criteria for transplantation and optimal utilization of a limited organ supply. If the basic ethical issue remains that of "saving the largest number of lives, and utilizing organs that have the greatest chance for a long-term function" [4], the present paper demonstrates, in our opinion, that there is the potential for increasing the donor pool by up to 25 % with the use of anomalous kidneys, without loosing the quality of post-implant function.

Last, but not least, the allocation system now being assessed, maximizing outcome and minimizing costs and risk for transplantation, has a valuable financial benefit to society and to the patient.

References

1. Benoit G, Jaber N, Jaber N, Moukarzel M (1994) Incidence of arterial and venous complications in kidney transplantation: role of the kidney preservation solution. Transplant Proc 26: 295–296
2. Berardinelli L, Vegeto A (1978) A simple vascular shield for microanastomoses. Am J Surg 134: 127
3. Berardinelli L, Vegeto A (1995) Twenty-five years of transplant experience at the Policlinico University Hospital of Milan. In: Terasaki PI, Cecka JM (eds) Clinical transplant 1994. UCLA Tissue Typing Laboratory, Los Angeles, pp 243–253
4. Halasz NA (1991) Medicine and ethics: how to allocate transplantable organs. Transplantation 52: 43–46
5. Nghiem DD (1994) Donor aortoplasty for transplantation of kidneys with multiple arteries. J Urol 152: 2055–2056
6. Shokeir AA, El-Diasty TA, Shaaban AA (1993) Evaluation of potential kidney donors using digital subtraction angiography. Transplant Proc 25: 2272–2273
7. Transplant News (1992) 2: 1
8. Vegeto A, Berardinelli L, Beretta C (1982) Outcome of renal grafts with multiple or damaged vessels. Proc Eur Dial Transplant Assoc 19: 477–481
9. World Transplant Records 1994 (1995) Terasaki PI, Cecka JM (eds) Clinical transplant 1994. UCLA Tissue Typing Laboratory, Los Angeles, p 567

Organ Procurement

Transpl Int (1996) 9 [Suppl 1]: S 409–S 413
© Springer-Verlag 1996

T. Auer
W. Weihs
B. Grasser
B. Schmidt
B. Petutschnigg
A. Wasler
F. Iberer
K. H. Tscheliessnigg

Donor heart quality control. Analysis of echocardiographic (EC) findings and patient outcome

T. Auer (✉) · B. Grasser · B. Schmidt ·
B. Petutschnigg · A. Wasler · F. Iberer ·
K. H. Tscheliessnigg
Department of Surgery, University of Graz,
Auenbruggerplatz 29, A-8036 Graz,
Austria

W. Weihs
2nd Department of Medicine, University of
Graz, Auenbruggerplatz, A-8036 Graz,
Austria

Abstract In a retrospective analysis, 149 echocardiographic (EC) evaluations were compared with conventional clinical parameters for donor heart selection. Of these cases, 12 % were found with severe impairment of ventricular wall motion or with morphological abnormalities. Nearly half of the echocardiographically diagnosed pathological findings in donor hearts were not detected by conventional standards for heart screening. Analysis of EC-screened donor heart outcome showed a primary graft nonfunction rate of 3.1 %. We suggest EC as an additional screening instrument for further dynamic and morphological information about donor heart condition. Potential donors can be saved for transplantation and severe complications can be avoided by detecting occult cardiac dysfunction. Early detection of cardiac dysfunction may have an impact on donor therapy and can avoid unnecessary and expensive transportation of the surgical team to the harvest site.

Key words Echocardiography ·
Donor heart Selection ·
Occult donor heart diseases

Introduction

Selection of donor hearts (DH) is one of the most important and difficult parts of heart transplantation and must be carried out with care to minimize the risk of primary graft nonfunction (PGNF) and to preserve high standards of outcome. Optimal donor management includes comprehensive hemodynamic monitoring, such as can be provided in highly specialized intensive care units only. However, a part of donor management takes place in regional hospitals. Usually, the results of conventional procedures such as chest X-radiograph, electrocardiogram (ECG), arterial and central venous blood pressure, and blood chemistry are available at the time of decision for DH harvesting. Dynamic parameters such as electrocardiographic (EC) evaluation, are generally not available. Additional to the problems of DH selection using classical criteria, the DH shortage has urged some centers to extend the classical donor criteria with respect to age, trauma history, inotropic support needs, donor size matching, resuscitation and hemodynamic status [6, 8].

In our donor procurement program, EC is used as a screening method for dynamic function and morphological status of DH for each donor scheduled for multiorgan harvesting at the time of the onset of specific donor therapy. Our data, from $7^1/_2$ years experience, were analyzed to find out whether EC can give additional information on the DH in comparison with conventional parameters. All DH used for transplantation were investigated in follow-up to find out the primary function result.

Material and methods

Between January 1987 and August 1994, 182 organ donors were registered at the University Hospital of Graz, Austria. In a retrospective analysis, donors scheduled for or excluded from heart transplantation (HTX) were analyzed with respect to EC results and conventional DH criteria. Donor-specific therapy consisted of the usual management [1, 4]. Conventional parameters for the evaluation of DH quality were evaluated. Standard ECG was analyzed by the same cardiologist who performed the EC. Standard

Table 1 Criteria for acceptance of donor hearts for transplantation

1. Age below 55 years
2. No drug abuse (including alcohol)
3. No history of systemic disease
4. Circulation maintenance without high doses of catecholamines
5. No episodes of sustained resuscitation or hypotension
6. Chest X-radiograph normal
7. ECG without specific changes
8. Echocardiography indicates normal function and morphology

Table 2 Causes of exclusion from multiorgan and/or heart donation

Reason of exclusion	Number of donors
Age exceeded 55 years	8
Severe polytrauma with unstable circulation	12
Unstable circulation without trauma	16
Systemic disease	4
Pathological findings on echocardiography	18

Table 3 Early graft function analysis

	Patients
Normal EC (total)	130
No response from Tx center	20
Good primary function	87
Donor age exceeded	8
Not transplanted	12
Primary graft nonfunction	3 (3.1 %)

chest X-radiographic (anterior–posterior) results were reported by the radiologist on duty. Levels of creatinine phosphokinase (CPK) and its isoenzyme MB, indicated as units per liter (U/l), were obtained. We considered the normal range of CPK to be 0–80 U/l and of MB to be 0–10 U/l.

According to the donor's circulation status, the inotropic support needs were categorized into a low-dose group (dopamine < 6 µg/kg per min) and a high-dose group (dopamine in combination with one or more additional inotropics). Hypotensive episodes were defined as a drop of systolic blood pressure to 80 mm Hg or less lasting for more than 15 min. Spontaneous or traumatic cerebral affection or any trauma as the cause of death was also included in the analysis.

EC examinations were carried out in all donors judged suitable for transplantation, performed on the occasion of the first O-EEG. At this time, specific brain edema therapy was usually replaced by donor-specific therapy (i.e. excessive volume and electrolytes replacement). In a left elevated position, standard EC parameters were taken parasternally, apically, subcostally, and optionally suprasternally (longitudinally and crossectionally). In cases of doubtful results, transesophageal EC was also performed. In the M-mode, the ventricles and atria were measured. The global and regional left ventricular (LV) function was estimated by B-pictures in two dimensions. The LV was measured across the short axes at the end of diastole (LVED) and of systole (LVES). Using the formula of Teichholz, the fractional shortening (FS) and the ejection fraction (EF) were calculated. The width of the right ventricle (RV) and the left atrium (LA), as well as the myocardial wall thickness of the septum (IVS) and of the posterior wall (LVPW) were deter-

mined. The two- and four-chamber views were examined from the apical cross point and from the longitudinal section. All valves were examined with continuous wave, pulsed wave, and the color Doppler technique Examinations were carried out with a Hewlett Packart Sonos 1000 3.5 MHz sectorsonde by a small number of experienced investigators.

DH were offered for HTX according to the criteria listed in Table 1. Outcome analysis was performed for DHs transplanted in our center and for exported DHs (a questionnaire was sent to each transplant center). PGNF was defined as loss of cardiac function within 3 days of HTX. Excluded were cases of RV failure due to pulmonary hypertension, acute rejection and death from other noncardiac causes.

Results

The mean age of the 183 donors was 33 years (range 2–66), 122 were males and 142 (77.6 %) were multiorgan donors (explantation of two or more different organs). Reasons for exclusion from multiorgan and/or heart donation are listed in Table 2.

EC findings were obtained from 149 donors, of which 130 had normal global and regional LV contractility, normal valve functions and normal morphology. LVED mean score was 46.1 ± 3.2 mm, LVES mean score 28.4 ± 2.1 mm and the FS mean score 37.8 ± 4.2 %. Of the DHs with normal EC transplanted in our institution, 48 had good primary graft function, and there was one case of PGNF. The remaining 81 DHs with normal EC were offered to heart transplant centers linked to the Eurotransplant network. Results from 90 transplanted DHs were analyzed; PGNF was 3.1 %, and 12 with normal parameters and function were not transplanted because of virus infection, drug abuse, risk group or were not able to coordinate with a recipient (Table 3).

Pathological EC results were obtained in 19 donors (12.7 %). The detailed results are listed in Tables 4 and 5. Of these hearts, 18 were excluded from transplantation and the detailed description of the relationship between EC and conventional parameters are described below.

Pathological ECs with normal conventional findings

Nine DHs (6 % of all potential DHs) were diagnosed normal according to conventional parameters. However, using EC, significant pathologies were detected (Table 4). Hypokinesis and akinesis of the LV were the main pathological findings by EC. Occult heart diseases were found in three cases. Case no. 6, a 9-year-old female donor with a spontaneous ICH, suffered from bivalve insufficiency (mitral, tricuspidal). In case no. 8 (48-year-old female) an unknown HOCM was diagnosed, and in case no. 9 an atrial septal defect was diagnosed. All hearts except case no. 9 were excluded from

Table 4 Pathological EC findings listed with conventional parameters for donor heart screening. Conventional parameters are not considered to be a contraindication for transplantation (*Hypokin* Hypokinesis, *Akin* Akinesis, *MINS* Mitral valve insufficiency, *TRINS* Tricuspital valve insufficiency, *LV* left ventricle, *RV* right ventricle, *HOCM* hypertrophic obstructive CMP, *PV* pulmonary vein, *Pneumoth* pneumothorax, *ASD 2* septum secundum defect of the atrium)

No.	Age (years)	Echocardiography	ECG	Chest X-ray	CPK	MB	Hypo-tension	Resus-citation	Inotropic support	Trauma
1	21	Akin anterior wall	Nonspecific	0 pathol	82	5	No	No	Low	Yes
2	27	Akin diffuse, LV EF = 30 %	Nonspecific	0 pathol	119	17	No	No	Low	No
3	16	Hypokin diffuse, LV	Nonspecific	0 pathol	279	21	No	No	0	Yes
4	24	Hypokin LV EF = 76 %	Nonspecific	0 pathol	333	4	Yes	Yes	Low	Yes
5	34	Hypokin diffuse, LV, RV EF = 30 %	Nonspecific	0 pathol	112	15	Yes	Yes (10 min)	Low	No
6	9	Hypokin LV MINS TRINS EF = 33 %	Nonspecific	0 pathol	110	13	No	No	0	No
7	22	Hypokin LV, RV	Sinus tachycardia	Pneumoth unilateral	218	4	No	No	Low	No
8	48	HOCM	Nonspecific	0 pathol	341	8	No	No	Low	No
9	42	ASD 2	Nonspecific	0 pathol						

Table 5 Pathological EC findings listed with pathological findings of the conventional parameters for donor heart screening (*Hypokin* hypokinesis, *Akin* akinesis, *Dyskin* dyskinesis, *CMP* cardiomyopathy, *LA* left atrium, *RV* right ventricle)

No.	Age (years)	Echocardiography	ECG	Chest X-ray	CPK	MB	Hypo-tension	Resus-citation	Inotropic support	Trauma
10	54	Hypokin LV Hypertrophy LV LA dilatation Sclerosis aortae EF = 50 %	Pathological findings	Hypertrophy LV	62	11	Yes	Yes (10 min)	Low	No
11	47	Hypokin global EF = 45 %	Tachycardia Repolarization changes	0 pathology	74	67	No	No	Low	Yes
12	17	Hypokin posterior wall, LV	Nonspecific	Lung contusion	89	902	Yes	No	High	Yes, severe
13	24	Dyskin septum EF = 56 %, Dilatation	Nonspecific	Cardiac dilatation	146	54	Yes	No	High	Gun shot
14	21	Hypokin LV LVEDP elevated	Nonspecific	PV congestion	109	8	No	No	High	Yes
15	36	Hypokin LV Hypertrophy LV	T-wave elevated	Hypertrophy LV	69	16	No	No	High	No
16	33	Hypokin LV Hypertrophy LV EF = 45 %	Nonspecific	Hypertrophy LV	465	11	No	No	Low	No
17	13	Dilat LV Hypokin LV Dilatative CMP	Sinus tachycardia	Heart dilatation	133	95	No	No	High	Gun shot
18	17	Hypokin LV LVEDP elevated Dilatative CMP	Pathological findings	Heart dilatation	631	29	No	No	High	Yes
19	46	Hypokin diffuse	Arrhythmia	0 pathology	73	14	Yes	Yes	High	No

HTX; case no. 9 was used. The ASD 2 was closed by a running suture before implantation without complications.

In case no. 7 ECG indicated a sinus tachycardia and chest X-radiograph indicated a unilateral pneumothorax (due to central venous catheterization). Discreet elevation of the CPK/MB value was observed in two cases. One was associated with a 10-min resuscitation (case no. 5) and the other with trauma (case no. 3). Neither needed inotropics. Trauma was the cause of death in four cases. None of these conventional findings was a definite cause for exclusion of DHs from HTX.

Pathological ECs and pathological conventional findings

In ten cases (6.7 % of the potential DHs) pathological ECs were associated with significant pathological findings of conventional parameters. In five of these ten donors pathological ECG signals were observed. Chest X-radiographs were free from pathological findings of the heart in two cases only (no. 11 and no. 19). CPK/MB values were elevated in seven cases. Mechanical resuscitation had occurred in two and hypotension in four cases. A high inotropic drug support was required in seven cases. Trauma was the cause of death in six cases, two of them gun shots (to the head).

EC findings were mainly hypo- and akinesis. Hypertension was found in the history of one case out of three LV hypertrophies detected by EG and chest X-radiograph. Two cases of dilatative CMP, 13 and 17 years of age, were not reported in the patients' history.

Discussion

To select a DH for HTX can be a very delicate decision. As reported by the International Society of Heart and Lung Transplantation [5], approximately 26 % of deaths in HTX are accounted for by early donor heart failure, affirming the need for careful selection. In our analysis, nearly one-half of the hearts rejected on the basis of pathological findings by EC, such as LV dysfunction, valve insufficiency and occult heart disease, would been accepted by conventional standards and, if transplanted, would have led to deleterious complications. A recent report suggests a 22 % probability of death after HTX if diffuse wall-motion abnormalities are detected with EC [10]. In relation to a rate of 67 % acceptance of DHs previously reported [8], our data suggest a high rate (71 %) of acceptance of DHs using conventional screening parameters combined with EC screening. However, the overall Eurotransplant acceptance, rate is 38.3 % [6]. Potential DHs which have been rejected by conventional criteria, for example a history of

chest trauma, short episodes of resuscitation and hypotension and age over 50 years, could be considered for HTX when EC indicates normal function and none of the clinical findings not related to the heart provides a contraindication. Consistent with our own findings, a recent study suggests a 32 % increase in DHs for HTX when screened with EC despite exclusion by the usual clinical criteria [2]. Nevertheless, at least 12 of our donors found to have impaired ventricular function were previously healthy young people.

Experimental studies of brain death in baboons [7] have shown that severe myocardial cell damage is directly related to extreme autonomic nervous system activity which occurs during the agonal period. Additionally, significant reduction in the circulating levels of triiodothyronine, cortisol and insulin lead to increased anaerobic metabolism and depletion of myocardial high energy stores. Replacement of these hormones is accompanied by an improvement in myocardial function. A clinical investigation suggested the potential for increasing the donor pool by up to 30 % and for significantly improving the function of initially unsuitable DHs by hormone replacement and optimal donor management [9]. Early detection by EC may have an impact on therapy [3], which can avoid the exclusion of potentially usable organs.

Trauma had occurred in approximately 40 % of our EC-screened donors with impaired cardiac function. In all cases circulation was maintained by volume replacement or with additional inotropic support. Organs of donors who died from trauma can be affected by different impacts such as volume loss, hypoxemia and the previously described agonal trauma. These factors can cloud the real cause of heart damage. A unique case has been studied in our department recently. An ice-hockey professional, 31 years of age, experienced an isolated cardiac contusion in a high speed collision with a another player. Cardiac dilatation was primarily diagnosed on the following day from a chest X-radiograph. EC parameters were characterized by diffuse LV hypokinesis with a drop of the EF to 35 % and LV dilatation. All parameters recovered to normal within 7 days with strict rest and cardiac protective therapy. This case teaches us that traumatically impaired donor hearts could possibly be saved for transplantation by prolonging the special care period on condition that dynamic function and morphology of the heart is investigated repeatedly.

Hearts from donors over 50 years of age with normal EC were transplanted without complications in eight cases. These results are in accordance with those of studies with donors aged up to 54 years [8] and up to 49 years [6]. Two donors over 55 years were not used for HTX only because of their age, despite all cardiac parameters including EC being normal. In selected cases, this part of the donor pool can probably be considered for transplantation with optimal donor management and careful EC screening. EC can be considered a standard method used in nearly all hospitals that treat cardiac diseases in the Eurotransplant-associated countries. As HTX is a highly specialized treatment, good results can only be obtained with careful monitoring after HTX, but the same careful screening should also be applied in the selection of the donor organ.

References

1. English Ta, Spratt P, Wallwork J, Cory-Pearce R, Wheeldon D (1984) Selection and procurement of hearts for transplantation. B M J 288: 1889–1891
2. Gilbert ED, Krueger SK, Murray JL (1988) Echocardiographic evaluation of potential cardiac transplant donors. J Thorac Cardiovasc Surg 95: 1003–1007
3. Hauptmann PJ, Gass A, Goldman ME (1993) The role of echocardiography in heart transplantation. J Am Soc Echocardiogr 6: 496–509
4. Jordan CA, Snyder JV (1987) Intensive care and intraoperative management of the brain dead organ donor. Transpl Proc 19(4) [Suppl 3]: 21–25
5. Kaye MP (1992) The registry of the international society of heart transplantation. J Heart Lung Transplant 11 [Suppl 4]: 599–606
6. Mulvagh SL, Thompton B, Frazier OH, Radovancevic B, Norton HJ, Noon GP, Young JB (1989) The older cardiac transplant donor. Circulation 80(5) [Suppl III]: 126–132
7. Novitzky D, Wicomb WN, Cooper DKC, Reichard B (1984) Electrocardiographic, hemodynamic and endocrine changes occurring during experimental brain death in the chacma baboon. J Heart Transplant 4: 63–69
8. Schüler S, Warnecke H, Loebe M, Fleck E, Hetzer R (1989) Extended donor age in cardiac transplantation. Circulation 80 [Suppl III]: 133–139
9. Wheeldon DR, Potter CDO, Jonas M, Wallwork J, Large SR (1994) Using "unsuitable" hearts for transplantation. Eur J Cardiothorac Surg 8: 7–10
10. Young Jb, Naftel DC, Bourge RC (1994) Matching the heart donor and heart transplant recipient. Clues for successful expansion of the donor pool. J Heart Lung Transplant 13: 353–165

Transpl Int (1996) 9 [Suppl 1]: S414–S417
© Springer-Verlag 1996

L. De Carlis
C. V. Sansalone
G. F. Rondinara
G. Colella
A. O. Slim
O. Rossetti
P. Aseni
A. Della Volpe
L. S. Belli
A. Alberti
R. Fesce
D. Forti

Is the use of marginal donors justified in liver transplantation? Analysis of results and proposal of modern criteria

L. De Carlis (✉) · C. V. Sansalone ·
G. F. Rondinara · G. Colella · A. O. Slim ·
O. Rossetti · P. Aseni · A. Della Volpe ·
D. Forti
Department of Surgery and
Abdominal Transplantation,
"Pizzamiglio 2°", Niguarda Hospital,
I-20162 Milan, Italy

L. S. Belli · A. Alberti
Department of Hepatology,
Niguarda Hospital, Milan, Italy

R. Fesce
CNR DIBIT IRCCS San Raffaele, Milan,
Italy

Abstract A discrepancy exists worldwide between the number of suitable liver donors and the increasing demand for transplantation. Thus many centers have considered widening their liver donor acceptance criteria and this may increase the incidence of primary dysfunction (PD) with negative effect on the results of transplantation. In order to reduce the incidence of PD and improve patient and graft survival it becomes important to identify those risk factors associated with its occurrence. In a retrospective univariate and multivariate analysis we evaluated several donor, preservation and recipient parameters and their correlation with PD. In our Department 282 orthotopic liver transplantations (OLT) were performed on 256 adult patients over a 10-year period. Excluded were 15 cases with early vascular problems and 4 intraoperative deaths. A complete series of donor, recipient and procedure-related data were analyzed. About 30 % of donors showed abnormal values. In 70 cases of PD (26 %) there was a 61.4 % graft failure rate compared with 15 % in the group with immediate function (P < 0.05). Univariate analysis showed donor age, steatosis, ischemia time, amines, oliguria, hypotension and ICU stay to be significantly associated with PD. Multivariate analysis showed steatosis, ischemia time and amine dosage to be independent risk factors for the development of primary non function. In conclusion, the acceptance of marginal donors worsened the results of transplantation, but the rejection of these donors would reduce by about 30 % our transplant activity resulting in increased mortality in the waiting list. Combinations of risk factors when possible should be avoided, and ischemia time, as the only variable that can be controlled, should be kept as short as possible.

Key words Liver transplantation · Liver donor selection · Donor criteria

Introduction

The current selection criteria for liver donation are the subject of great controversy at different centers as they are considered of little value in the prediction of transplant outcome. The discrepancy between the increasing number of candidates for liver transplantation (OLT) and the number of available organs is largely attributed to the fact that many potential suitable donors are not harvested because they do not fulfil predefined criteria. To remedy this deficit, many centers have considered widening their liver donor acceptance criteria. Thus abnormal liver tests, hemodynamic instability, older age and steatosis are no longer absolute contraindications to organ retrieval [5, 9].

On the other hand, primary dysfunction (PD) of the harvested liver may lead to significant morbidity and mortality after OLT. Primary non function (PNF) is the

Table 1 Univariate analysis: donor variables significantly associated with PD

	Immediate function (n = 193)	IPF (n = 48)	PNF (n = 22)	P-value
Donor age				
< 55 years (n = 229)	78 %	16.5 %	5.5%	
> 55 years (n = 34)	41 %	32 %	27 %	< 0.001
Steatosis				
No (n = 189)	81 %	14.5 %	4.5 %	
slight to moderate (n = 59)	68 %	27 %	5 %	
Severe (n = 15)	0 %	33 %	66 %	< 0.001
Ischemia time				
< 10 h (n = 185)	84.5 %	10 %	4.5 %	
> 10 h (n = 78)	46.5 %	37 %	16.5 %	< 0.05
Amines (Dopamine)				
< 10 µg/kg/min (n = 168)	81 %	13.5 %	5.5 %	
> 10 µg/kg/min (n = 95)	60 %	27 %	13 %	< 0.05
Oliguria				
No (n = 226)	79.5 %	14 %	6.5 %	
Yes (n = 37)	35 %	46 %	19 %	< 0.05
Hypotension				
< 60 min (n = 184)	82 %	13 %	5 %	
> 60 min (n = 79)	53 %	30.5 %	16.5 %	< 0.03
ICU stay				
< 5 days (n = 191)	84 %	11.5 %	4.5 %	
> 5 days (n = 72)	46 %	36 %	18 %	< 0.03

most serious form of PD occurring in 10–23 % and resulting in rapid death of the patient unless an urgent retransplantation is performed. In other cases the graft shows a borderline function immediately after OLT and in these cases the graft may recover after a variable period of dysfunction, retransplantation may be required or the patient may die. These forms are defined as 'delayed function' (DGF) or 'initial poor function' (IPF) and are characterized, in the first week, by high transaminase levels, prolonged prothrombin time and nearly absent bile production. The genesis of these conditions are most likely multifactorial including donor- and recipient-related factors as well as various surgical events [4, 7, 8]. In the present study, a number of variables widely associated with the entire procedure and their correlation with graft dysfunction were analyzed with the aim of defining modern criteria for liver donation and their impact on the results of transplantation.

Materials and methods

Between 1985 and 1995, 282 orthotopic liver transplants (OLT) were performed in our department on 256 adult patients, and of these 32 were urgent cases (acute hepatic failure, urgent retransplantation, ICU patients). Organs were harvested according to the rapid or standard techniques of Starzl et al. [10, 11]. UW solution was used in all except the first 30 procedures. All organs were ABO identical or compatible with the recipients. No reduced or 'split' livers were transplanted. The majority of donor livers were procured by the Niguarda team, only three being procured by oth-

ers and sent to our institution. All livers had biopsies which were evaluated retrospectively or immediately before surgery, when required. The OLT operations were performed using standard techniques and venovenous bypass (234 cases) or the 'piggy-back' technique (48 cases). Quadruple induction immunosuppression (RATG, azathioprine, cyclosporine and steroids) and cyclosporine monotherapy after the 6th month were routinely adopted.

The following donor parameters were considered: age, sex, cause of death, hospital of procurement, amines, days in ICU, hypotension, oliguria, transaminases, protime, grade of steatosis, macroscopic appearance of the liver, MEGx test (100 cases) and type of cold storage solution. Other parameters considered were recipient age, sex, UNOS and Child status, preservation time, time of anastomosis, blood losses and number of donor/recipient mismatches. These data were compared with patient survival during the 3 months posttransplant and with immediate graft function. In particular IPF was defined as a form of dysfunction with AST > 1500 U/l, AP 20–30 %, and nearly absent bile flow; PNF was defined as an irreversible dysfunction causing death or retransplantation within 8 days. Excluded from the analysis were 4 cases of early death and 15 cases of vascular complications.

Statistical univariate analysis was carried out using the Chisquared, log-rank and Mantel-Haenzel tests (significance assumed for $P < 0.05$). Multivariate analysis was carried out using a multiple linear regression model (MS-BMDP vers. 1.0) and significance assumed for $P < 0.02$.

Results

Median donor age was 33 years (range 4–66); 34 (12.9 %) were older than 55 years. Steatosis was absent in 189 livers; mild to moderate steatosis was present in 59 grafts (22.4 %) and severe steatosis in 15 (5.7 %). Median ischemia time was 480 min (range 180–1320) and 78 livers (29.6 %) had an ischemia time longer than 10 h. Median ICU stay was 3 days (range 1–24) and 72 donors (27.3 %) had a prolonged ICU stay of more than 5 days. Donor dosage of amines of more than 10 µg/kg/min of dopamine or oliguria were present, respectively, in 95 (36.1 %) and 37 (14.1 %) cases (Table 1). PD occurred in 70 cases (26.6 %) including 22 PNF (8.4 %) and 48 IPF (18.2 %) and within 3 months of transplantation, 43 of these 70 PD grafts (61.4 %) failed (22/22 PNF and 21/48 IPF) compared with 29 of 193 (15 %) with immediate function ($P < 0.05$; Table 2).

Univariate analysis of IPF grafts performed with both discrete and continuous variables showed the following factors to have a statistically significant effect: donor age, ICU stay, amines, hypotensive episodes, steatosis, ischemia time, oliguria, appearance of the liver, blood losses and UNOS status (Table 1). Multivariate analysis of IPF grafts showed donor age, steatosis, ischemia time, hypotensive episodes and amine dosage to be significant independent variables.

Univariate analysis of PNF grafts showed donor age, amines, hypotension, steatosis, ischemia time, oliguria and UNOS status to be significant (Table 1). Multivariate analysis of PNF grafts showed steatosis, ischemia time and amine dosage to be independent risk factors (Table 3).

Discussion

The selection of liver donors is a process in which several parameters have to be weighed in order to maximize the chances of success to the procedure. Currently used criteria are not well defined and it is difficult to establish how much each individual parameter contributes to graft function within the context of all the available parameters [1, 4, 9]. The clarification of this dilemma is critical, as the demand for OLT is increasing in the face of a constant donor pool. To remedy the shortage of suitable donors many centers have widened their acceptance criteria. It is crucial to define how much this is possible and what its impact is on the results of transplantation [1, 4, 8, 9]. From our data, PD occurred in a relevant percentage of cases as in other series (20 %). Together with PNF which by definition resulted in failure of the graft, IPF is also a major complication of OLT and is associated with a significantly higher mortality, graft insufficiency and retransplantation rate than observed in patients with immediate liver function.

Several historical parameters [3, 7, 13] are associated with the occurrence of dysfunction, such as the donor hemodynamic instability (amine dosage, hypotension, oliguria), preexisting or death-induced conditions (donor age, steatosis, appearance of the liver, ICU stay)

Table 2 Incidence of primary dysfunction in 263 OLT (*PNF* primary non function, *IPF* initial poor function)

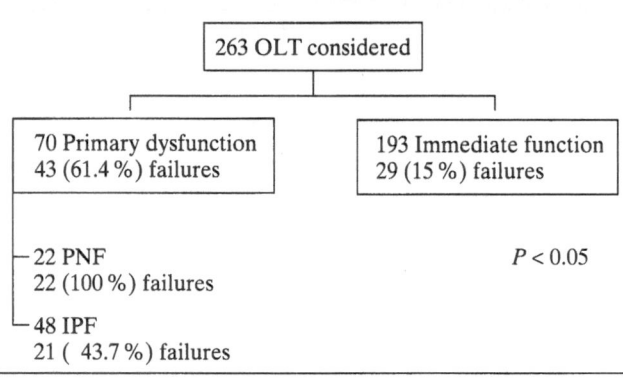

Table 3 Multivariate analysis: variables independently corelated with PNF

	Correlation coefficient	*P*-value
Steatosis	0.72	0.0002
Ischemia time	0.29	0.001
Amine dosage	0.03	0.02

and recipient variables (UNOS status, blood losses). All these parameters can induce different grades of damage to the liver that may result in dysfunction after harvesting, cold storage and transplantation. However, multivariate analysis showed only steatosis, amines and ischemia time to be significant as independent variables associated with PNF. Donor age was independently correlated with IPF and not with PNF [1, 7, 13], reflecting the fact that an old but healthy donor should not routinely be rejected. A long ischemia time, even since the introduction of UW solution, has a detrimental effect on graft function, and this is especially evident with poor condition donors in whom different parameters are altered [4, 7]. Undoubtedly UW solution has had an invaluable effect in improving the results of OLT, but care must be taken not to overextend preservation time when this is not necessary [3, 7].

Moderate to severe fatty changes in the liver graft, as in previous studies, was significantly related to PD [2, 12]. Since steatosis is not easily evaluable macroscopically, biopsies have to be obtained in every uncertain case [2]. The MEGx test was not predictive in our experience of graft function [6].

In conclusion, the acceptance of marginal donors increases the risks of PD and negatively influences the results of OLT. Their rejection, however, would reduce by about 30 % the actual transplantation rate in our center leading to unacceptable increases in mortality in the waiting list. The data should be used as background information to facilitate clinical judgement for an individual case. The combination of significant factors should be avoided when possible. Preservation time, as the only variable that can be controlled, shoul be kept as short as possible.

References

1. Alexander JW, Vaughn WK (1991) The use of marginal donors for organ transplantation: influence of donor age on outcome. Transplantation 51: 135–137
2. D'Alessandro AM, Kalayoglu M, Sollinger HW, Hoffmann RM, Reed A, Knechtle SJ, Pirsch JD, Hafez GR, Lorentzen D, Belzer FO (1991) The predictive values of donor liver biopsies for the development of primary non function after orthotopic liver transplantation. Transplantation 51: 157–163
3. Kalayoglu M, Sollinger HW, Stratta RJ, D'Alessandro AM, Hoffmann RM, Pirsch JD, Belzer FO (1988) Extended preservation of the liver for clinical transplantation. Lancet i: 617–619
4. Makowka L, Gordon RD, Todo S, Ohkohchi N, Marsh JW, Tzakis AG, Yokoi H, Ligush J, Esquivel CO, Satake M, Iwatsuki S, Starzl TE (1987) Analysis of donor criteria for the prediction of outcome in clinical liver transplantation. Transplant Proc 19: 2378–2382
5. Mirza DF, Gunson BK, Da Silva RF, Mayer DA, Buckels JAC, McMaster P (1994) Policies in Europe on marginal quality donor livers. Lancet 344: 1480–1483
6. Oellerich M, Burdelski M, Ringe B, Lamesh P, Gubernatis G, Bunzendhal H, Pichlmayr R, Herrmann H (1989) Lignocaine metabolite formation as a measure of pretransplant liver function. Lancet i: 640–642
7. Ploeg RJ, D'Alessandro AM, Knechtle SJ, Stegall MD, Pirsch JD, Hoffmann RM, Sasaki T, Sollinger HW, Belzer FO, Kalayoglu M (1993) Risk factors for primary dysfunction after liver transplantation – a multivariate analysis. Transplantation 55: 807–813
8. Pruim J, van Woerden WF, Knol E, Klompmaker IJ, de Bruijn KM, Persijn GG, Sloff MJH (1989) Donor data in liver graft with primary non-function: a preliminary analysis by the European Liver Registry. Transplant Proc 21: 2383–2384
9. Pruim J, Klompmaker IJ, Haagsma EB, Bijleveld CMA, Slooff MJH (1993) Selection criteria for liver donation: a review. Transplant Int 6: 226–235
10. Starzl TE, Hakala TR, Shaw BW, Hardesty RL, Rosenthal TJ, Griffith BP, Iwatsuki S, Bahnson HT (1984) A flexible procedure for multiple cadaveric organ procurement. Surg Gynecol Obstet 158: 223–228
11. Starzl TE, Miller C, Broznick B, Makowka L (1987) An improved technique for multiple organ harvesting. Surg Gynecol Obstet 165: 343–347
12. Todo S, DeMetris AJ, Makowka L (1990) Primary non function of hepatic allografts with pre-existing fatty infiltration. Transplantation 47: 903–905
13. Wall WJ, Mimeault R, Grant DR, Bloch M (1990) The use of older donors for hepatic transplantation. Transplantation 49: 377–381

Transpl Int (1996) 9 [Suppl 1]: S418–S419
© Springer-Verlag 1996

C. Tielemans
J. Decruyenaer
H. Kerremans
P. Pattyn
U. Hesse
B. de Hemptinne

The impact of donor age on graft outcome after liver transplantation

C. Tielemans · J. Decruyenaer ·
H. Kerremans · P. Pattyn · U. Hesse
B. de Hemptinne (✉)
Surgery, 185 De Pintelaan, B-9000 Gent,
Belgium

Key words Liver transplantation ·
Donor age

Introduction

Increasing demand for organs for transplantation together with a stable or even decreasing quantity of donor livers offered has urged the need to increase the donor pool by expanding the criteria for donor selection. Liver transplant teams are consequently confronted with the need to use second choice donors. In the early days, an age of 40 years for donors was considered the upper limit. This limit moved to 50 years with time and has moved even higher more recently. It has been reported by several groups that livers from donors of 55 years of age may be transplanted with success [1]. This study evaluated the impact of acceptance of even older donors on liver function and outcome after transplantation.

Patients and methods

Between May 1991 and May 1995, 83 orthotopic liver transplants (OLT) were performed in an elective manner in ABO-compatible patients. The age distribution of the donors ranged from 16 to 75 years, with 37 grafts from donors < 30 years of age (group I), 28 from donors between 30 and 50 years of age (group II) and 18 from donors > 50 years of age (group III). The mean age of the donors of group III was 65 years. Grafts with > 75 % steatoses as evaluated by pretransplant biopsy were routinely discarded. All grafts were preserved with UW solution and all groups were treated with standard triple immunosuppression (cyclosporin A, prednisolone and azathioprine). During to a more restrictive policy of selection of older donors, the mean ICU stay, GGT, bilirubin, cold ischemic time, ALT, AST and prothrombin time (PT) were all lower in group III donors (the oldest group) than in group II donors.

These differences were, however, not statistically significant (Table 1).

Recipient data, including conventional liver function tests and indications for OLT, were similar in all groups, but there was a clear tendency for livers from older donors to be transplanted into older recipients. The function and outcome of grafts from the three groups were compared.

Results

Liver biochemistry early after transplantation (Table 2) showed a significantly higher degree of hepatocellular injury during the first 48 h for group III. The increased levels of cytolysis during the first 6 h for group II were not significant and not recorded later during the postoperative evolution.

Postoperative PT was also clearly lower during the first 48 h in grafts from group III donors. Metabolism of lactate was, however, similar in grafts from all groups

Table 1 Characteristics of the donor groups

	Group I	Group II	Group III	
Number *(n)*	37	28	18	NS
ICU stay (days)	2.5	5	2.5	NS
GGT (IU/l)	29.4	50.6	22.6	NS
Bilirubin (mg/dl)	1	1.5	0.95	NS
Cold ischemic time (h)	797.5	845.4	707.4	NS
Sodium (mEq/l)	145	142.4	147.7	NS
ALT (IU/l)	46.8	43.3	32.5	NS
AST (IU/l)	33.0	47.3	17.0	NS
PT (%)	51.4	66.5	62.6	NS

Table 2 Posttransplant ALT tests and prothrombin time (PT)

	Hours posttransplant						
	0	6	12	24	48	72	120
ALT (IU/l)							
Group I	633	619	615	709	795	617	273
Group II	814	750	578	421	508	764	178
Group III	970*	988*	1189*	1674*	1409*	839	410
PT (%)							
Group I	48	46	48	51	60	67	67
Group II	39	47	50	53	77	74	78
Group III	36	34*	34*	39*	49*	62	71

* $P < 0.05$

Table 3 Posttransplant lactate levels

	Hours posttransplant			
	0	6	12	24
Group I	40	31	22	16
Group II	24	17	17.5	12.5
Group III	43	36	26	22

over the first 24 h (Table 3). The incidence of rejections showed no significant differences between grafts from the three groups, and 6-month graft survivals were 88 %, 85.8 %, and 74 % for group I, II and III grafts, respectively (Tables 2, 3).

No difference was observed in terms of primary nonfunction, retransplantation and graft survival up to 6 months posttransplant.

Discussion

The increasing demand for organs for OLT has forced us to accept older donors. Our results show that grafts from older donors had substantial differences in function during the first 48 postoperative hours, despite a stricter donor selection which compensated for the preferential transplantation of these livers into older recipients. This difference in liver function was probably caused by a higher sensitivity to preservation in-

jury. However, graft outcome, as shown by the incidence of graft failure and graft survival demonstrate that the impaired initial graft function was transitory and did not lead to a significantly higher proportion of grafts lost.

It is important to stress the fact that the selection of older donors was more rigorous than that for the younger donors and that all measures were taken to minimize accumulation of risk factors. In the two cases in which ischemic time was prolonged for logistical reasons for more than 14 h, the immediate price to pay was primary nonfunctioning.

A review of recent literature concerning donor age in OLT [2] suggests that donor age is a risk factor for poor function after OLT. The effect of age on OLT outcome appears much more evident when the medical status of the recipient is poor (old UNOS grades 5 and 6) [3]. The age at which the risk begins to increase is not yet established, and results of long-term survival are still not available. Both of these aspects need further study and will be analysed in the future. Indeed, donors over 70 years of age (in our own experience the maximum is 75 years) are being used more frequently for OLT.

In summary, we found that provided preservation times were kept short, grafts from older donors who did not present other risk factors, showed only a transitorily impaired initial graft function. Older livers recovered their full function after 48 h without affecting short-term graft and patient survival.

References

1. Wall WJ, Mimeault R, Grant et al (1990) Transplantation 49: 377
2. Strasberg SM, Howard T, Molmanti E et al (1994) Hepatology 20: 829
3. Buckel L, Sanchez-Urdazpol L, Steers J et al (1993) Transplant Proc 25: 1558

Transpl Int (1996) 9 [Suppl 1]: S 420–S 424
© Springer-Verlag 1996

ORGAN PROCUREMENT

F. Pellegatta
E. Ferrero
A. Marni
S. Chierchia
D. Forti
M. E. Ferrero

The anti-ischemic drugs defibrotide and oligotide analogously inhibit leukocyte-endothelial cell adhesion in vitro

F. Pellegatta · E. Ferrero · S. Chierchia
Cardiovascular Physiopathology and
Adoptive Immunotherapy Laboratory,
Ospedale San Raffaele, Milan, Italy

A. Marni · D. Forti
II Department of Surgery Pizzamiglio,
Ospedale Niguarda, Milan, Italy

M. E. Ferrero (✉)
Instituto di Patologia Generale
e Centro di Studio
Sullo Patologia Cellulare
del CNR,
Università di Milano, Via Mangiagalli 31,
I-20133 Milan, Italy
Fax +39 2 26681092

Abstract Defibrotide (a polydeox-yribonucleotide) and oligotide (an oligodeoxyribonucleotide) obtained from mammalian single-stranded DNA, have been demonstrated to have anti-ischemic activity in some experimental models of ischemia/reperfusion of kidney in rats. We hypothesized that their anti-ischemic activity could be related to an inhibition of leukocyte-endothelial cell adhesion and also the consequent generation of oxygen free radicals by leukocytes. We studied the in vitro adhesion of neutrophils to human umbilical vein endothelial cells under basal conditions and following neutrophil or endothelial cell activation (using 10^{-7} fMLP and 500 U/ml TNF-α, respectively). De-fibrotide and oligotide significantly inhibited neutrophil adhesion to endothelial cells (after only 1 min of drug treatment). When the anti-LFA-1 70H12 F(ab)$_2$ monoclonal antibody was used, the drugs exerted only slight additional inhibition of the adhesion of fMLP-activated neutrophils to endothelium. These results, confirmed in NIH/3T3-ICAM-1-transfected cells, demonstrate that defibrotide and oligotide interfere with leukocyte adhesion to endothelial cells by an LFA-1-dependent mechanism.

Key words Endothelial cells · Neutrophils · Anti-LFA-1 · Defibrotide · Oligotide

Introduction

There is substantial evidence that myocardial ischemia provokes an acute inflammatory response that is augmented by reperfusion [5]. In the inflammatory reactions occurring during the ischemia/reperfusion process, neutrophils play the major role. Polymorphonuclear leukocyte intervention contributes to tissue injury [1] through the release of proteases and leukotrienes. Furthermore, activation of the neutrophil membrane-associated NADPH oxidase system by appropriate stimuli induces a respiratory burst characterized by an increase in cellular oxygen consumption and production of oxygen free radicals [14], which have cytotoxic properties [13]. Indeed, the inhibition of neutrophil respiratory burst activity and the use of antioxidants can limit oxygen free radical-mediated tissue damage [5]. However, an inhibition of neutrophil extravasation could prevent the effects due to such cell accumulation and degranulation.

Neutrophil extravasation is mediated by three sequential steps: (1) rolling of polymorphonuclear leukocytes along the endothelium, (2) strong adhesion of the same cells following their activation, and (3) transendothelial migration. Leukocyte rolling is mediated by the selectin family of adhesion molecules (L-selectin, constitutively expressed on the surface of leukocytes, E-selectin, expressed on endothelial cells, and P-selectin, stored in Weibel-Palade bodies of endothelial cells). Firm attachment of neutrophils to endothelium and subsequent diapedesis are mediated by some integrins (which are heterodimeric molecules consisting of non-covalently associated α and β subunits). The integrin CD11a/CD18 is an adhesion molecule, known as LFA-

1 (leukocyte function-associated antigen-1), constitutively expressed on neutrophils; it is involved in the mechanism of strong adhesion of leukocytes to endothelial cells, where its principal ligand ICAM-1 (intercellular adhesion molecule-1, of the immunoglobulin superfamily) is located. Administration of monoclonal antibodies against CD11b/CD18 before reperfusion has been shown to induce a reduction in myocardial infarct size and neutrophil accumulation in a dog model [11].

We have previously been able to limit ischemia/reperfusion damage in rat kidney by the use of defibrotide (a polydeoxyribonucleotide) and oligotide (an oligodeoxyribonucleotide) which are obtained from mammalian single-stranded DNA (Marni et al., submitted for publication). Defibrotide has been demonstrated by us to be a useful anti-ischemic drug in many experimental models in rat heart and kidney [4, 7]. We hypothesized that the anti-ischemic activity of defibrotide and oligotide could be related to their capacity to inhibit leukocyte-endothelial cell adhesion, and also to the consequent production of oxygen free radicals, proteases and leukotrienes by leukocytes.

In the present work, we tested such a hypothesis by studying the in vitro adhesion of neutrophils to endothelial cells, under basal conditions and following neutrophil or endothelial cell activation, in the presence of the two drugs.

Materials and methods

Endothelial cell cultures

Primary cultures of human umbilical vein endothelial cells (HUVEC) were derived from umbilical cords and maintained as previously described [6]. HUVEC were found to express endothelial-related antigens such as PECAM (platelet endothelial cell adhesion molecule, or CD31) and factor VIII.

NIH/3T3-ICAM-1-transfected cells were kindly provided by Dr. R. Pardi (Human Immunology Unit, Scientific Institute San Raffaele, Milan, Italy). ICAM-1$^+$-transfected cells were obtained from NIH/3T3 murine fibroblasts with ICAM1 and neomycin resistance on the same plasmid. ICAM-1 subcloned into pcDNA I/Neo (Invitrogen, San Diego, Calif.) at the XbaI site was kindly provided by Dr. R. Pardi. Transfection was performed by calcium phosphate-DNA coprecipitation. Stable transfectants were selected by the addition of the neomycin analogue G418 to a final concentration of 0.8 mg/ml. Neomycin-resistant colonies were picked 10 days later, expanded and tested for ICAM-1 expression by immunofluorescence using the 84H10-IO154 monoclonal antibody (Immunotech, Luminy-Marseille, France). For the adhesion assay, endothelial cells, detached by a brief exposure to 0.25 % trypsin and 0.22 % EDTA, were plated and grown to confluence in 24-well plates.

Preparation of neutrophils

Venous blood from healthy donors who had not received any medication for at least 2 weeks was anticoagulated with 0.065 M citric acid (Riedel, Hannover, Germany), 0.085 M sodium citrate (Far-

mitalia, Milan, Italy), and 2 % glucose monohydrate (Riedel) in a blood-anticoagulant ratio of 7:1. Neutrophils were isolated by dextran (Sigma, Milan, Italy) sedimentation, followed by Lymphoprep (Nycomed, Oslo, Norway) gradient and hypotonic lysis of erythrocytes [3]. Neutrophils were washed with phosphate-buffered saline without calcium or magnesium (Gibco, Paisley, UK) and resuspended in ice-cold HEPES-Tyrode's buffer (pH 7.4) containing 129 mM NaCl, 9.9 mM NaHCO$_3$, 2.8 mM KCl, 0.8 mM KH$_2$PO$_4$, 0.8 mM MgCl$_2 \cdot$ 6H$_2$O, 5.6 mM glucose monohydrate, 1 mM CaCl$_2$, and 10 mM HEPES. Cell suspensions contained more than 97 % viable neutrophils as evaluated by the Trypan blue dye exclusion test. Neutrophils were used within 2 h of their isolation. Cell suspensions contained 95 % neutrophils; an average of one platelet per 10–20 neutrophils was usually observed.

Measurement of neutrophil adhesion to endothelial cells

Neutrophils were radiolabelled for 1 h at room temperature with Na$_2$^{51}CrO$_4$ (1 mCi/10^6 cells, Amersham, Milan, Italy), washed twice, and resuspended at 5×10^6/ml in HEPES-Tyrode's buffer. Their viability was assessed by the Trypan blue dye exclusion test. The radiolabelled neutrophil suspension (100 µl) was layered on endothelial cells in the presence or absence of the drugs and was incubated for 15 min at 37 °C. In resting conditions, neutrophil adhesion was about 6 % of added neutrophils, and neutrophil radioactivity was about 0.05 cpm/neutrophil. The loss of radioactivity from neutrophils during the course of the experiment was < 5 %.

Treatments were performed for 1 min before leukocyte addition to monolayers of endothelial cells. Neutrophils were activated by preincubation (3 min) with 10^{-7} fMLP (formyl-methionyl-leucyl-phenylalanine), and endothelial cells were activated by overnight treatment with 500 U/ml TNF-α (Endogen, Boston, Mass.). In adhesion blockage experiments, neutrophils were preincubated with monoclonal F(ab)$_2$ antibodies (anti-LFA-1 [70H12] and anti-CD31 [M89D3], 5 µg/ml for 20 min at 4 °C). The anti-LFA-1 α 70H12 monoclonal antibody was kindly provided by Dr. A. Poggi (Laboratory of Immunopathology, Italian National Institute for Cancer Research, Genova). The specificity for the α chain was assessed using LFA-1 α-expressing cos-7-transfected cells. The antibody was purified by affinity chromatography and the F(ab)$_2$ fragment prepared by pepsin digestion according to the method of Parham [9]. At the end of the incubation time, the wells were washed three times to remove nonadherent cells, the remaining bound cells were lysed with Triton X-100 (1 %; BDH, Poole, UK), and the individual lysates were counted in a gamma counter (model 500, Packard, Sterling, Va.).

Pharmacological treatment

Defibrotide and oligotide were gifts from Crinos Biological Research Laboratories (Villa Guardia, Como, Italy). The drugs are, respectively, a polydeoxyribonucleotide and an oligodeoxyribonucleotide, and are obtained by controlled hydrolysis of DNA from mammalian lungs; they have a molecular weight of approximately 20 and 6 kDa, respectively. The drugs were added to endothelial cells at a dose of 1000 µg/ml medium, which was shown to be the maximal inhibiting dose for endothelial-neutrophil adhesion.

Statistical analysis

Statistical analyses were performed with the Mann-Whitney and Wilcoxon tests for nonparametric results, and the data were considered statistically significant for P < 0.05.

S 422

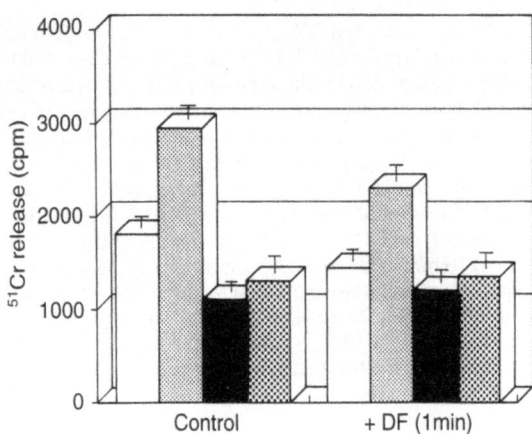

Fig. 1 Effect of defibrotide (1000 µg/ml) on neutrophil adhesion to HUVEC. The data represent neutrophil adhesion under basal conditions *(white bars)*, after neutrophil activation by 10^{-7} fMLP *(gray bars)*, in the presence of monoclonal antibodies anti-CD31 and anti-LFA-1 $(F(ab)_2$, 5 µg/ml) *(black bars)* and in the presence of the same antibodies after neutrophil activation by fMLP *(stippled bars)*. The data are expressed as the means ± SEM of five experiments, each done in triplicate

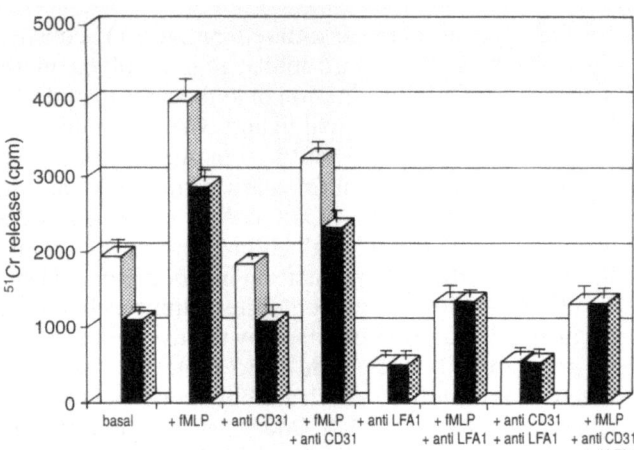

Fig. 2 Effect of oligotide (1000 µg/ml) on neutrophil adhesion to NIH/3T3-ICAM-1-transfected cells *(white bars* control, *black bars* oligotide). fMLP $(10^{-7} M)$ was used to activate neutrophils. Monoclonal antibodies anti-CD31 and anti-LFA-1 $(F(ab)_2$, 5 µg/ml) were also used. The data are expressed as the means ± SEM of five experiments, each done in triplicate

Results

We performed preliminary dose-response experiments using different concentrations of defibrotide and oligotide (100, 250, 500 and 1000 µg/ml medium), and demonstrated (data not shown) that the most efficient concentration of the two drugs was 1000 µg/ml. Under basal conditions, defibrotide and oligotide significantly reduced neutrophil adhesion to HUVEC or NIH/3T3-ICAM-1-transfected cells after only 1 min of treatment (Figs. 1, 2). TNF-α increased neutrophil adhesion to HUVEC (data not shown). Both defibrotide and oligotide added for 1 min after endothelial cell stimulation (TNF-α overnight) significantly inhibited neutrophil adhesion (data not shown).

Using $10^{-7} M$ fMLP to activate neutrophils, maximal leukocyte adhesion to HUVEC was obtained after 15 min of neutrophil-endothelial cell incubation (data not shown). After fMLP stimulation, defibrotide and oligotide (added 1 min before fMLP) significantly inhibited neutrophil adhesion to HUVEC and NIH/3T3-ICAM-1-transfected cells (Figs. 1, 2). The efficacy of the two drugs was found to be similar under our experimental conditions. Indeed, we showed in the adhesion blockage experiments the efficacy of defibrotide in limiting adhesion of neutrophils to HUVEC and the efficacy of oligotide in limiting neutrophil adhesion to NIH/3T3-ICAM-1-transfected cells.

Figure 1 shows neutrophil adhesion (expressed as ^{51}Cr release) to HUVEC in controls and after 1 min of defibrotide treatment. Under basal conditions, defibrotide significantly inhibited neutrophil adhesion to HUVEC, while fMLP significantly increased neutrophil ad-

hesion to HUVEC. Defibrotide treatment significantly reduced adhesion to HUVEC of activated neutrophils. In the presence of monoclonal antibodies directed towards CD31 and LFA-1 adhesion molecules used together, neutrophil adhesion to HUVEC was significantly inhibited. Under these conditions, the addition of defibrotide did not modify inhibition. Similar results were obtained when neutrophils were activated by the addition of fMLP.

Figure 2 shows neutrophil adhesion (expressed as ^{51}Cr release) to NIH/3T3-ICAM-1-transfected cells in controls and after 1 min of oligotide treatment. Under basal conditions, oligotide significantly inhibited neutrophil adhesion to transfected cells. In the presence of fMLP, neutrophil adhesion to transfected cells was significantly increased, but oligotide treatment significantly reduced adhesion to transfected cells of activated neutrophils. When anti-CD31 monoclonal antibodies were used, adhesion of neutrophils was not inhibited under basal conditions and was only slightly inhibited after fMLP stimulation. Oligotide treatment, in the presence of anti-CD31 antibodies, exerted its inhibitory action. When anti-LFA-1 antibodies were used, neutrophil adhesion to transfected cells was highly inhibited, and oligotide did not further exert an inhibitory action under basal conditions or after fMLP stimulation. When anti-CD31 and anti-LFA-1 antibodies were used simultaneously, the results were the same as when only anti-LFA-1 was used.

Discussion

Cellular adhesion molecules mediate the diapedesis of leukocytes from blood to the subendothelial regions. Firstly, selectins favor neutrophil rolling along endothelial cells. A rapid mobilization of P-selectin from endothelial Weibel-Palade bodies to the cell surface has been observed following many inflammatory stimuli such as thrombin, histamine or oxygen free radicals [10]. Similar translocation of P-selectin to the endothelial cell membrane has been shown in myocardial microvasculature after heart ischemia and reperfusion [15]. The subsequent firm adhesion of leukocytes to endothelium is mediated by their integrins such as LFA-1, which binds to its endothelial cell immunoglobulin-like counter-receptor ICAM-1. ICAM-1 is upregulated by cytokine stimulation [2], and it regulates neutrophil adherence to the endothelium after exposure to oxygen free radicals or after anoxia-reoxygenation [16]. The inhibition of selectins, integrins or ICAM-1 could reduce leukocyte adhesion to endothelium and thus limit tissue damage due to cell activation and migration. The use of monoclonal antibodies against LFA-1 and ICAM-1 prolongs the survival of cardiac xenografts [8], which represent the most complex model of ischemia/reperfusion.

We have previously demonstrated the usefulness of defibrotide treatment, and recently of oligotide treatment, in some experimental models of ischemia/reperfusion. We tested and compared the activity of the two drugs in inhibiting neutrophil-endothelial cell adhesion in vitro. Our results demonstrated that defibrotide and oligotide were analogously able to rapidly inhibit neutrophil adhesion to HUVEC under basal conditions and following neutrophil or endothelial cell stimulation (using fMLP or TNA-α, respectively). In addition, we showed that the use of anti-LFA-1 monoclonal antibodies significantly inhibited neutrophil adhesion to endothelial cells by demonstrating the efficacy of the adhesion molecule LFA-1 in favoring neutrophil attachment to the endothelium. The addition to the two drugs in the presence of anti-LFA-1 antibodies did not further inhibit leukocyte adhesion to endothelial cells. Such results indicate that defibrotide and oligotide could act by inhibiting the adhesion molecule LFA-1.

When we used anti-CD31 monoclonal antibodies (CD31 amplifies integrin-mediated adhesion of neutrophils to endothelium [12]), no inhibitory effect of leukocyte adhesion to endothelial cells was seen under basal conditions, and only a slight inhibition was seen following neutrophil stimulation. In these experiments, defibrotide and oligotide produced a slight inhibition of neutrophil adhesion only after their stimulation.

When we used NIH/3T3-ICAM-1-transfected cells (in which the only adhesion system involved was ICAM-1/LFA-1), defibrotide and oligotide inhibited neutrophil adhesion in a manner similar to that obtained when anti-LFA-1 antibodies were used. The use of anti-LFA-1 and anti-CD31 antibodies together did not produce significantly different results. Oligotide and defibrotide exerted their inhibitory action in a similar manner. Our results show that the two anti-ischemic drugs inhibited neutrophil adhesion to endothelial or other cells by interfering with the adhesion system ICAM-1/LFA-1. Such properties could explain the anti-ischemic activity of the two drugs.

Acknowledgements We thank B. Johnston for editing the manuscript. This work was supported by grants Regione Lombardia, project no. 1364

References

1. Baumann H, Gauldie J (1994) The acute phase response. Immunol Today 15: 74–80
2. Bevilacqua MP, Pober JS, Wheeler ME, Cotran RS, Gibrone MA Jr (1985) Interleukin 1 acts on cultured human vascular endothelium to increase the adhesion of polymorphonuclear leukocytes, monocytes, and related leukocyte cell lines. J Clin Invest 76: 2003–2011
3. Boyum A (1968) Isolation of mononuclear cells and granulocytes from human blood. Scand J Clin Lab Invest 297: 77–89
4. Ferrero ME, Marni A, Parise M, Salari PC, Gaja G (1991) Protection of rat heart from damage due to ischemia-reperfusion during procurement and grafting by defibrotide. Transplantation 52: 611–615
5. Hansen PR (1995) Role of neutrophils in myocardial ischemia and reperfusion. Circulation 91: 1872–1885
6. Jaffe EA (ed) (1984) Biology of endothelial cells. Martinus Nijhoff, Boston
7. Marni A, Ferrero ME, Rovati M, Salari PC, Gaja G (1990) Protection of kidney from postischemic reperfusion injury in rats treated with defibrotide. Transplant Proc 22: 2226–2229
8. Miwa S, Kawasaki S, Makuuchi M, Miyasaka M, Yamazaki S, Sekiguchi M, Isobe M (1995) Role of ICAM-1 and LFA-1 in a cardiac xenograft rejection model. Transplant Proc 27: 111–112
9. Parham P (1983) On the fragmentation of monoclonal IgG1, IgG2a, and IgG2b form BALB/c mice. J Immunol 131: 2895–2902
10. Patel KD, Zimmerman GA, Prescott SM, McEver RP, McIntyre TM (1991) Oxygen radicals induce human endothelial cells to express GMP-140 and bind neutrophils. J Cell Biol 112: 749–759
11. Simpson PJ, Todd RF III, Mickelson JK, Fantone JC, Gallagher KP, Lee KA, Tamura Y, Cronin M, Lucchesi BR (1990) Sustained limitation of myocardial reperfusion injury by a monoclonal antibody that alters leukocyte function. Circulation 81: 226–237
12. Tanaka Y, Albelda SM, Horgan KJ, van Seventer GA, Shimizu Y, Newman W, Hallam J, Newman PJ, Buck CA, Shaw S (1992) CD31 expressed on distinctive T cell subsets is a preferential amplifier of $\beta 1$ integrin-mediated adhesion. J Exp Med 176: 245–253

13. Varani J, Ginsburg I, Schuger L, Gibbs DF, Bromberg J, Johnson KJ, Ryan US, Ward PA (1989) Endothelial cell killing by neutrophils: synergistic interaction of oxygen radical products and proteases. Am J Pathol 135: 435–438

14. Weiss SJ (1989) Tissue destruction by neutrophils. N Engl J Med 320: 365–376

15. Weyrich AS, Ma X-L, Lefer DJ, Albertine KH, Lefer AM (1993) In vivo neutralization of P-selectin protects feline heart and endothelium in myocardial ischemia and reperfusion injury. J Clin Invest 91: 2620–2629

16. Yoshida N, Granger DN, Anderson DC, Rothlein R, Lane C, Kvietys PR (1992) Anoxia/reoxygenation-induced neutrophil adherence to cultured endothelial cells. Am J Physiol 262: H1891–H1898

Transpl Int (1996) 9 [Suppl 1]: S 425–S 428
© Springer-Verlag 1996

Th. Minor*
W. Isselhard
H. Klauke

Reduction in nonparenchymal cell injury and vascular endothelial dysfunction after cold preservation of the liver by gaseous oxygen

T. Minor (✉) · W. Isselhard · H. Klauke
Institute for Experimental Medicine,
University of Cologne,
Robert-Koch-Str. 10,
D-50931 Cologne, Germany
Fax +49 221 478-6264

Abstract Reintroduction of oxygen to previously anoxic tissue may result in severe cell injury (oxygen paradox) and contribute to the so-called reperfusion damage of ischemic organs. Our study investigated the influence of simple gaseous oxygen supply during ischemia on nonparenchymal cell alterations upon reperfusion of the liver. Livers from male Wistar rats were isolated, rinsed blood-free and stored for 48 h at 4 °C in UW-preservation solution (group 1; $n = 6$). Gaseous oxygen was insufflated into a second group of livers (group 2; $n = 6$) during the storage period via the inferior caval vein at a pressure limited to 18 mmHg. To simulate the period of slow rewarming of the organ during surgical implantation in vivo, all livers were incubated at 25 °C in saline solution for 30 min prior to reperfusion. Reperfusion was carried out in vitro in a recirculating system with Krebs-Henseleit buffer. A control group was perfused immediately after harvest. The technique of aerobic storage (group 2) resulted in normal vascular perfusion characteristics without elevation of portal venous pressure (PVP) above control values, in contrast to group 1 livers which showed a significantly elevated PVP, averaging between 1.5 and 2 times the values of the control. Hepatic efflux of NO (nmol/ml) after 10 min of reperfusion was massively increased in group 1, while only low concentrations were found in group 2 and in control livers. Kupffer cell activation after ischemia was shown by a huge increase in acid phosphate release upon reperfusion compared with the control, with significantly lower values in group 2 after 10 min of reperfusion than in group 1. Thus, aerobic ischemia by gaseous oxygen persufflation seems an appropriate tool for long-term organ preservation, preventing vascular and parenchymal dysfunction upon reperfusion.

Key words Persufflation · Aerobic ischemia · Oxygen · Preservation · Liver

* Supported by a grant from the Deutsche Forschungsgemeinschaft (Mi 470/2-1)

Introduction

Previous data from our laboratory have shown that gaseous oxygen insufflation into the venous system of cold-stored livers prevents anaerobic breakdown by hepatic parenchymal energy metabolism during preservation and improves the metabolic recovery of the organ upon postischemic reperfusion [16]. Moreover, circulatory disturbances are also significantly reduced after aerobic liver preservation by oxygen insufflation. Thus the purpose of this study was to determine the effects of the administration of gaseous oxygen during cold preservation on nonparenchymal tissue and on the functional and morphological integrity of the vascular system during postischemic reperfusion.

Materials and methods

Livers from male Wistar rats were isolated, rinsed blood-free and stored for 48 h at 4°C in UW-preservation solution (group 1; $n = 6$). Gaseous oxygen was insufflated into a second group of livers (group 2; $n = 6$) during the storage period via the inferior caval vein at a pressure limited to 18 mmHg. The gas escaped through small pinpricks at the margin of the liver lobes [15]. To simulate the period of slow rewarming of the organ during surgical implantation in vivo [3, 18], all livers were incubated at 25°C in saline solution for 30 min prior to reperfusion. Reperfusion was carried out in vitro in a recirculating system at a constant flow of approximately 3 ml/g liver per min with Krebs-Henseleit buffer, and no perfusate leakage was observed via the venous pricks. A control group ($n = 3$) was perfused immediately after harvest.

Effluent was collected during the in vitro perfusion by means of a short tube telescoped over a splint in the suprahepatic caval vein, allowing effluent perfusate samples to be taken for the determination of oxygen partial pressure with exclusion of room air contamination.

The following assays of enzyme activities in the perfusate were carried out. Alanine-aminotransferase (ALT) was determined photometrically using commercial standard kits (Fa. Boehringer, Mannheim, Germany). Purine-nucleoside-phosphorylase (PNP), which has been shown to be indicative of vascular endothelial lesions [21], was measured in frozen perfusate samples by high-performance liquid chromatography as described elsewhere [17].

The activity of acid phosphatase (ACP) in the effluent perfusate has been shown to provide an estimate of Kupffer cell activation during reperfusion of isolated livers [2] and was measured using a commercial kit (Fa. Boehringer).

The functional ability of the vascular endothelium to release the endogenous vasodilator NO was estimated by measurement of the stable oxidation products nitrate and nitrite ($NO_3 + NO_2$) in the effluent, based on the method described by Evans et al. [4].

Hepatic oxygen consumption was calculated from perfusate samples from the inflow and from the effluent which were immediately analysed using a pH blood gas meter (ABL 2 Acid-Base-Laboratory, Radiometer, Copenhagen). The results are expressed as means ± standard deviation (SD) if not otherwise indicated. Comparisons between multiple groups were performed with one way analysis of variance (ANOVA) and the Bonferroni t-test. Comparisons between two groups were done with the Mann-Whitney rank sum test or alternate t-test (GraphPad INSTAT); $P < 0.05$ was considered as significant.

Results

During postischemic reperfusion in vitro, untreated livers showed an increase in the portal venous perfusion pressure (PVP), which was about twice as high as in the control group and remained elevated throughout the observation period. In contrast, the PVP of livers persufflated with oxygen during the 48 h of ischemic storage did not differ from the values observed in the controls.

The endothelial release of NO was followed by the measurement of its stable oxidation products NO_x (Fig. 1). Interestingly, there was a large increase in NO_x production in untreated livers, corresponding to the elevated perfusion pressure in this group, while concentra-

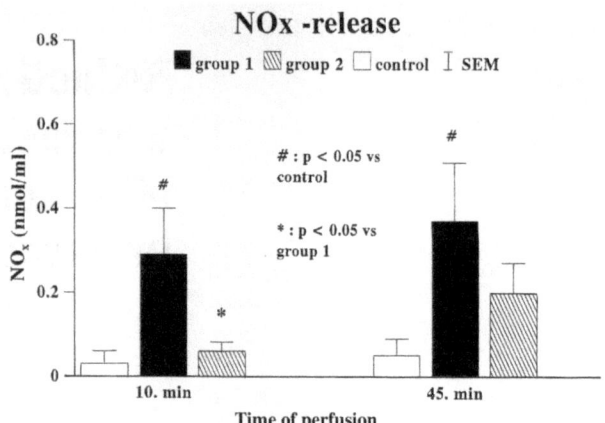

Fig. 1 Release of NO as approximated by its oxidation products NO_x after 10 min and after 45 min of isolated perfusion in vitro. Values are means ± SEM

tions of NO_x in the perfusate of oxygen-persufflated livers were only slightly increased as compared with the controls.

The time course of enzyme leakage from the hepatic parenchyma into the perfusate is shown in Fig. 2. Control preparations exhibited low basal activities of ALT in the perfusate, which did not rise throughout the observation period. Upon reperfusion of ischemically preserved livers (group 1) sixfold higher activities of the enzyme were found during the first 10 min, after which time a steep and ongoing increase in ALT activities in the effluent was found until the end of the experiment. Gaseous aerobiosis during ischemia (group 2) resulted in a significant reduction in the initial ALT activities in the perfusate and completely suppressed the steep rise during the later reperfusion period.

Nonparenchymal enzyme release was followed by the activities of PNP from the vascular endothelium and acid phosphatase from activated Kupffer cells. While PNP was merely detectable in the perfusate of control livers, a progressive increase in PNP activity was observed in group 1 during postischemic reperfusion (Fig. 3). Livers of group 2 exhibited lower activities of this enzyme in the perfusate during the whole experimental course as compared to group 1, the differences being significant after 45 min.

Kupffer cell activation after ischemia was indicated by a huge increase in acid phosphatase release upon reperfusion in both experimental groups compared with the control, but significantly ($P < 0.05$) lower values in group 2 after 10 min of reperfusion compared with group 2 (0.22 ± 0.07 group 2; 1.07 ± 0.41 group 1; 0.02 ± 0.01 U/g per h control).

Oxygen consumption at the end of the perfusion period averaged 2.53 ± 0.19 ml/100 g per min in the control group. It recovered only to 1.47 ± 0.17 ml/100 g per min ($P < 0.01$) in group 1, whereas liver of group 2 reached

Parenchymal enzyme release

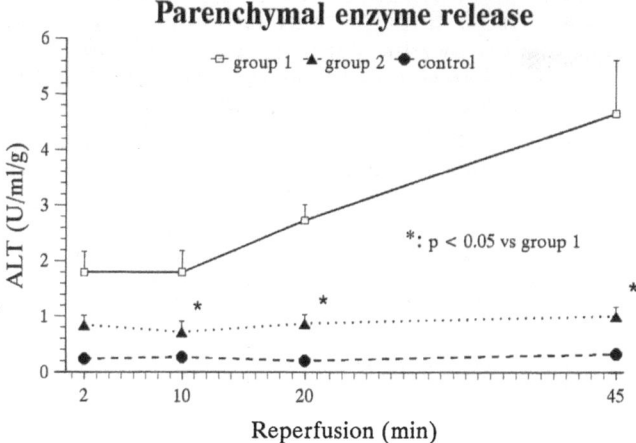

Fig. 2 Release of alanine aminotransferase (ALT) from livers during isolated perfusion in vitro. Values are means ± SEM

Endothelial enzyme release (PNP)

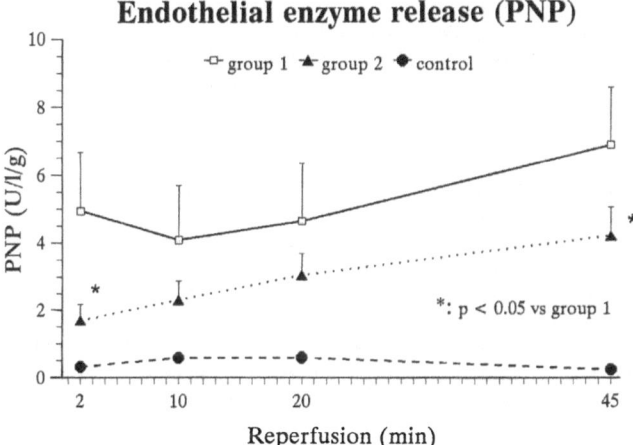

Fig. 3 Release of purine nucleoside phosphorylase (PNP) from livers during isolated perfusion in vitro. Values are means ± SEM

an average of 2.11 ± 0.24 ml/100 g per min, which was not significantly different from the controls.

Discussion

Artificial oxygenation of an ischemic organ has previously been tried in the early 1960s. Oxygen was applied at hyperbaric pressures to the nonperfused organ in order to achieve surface oxygenation of the tissue [12, 13]. However, the high oxygen partial pressures necessary to achieve sufficient supply to larger organs by diffusion require complicated devices and risk oxygen intoxication [24]. An alternative means to provide larger amounts of oxygen to a nonperfused organ has been developed using the arterial or venous vascular system, which avoids the inconvenience of hyperbaric pressure.

While orthograde oxygen persufflation, i.e. the application of oxygen via the arterial system, has been shown to achieve a highly significant improvement in the energy metabolism of ischemically preserved kidneys, this method does not result in functional recovery after reperfusion because of severe alterations in the arterial vascular system and the glomerula [10]. These side effects on the vascular system could be eliminated if the gas was introduced in a retrograde manner via the venous system. This method provides a sufficient aerobiosis of kidneys during ischemia as well as good postischemic function in vivo [5, 9, 22, 23]. Furthermore, no alteration in the portal vascular resistance have been observed upon reperfusion of livers which had previously been preserved in UW-solution using retrograde oxygen insufflation. On the contrary, livers in a persufflation group showed improved perfusion characteristics compared with untreated livers [16].

Endothelial cells play an important role in the regulation of vascular tone, producing and releasing several vasoactive substances including endothelium-derived vascular relaxing factor (EDRF), which has been identified as NO [19]. Alterations in the endothelial cells, which are most vulnerable in the sinusoidal and postsinusoidal veins [8, 25], may cause early microcirculatory disturbances and eventually result in early hepatocellular injury [8, 14].

In the present study we showed an increased production of NO in untreated postischemic livers, which was nevertheless not followed by an adequate reduction in vascular resistance. Endothelial NO is released in response to increased shear stress on the vascular wall [20] in order to normalize vascular flow characteristics. There was a strong stimulus for the release of NO in group 1, whereas only little or no need for vasodilative mediators was seen in control livers or livers kept oxygenated during ischemic storage. Since we did not measure the active form of NO, but only its oxidation products, it can be hypothesized that NO was rendered biologically inactive, e.g. by an excess of superoxide anion radicals [7], arising upon reoxygenation, thus preventing adequate vasorelaxation and an ensuing sustained stimulus to release NO.

Furthermore, it is known that the stress of ischemia/reperfusion can lead to an abnormal increase in endothelin production by the vascular endothelium [6, 11], leading to vasoconstriction and circulatory disturbances. We did not perform endothelin measurements and thus we cannot decided yet whether reduced stimulation of endothelin production or perhaps a simple reduction in endothelial cell swelling during preservation is the physiological mechanism responsible for the beneficial effect of aerobic ischemic storage on the hepatic vasculature. The significant improvement in the portal vascular conductance, however, underlines the overall protective effect of retrograde gaseous oxygen application on the vascular system.

Kupffer cell activation upon reperfusion occurs in response to factors released by injured endothelial cells [2], and eventually may contribute to microcirculatory disturbances in the liver [1]. Thus, the direct or indirect attenuation of hepatic activation of Kupffer cells obtained by oxygen persufflation during ischemic preservation is likely to be partially responsible for the improvement in hepatic perfusion characteristics in this group. In conclusion our findings show that aerobic ischemia by gaseous oxygen persufflation seems an appropriate and feasible tool for long-term liver preservation, preventing vascular and parenchymal dysfunction upon reperfusion.

References

1. Arii S, Monden K, Adachi Y, Zhang WH, Higashitsuji H, Furutani M, Mise M, Fujita S, Nakamura T, Imamura M (1994) Pathogenic role of Kupffer cell activation in the reperfusion injury of cold-preserved liver. Transplantation 58: 1072–1077
2. Caldwell-Kenkel JC, Currin RT, Tanaka Y, Thurman RG, Lemasters JJ (1991) Kupffer cell activation and endothelial cell damage after storage of rat livers: effects of reperfusion. Hepatology 13: 83–95
3. Dunne JB, Davenport M, Williams R, Tredger JM (1994) Evidence that S-adenosylmethionine and N-acetylcysteine reduce injury from sequential cold and warm ischemia in the isolated perfused rat liver. Transplantation 57: 1161–1168
4. Evans T, Carpenter A, Kinderman H, Cohen J (1993) Evidence of increased nitric oxide production in patients with the sepsis syndrome. Circ Shock 41: 77–81
5. Fischer JH, Czerniak A, Hauer U, Isselhard W (1978) A new simple method for optimal storage of ischemically damaged kidneys. Transplantation 25: 43–49
6. Grace PA (1994) Ischaemia-reperfusion injury. Br J Surg 81: 637–647
7. Gryglewski RJ, Palmer RMJ, Moncada S (1986) Superoxide anion is involved in the breakdown of endothelium-derived vascular relaxing factor. Nature 320: 454–456
8. Haba T, Hayashi S, Hachisuka T, Ootsuka S, Tanaka Y, Satou E, Takagi H (1992) Microvascular changes of the liver preserved in UW solution. Cryobiology 29: 310–322
9. Isselhard W, Berger M, Denecke H, Witte J, Fischer JH, Molzberger H (1972) Metabolism of canine kidneys in anaerobic ischemia and in aerobic ischemia by persufflation with gaseous oxygen. Pflügers Arch 337: 87–106
10. Isselhard W, Denecke H, Stelter W, Berger M, Sachweh D, Witte J, Fischer JH (1973) Function and metabolism of canine kidneys after aerobic ischemia by orthograde persufflation with gaseous oxygen. Res Exp Med 159: 288–297
11. Jin MB, Kobayashi Y, Ochiai T, Yasui J, Ohsada S, Nakano K, Yamagishi H, Hironaka T, Oka T (1994) Relationship between nitric oxide and endothelin-1 during the perioperative phase in canine orthotopic liver transplantation (abstract). Eur Surg Res 26 [Suppl 1]: 27
12. Lillehei RC, Manax WG, Bloch JH, Eyal Z, Hidalgo F, Longerbeam JK (1964) In vitro preservation of whole organs by hypothermia and hyperbaric oxygenation. Cryobiology 1: 182–193
13. Manax WG, Largiader F, Lillehei RC (1966) Whole canine organ preservation. Prolongation in vitro by hypothermia and hyperbaria. JAMA 196: 1121–1124
14. McKeown CMB, Edwards V, Philips MJ, Harvey PRC, Petrunka CN, Strasberg SM (1988) Sinusoidal lining cell damage: the critical injury in cold preservation of liver allografts on the rat. Transplantation 46: 178–191
15. Minor T, Isselhard W (1994) Venous oxygen insufflation to prevent reoxygenation injury after ischemia of a solid organ. Transplantation 58: 121–123
16. Minor T, Isselhard W (1996) Synthesis of high energy phosphates during cold ischemic rat liver preservation with gaseous oxygen insufflation. Transplantation 61: 20–22
17. Minor T, Osswald B, Krauss TW, July N, Isselhard W, Klar E (1995) Determination of plasma activities of purine nucleoside phosphorylase by high performance liquid chromatography: estimates of nonparenchymal cell injury after porcine liver transplantation. J Chromatogr B 670: 332–336
18. Minor Th, Yamaguchi Y, Isselhard W (1995) Effects of taurine on liver preservation in UW solution with consecutive rewarming in the isolated perfused rat liver. Transplant Int 8: 174–179
19. Palmer RMJ, Ferrige AG, Moncada S (1987) Nitric oxide release accounts for the biological activity of endothelium-derived relaxing factor. Nature 327: 524–526
20. Post S, Palma P, Gonzalez AP, Rentsch M, Menger MD (1994) Timing of arterialization in liver transplantation. Ann Surg 220: 691–698
21. Rao PN, Walsh TR, Makowka L, Rubin RS, Weber T, Snyder JT, Starzl TE (1990) Purine nucleoside phosphorylase: a new marker for free oxygen radical injury to the endothelial cell. Hepatology 11: 193–198
22. Rolles K, Foreman J, Pegg D (1989) A pilot clinical study of retrograde oxygen persufflation in renal preservation. Transplantation 48: 339–342
23. Ross H, Escott ML (1979) Gaseous oxygen perfusion of the renal vessels as an adjunct in kidney preservation. Transplantation 28: 362–364
24. VanZyl JJW, Groenewald JH, Murphy GP (1970) The influence of hyperbaric oxygen toxicity on renal preservation. Cryobiology 6: 493–499
25. Vaubourdolle M, Chazouilleres O, Poupon R, Ballet F, Braunwald J, Legendre C, Baudin B, Kirn A, Giboudeau J (1993) Creatine kinase-BB: a marker of liver sinusoidal damage in ischemia-reperfusion. Hepatology 17: 423–428

Transpl Int (1996) 9 [Suppl 1]: S 429–S 431
© Springer-Verlag 1996

Andreas Salat
Michael Rolf Mueller
Dagmar Boehm
Petra Stangl
Sad Pulaki
Friedrich Laengle

Influence of UW solution on in vitro platelet aggregability

A. Salat (✉) · P. Stangl · F. Laengle
University of Vienna,
Department of General Surgery,
General Hospital of Vienna,
Waehringer Gürtel 18–20, A-1090 Vienna,
Austria
Fax +43 14 04 00 56 41

M. R. Mueller
University of Vienna,
Department of Cardio-Thoracic Surgery,
General Hospital of Vienna, Austria

D. Boehm
University of Vienna,
Department of Anesthesiology,
General Hospital of Vienna, Austria

S. Pulaki
University of Vienna,
Center for Biomedical Research,
General Hospital of Vienna, Austria

Abstract Bleeding problems in orthotopic liver transplantation (OLT), starting immediately after reperfusion of the graft, are complicating the outcome of transplantation. Platelets may be involved in this situation, but there is still a lack of information about the influence of UW solution on platelet function. We evaluated the effect of UW solution on in vitro platelet aggregability in healthy volunteers using whole blood electrical aggregometry and concluded, that UW solution causes impaired platelet aggregability and may contribute to bleeding problems during OLT. The mechanism of impairment remains unclear, since central pathways as well as membrane receptors seem to be involved. Furthermore, our data support the necessity of extended flushing of the liver graft after reperfusion.

Key words Platelets · Whole blood electrical aggregometry · UW solution · Platelet function

Introduction

Bleeding is a significant contributory factor to the postoperative short- and long-term outcome in OLT [1, 3, 17]. Two major causes could be identified to be responsible for this phenomenon. Firstly, hyperfibrinolysis, mainly in the anhepatic phase, and secondly, disseminated intravascular coagulopathy (DIC), starting immediately after reperfusion [3, 4, 6, 13–15]. Another cause may be damage or alteration to the graft liver's vessel wall during the cold ischemic time, suspected because of the beneficial effect of prostaglandin E_1 in the reperfusion injury of the liver [8, 12]. However, other factors may be involved. Some studies have pointed out a decreased platelet aggregability to be one of these factors. Himmelreich et al. found a reduced platelet count and a reduced maximum amplitude of platelet aggregation in platelet rich plasma (PRP) 5 min post reperfusion compared to 5 min before reperfusion. Furthermore, samples taken from the perfusate were significantly lower than systemic samples [7, 9], partly explained by the influence of the UW solution [5].

Whole blood aggregometry (WBEA) was first described in 1980 [2], but did not reach clinical importance because of considerable interindividual differences due to the influences of hematocrit and platelet count. Furthermore, the interpretation of aggregation curves was more intuitive than quantitative. So this convincing method was reserved to a small group of experienced investigators. We established a software package with an A/D converter enabling a mathematical analysis of aggregation curves [16] and a correction for the influence of hematocrit and platelet count [11]. On the one hand, these improvements pushed the reliability of WBEA to an acceptable standard for a laboratory method, enabling reproducible information on in vitro platelet function, and on the other hand, the advantages of WBEA, quick information and easy handling, were enforced.

The aim of this study was to evaluate the influence of UW solution on in vitro platelet aggregability in whole blood.

Materials and methods

Five female and five male, healthy, non-smoking volunteers (mean age 28.4 ± 3.5 years), who denied intake of any medication throughout the 14 days prior to sampling, participated in this study. Following aseptic venipuncture of the cubital vein, blood was drawn directly into a 5 ml Vacutainer tube containing 0.5 ml of 0.129 M buffered sodium citrate (3.8 %). Samples were measured for red and white blood cells, mean cellular volume, and platelet count using an electronic particle counter (Coulter Counter, T-540). The hematocrit was calculated from the red blood cell count and mean cellular volume. Platelet counts, hematocrit, and white blood cell counts were within normal ranges for all probands.

One milliliter of citrated whole blood was transferred to special polystyrene tubes (Chrono-log Corporation, Haverton, Pa.) containing 0 µl (control), 50 µl (group B), 75 µl (group C), or 100 µl (group D) UW solution (supplied by Beltzer). Thereafter, samples were incubated at 37 °C and stirred at 700 rpm for 10 min. To avoid possible artefacts [10], platelet aggregation testing was performed within 1 h of blood collection using a whole blood aggregometer (Chrono-log Corporation, Haverton, Pa.). Aggregation was triggered using arachidonic acid (AA), adenosine diphosphate (ADP), and collagen (COL), AA at a final concentration of 500 µM, ADP at a final concentration of 10 µM, and COL at a final concentration of 5 µg/ml. [All trigger substances were from Chrono-log Corporation, Haverton, Pa. (Chrono-par)]. The original aggregation data were transferred to a PC/XT-386, the area under the aggregation curve (A-under) was calculated for each sample [16] and corrected for the influence of hematocrit and platelet count [11]. A-under reflects not only the maximum amplitude, but also the steepness of the curve, allowing the quantification of the complete aggregation process. Differences between groups were checked by means of a non-parametric t-test (Wilcoxon two-sample test).

Results

Platelet aggregability for each trigger substance, quantified by the parameter A-under, decreased with the addition of 50 µl UW solution. Samples stimulated with ADP showed a significant dose-dependent reduction of platelet aggregability compared to the control group, whereas for samples stimulated with AA or COL, no significant differences were found with higher concentrations of UW solution (75 or 100 µl). Detailed data for each group and trigger substance are given in Table 1.

Table 1 Area under aggregation curve (*AA* arachidonic acid, *ADP* adenosine diphosphate, *COL* collagen)

Trigger substance		Control	Group B	Group C	Group D
AA	Mean	5229	4736	5120	5198
	SD	867	1245	1049	1154
	P value (vs control)		< 0.049	n.s.	n.s.
ADP	Mean	6305	4526	4130	4060
	SD	1267	1209	1066	967
	P value (vs control)		< 0.046	< 0.0051	< 0.0038
COL	Mean	10042	8932	10603	10235
	SD	2341	1072	1856	1788
	P value (vs control)		< 0.036	n.s.	n.s.

Discussion

UW solution is widely used for the preservation of organs during orthotopic liver transplantation, since it allows an extension of the cold storage time with a lower incidence of thrombosis in the hepatic artery and higher survival rates. During liver transplantation, after flushing and reperfusion of the graft, bleeding complicates and influences the short- and long-term outcome of the transplantation procedure. Although other causes of impaired hemostasis have been identified previously, the role of platelets in this context is not well defined. Only one study was found in the literature reporting impaired platelet aggregation in platelet-rich plasma, at least partially caused by UW solution [5]. Therefore, we evaluated the influence of UW solution on in vitro platelet aggregability in ten healthy volunteers using whole blood electrical aggregometry, a method first described in 1980 [2] and modified by our group in recent years [11, 16]. Since testing is performed in citrated whole blood, this method offers a more physiological milieu than platelet aggregation in platelet-rich plasma, which has been used for most studies in this field.

Our results show an impaired AA-, ADP-, and COL-triggered platelet aggregation caused by the addition of 50 µl/ml UW-solution. The stimulation with ADP resulted in a dose-dependent impairment, whereas for aggregation triggered by AA and COL, no significant differences were found with higher concentrations of UW solution (groups C, D). This pattern of aggregation responses is in concurrence with the findings of Himmelreich et al. [5] and implies that UW solution may effect platelet aggregation not only via receptor inhibition, but probably also via a central mechanism. The individual ingredients of UW solution may influence platelet aggregation in one direction (inhibition or stimulation), but the interaction of all component may result in diverse action depending on the concentration. Platelet aggregation triggered with AA and COL was only reduced at a concentration of 50 µl/ml UW solution. At this concentration, inhibiting effects of UW solution may prevail. However, ADP-triggered aggregation showed a dose-dependent impairment, suggesting an additional competitive mechanism at the membrane receptor. Altogether, the mechanism of impaired platelet aggregation caused by UW solution is still unclear and needs further investigation.

We conclude that UW solution causes impaired platelet aggregation in whole blood, probably contributing to bleeding complications directly after reperfusion. To prevent this side effect, extensive flushing of the reperfused graft is necessary.

References

1. Bontempo FA, Lewis JH, Van Thiel D, Spero JA, Ragni MV, Butler P, Israel I, Starzl TE (1985) The relation of preoperative coagulation findings to diagnosis, blood usage and survival in adult liver transplantation. Transplantation 39: 532–536
2. Cardinal DC, Flower RC (1980) The electronical aggregometer: A novel device for assessing platelet behavior in blood. J Pharmacol Methods 3: 135–158
3. Dzik WH, Arkin CF, Jenkins RL, Stump DC (1988) Fibrinolysis during liver transplantation in humans. Role of tissue-type plasminogen activator. Blood 71: 1090–1095
4. Harper PL, Luddington RJ, Jennings I, Reardon D, Seaman MJ, Carrell RW, Klinik JR, Smith M, Rolles K, Calne R (1989) Coagulation changes following hepatic revascularisation during liver transplantation. Transplantation 48: 603–607
5. Himmelreich G, Riess H (1991) In vitro inhibition of platelet aggregation by the liver preservation fluid UW solution. Transplantation 52: 30–33
6. Himmelreich G, Kierzek B, Neuhaus P, Slama KJ, Riess H (1991) Coagulation changes and the influence of the early perfusate in the course of orthotopic liver transplantation (OLT) when aprotinin is used intraoperatively. Blood Coag Fibrinol 2: 51–59
7. Himmelreich G, Hundt K, Neuhaus P, Blumhardt G, Riess H (1992) Decreased platelet aggregation after reperfusion in orthotopic liver transplantation. Transplantation 53: 582–586
8. Himmelreich G, Hundt K, Bechstein WO, Rossaint R, Neuhaus P, Riess H (1993) Influence of prostaglandin E1 infusion on hemostasis in orthotopic liver transplantation. Semin Thromb Hemostas 19(3): 273–278
9. Himmelreich G, Riewald M, Rosch R, Bechstein WO, Gerlach H, Neuhaus P, Riess H (1993) Soluble thrombomodulin as a mediator of endothelial damage in orthotopic liver transplantation? Semin Thromb Hemostas 19(3): 246–249
10. Mueller MR, Schreiner W, Wohlfahrt A, Salat A, Wolner E (1990) The influence of sample age on collagen-induced platelet aggregation in whole blood. Thromb Res 60: 477–487
11. Mueller MR, Salat A, Pulaki S, Stangl P, Erdem E, Schreiner W, Wolner E (1995) The influence of hematocrit and platelet count on whole blood electrical aggregometry J Pharmacol Methods 34(1): 17–22
12. Otto G, Wolff H, Uerlings I, Gelbert K (1986) Preservation damage in liver transplantation. Transplantation 42: 122–124
13. Palareti G, De Rosa V, Fortunato G, Grauso F, Legnani C, Maccaferri M, Poggi M, Bianchini B, Bellusci R, Franceschelli N, Cocheri S (1988) Control of hemostasis during orthotopic liver transplantation. Fibrinolysis 2: 61–66
14. Porte RJ, Bontempo FA, Knot EAR, Lewis JH, Kang YH, Starzl TE (1989) Systemic effects of tissue plasminogen activator-associated fibrinolysis and its relation to thrombin generation in orthotopic liver transplantation. Transplantation 47: 978–984
15. Porte RJ, Knot EAR, Bontempo FA (1989) Hemostasis in liver transplantation. Gastroenterology 97(2): 488–501
16. Schreiner W, Mueller MR, Premauer W, Wolner E (1991) Computerized acquisition and evaluation of whole blood aggregometry data. Comput Biol Med 21(6): 435–441
17. Starzl TE, Demetris AJ, Van Thiel D (1984) Liver transplantation. N Engl J Med 311: 1658–1664

Transpl Int (1996) 9 [Suppl 1]: S432–S436
© Springer-Verlag 1996

Kazuhiko Seya
Nobuhiro Ohkohchi
Shigeki Tsukamoto
Susumu Satomi

Why is liver preservation performed at 4 °C?

K. Seya (✉) · N. Ohkohchi · S. Tsukamoto ·
S. Satomi
Second Department of Surgery,
Tohoku University School of Medicine
1-1 Seiryo-machi, Aoba-ku, Sendai 980-77,
Japan

Abstract To establish the most suitable temperature for liver preservation, we preserved rat livers at various temperatures (0, 5, 10, and 15 °C) in UW solution and investigated, biochemically, the proton ATPase activity, ATP metabolites in mitochondria, and phosphatidylcholine hydroperoxide (PC-OOH) in liver tissue. Liver specimens were taken every 6 h up to 24 h. The proton ATPase activity and the concentration of ATP, ADP, AMP, and adenosine in livers preserved at 0 °C showed the best results. The total adenine nucleotide (TAN) in livers preserved for 18 and 24 h had significantly higher concentrations compared with those at other temperatures (5, 10, and 15 °C). In the livers preserved at 5 °C, TAN was degraded to hypoxanthine. On the other hand, those preserved at both 10 and 15 °C showed changes from hypoxanthine to xanthine. The concentration of xanthine in both groups preserved at 10 and 15 °C showed high values at 6 and 12 h, respectively, and similar changes in PC-OOH concentrations at both 10 and 15 °C were observed. However, the changes in PC-OOH concentration at various temperatures were not significant for any length of preservation time. In light microscopical examinations, there were no morphological changes in the hepatocytes. From these results, we conclude that the capability of ATP synthesis of mitochondria in livers preserved at 0 °C keep them in the best condition compared with livers preserved at 15, 10, and 5 °C.

Key words Liver preservation ·
Low temperature · Mitochondrial
proton ATPase activity ·
Mitochondrial ATP metabolites ·
Phosphatidylcholine hydroperoxide

Introduction

One of the most vital problems in liver transplantation is the preservation of the liver in the best condition. At present, the liver for transplantation is generally preserved at 0–4 °C to inhibit its metabolism. Some investigators have studied the optimal temperature for liver preservation. Attenburrow et al. [1] measured the tissue adenosine nucleotide level in the rat liver and concluded that the optimal temperature was 10 °C. On the other hand, Okouchi et al. [2] investigated the bile flow rate after liver transplantation in the rat at various temperatures and suggested that preservation at 0–5 °C is optimal. The most appropriate temperature, however, for liver transplantation is not clear because of a lack of information concerning the changes in biochemical values at various temperatures during the liver preservation.

Recently, we reported that the deterioration of ATP synthesis in the mitochondria of hepatocytes and the disruption of sinusoidal endothelial cells contributed greatly to liver injury during preservation [3, 4]. Therefore, it is important to prevent these injuries before liver transplantation. To elucidate the optimal temperature for liver preservation, we studied the changes in mitochondrial function and in the sinusoidal endothelial cells in livers preserved at various temperatures. We have already measured the proton ATPase activity [5] and ATP concentration in mitochondria using livers preserved in UW solution at various temperatures and have considered that the optimal temperature for liver preservation should be 0 °C [6]. To confirm our hypothesis, however, more biochemical information was necessary; for example, the capability of ATP synthesis, the degradation of TAN, and the possibility of phospholipid peroxidation of cell membranes by a generated free radical in the liver.

In this report, we further investigated the consequences of liver preservation at low temperatures by measuring the levels of ATP metabolites in mitochondria and phosphatidylcholine hydroperoxide (PC-OOH) in liver tissue in order to clarify the optimal temperature for liver preservation from the viewpoint of ATP production and phospholipid peroxidation.

Materials and methods

Preservation method

Male Wistar rats weighing 250–300 g were used. Under anesthesia with ether, the liver was flushed with Ringer's lactate solution and then with UW solution via the portal vein. The Ringer's lactate and UW solutions were cooled to various temperatures (0, 5, 10, and 15 °C). The liver was then immediately excised and preserved in UW solution at 0, 5, 10, and 15 °C ($n = 4$ in each group). Liver specimens were examined every 6 h from 0 h to 24 h.

Isolation of mitochondria

Mitochondria were isolated from the liver by the "high-yield" differential centrifugation method [7]. The isolation medium consisted of 0.25 M sucrose buffer (pH 7.4).

Measurement of mitochondrial proton ATPase activity

ATPase activity was measured by a Jasco FP-777 fluorometer (Tokyo, Japan) at 23 °C at an excitation of 625 nm and an emission of 670 nm using 100 μl of mitochondria (4–10 mg/ml protein) isolated by our previously described method [8]. We used diS-C$_3$ (5) as the fluorescence reagent.

Measurement of concentrations of ATP, ADP, and AMP

The isolated mitochondria in 0.5 N aqueous perchloric acid were smashed by sonication. The extracted medium was injected to a high performance liquid chromatography (HPLC) system using a reverse phase column (Wakosil-II 5C18 HG, 4.6 mm i. d. × 15 cm) using a UV detector (260 nm, Shimadzu SPD-6AV). The eluent was 60 mM phosphate buffer (pH 5.0) and the flow rate was 0.5 ml/min. Protein concentration in the mitochondria was determined by the Bradford method [9].

Measurement of concentrations of adenosine, inosine, xanthine, and hypoxanthine

The extracted medium, obtained by pretreating mitochondria, was injected to the HPLC system using a reverse phase column (Tosoh TSKgel ODS 80TM, 4.6 mm i. d. × 25 cm). The eluent was 3.5 % acetonitrile in 50 mM phosphate buffer (pH 3.0) and the flow rate was 0.7 ml/min.

Measurement of PC-OOH concentration

PC-OOH in the liver tissue was measured by a chemiluminescence high performance liquid chromatography (CL-HPLC) system applying our improved method. The homogenized solution was centrifuged and extracted with dichloromethane-methanol (2:1) containing 0.002 % 2,6-di-tert-butyl-4-methylphenol [10]. Removal of the dichloromethane phase gave a residue, the total lipids, which was supplemented with methanol. The solution, filtered through a 0.5 mμ Millipore filter, was injected into the CL-HPLC system.

The CL-HPLC system was equipped with a TSK-gel Silica-60 column (5 mμ, 4.6 mm i. d. × 25 cm, Tosoh). Using a Jasco 875-CE UV detector, the flow rate of the mobile phase, dichloromethane-methanol (1:4, v/v), was 1.0 ml/min. After passing through the UV detector, the eluate was mixed with a CL reagent by using a mixing cell. The flow rate of the CL reagent was 1.0 ml/min using a Jasco PU-980i pump. The generated CL was monitored with a single photon counting apparatus, Jasco 825-CL, equipped with a flow spiral quartz cell. The CL reagent was prepared by dissolving 4 μM 2-methyl-6-[p-methoxyphenyl]-3,7-dihydroimidazo [1,2-a] pyrazin-3-one (MCLA) and 10 μM FeSO$_4$ in methanol.

Histological examination

For light microscopy, the rat liver was fixed in 10 % aqueous formalin for 24 h at room temperature, dehydrated, and embedded in paraffin. Sections were stained by hematoxylin and eosin.

Statistical data

All results were expressed as the mean ± standard deviation. Statistical analysis was performed by Student's t-test.

Results

Concentration of ATP metabolites

In our previous paper we reported that the deterioration of proton ATPase activity had a close relationship with the decrement of ATP concentration [6]. The changes in the total adenine nucleotide (TAN) are shown in Fig. 1. The levels of ATP, ADP, and AMP preserved at various temperatures all decreased during preservation. The TAN level in livers preserved at 0 °C kept significantly high values at 18 and 24 h, 10.44 ± 2.19 nmol/mg of mitochondrial protein at 18 h ($P < 0.05$ versus preservation at 5 °C), and 7.38 ± 1.18 nmol/mg at 24 h ($P < 0.05$ versus preservation at 5 °C). The levels of TAN in mitochondria in livers preserved at 5 °C remained the same

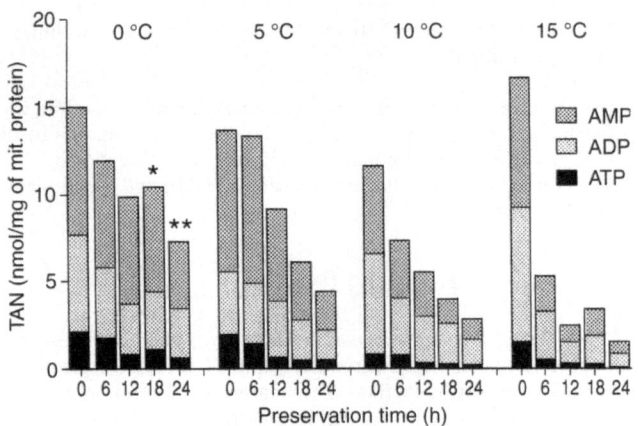

Fig. 1 TAN (ATP + ADP + AMP) in mitochondria during rat liver preservation in UW solution at various temperatures (0, 5, 10, and 15 °C). (* $P < 0.05$ vs other temperatures for 18 h, ** $P < 0.05$ vs other temperatures for 24 h)

6 h (3.67 ± 0.64 nmol/mg of mitochondrial protein, $P < 0.05$ versus at 0 h). On the other hand, the concentration of xanthine in these livers showed significant increments at 6 and 12 h. The level of xanthine in livers preserved at 10 °C also showed significant increments at 12 h (Fig. 2).

The concentration of PC-OOH (Fig. 3)

The concentrations of PC-OOH remained at low values without significant changes for various preservation times and at all temperatures. The PC-OOH concentration at 0 °C was, however, slightly lower for all lengths of preservation time (0.44 ± 0.62 nmol/100 mg of total lipids in the liver at 0 h, 0.64 ± 0.21 at 12 h, and 0.21 ± 0.29 at 18 h).

Histological findings

The 24-h-preserved livers at any temperature showed increments of intracellular space in comparison with the specimens just after graftectomy. There were, however, no morphological changes in the hepatocytes for any length of preservation times.

as those preserved at 0 °C up to 12 h, but these values deteriorated at 18 h (6.07 ± 1.73 nmol/mg of mitochondrial protein). In livers preserved at both 10 and 15 °C, the level of the energy charge became significantly worse at 12 h.

The level of adenine in livers preserved at 0 °C also remained unchanged for 18 h (1.48 ± 0.66 nmol/mg of protein at 18 h, $P < 0.05$ versus preservation at 5 °C). At other temperatures, the decrement of the adenosine levels was observed. The concentration of inosine remained unchanged at any temperature and for any length of preservation time (Table 1, 2). The concentration of hypoxanthine in livers preserved at 5 °C remained at a high value for any length of preservation time and showed significant change at 12 h, 6.08 ± 2.20 nmol/mg of mitochondrial protein ($P < 0.05$ versus other temperatures). The hypoxanthine level in livers preserved at 15 °C showed a significant increment at

Discussion

It is well known that livers are injured by the reperfusion after preservation. We confirmed from our investigations that the mitochondria and sinusoidal lining cells are especially susceptible to injury during preservation [3, 4]. Accordingly, it is important to prevent injury to the mitochondria and sinusoidal cells during liver preservation before liver transplantation. Investigations to develop a preservation solution are constantly being

Table 1 Adenosine in mitochondria during preservation ($n = 4$), measured in nmol/mg mitochondrial protein

Preservation temperature (°C)	0	6	Preservation time (h)		
			12	18	24
0	1.53 ± 0.83	1.66 ± 0.40	1.38 ± 0.74	1.48 ± 0.66	0.84 ± 0.32
5	2.61 ± 1.04	2.36 ± 0.72	1.07 ± 0.90	0.41 ± 0.41	0.48 ± 0.34
10	0.83 ± 0.58	0.71 ± 0.39	0.51 ± 0.22	0.38 ± 0.21	0.18 ± 0.19
15	1.73 ± 0.27	0.71 ± 0.08	0.41 ± 0.09	0.38 ± 0.08	0.29 ± 0.13

Table 2 Inosine in mitochondria during preservation ($n = 4$), measured in nmol/mg mitochondrial protein

* $P < 0.001$ versus 15 °C preservation at 6 h; ** $P < 0.05$ versus 15 °C preservation at 6 h

Preservation temperature (°C)	0	6	Preservation time (h)		
			12	18	24
0	3.64 ± 1.58	4.52 ± 1.13	5.59 ± 1.10	3.72 ± 1.60	5.90 ± 1.69
5	6.80 ± 2.51	6.44 ± 1.76	6.24 ± 1.41	6.99 ± 1.39	6.92 ± 1.30
10	5.49 ± 1.06	5.48 ± 1.65	5.70 ± 0.92	5.41 ± 1.13	4.97 ± 1.25
15	3.57 ± 0.50*	6.83 ± 1.02	5.88 ± 1.32	4.88 ± 0.93	4.41 ± 0.57**

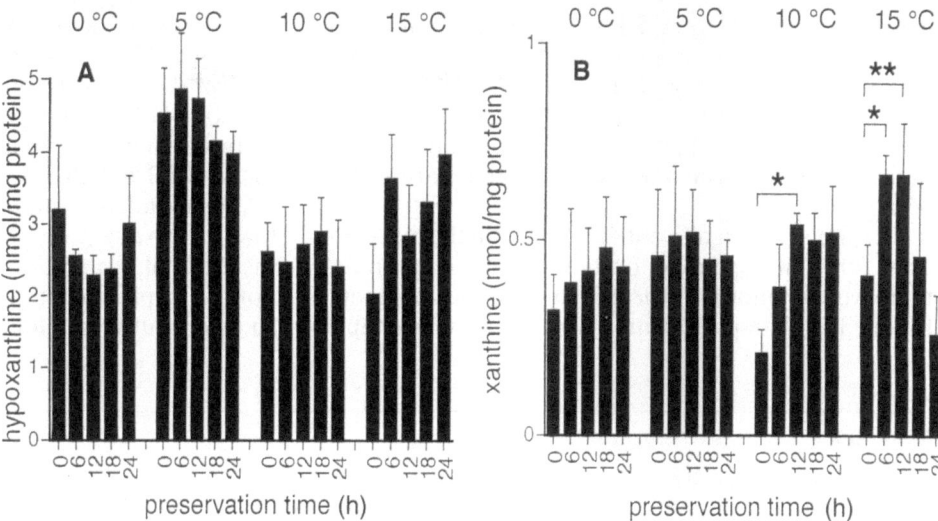

Fig. 2 A, B Hypoxanthine (**A**) and xanthine (**B**) in mitochondria during rat liver preservation in UW solution at various temperatures (0, 5, 10, and 15 °C). (* $P < 0.01$, ** $P < 0.05$)

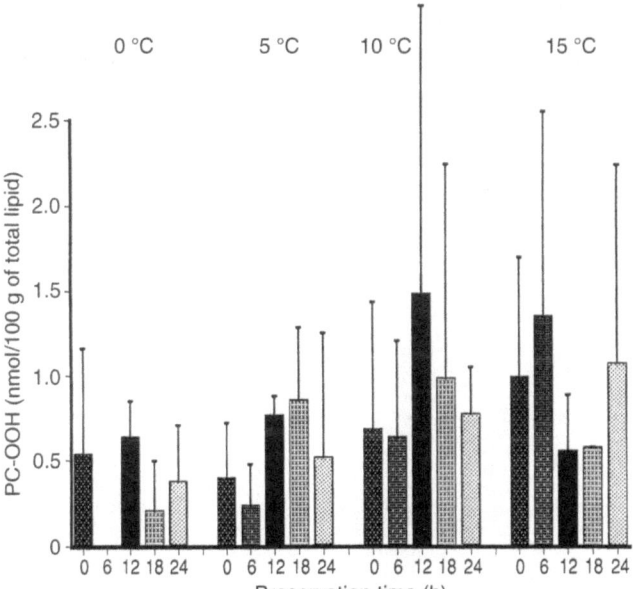

Fig. 3 Phosphatidylcholine hydroperoxide (PC-OOH) in liver tissue during rat liver preservation in UW solution at various temperatures (0, 5, 10, and 15 °C)

preformed. However, we considered the influence of temperature on preservation and investigated the change of mitochondrial function under various temperatures to clarify the best temperature for liver preservation.

The decrement of TAN is generally attributed to the natural degradation of ATP. We suspected that the TAN level in livers preserved at 0 °C remained high in comparison with those at other temperatures because the lowest temperature for preservation will slow the rate of its degradation. We also measured the change in the levels of adenosine, inosine, hypoxanthine, and xan-

thine to elucidate the limit of TAN degradation at the various temperatures during preservation. In livers preserved at 0 °C, the degradation of TAN was limited to adenosine; the values of the other components remained low. In those preserved at 5 °C, the degradation of TAN was limited to hypoxanthine because the levels of inosine and hypoxanthine were higher than at other temperatures and the levels of xanthine were very low. On the other hand, the levels of xanthine in livers preserved at 10 °C increased at 12 h, and in those preserved at 15 °C increased at 6 h. From these results, we suggested that the ATP degradation is prevented at a lower temperatures and the best temperature for liver preservation is 0 °C.

To clarify the possibility of free radical generation induced by abundant oxygen in the UW solution, we measured PC-OOH in the liver tissue. Measurement of PC-OOH by CL-HPLC has been developed by Miyazawa et al. [11]. In this system, however, since the eluent (methanol-chloroform) and reaction solution (borate buffer) when mixed generate chemiluminescence, so the reproducibility of this system is disrupted by the generation of foam. Consequently, we investigated and developed an improved method which uses methanol medium including a highly sensitive chemiluminescence reagent, MCLA, and $FeSO_4$ as the reagent for the Fenton reaction. The non-metallic pump was used for the elution of reactive solution. The detection limit of PC-OOH using our improved method was 50 pmol (S/N ratio > 3). Thus, we utilized our improved method to measure the concentration of PC-OOH because of its high sensitivity.

The phospholipid peroxidation by oxygen-derived free radicals is well investigated and it is well known that the microsomal membrane is easily injured by free radicals. Although a significant change of PC-OOH concentration for any length of preservation at various temperatures was not observed, it was shown that the the change of xanthine levels is similar to the change of PC-OOH concentration at 10 and 15 °C. However, the degree of these changes was small and we suggest that the influence of the phospholipid peroxidation by free radicals is little during the preservation at various temperatures.

In spite of the significant differences in the mitochondrial function depending on the various temperatures, there were no morphological changes to the hepatocytes for any length of preservation time. Light microscopical study is incapable of demonstrating the condition of the sinusoidal endothelial cells precisely [4]. It is necessary to scan the microstructure of sinusoidal cells by transmission of electron microscopy.

In summary, we confirm that the deterioration of mitochondrial function in liver preservation is caused by TAN degradation and of proton ATPase activity by low temperature. In this study, we can conclude that the optimal temperature for liver preservation is 0 °C. For more precise information, electron microscopical study of sinusoidal endothelial cells is required.

References

1. Attenburrow VD, Fuller BJ, Hobbs KEF (1981) Cryo-Lett 2: 15
2. Okouchi Y, Tamaki T, Kozaki M (1992) Transplantation 54: 1129
3. Sakurada M, Ohkohchi N, Katoh H, Koizumi M, Fujimori K, Satomi S, Sasaki T, Taguchi Y, Mori S (1989) Transplant Proc 21: 1321
4. Koizumi M, Ohkohchi N, Katoh H, Koyamada N, Fujimori K, Sakurada M, Andoh T, Satomi S, Sasaki T, Taguchi Y, Mori S, Kataoka S, Yamamoto T (1989) Transplant Proc 21: 1323
5. Seya K, Ohkohchi N, Watanabe N, Shibuya H, Taguchi Y, Mori S (1995) Transplant Proc 27: 736
6. Seya K, Ohkohchi N, Tsukamoto S, Satomi S, Taguchi Y, Mori S (1996) Transplant Proc 28: (in press)
7. Schneider WC, Hogeboon GH (1948) J Biol Chem 183: 123
8. Seya K, Ohkohchi N, Watanabe N, Shibuya H, Taguchi Y, Mori S (1994) J Clin Lab Anal 8: 418
9. Bradford M (1976) Anal Biochem 72: 248
10. Folch J, Ascoli I, Lees M, Meath JA, LeBaron FN (1951) J Biol Chem 191: 833
11. Miyazawa T, Yasuda K, Fujimoto K, Kaneda T (1987) Anal Lett 20: 915

Transpl Int (1996) 9 [Suppl 1]: S437–S441
© Springer-Verlag 1996

R. Prestel
M. Storck
R. Pooth
G. Steinbach
C. Hammer
D. Abendroth

Na-K/2Cl transporter inhibition for reduction of postischemic kidney failure tested in autologous reperfusion

R. Prestel · C. Hammer
Institute for Surgical Research,
LM University Munich, Germany

M. Storck (✉) · R. Pooth · D. Abendroth
Department of Surgery II,
University of Ulm, Steinhövelstrasse 9,
D-89075 Ulm, Germany
Tel. +49 7 31 5 02 73 00;
Fax +49 7 31 5 02 72 89

G. Steinbach
Institute for Clinical Chemistry,
University of Ulm, Ulm, Germany

Abstract Postischemic kidney function may be influenced by donor conditioning. The sulfamoylbenzoate "piretanide" (P) is a diuretic agent with an inhibitory effect on the luminal Na-K-2CL-transporter system in the ascending part of the loop of Henle. A clinical pilot study demonstrated a lower rate of organ dysfunction following transplantation in humans when the donor organs were pretreated with piretanide. In an experimental ex vivo model the effect of piretanide on immediate organ function following long or short cold ischemia was studied. Porcine kidneys ($n = 36$) were removed after in situ transaortal hypothermic flushing with 2 l Eurocollins solution. Following short storage (1 h, $n = 18$) or long storage (24 h, $n = 18$) the kidneys were reperfused with intraoperatively drawn heparinized autologous blood diluted with Ringer's lactate to a hematocrit of 25 %. Urine flow was higher in the piretanide-pretreated group (p), especially after long storage. The electrolyte loss was comparable in both groups. Postischemic endogenous creatinine clearance was significantly elevated in the treatment group (4.45 ± 0.6 ml/min per 100 mg in P vs 1.91 ± 0.4 ml/min per 100 mg, in control, $P < 0.05$ Mann-Whitney test). Renal hemodynamics were improved by piretanide, resulting in significantly lower resistance and allowing higher flow during pressure-controlled perfusion. O_2 consumption, representing general metabolic activity, was higher after long storage, indicating an earlier recovery from cold ischemia. In this ex vivo model, autologous reperfusion of porcine kidneys could be improved by piretanide pretreatment. Autoregulation of kidney vasculature was maintained as well as functional parameters such as creatinine clearance or gluconeogenesis. Therefore, piretanide may be used in larger clinical trials to further improve organ quality in times of donor shortage.

Key words Piretanide · Kidney transplantation · Donor conditioning · Ex vivo hemoperfusion

Introduction

The concept of improving organ quality by donor pretreatment has gained importance in clinical transplantation. The incidence of early graft failure (ARF) following allogeneic cadaver kidney transplantation is an important clinical parameter [12] independent of immunological aspects such as HLA mismatch or antibody status of the recipient. Piretanide (P), a loop diuretic with a similar chemical structure to furosemide but different pharmacodynamic properties [3], inhibits the energy dependent luminal Na-K/2Cl ion transportation in renal tubular cells and thus contributes to higher ATP concentrations during and after the cold ischemia period [8]. In addition, piretanide influences arachidonic acid metabolism resulting in vascular effects that attenuate postischemic vasoconstriction [9]. Both effects may be of advantage in kidney conservation if piretanide is given to the donor. In a clinical pilot study, a beneficial effect of this concept could be demonstrated through a reduction of the ARF rate in patients receiving piretanide-pretreated donor organs [1]. Because of these direct clinical implications, it was the aim of this experimental study to verify these preliminary results and to describe early functional characteristics of piretanide-pretreated kidneys after short and long cold ischemia time in a standardized autologous perfusion model.

Material and methods

Thirty-six kidneys from German Landrace pigs (mean weight 22.7 ± 3 kg) were studied. The experiments were approved by the local board of animal protection, as required. Under deep anesthesia following arterial and venous catheterization, a laparotomy was performed and the bladder canulated. Mean arterial pressure, heart rate and PO$_2$ were continuously monitored. The treatment group ($n = 18$) received 1.6 mg/kg body weight i. v. piretanide for 30 min before organ removal, followed by systemic heparin administration (3000 I. E.). Transaortal in situ hypothermic perfusion with 3000 ml Eurocollins (EC) solution was used and warm ischemia was avoided.

Half the organs (mean weight 63 ± 5 g) were stored for 1 h on ice and the other half for 24 h, resulting in four groups: piretanide short storage, piretanide long storage, control short storage and control long storage (each $n = 9$) (P = piretanide, C = control, SS = short storage, LS = long storage).

Intraoperatively drawn autologous heparinized blood was diluted and kept at a constant hematocrit of 25 %, resulting in a volume of 450 ml per experiment. The pH value was maintained at physiological values using bicarbonate titration. PO$_2$/PCO$_2$ were adjusted by changing the gas flow to the system (resulting in PO$_2$ of > 200 mm Hg and PCO$_2$ of 37–40 mm Hg). The perfusion system (Fig. 1) consisted of two separate precision pumps, one to control oxygenator circulation into a reservoir and one to control pulsatile kidney perfusion at a defined pressure of 100 mm Hg. White blood cell counts did not significantly decrease during oxygenator passage as controlled by washout experiments. Perfusate flow was recorded on-line using a digital interface. The ratio of flow:pressure was calculated as whole organ resistance (R).

The kidney was positioned in the system following arterial canulation and ureteral canulation. The first fraction of 70 ml venous outflow was separately collected as effluate (high potassium, EC solution), the experiment was then continued in a closed circulation. Changes in hematocrit were substituted with 0.9 % NaCl solution according to the amount of collected urine and according to the measured hematocrit. The experimental period was limited to 1 h.

At 0, 5, 15, 30, and 60 min blood samples were taken and at the end the kidney was removed for weight determination and prepared for histological examination.

For statistical purposes, Student's t-test or the Mann-Whitney test was used for the comparison of the numerical data of two independent groups.

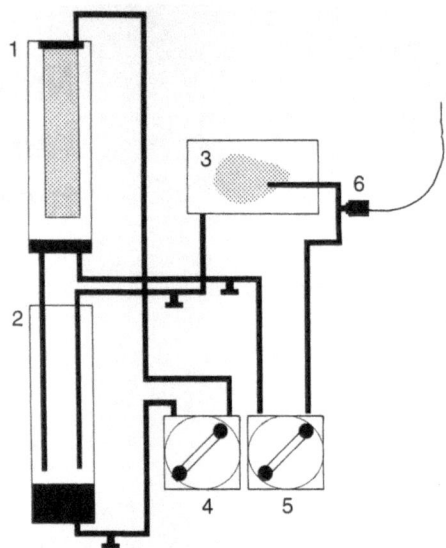

Fig. 1 Depiction of perfusion system. (*1* oxygenator, *2* reservoir, *3* perfusion chamber, *4* oxygenation pump, *5* perfusion pump, *6* pressure monitoring)

Results

Weight

Significant differences in weight increase were found only following short storage (9.5 ± 2.9 g P vs 23.4 ± 7.1 g C; $P < 0.01$). Long storage resulted in comparable weight increases (24.8 ± 6.1 g C vs 25.1 ± 4.2 g P; n.s.).

Urine flow

There were no statistical differences in urine flow or osmolarity with or without piretanide pretreatment. However, following SS, urine flow was about 50 % higher (3 ml/min) compared to LS (2 ml/min).

Creatinine clearance

Creatinine clearance was improved by P in both SS and LS, reaching statistical significance. Clearance of control organs in situ before surgical manipulation of the donor animal was 40 ml/min per 100 g.

Resistance

Piretanide lowered whole-organ resistance in both SS and LS (Fig. 2). After SS, P led to a decrease to 52 % of baseline value, whereas in C resistance values remained significantly higher after 20 min until the end of the experiments. Similar results were seen in the LS group,

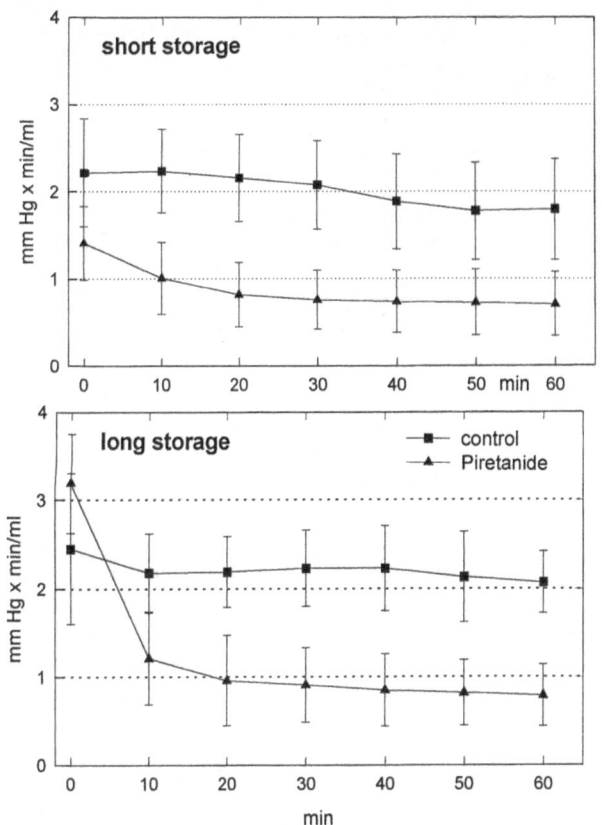

Fig. 2 Whole-organ resistance of kidneys, a recorded during perfusion. $P < 0.05$, Mann-Whitney test P vs C)

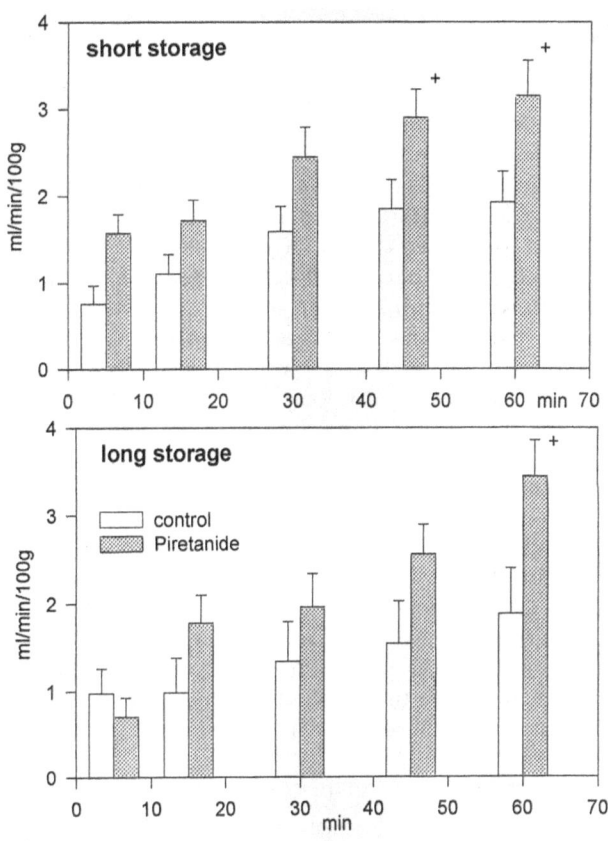

$^+$ p < 0.05 control vs. Piretanide (Whitney-Mann-Test)

Fig. 3 Oxygen consumption ($AVDO_2$) of reperfused kidneys

with the difference that P kidneys needed 10 min of low-flow perfusion before reaching physiological resistance values of $< 1.5 \, mm \, Hg \times min/ml$. When calculating flow:GFR (vascular resistance), the differences were more obvious, but due to large SD values did not reach significance.

Oxygen consumption

Oxygen consumption was quantified by the $AVDO_2$ measured in the arterial inflow line and in the venous outflow of the organ (Fig. 3). All kidneys of the treatment group exhibited a higher $AVDO_2$, reaching statistical significance in SS after 30 min of reperfusion and in LS after 45 min ($P < 0.05$, Mann-Whitney test).

Serum blood glucose levels

No glucose was added to the blood during the experimental closed circulation. P kidneys led to significantly lower glucose levels in both SS and LS at all time points, thus effectively reducing gluconeogenesis.

Cumulative electrolyte excretion

Special attention was paid to electrolyte excretion in the urine. Even though creatinine clearance was higher in P, the cumulative electrolyte loss was equal in P and C. Depending on the total urine flow, there were differences between SS and LS. All electrolytes showed a similar linear profile of excretion (potassium excretion was higher in LS compared to SS) thus P showed, despite an increased creatinine clearance, a relative sodium and potassium sparing effect.

Histology

In paraffin-embedded sections, differences were observed between the two groups which became more pronounced following LS. In the treatment group, medullary edema and tubular damage, such as epithelial disruption and cell debris in the tubular lumen, was reduced. Glomerula of untreated kidneys showed retraction of capillaries, loose cytoplasm, and flat epithelium with vacuolisation. These changes were not seen in the piretanide group.

Discussion

This study was undertaken to investigate kidney function following donor pretreatment with piretanide in a transplantation model. Autologous blood rather than allogeneic blood was used for reperfusion to exclude immunological, antibody-mediated reactions, e.g., isoagglutinin-associated blood group incompatibility. The pig is known to have 15 blood groups, with occasional isoagglutinins [5] that might interfere with mere reperfusion phenomena. Another advantage of ex vivo hemoperfusion, as developed by our group, is the possibility of pressure-controlled perfusion, which is not possible in other transplantation models. To judge kidney protection during ischemia, physiological parameters of reperfusion are accepted as being most adequate.

In our experiments, the plasma filtration of the reperfused kidneys was sufficient, as judged by the amount of urine produced. The observed creatinine clearance was lower than expected (1–5 ml/min), but no data exist for comparing how isolated porcine kidneys function in the first hour of hemoperfusion. However, our results are comparable with the results of Bretschneider obtained from canine kidneys after in situ ischemia with EC or HTK solution [6].

A positive effect of piretanide pretreatment could nevertheless be demonstrated, since in both groups (short and long storage) creatinine clearance was increased. Another very important parameter is the profile of renal hemodynamics, because kidney microvasculature is subject to autoregulation. The calculated whole-organ resistance reflects the quality of reperfusion; in our system pressure-controlled perfusion was used at 100 mm Hg mean arterial pressure, which resembles the physiological situation. Microcirculation of the renal cortex is difficult to monitor. Intravital microscopy can only visualize capsular capillaries which do not necessarily reflect the situation in vessels of the renal cortex [2]. A new possible way to assess cortical perfusion is the use of a laser doppler perfusion imaging system that allows continuous scanning of the organ surface [15].

In our study, whole-organ resistance was significantly reduced by piretanide in the reperfusion period, thus allowing a higher renal blood flow with higher glomerular filtration. This mechanism is probably due to altered arachidonic acid metabolism [9]. Postoperative vasoconstriction can also be reduced by direct cyclooxygenase inhibition, which leads to a decrease in thromboxane release in the venous effluate directly after declamping [16]. It can be speculated, that piretanide acts in a similar way.

Improved capacity to consume oxygen is a further important parameter reflecting early recovery after nephroplegia. During cold ischemia, anaerobic glucolysis maintains structural metabolism, and, at reperfusion,

the organ switches again to aerobic metabolism. Considering their relative weight in the organism, kidneys are the organs with the highest potential for gluconeogenesis [13]. In our experiments, there was an improved blood glucose regulation in piretanide-pretreated kidneys, in the sense of reduced hyperglycemia in the perfusate. In transplantation, this effect is difficult to observe, since released glucose is immediately metabolized by other organs (liver, muscle and brain). To our knowledge, not much attention has been paid to the phenomenon of glucose release by reperfused kidneys. The mechanism, by which piretanide influences glucose release, can only be speculated upon. A link to improved ATP content in the distal tubular cells and the reduced need for anaerobic glucolysis is a possible hypothesis that should be the object of further investigation.

All the observed parameters of kidney function suggest an advantage in using piretanide over no treatment. A direct comparison with furosemide was not done, because furosemide pretreatment does not seem to influence subsequent renal allograft function [7, 14]. Piretanide has a higher potential for diuresis and electrolyte excretion than furosemide [10], as has been shown in patients with renal insufficiency [11]. Another advantage is the reduced ototoxicity of piretanide [4]. In the clinical setting, the transplanted patient is treated with high doses of furosemide and dopamine in the postoperative phase. These measures were not used in our experimental study, but, in the already mentioned clinical pilot study, there was an effect of piretanide on the ARF rate [1].

For further investigation of the multiple effects of piretanide pretreatment for postischemic kidney function independent of the postoperative treatment, transplantation studies must be carried out, since in an ex vivo model it is not possible to imitate the ARF situation. Different dosages and combinations of pre- and postischemic treatment should also result in improved organ protection in humans.

References

1. Abendroth D, Pooth R, Schneeberger H, Land W (1993) Effects of piretanide on early graft function in kidney transplantation – a pilot study. Transplant Proc 25: 2626–2627

2. Booster M, Yin M, Kurvers HAJM, et al (1995) Inhibition of CD18-dependent leukocyte adherence by mAb 6.5 E does not prevent ischemia-reperfusion injury as seen in grafted kidneys. Transplant Int 8: 126–132

3. Clissold SP, Brogden RN (1985) Piretanide – a preliminary review of its pharmacodynamic and pharmacokinetic properties, and therapeutic efficacy. Drug 29: 489–530

4. Göttl KH, Roesch A, Klinke R (1985) Quantitative evaluation of ototoxic side effects of furosemide, piretanide, bumetanide, azosemide and ozolinone in the cat – a new approach to the problem of ototoxicity. Naunyn Schmiedeberg's Arch Pharmacol 331: 275–282

5. Hammer C (1994) Nature's obstacles to xenotransplantation. Transplant Rev 8: 174–184

6. Kallerhoff M, Blech M, Kehrer G, et al (1987) Kidney function parameters after ischemic stress under Euro-collins or under HTK protection according to Bretschneider. Urologe 26: 96–103

7. Kaplan MP, Toledo-Pereya LH, Pietroski R, et al (1986) Transplant Proc 18: 504–505

8. Kirsten R, Alexandridis T, Heintz B, et al (1987) Elsevier 365–368

9. Klaus E, Alpermann MG, Caspritz G, Linz W, Scholkens B (1983) Vascular effects of piretanide. Studies on extrarenal action in several animal models. Arzneim Forsch 33: 1273–1276

10. Lawrence JR, Ansari AF, Elliot HL, et al (1978) Kinetic and dynamic comparison of piretanide and furosemide. Clin Pharmacol Ther 23: 558–565

11. Marone C, Reubi FC, Lahn W (1984) Comparison of the short-term effects of the loop diuretic piretanide and furosemide in patients with renal insufficiency. Eur J Clin Pharmacol 26: 413–418

12. Rocher LL, Landers C, Dafoe DC, et al (1987) The importance of prolonged post-transplant dialysis requirement in cyclosporine-treated renal allograft recipients. Clin Transplant 1: 29–36

13. Ross BD, Espinal J, Silva P (1986) Glucose metabolism in renal tubular function. Kidney Int 29: 54–67

14. Schneeberger H, Schleibner S, Schilling M, et al (1990) Prevention of acute renal failure after kidney transplantation by treatment with rh-SOD: interim analysis of a double-blind placebo controlled trial. Trnasplant Proc 22: 2224–2225

15. Storck M, Sirsjö A, Abendroth D, Hammer C (1995) Laser perfusion imaging (LPI) – a new method of monitoring microcirculation in postischemic organ reperfusion. (submitted)

16. Storck M, Schilling M, Steinbach G, Abendroth D Influence of systemic cyclooxygenase inhibition with single dose aspisol (ASA) on kinetics of arachidonic acid metabolism in the venous effluate of transplanted kidney grafts in humans. Transplant Proc (in press)

Transpl Int (1996) 9 [Suppl 1]: S 442–S 446
© Springer-Verlag 1996

J. H. Fischer
S. Jeschkeit

Minimal amounts of hyaluronidase in HTK or UW solution substantially improve the recovery of preserved hearts

J. H. Fischer (✉) · S. Jeschkeit
Institut für Experimentelle Medizin der
Universität zu Köln,
Robert-Koch-Strasse 10, D-50931 Köln,
Germany

Abstract Rat hearts were preserved by simple storage for 18 h at 0–1 °C and reperfused parabiotically with whole blood from a host rat. The preservation solutions used for flush perfusion and storage were the commercial solutions EuroCollins, HTK, or UW with or without adding 40 mg/l hyaluronidase or Euro-Flush-Glutathione (EFG) solution, especially designed for prolonged heart storage. All solutions were filtered (0.45 µm) before use. The functional recovery was measured using a latex balloon in the left ventricle for LVP, dp/dt, and isotonic stroke volume. The metabolic recovery as well as the edema formation was determined from freeze-clamped myocardium at the end of reperfusion. In hearts preserved with hyaluronidase-containing solutions, the edema formation during reperfusion was reduced combined with an improvement in the coronary flow. Functional and metabolic recovery were improved in these hearts with significant increase in the stroke volume and ECP in all groups versus hearts preserved in the hyaluronidase-free basic solutions. The effectiveness of HTK preservation was significantly improved by hyaluronidase in all parameters measured in our study. The best functional and metabolic recovery was found in hearts preserved by HTK + H- or EFG-solution. Thus, preservation solutions containing hyaluronidase, especially HTK + H and EFG, seem best suited for the prolonged storage preservation of the heart.

Key words Heart preservation · Hyaluronidase · Hypothermic storage · Parabiotic perfusion · Transplant recovery

Introduction

EuroCollins, Bretschneider's HTK, or the University of Wisconsin organ preservation (UW) solution have been used clinically for up to 4 h storage preservation of hearts [1]. Successful prolonged storage (from 4.2 h [2] to 8 h [3]) has been reported only in a few isolated single cases. The problems resulting from prolonged heart storage are mainly contracture and reduced coronary flow which inhibit sufficient recovery of cardiac function in a reasonable time to guarantee the survival of the recipient. Many attempts have been made in animal experiments to improve the outcome of prolonged-stored hearts including continuous perfusion systems [4], modifications of the storage solution [5], "refreshment" of ageing commercial solutions [6], or development of new preservation solutions [7]. The newly developed solutions "EuroFlush" (EF) [7] or "Euro-Flush-Glutathione" (EFG) [6] contain a component, hyaluronidase, which is well known for preventing ischemically induced increase in vascular resistance [8], but has never been used in preservation solutions before.

Hyaluronidase acts by specifically reducing the hyaluronate content of tissues, which is the principal glycosaminoglycan of the interstitium, has a high water-binding capacity and exerts a strong osmotic force [9]. Application of hyaluronidase decreases the interstitial volume of edematous tissues and prevents ischemically induced increase in vascular resistance, but does not change the microvascular permeability. It, thus, reduces edema formation and improves the reflow in ischemically damaged organs. Applied intravenously for the treatment of acute myocardial infarction, the cardioprotective effect of hyaluronidase could be shown in many clinical and experimental studies [10–15], demonstrating reduction of edema and vascular resistance or better maintenance of myocardial lymph flow. Hyaluronidase was shown to improve the poststorage reflow in hearts preserved for 24 h at 0–1 °C in our previous asanguinous electrolyte reperfusions. Hearts preserved in EC or EF solution with hyaluronidase [7], also resulted in a higher functional recovery than HTK- or UW-preserved hearts. Experiments with parabiotic reperfusions comfirmed this excellent effect in 18-h-preserved hearts using EFG solution, but the effectiveness of combining hyaluronidase with the commercial solutions was not evaluated in these investigations.

Here we present results from rat hearts stored for 18 h in commercial solutions, the same solutions with hyaluronidase added or EFG solution, developed for prolonged heart preservation and which also contains hyaluronidase. The organs were reperfused with whole blood in a parabiotic system – a technique, which combines the reperfusional effects of a transplantation with the possibility of continuous functional testing.

Table 1 Components (mmol/l) of preservation solutions used in this study

	EC	EFG	HTK	UW
Na^+	10	15	15	30
K^+	115	90	10	125
Ca^{++}	–	0.05	–	–
Mg^{++}	–	35	4	5
Cl^-	15	0.1	50	–
HCO_3^-	10	15	–	–
SO_4^-	–	80	–	5
Phosphate	57.5	–	–	25
Glutarate	–	–	1	–
Histidine	–	–	198	–
Lactobionate	–	–	–	100
Tryptophane	–	–	2	–
Glucose	194.3	–	–	–
Mannitol	–	–	30	–
Sucrose	–	100	–	–
Raffinose	–	–	–	30
Adenosine	–	–	–	5
Allopuriol	–	0.5	–	1
Glutathione	–	–	–	3
Hepes	–	1	–	–
Pentastarch	–	–	–	50 g/l
Fresh additives before use:				
Dexamethasone	–	–	–	16 mg/l
Glutathione red.	–	3 mmol/l	–	–
Hyaluronidase	–	40 mg/l	–	–
Insulin	–	–	–	40 U/l
Penicillin	–	–	–	2×10^5 U/l
Verapamil	–	2 mg/l	–	–

Materials and methods

All animals were housed, fed, and handled in compliance with German legislation on protection of animals and the "Guide for the Care and Use of Laboratory Animals" published by the NIH (Publication number 86–23, 1985).

Hearts of male inbred Lewis rats (220–260 g body weight) were grafted under ether anesthesia. Pressure-controlled flush perfusion with cold (0–1 °C) preservation solution started in situ via an aortic catheter without ischemic damage to the heart. It was performed at 75 mm Hg for 5 min in all groups except the HTK groups, where it lasted for 10 min with reduction of the perfusion pressure to 50 mm Hg after 1 min with respect to the special HTK application rules [16].

The preservation solutions were as follows ($n = 6$ in all groups):
A. Three commercially available original solutions, EuroCollins solution (EC, Fresenius AG, Bad Homburg, Germany), HTK solution (Custodiol, Dr. F. Köhler Chemie, Alsbach-Hähnlein, Germany), or UW solution (ViaSpan, Du Pont Pharma, manufactured by NPBI, The Netherlands)
B. Hyaluronidase-containing solutions, i. e., the original solutions with hyaluronidase (40 mg/l) added (EC + H, HTK + H, UW + H) or EuroFlush-Glutathione solution (EFG) prepared in our laboratory (Table 1)
All perfusates were filtered (0.45 µm) before use. This pore size guaranteed the extraction of all damaging particles without having any influence on the crystalloid or colloidal components of the solutions.

After flushing, the organs were stored for 18 h in 5 ml of the respective preservation solution at 0–1 °C in small, safely sealed vessels. The vessels were continuously gassed with purest nitrogen (purity > 99.9993 vol%), to guarentee real ischemia of the organs during the storage period without oxygenation from the surface. Control hearts were arrested by surface cooling and immediately reperfused similar to the preserved hearts.

Reperfusion started after a 5 min warm reflush (37 °C) using oxygenated modified Krebs-Henseleit solution (only 50 µmol/l calcium, but containing 15 µmol/l adenosine and 1 mmol/l uric acid) at a pressure of 50 mm Hg (non-recirculating Langendorff mode). The reperfusion was performed for 30 min parabiotically using whole blood from the carotid artery of an anesthetized host rat (pentobarbital anesthesia) of the same inbred Lewis strain with the graft maintained at 37 °C in a water-jacketed constant temperature chamber. The blood retured from the pulmonary artery into the jugular vein of the host. Adenosine was infused up to the 20th min of reperfusion in declining concentrations, resulting in an initial blood pressure of about 50 mm Hg, similar to the warm reflush, with continuous increase to normal values (> 80 mm Hg) within a few minutes.

The coronary effluent was determined by timed collection. Functional recovery was measured with the aid of a latex balloon in the left ventricle and continuously recorded on a thermo-oscillographic recorder. Isometric left ventricular pressure amplitude (LVP) at end-diastolic pressures of 10 mm Hg with or without pacing to a heart rate of 300/min, dp/dt, and serial measurements of isotonic stroke volume were recorded.

At the end of reperfusion the hearts were immediately frozen in liquid nitrogen using the freeze-stop technique. The energy metabolism was determined in the lyophilized myocardium using enzymatic [17] and HPLC techniques [18].

Table 2 Myocardial water content (ml/g dry weight) at the end of storage or after 18 h storage and 30 min parabiotic reperfusion, determined from freeze-clamped rat heart ventricles. Mean ± SD, $n = 6$ per group, C: hearts in situ or after control reperfusion without storage

	After storage	After reperfusion
Control	3.42 ± 0.08	4.04 ± 0.23
EC	3.97 ± 0.16	4.36 ± 0.49
EC + H		3.80 ± 0.28
HTK	3.48 ± 0.04	4.61 ± 0.47
HTK + H		4.44 ± 0.10
UW	3.15 ± 0.13	5.14 ± 0.88
UW + H		4.07 ± 0.27
EFG	3.68 ± 0.08	4.15 ± 0.42

Table 3 Coronary flow (ml/min) during initial 5 min warm reflush (mean of 2–5 min) or at the end of 30 min parabiotic reperfusion after 18 h storage preservation. Mean ± SD, $n = 6$ per group

	2–5 min KH	30 min blood
Control	11.7 ± 1.4	6.1 ± 0.8
EC	3.6 ± 0.6*	1.4 ± 0.5
EC + H	5.4 ± 0.5*	1.6 ± 0.3
HTK	4.4 ± 0.8*	1.8 ± 1.2
HTK + H	7.3 ± 1.0*	2.6 ± 0.7
UW	4.2 ± 0.3*	1.3 ± 0.3
UW + H	5.5 ± 1.4*	2.2 ± 1.1
EFG	7.0 ± 0.5	2.3 ± 0.7

* $P < 0.05$

Energy charge potential (ECP) was calculated according to Atkinson [19] from the formula $ECP = (ATP + \frac{1}{2} ADP)/(ATP + ADP + AMP)$.

Mean values and standard deviations of the parameters are given in Fig. 3. The Mann-Whitney test was used for the comparison of two groups and differences were considered significant when $P < 0.05$. For multiple comparison, adjustment of the Mann-Whitney test was by the Bonferroni method.

Results

After 18 h preservation of rat hearts in one of the commercially available solutions, EC, HTK, or UW solution, parabiotic whole blood reperfusion resulted in edema formation and impaired recovery. The amount of fluid accumulation during reperfusion as well as the total water content at the end of reperfusion was highest in the group with the lowest poststorage edema (UW).

In combination with each of these solutions, hyaluronidase improved the recovery of the hearts. In the hyaluronidase-containing solutions the reperfusion edema was reduced, reaching the level of the control group after EC + H, UW + H, and EFG preservation (Table 2). The coronary flow was already significantly increased during the warm reflush (Table 3), resulting in an increase of several functional and metabolic parameters

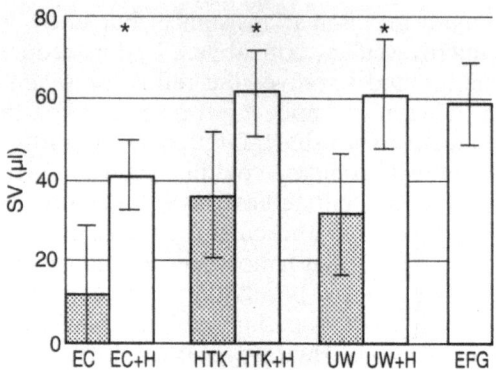

Fig. 1 Left ventricular isotonic stroke volume *(SV)* of 18-h-preserved rat hearts, ejected from the intraventricular balloon. Highest values after 20–30 min of parabiotic reperfusion. Mean ± SD, $n = 6$ per group. (* $P < 0.05$ versus basic solution without hyaluronidase)

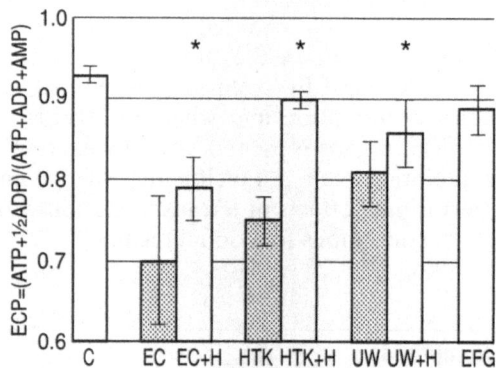

Fig. 2 Energy charge potential after 30 min of parabiotic reperfusion of 18-h-preserved rat hearts. Mean ± SD, $n = 6$ per group. (*C* control reperfusion, * $P < 0.05$ versus basic solution without hyaluronidase)

during further reperfusion compared to hearts preserved in solutions without hyaluronidase. The ventricular isotonic stroke volume increased significantly in all groups (Fig. 1), as well as the myocardial energy charge potential at the end of reperfusion (Fig. 2). For most other functional and metabolic parameters of the hearts, hyaluronidase content of the storage solution resulted in a more or less pronounced improvement. This improvement was always significant in HTK + H- versus HTK-preserved hearts, but for EC + H- or UW + H-preserved hearts it did not reach the level of significance versus the basic solution in all of the remaining parameters (see Fig. 3, Tables 4, 5).

Optimal recovery – substantially higher than after storage in any of the commercial solutions – was reached with the preservation solutions HTK + H and EFG and, in some parameters (stroke volume, ATP content, and total adenine nucleotide content), for UW + H also. The recovery after storage in the commer-

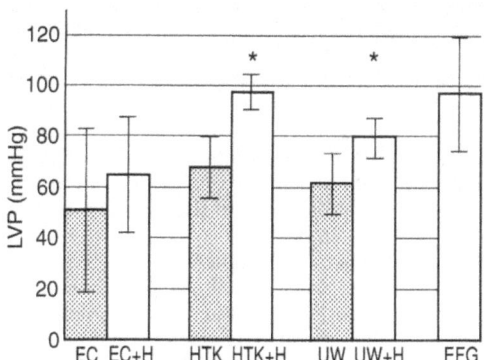

Fig. 3 Left ventricular pressure amplitudes (LVP) (isovolumetric) of 18-h-preserved rat hearts at the end of parabiotic reperfusion. Spontaneously beating hearts at heart rates between 74 and 135/min, except HTK (176/min) and HTK + H (226/min). Mean ± SD, $n = 6$ per group. (* $P < 0.05$ versus basic solution without hyaluronidase)

cial solutions EC, HTK, or UW without hyaluronidase was insufficient. Damage by the particles, which have been shown to be typical for UW solution [6], could be prevented by the filtering procedure used in our experiments for all solutions and, thus, did not influence these results. Under these conditions the effectiveness of the commercial solutions was for functional parameters UW = HTK > EC, for metabolic parameters UW > HTK > EC, while the use of unfiltered UW solution did not allow recovery of 18 h preserved rat hearts.

Discussion

Eighteen hour storage preservation using commercial EC, HTK, or UW solution, did not allow acceptable recovery of rat hearts in our experiments. However, the addition of 40 mg/l hyaluronidase to these solutions enhanced the functional recovery in rat hearts with increase in the energy charge potential, obviously caused by reduced fluid accumulation and hereby improved coronary flow. Thus, the effectiveness of HTK solution could be significantly improved by the addition of hyaluronidase. Hearts preserved in HTK + H solution had an optimal recovery during parabiotic reperfusion similar to those stored in EFG. EC + H-preserved hearts did not reach a comparable level and UW + H-

Table 4 ATP, total adenine nucleotide (TAN = ATP + ADP + AMP) or creatine phosphate (CP) content of ventricular myocardium (µmol/g dry weight) after 18 h storage and 30 min parabiotic reperfusion. Mean ± SD, $n = 6$ per group.

	ATP	TAN	CP
Control	21.9 ± 1.1	25.1 ± 1.5	39.4 ± 3.4
EC	4.7 ± 1.6*	8.0 ± 1.7*	4.2 ± 2.3
EC + H	6.9 ± 1.6*	10.1 ± 1.9*	6.5 ± 2.1
HTK	6.2 ± 1.0*	10.2 ± 1.5*	5.4 ± 1.3*
HTK + H	12.5 ± 1.1*	15.2 ± 1.1*	20.3 ± 3.6*
UW	9.2 ± 3.0	13.1 ± 3.1	10.9 ± 6.5
UW + H	11.9 ± 2.6	15.2 ± 2.8	15.2 ± 4.5
EFG	11.7 ± 2.7	14.2 ± 2.6	19.4 ± 6.9

* $P < 0.05$ for difference between basic solutions and modification with hyaluronidase

Table 5 Left ventricular pressure amplitude, contractility (+ dp/dt_{max}) and relaxation velocity (– dp/dt_{max}) at a paced heart rate of 300/min after 25–30 min parabiotic reperfusion. Mean ± SD, $n = 6$ per group.

At 5 Hz pacing	LVP	+ dp/dt_{max}	– dp/dt_{max}
Control	139 ± 39	3293 ± 976	2187 ± 658
EC	24 ± 30	527 ± 668	393 ± 506
EC + H	41 ± 18	920 ± 419	670 ± 275
HTK	58 ± 15*	1355 ± 310*	980 ± 231*
HTK + H	97 ± 13*	2153 ± 297*	1600 ± 209*
UW	56 ± 15	1253 ± 339	900 ± 222
UW + H	72 ± 19	1607 ± 454	1163 ± 299
EFG	87 ± 22	1999 ± 492	1398 ± 382

* $P < 0.05$ for difference between basic solutions and modification with hyaluronidase

hearts reached an optimal recovery only in a few parameters. Here, especially for UW and UW + H solution, a better improvement seems to be hindered by the oxidation of GSH in commercial UW solution (as shown in our previous study [6]).

Thus, for prolonged 18 h heart storage preservation, the commercial solutions EC, HTK, or UW should not be used without the addition of hyaluronidase and, in the case of UW solution, in combination with filtration and refreshing procedures.

Acknowledgements We gratefully acknowledge the technical assistance of Corinna July. The experiments were supported by a grant from the Maria Pesch Stiftung, Universität zu Köln.

References

1. Reichenspurner H, Russ C, Überfuhr P, Nollert G, Schlüter A, Reichart B et al (1993) Myocardial preservation using HTK-solution for heart transplantation – a multicenter study. Eur J Cardiothorac Surg 7: 414–419

2. Jeevanandam V, Auteri JS, Sanchez JA, Barr ML, Ott GY, Hsu D, Marboe C, Smith CR, Rose EA (1991) Improved Heart Preservation with University of Wisconsin Solution – Experimental and Preliminary Human Experience. Circulation 84: 324–328.

3. Drinkwater DC, Stein DG, Permut LC, Laks H (1991) Clinical Trial of University of Wisconsin Solution for Cardiac Transplantation – Preliminary Results. J Thorac Cardiovasc Surg 102: 798–799

4. Mendler N, Struck E, Sebening F (1984) Orthopic canine heart transplantation after 24 hours cold perfusion. Transplant Proc 16 (Suppl 1): 173–176

5. Konertz WF, Saka B, Bernhard A (1988) Eurocollins solution for heart preservation: Experimental and clinical experience. Transplant Proc 20 (Suppl 1): 984–986

6. Fischer JH, Jeschkeit S (1995) Effectivity of freshly prepared or refreshed solutions for heart preservation versus commercial EuroCollins, Bretschneider's HTK, or University of Wisconsin solution. Transplantation 59: 1259–1262

7. Fischer JH, Jeschkeit S, Klein P (1994) Adding a new principle to hypothermic storage preservation – Reduction of edema formation by hyaluronidase. Transplantation 58: 748–753

8. Sunnergren KP, Rovetto MJ (1985) The effects of hyaluronidase on interstitial hydration, plasma protein exclusion, and microvascular permeability in the isolated perfused rat heart. Microvasc Res 30: 286–297

9. Ogston AG (1970) The biologic functions of the glycosaminoglycans. In: Balazs EA (ed) Chemistry and molecular biology of the intercellular matrix. Academic Press, New York, pp 1231–1240

10. Maroko PR, Libby P, Bloor CM, Sobel BE, Braunwald E (1972) Reduction by hyaluronidase of myocardial necrosis following coronary artery occlusion. Circulation 46: 430–437

11. Kloner RA, Braunwald E, Maroko PR (1978) Long-term preservation of ischemic myocardium in the dog by hyaluronidase. Circulation 58: 220–226

12. Flint EJ, De Giovanni J, Cadigan PJ, Lamb P, Pentecost B (1982) Effect of GL enzyme (a highly purified form of hyaluronidase) on mortality after myocardial infarction. Lancet 1: 871–874

13. Saltissi S, Robinson PS, Coltart DJ, Webb Peploe MM, Croft DN (1982) Effects of early administration of a highly purified hyaluronidase preparation (GL enzyme) on myocardial infarct size. Lancet 1: 867–871

14. Roberts R, Braunwald E, Muller JE, Croft C, Gold HK, Hartwell TD, et al (1988) Effect of hyaluronidase on mortality and morbidity in patients with early peaking of plasma creatine kinase MB and nontransmural ischaemia. Multicentre investigation for the limitation of infarct size (MILIS). Br Heart J 60: 290–298

15. Taira A, Uehara K, Fukuda S, Takenada K, Koga M (1990) Active drainage of cardiac lymph in relation to reduction in size of myocardial infarction: an experimental study. Angiology 41: 1029–1036

16. Preusse CJ (1991) Cardioplegia in neonatal heart. J Thorac Cardiovasc Surg 101: 170–171

17. Bergmeyer HU (1985) (ed) Methods of enzymatic analysis. Weinheim, Verlag Chemie

18. Fischer JH (1995) Specific detection of nucleotides, creatine phosphate and their derivatives from tissue samples in a simple, isocratic, recycling, low-volume system. LC-GC International 8: 254–264

19. Atkinson DE (1968) The energy charge of the adenylate pool as a regulatory parameter. Interaction with feedback modifiers. Biochemistry 7: 4030–4034

Transpl Int (1996) 9 [Suppl 1]: S447–S451
© Springer-Verlag 1996

Hideki Ohdan
Yasuhiko Fukuda
Takashi Urushihara
Ryo Sumimoto
Toshimasa Asahara
Hisao Ito
Kiyohiko Dohi

Synergistic effects of nafamostat mesilate rinse and Kupffer cell blockade for rat liver preservation

H. Ohdan (✉) · Y. Fukuda · T. Urushihara ·
R. Sumimoto · T. Asahara · K. Dohi
Second Department of Surgery,
Hiroshima University, School of Medicine,
1-2-3 Kasumi, Minami-ku, Hiroshima 734,
Japan
Tel. +81 822 57 52 22; Fax +81 822 57 52 24

H. Ito
First Department of Pathology,
Tottori University, School of Medicine,
86 Nishi-machi, Yonago 683, Japan

Abstract We investigated the efficacy of a new rinse solution containing nafamostat mesilate (NM) (a serine protease inhibitor) for liver preservation with modulation of Kupffer cell function. Orthotopic liver transplantation (OLT) was performed in male Lewis rats after 24 h of cold storage in University of Wisconsin organ preservation solution. After OLT, survival was determined, together with assays of blood chemistry, tissue NM metabolites, and histology 3 h after OLT. NM rinse was found to have a cytoprotective effect on liver parenchymal cells, based on enzyme data showing that NM rinse reduced the release of serum alanine aminotransferase significantly in comparison with saline rinse ($P < 0.05$). However, the effect was not sufficient to improve the survival rate. In contrast, when the donor was treated with gadolinium chloride 24–30 h before graft harvest, NM rinse improved the survival rate to around 80 % compared with 25 % for saline. The assay of NM metabolites in grafted liver tissue showed that pretreatment of the donor rats with $GdCl_3$ delayed the degeneration of NM in the liver tissue. These data demonstrate that NM rinse and Kupffer cell blockade exert synergistic effects, leading to increased survival after cold-preserved liver transplantation.

Key words Liver transplantation · Nafamostat mesilate · Preservation · Kupffer cell · Gadolinium chloride

Introduction

Nafamostat mesilate (NM; 6-amidino-2-naphthyl p-guanidinobenzoate dimethanesulfonate), is a synthetic serine protease inhibitor used for the treatment of pancreatitis and disseminated intravascular coagulation. Its main actions are: 1) the suppression of proteases such as thrombin, activated coagulation factors (XII a, X a), plasmin, complements (Clr̄, Cls̄), trypsin, and phospholipase A_2, 2) the inhibition of platelet aggregation, and 3) the stabilization of lysosomal and cellular membranes [1, 3, 4, 17]. We have recently demonstrated that a cocktail of NM added to a prereperfusion rinse solution (NM rinse) can improve graft survival dramatically after transplantation of a long-term-preserved pancreas in the rat [16]. This new strategy is also expected to be po-

tentially useful for attenuating reperfusion injury in cold-preserved liver transplantation, because several reports have shown that proteases are involved in the development of liver ischemia-reperfusion injury [2, 8, 9, 12, 15]. Considering NM can be easily hydrolyzed, however, it is anticipated that hydrolases from activated Kupffer cells would facilitate the degradation of NM in the graft tissue if an NM rinse were used in cold-preserved liver transplantation. Therefore, in the present study, we investigated the efficacy of an NM rinse solution for extended liver preservation together with modulation of Kupffer cell function.

Table 1 Composition of UW solution and NM rinse. Values in mmol/l, unless otherwise stated

	UW	NM rinse
Potassium lactobionate	100	
Sodium lactobionate		110
NaKH$_2$PO$_4$	25	
NaH$_2$PO$_4$		25
Raffinose	30	30
MgSO$_4$	5	
Glutathione	3	3
Adenosine	5	
Allopurinol	1	1
Insulin (IU/l)	100	
Hydroxyethyl starch (g%)	5	
Nafamostat mesilate		0.8
β-Cyclodextrin		3
γ-Cyclodextrin		10
Osmolarity	320–330	273
pH	7.4	7.4

Materials and methods

Composition of the NM rinse

The composition of the University of Wisconsin organ preservation (UW) solution used for preservation and that of the NM rinse solution are listed in Table 1. The NM rinse is potassium-free to avoid potassium loading after reperfusion, and contains cyclodextrin as a solubilizer of NM. Immediately before use, NM (Torii Pharmaceutical Company, Tokyo, Japan) was added.

Liver transplantation

Syngeneic orthotopic liver transplantation (OLT) without rearterialization was performed in male Lewis rats weighing 180–280 g (Japan Charles River Laboratory, Osaka, Japan) as described previously [7]. Donor livers were flushed in situ through the portal vein with 10 ml of UW solution at 4°C. Grafts were preserved for 24 h in UW solution at 4°C. Immediately before implantation, grafts were rinsed with 12–15 ml of test solution at 4°C via the portal vein under a pressure of 10–15 cmH$_2$O. After revascularization of the graft, each recipient was given 1 ml of lactate Ringer's solution through the penile vein and 100 mg/kg cefazolin sodium was administered intramuscularly. Implantation surgery required less than 50 min, during which time the portal vein was clamped for 11–15 min.

Experimental groups

Experimental animals were divided into four groups, which differed according to the presence or absence of donor pretreatment with Kupffer cell blockade and the type of rinse solution used. In groups 1 ($n = 9$) and 2 ($n = 8$), donor animals received no pretransplant treatment. In donor animals of groups 3 ($n = 8$) and 4 ($n = 9$), gadolinium chloride (GdCl$_3$) (GdCl$_3$.6H$_2$O, Nacalai Tesque, Kyoto, Japan) was administered intravenously, at a dose rate of 10 mg/kg body weight 24–30 h before harvest, to destroy the Kupffer cells [13]. Immediately before implantation, the preservation solution was flushed out with the test rinse solution. Saline was used for this purpose in groups 1 and 3, whereas NM rinse was used in

groups 2 and 4. One-week survival rates were compared and an autopsy was performed on all recipient animals that died before 7 days to determine the cause of death. Five additional recipients in each group were sacrificed 3 h after liver graft reperfusion for the determination of blood chemistry, measurement of tissue NM metabolite concentration in the liver, and histology.

Blood chemistry

Blood samples were collected via the inferior vena cava 3 h after reperfusion. Serum levels of alanine aminotransferase (ALT) were measured using the standard enzymatic procedure to evaluate the degree of liver parenchymal cell damage. Serum levels of hyaluronic acid (HA) were measured with the aid of a radiometric kit (FML Laboratories, Hiroshima, Japan) to evaluate the degree of liver endothelial cell damage [14].

Determination of tissue NM metabolite concentrations

The tissue concentrations of intact NM and its hydrolysis product, 6-amidino-2-naphthol (AN), were measured in grafted livers by fluorometric detection as described previously [11].

Histology

Histological specimens of rat livers were stored in 10% formalin and embedded subsequently in paraffin, followed by sectioning and staining with hematoxylin and eosin.

Statistics

Statistical evaluation was made by the unpaired t-test. Differences were considered significant at a P value of less than 0.05.

Results

Survival

Survival curves following transplantation surgery are shown in Fig. 1. One-week survival rates in groups 1, 2, 3, and 4 were 22.2% (2/9), 25.0% (2/8), 25.0% (2/8) and 77.7% (7/9), respectively. Survival rate was not improved when the NM rinse and the pretreatment of donor rats with GdCl$_3$ were employed separately. However, a combination of the two strategies improved the 1-week survival rate.

Blood chemistry

The results of the blood chemical assays are shown in Table 2. The elevation of serum ALT was significantly suppressed in group 2 compared with group 1 ($P < 0.05$), and was more suppressed in group 4. The elevation of serum HA was significantly suppressed in groups 3 and 4 compared with group 1 ($P < 0.05$) (Table 2).

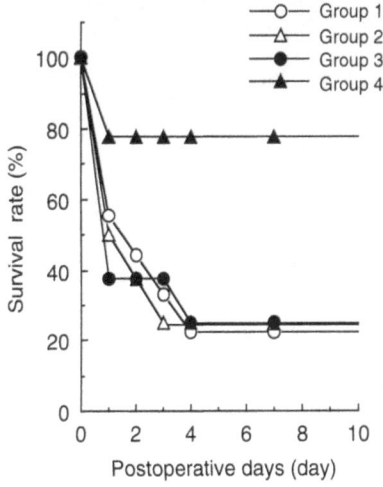

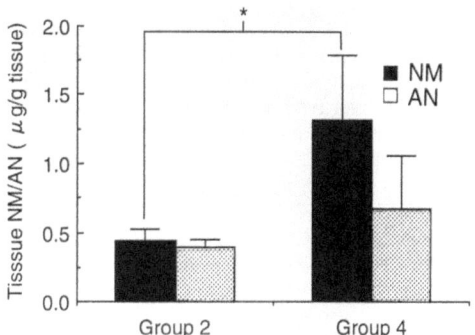

Fig. 1 Postoperative survival rate. Data expressed as percentages (n = 8–9/group)

Fig. 2 NM metabolite concentrations in graft liver tissues 3 h after OLT. The tissue concentrations of intact nafamostat mesilate *(NM)* and its hydrolyzed product, amidino-naphthol *(AN)*, were measured in liver tissues. Data expressed as mean ± SEM (n = 3–5/group, $^*P < 0.05$)

Table 2 Serum levels of alanine aminotransferase (ALT) and hyaluronic acid (HA) 3 h after OLT in each group. Data expressed as mean ± SE

Group	n	ALT (IU/l)	HA (ng/ml)
1. (Saline rinse)	5	3134 ± 1037	936 ± 272
2. (NM rinse)	5	1069 ± 225*	634 ± 383
3. (GdCl$_3$ + saline rinse)	5	1645 ± 304	303 ± 36*
4. (GdCl$_3$ + NM rinse)	5	814 ± 251*·**	196 ± 52*

$^* P < 0.05$ vs group 1; $^{**} P < 0.05$ vs group 3

Liver tissue NM metabolite concentrations

After 3 h of reperfusion, the concentration of intact NM in the liver tissue was significantly higher in group 4 than in group 2 ($P < 0.05$). Tissue AN concentration in the liver did not differ significantly between groups 2 and 4 (Fig. 2).

Histology

After 3 h of reperfusion in groups 1, 2, and 3, severe congestion and extensive vacuolization of hepatocytes were observed. Hyaline inclusion bodies were frequently recognized in the hepatocytes of the congested areas. In contrast, in group 4, mild injury consisting only of some centrilobular vacuolation was observed, but hyaline inclusion bodies were not evident (Table 3).

Discussion

It has been suggested that ischemia-reperfusion injury to the liver is mediated, at least in part, by graft proteases released immediately after graft revascularization [2, 8, 9, 12, 15]. Proteases appear to be involved in the development of liver ischemia-reperfusion injury and some protease inhibitors have been shown to be cytoprotective in various models of liver transplantation. Aprotinin has been reported to have significant impact on survival when administered continuously to the recipient animal for 6 h following revascularization in a pig OLT model [12], and when given to the donor and added to the preservation solution in a rat OLT model [9, 15]. It has been recently indicated that rat liver ischemia-reperfusion injury is attenuated by pretreatment with urinary trypsin inhibitor, which suppresses neutrophil elastase and cathepsin G, and stabilizes lysosomal and cellular membranes [8]. Thus, protease inhibitors have a beneficial effect on liver preservation by protecting against ischemia-reperfusion injury.

NM is a synthetic serine protease inhibitor, whose main actions include the suppression of various proteases, the inhibition of platelet aggregation, and the stabilization of lysosomal and cellular membranes, these actions being more potent than those of other protease inhibitors such as aprotinin and gabexate mesilate [1, 3, 4, 17]. Recently, we have devised a new strategy that involves the use of a cocktail of NM added to a prereperfusion rinse solution, for extended organ preservation. This strategy seems reasonable because it can deliver a high concentration of the cytoprotective agent to graft tissues during reperfusion; otherwise the agent may be degraded during prolonged storage and may be removed from grafts by prereperfusion rinsing when the agent is added to the preservation solution. In our recent study, NM rinse has been shown to dramatically improve the graft survival rate of rat pancreas, cold-preserved for 48 or 72 h in UW solution [16].

In the present study, NM rinse exerted some beneficial effects on 24 h rat liver preservation, although it did not prolong the survival of liver-transplanted recipients. It obviously reduced the release of ALT from hep-

Table 3 Number of intracytoplasmic hyaline bodies per field in histological specimens of 24 h cold-preserved livers. The number of intracytoplasmic hyaline bodies was determined in a randomly selected field of liver from rats killed 3 h after OLT. The number per field ($\times 200$) was classified as follows: – no hyaline bodies, + $1 \leq$ hyaline bodies < 3, ++ $3 \leq$ hyaline bodies < 6, +++ $6 \leq$ hyaline bodies

Group	Number of hyaline bodies
1. (Saline rinse)	+, +, +, ++, ++
2. (NM rinse)	+, +, ++, +++, +++
3. (GdCl$_3$ + saline rinse)	–, +, ++, ++, +++
4. (GdCl$_3$ + NM rinse)	–, –, –, –, –

Fig. 3 Structural formula of nafamostat mesilate *(NM)* and its hydrolysis products, 6-amidino-2-naphthol *(AN)* and *p*-guanidino benzoic acid *(PGBA)*

atocytes into the serum after 3 h of reperfusion. In contrast, the elevation of serum HA after 3 h of reperfusion was not substantially suppressed by the use of NM rinse. These findings indicate that NM rinse acts on liver parenchymal cells rather than on endothelial cells.

The liver has resident macrophages, Kupffer cells, that are known to be the predominant source of reactive oxygen formed during the initial reperfusion period. Kupffer cell activity, including reactive oxygen formation, contributes to reperfusion injury in the liver. Previous reports have documented that inactivation of Kupffer cells by blockade with agents such as GdCl$_3$ and methyl palmitate protects the liver against ischemia-reperfusion injury [5, 10]. In the present study, pretreatment of donor rats with GdCl$_3$ prevented endothelial cell damage during reperfusion, as shown by assay of serum HA, although it did not prolong the survival of recipients that received transplants of 24 h cold-preserved liver.

It has been suggested that Kupffer cells, activated by transplantation, release mediators that stimulate the mitochondria of parenchymal cells and enhance drug metabolism by increasing the supply of cofactors [13]. Considering that NM can be easily hydrolyzed by certain cofactors [11], this hypothesis is of particular interest, since the increase of hydrolase supplied by activated

Kupffer cells might facilitate the degradation of NM in grafted liver tissue (Fig. 3). In the assay of liver tissue NM metabolites, we observed that pretreatment of donor rats with GdCl$_3$ delayed the degradation of NM in the grafted liver tissue and maintained an effective concentration of intact NM after 3 h of reperfusion. Furthermore, combined treatment with NM rinse and pretreatment with GdCl$_3$ produced a marked improvement in the survival rate of rats that received transplants of 24 h cold-preserved livers. This finding is in good agreement with the histological data that showed obvious prevention of hyaline inclusion body formation due to an increase in membrane permeability caused by hypoxia and excessive inhibition of serum protein [6]. These results are the first documented evidence of a synergistic effect of protease inhibitor and Kupffer cell blockade in preventing ischemia-reperfusion injury in cold-preserved liver transplantation.

Acknowledgements The authors gratefully thank Torii Pharmaceutical Co. (Tokyo, Japan) for their support in this work, and M. Iwata (Research Laboratories, Torii and Co., Chiba, Japan) for technical assistance with assays for tissue NM metabolites.

References

1. Aoyama T, Ino Y, Ozeki M, Oda M, Sato T, Koshiyama Y, Suzuki S, Fujita M (1984) Pharmacological studies of FUT-175, nafamostat mesilate. I. Inhibition of protease activity in in vivo and in vitro experiments. Jpn J Pharmacol 35: 203–227

2. Himmelreich G, Muser M, Neuhaus P, Bechstein WO, Slama KJ, Jochum M, Riess H (1992) Different aprotinin applications influencing hemostatic changes in orthotopic liver transplantation. Transplantation 53: 132–136

3. Hitomi Y, Ikari N, Fujii S (1985) Inhibitory effect of a new synthetic protease inhibitor (FUT-175) on the coagulation system. Haemostasis 15: 164–168

4. Iwaki M, Ino Y, Motoyoshi A, Ozeki M, Sato T, Kurumi M, Aoyama T (1986) Pharmacological studies of FUT-175, nafamostat mesilate. V. Effects on the pancreatic enzymes and experimental acute pancreatitis in rats. Jpn J Pharmacol 41: 155–162

5. Jaeschke H, Farhood A (1991) Neutrophil and Kupffer cell-induced oxidant stress and ischemia-reperfusion injury in rat liver. Am J Physiol 260: G 355–362

6. Kajihara H, Yamamoto M, Yamada H, Mochizuki T, Taguchi (1981) Intracytoplasmic inclusion bodies in hepatocytes during prolonged extracorporeal circulation. Path Res Pract 172: 349–362

7. Kamada N, Calne RY (1983) A surgical experience with five hundred and thirty liver transplants in the rat. Surgery 93: 64–69

8. Li XK, Matin AFM, Suzuki H, Uno T, Yamaguchi T, Harada Y (1993) Effect of protease inhibitor on ischemia/reperfusion injury of the rat liver. Transplantation 56: 1331–1336

9. Lie TS, Seger R, Hong GS, Preissinger H, Ogawa K (1989) Protective effect of aprotinin on ischemic hepatocellular damage. Transplantation 48: 396–399

10. Lindert KA, Caldwell-Kenkel JC, Nukina S, Lemasters JJ, Thurman RG (1992) Activation of Kupffer cells on reperfusion following hypoxia: particle phagocytosis in a low-flow, reflow model. Am J Physiol 262: G 345–350

11. Nanpo T, Ohtuki T, Jin Y, Matunaga K, Takahashi M (1984) Pharmacokinetic studies of FUT-175 (nafamostat mesilate) (1) – blood level profiles, tissue distribution, metabolism and excretion in rats after intravenous administration (in Japanese). Kiso to Rinsho 18: 467–488

12. Oldhafer KJ, Schuttler W, Wiehe B, Hauss J, Pichlmayr R (1991) Treatment of preservation/reperfusion liver injury by the protease inhibitor aprotinin after cold ischemia storage. Transplant Proc 23: 2380–2381

13. Qu W, Savier E, Thurman RG (1992) Stimulation of monooxygenation and conjugation after liver transplantation in the rat: involvement of Kupffer cells. Mol Pharmacol 41: 1149–1154

14. Shimazu H, He W, Guo P, Dziadkoviec I, Miyazaki M, Falk RE (1994) Serum hyaluronate in the assessment of liver endothelial cell function after orthotopic liver transplantation in the rat. Hepatology 20: 1323–1329

15. Takei Y, Marzi I, Kauffman FC, Currin RT, Lemasters JJ, Thurman RG (1990) Increase in survival time of liver transplants by protease inhibitors and a calcium channel blocker, nisoldipine. Transplantation 50: 14–20

16. Urushihara T, Sumimoto K, Sumimoto R, Ikeda M, Fukuda Y, Dohi K (1994) Rinse solution containing a protease inhibitor and Na lactobionate increases graft survival after acute rat pancreas preservation. Transplant Proc 26: 559–560

17. Yoshikawa T, Murakami M, Furukawa Y, Kato H, Takemura S, Kondo M (1983) Effects of FUT-175, a new synthetic protease inhibitor on endotoxin-induced disseminated intravascular coagulation in rats. Haemostasis 13: 374–378

Transpl Int (1996) 9 [Suppl 1]: S452–S454
© Springer-Verlag 1996

J. A. B. van der Hoeven
I. J. de Jong
R. F. E. Wolf
R. L. Kamman
R. J. Ploeg

Tissue hydration in kidneys during preservation: a relaxometric analysis of time-dependent differences between cortex and medulla

J. A. B. van der Hoeven (✉) · I. J. de Jong ·
R. J. Ploeg
Department of Surgery,
University Hospital Groningen,
Hanzeplein I, PO Box 30.001,
NL-9700 RB Groningen,
The Netherlands

R. F. E. Wolf · R. L. Kamman
Department of Radiology,
University Hospital Groningen,
Hanzeplein 1, PO Box 30.001,
NL-9700 RB Groningen,
The Netherlands

Abstract Cold preservation of donor organs induces hypothermia-related tissue edema as a result of a reduced activity of the ATP-dependent sodium pump at low temperatures. Hypothermia-induced tissue edema occurs in kidney preservation and is a significant risk factor for delayed graft function (DGF) after transplantation. DGF remains a major problem in kidney transplantation and is significantly associated with preservation injury. The state of hydration of cold-stored organs can be assessed from a biopsy for determination of the wet/dry weight ratio. As a non-invasive method to determine tissue hydration MRI T_1 and T_2 relaxometry can be used. In this study we have compared changes in tissue hydration in UW-preserved porcine kidneys with increasing cold ischemia times (CIT) using wet/dry weight ratio and MR ralaxometry.

The results of the two techniques were correlated to evaluate the use of MR relaxometry. Wet/dry weight ratios of the renal cortex decreased with prolonged CIT ($P < 0.01$) whereas those of the medulla did not change significantly. T_1 values of the cortex decreased with prolonged CIT ($P < 0.01$). T_2 values of the cortex showed a non-significant decline with increased CIT. No significant changes in T_1 and T_2 were found in the medulla. The correlation between T_1 and the wet/dry weight ratio of the cortex was significant ($P = 0.05$, linear correlation coefficient 0.8698). We conclude that MR relaxometry can be a valuable non-invasive technique to assess tissue hydration in cadaveric donor kidneys before transplantation.

Key words Preservation · Kidney · Tissue hydration, MRI

Introduction

During cold-storage preservation of donor organs reduced activity of the ATPase-dependent sodium pump causes sodium and water influx into the cell [1, 2]. With longer cold ischemia times (CIT) more edema in the tissue is expected. The hypothermia-induced tissue edema is a potential factor contributing to the incidence of delayed graft function (DGF) after kidney transplantation. DGF remains a major problem in kidney transplantation and is associated with preservation injury [3, 4, 6]. The state of hydration of the cold-stored organ can be determined with a surgical biopsy. The difference between the wet weight and the dry weight of the biopsy represents the hydration state of the tissue, the wet/dry weight ratio. MRI offers a non-invasive alternative method to assess tissue hydration by measuring the T_1 and T_2 relaxometric characteristics. In previous reports, MR relaxometry has been used to evaluate changes in tissue hydration of ischemic reperfused kidneys in an experimental model and in human cold-stored donor livers [5, 6]. In this study we have looked at the changes in tissue edema in UW-preserved porcine kidneys with increasing CIT. MR relaxometry was compared to the standard wet/dry weight ratios.

Table 1 Wet/dry weight ratio and T_1 and T_2 relaxometric data. Data are shown as means ± SD ($n = 20$) per cold ischemia time *(CIT)* group

	6 h CIT	12 h CIT	24 h CIT	36 h CIT	72 h CIT	P values
Mean T_1 cortex	491.56 ± 28.00	474.20 ± 27.37	470.85 ± 31.50	460.93 ± 27.63	463.59 ± 28.64	< 0.01
Mean T_2 cortex	64.22 ± 5.55	63.79 ± 6.18	62.62 ± 6.67	61.97 ± 5.46	60.63 ± 4.74	NS
Mean T_1 medulla	745.32 ± 54.31	738.62 ± 52.72	734.20 ± 57.53	712.03 ± 48.06	739.04 ± 38.64	NS
Mean T_2 medulla	105.89 ± 13.43	108.93 ± 16.58	104.61 ± 17.80	104.97 ± 14.76	105.69 ± 10.39	NS
Wet/dry weight ratio cortex	0.8058 ± 0.009	0.8018 ± 0.010	0.7878 ± 0.013	0.7829 ± 0.011	0.7752 ± 0.010	< 0.01
Wet/dry weight ratio medulla	0.8553 ± 0.022	0.8621 ± 0.009	0.8595 ± 0.007	0.8479 ± 0.008	0.8579 ± 0.013	NS

Materials and methods

Twenty porcine kidneys were harvested from 6-month-old female Dutch pigs. After a warm ischemic period of 20 min, the kidneys were flushed with 250 ml of UW solution (0–4 °C) on a backtable. After the UW flush, the kidneys were divided into a caudal and a cranial part. Both parts were stored in UW-filled dishes and placed in seperate ice-filled styrofoam containers. At 6, 12, 24, 36, and 72 h CIT, MR relaxometry was performed on the cranial segments of the kidneys. At the same time, biopsies were taken from the cortex and the medulla of the caudal segments for wet/dry weight radio determination.

Wet/dry weight ratio

The surgical biopsies were taken from the caudal segment of the kidneys. Both medullary and cortical biopsies were obtained in a room with constant relative humidity. The biopsies were blotted twice on blotting paper before they were weighted. After the wet weight was established, the biopsies were stored in biofreeze vials (Co-Star 2 ml) in liquid nitrogen. The dry weight was determined after dry freezing for 120 h. To ascertain that the tissue was completely dry, five samples were freeze-dried for another 120 h in which they did not loose additional weight. Then the wet/dry weight ratio was calculated.

MRI and relaxometry

Images were obtained with a 1.5 Tesla whole-body system (Gyroscan S15/HP, Philips Medical Systems, Best, The Netherlands). Scoutview image allowed exact determination of the kidneys in the container and also allowed planning of the relaxometric imaging series. Images were obtained using a 'mixed pulse sequence' which is a combination of a spin echo (SE) and an inversion recovery (IR) pulse sequence. Both sequences were applied with eight echos and echo times of 30 msec. One average was made of a single 5-mm-thick slice with a scan matrix resolution of 256×256 in a 500 mm field of view. The repetition time for the SE sequence was 100 msec and for the IR sequence 1400 msec, with an inversion time of 400 msec. With standard system software features, images with signal intensities directly proportional to T_1 and T_2 (relaxometric images) were calculated. The two-dimensional fast Fourier technique (2D-FFT) was used for image reconstruction.

Image analysis

Reconstructed images were presented in a 256×256 pixel matrix and studied on a viewing console (Philips Medical Systems, Best, The Netherlands). Relaxation parameters, T_1 and T_2, were calculated as follows: in every calculated T_1 and T_2 image six regions of interest (ROI) of 0.1 cm^2 were positioned, three ROI in the cortex and three ROI in the medulla. The ROI were positioned in such a way that the contribution of UW in the vessels was minimal and there was no partial volume effect. In this way, information about T_1 and T_2 characteristics was obtained from 0.05 cm^3 renal parenchyma with each ROI. A mean T_1 and T_2 of cortex and medulla was calculated for each kidney.

Data analysis

Statistical analysis was performed using the paired Student's t-test and a linear correlation coefficient with $P < 0.05$ considered significant.

Results

The results of the determination of the tissue hydration state with wet/dry weight ratios and T_1 and T_2 relaxometry are shown in Table 1. The wet/dry weight ratio of the renal cortex decreased significantly from a mean of 0.8058 at 6 h CIT to a mean of 0.7752 at 72 h CIT ($P < 0.01$, paired Student's t-test). The wet/dry weight ratios of the renal medulla did not change during the same period. The MR relaxometric data showed a significant decline of T_1 and T_2 values of the cortex with longer CIT from 6 to 72 h ($P < 0.01$, paired Student's t-test). No significant changes in T_1 and T_2 were measured in the medulla although T_1 declined. The correlation between T_1 and the wet/dry weight ratio of the cortex was significant (linear correlation coefficient 0.8698, $P < 0.05$) (Table 1).

Discussion

The decrease in the wet/dry weight ratio of the cortex demonstrates the dehydrating properties of UW solution due to the impermeants lactobionate and raffinose. In our model, UW solution protected against the development of tissue edema in the medulla since the wet/dry weight ratio did not change. The dehydrating properties of the UW solution have been reported to exceed those of Eurocollins or phosphate-buffered sucrose in experimental models [5]. A significant correlation was seen between MR relaxometric data and wet/dry weight ratios. This indicates that MR relaxometry could be a valuable non-invasive alternative technique to assess tissue hydration in cadaveric donor kidneys during cold storage. Further studies are in progress to investigate the clinical value of MR relaxometry in human cadaveric donor kidneys and its relation to the incidence of posttransplant delayed graft function.

References

1. Belzer FO, Southard JH (1988) Principles of solid organ preservation by cold storage. Transplantation 45: 673–676
2. Martin DR, Scott MDF, Downes GL, Belzer FO (1972) Primary cause of unsuccesful liver and heart preservation: cold sensitivity of the ATPase system. Ann Surg 175: 111
3. Ploeg RJ, Bockel H van, Langendijk PTH, et al (1992) A randomized controlled clinical trial comparing preservation with UW solution and Eurocollins in cadaveric renal transplantation. Lancet 340: 129–137
4. Thiel G et al (1982) The role of reduced medullary perfusion in the genesis of acute ischaemic renal falure. Nephron 31: 321
5. Walhberg JA, Southard JH, Belzer FO (1986) Development of a cold storage solution for pancreas preservation. Cryobiology 23: 477
6. Yamamoto K, Wilson DR, Baumal R (1984) Outer medullary circulatory defect in ischaemic acute renal failure. Am J Pathol 116: 253

Transpl Int (1996) 9 [Suppl 1]: S455–S459
© Springer-Verlag 1996

J. Torras
K. Soto
M. Riera
I. Herrero
J. Valles
J. M. Cruzado
J. Alsina
J. M. Grinyo

Changes in renal hemodynamics and physiology after normothermic ischemia in animals supplemented with eicosapentaenoic acid

J. Torras · K. Soto · M. Riera · I. Herrero ·
J. M. Cruzado · J. Alsina
Nephrology Service, Hospital of Bellvitge,
Fundació August Pi i Sunyer, Department
of Medicine, University of Barcelona,
Ciutat Sanitària i Universitària de Bellvitge

J. Valles
LASA Laboratories, Barcelona, Spain

J. M. Grinyo (✉)
Nephrology Service, Hospital of Bellvitge,
Ciutat Sanitària i Universitària de
Bellvitge, Feixa Llarga s/n, 08097
L'Hospitalet de Llobregat, Barcelona,
Spain
Tel. +34-3-3356111-2405
Fax +34-3-2631595

Abstract In order to determine whether treatment of animals with an n-3 fatty acid, eicosapentaenoic acid (EPA), could modify renal hemodynamics and physiology after normothermic ischemia, we studied 42 Spraque Dawley rats orally supplemented with either olive oil or a purified lysine salt of EPA for 4 weeks. Four experimental groups were established. Three groups were treated with increasing doses of EPA: 20 mg/kg per day (EPA 20), 40 mg/kg per day (EPA 40) and 80 mg/kg per day (EPA 80), and one group was supplemented with isovolumetric olive oil (OLI). A control group that received neither EPA nor ischemia was also studied. On day 28, right nephrectomy was performed, followed by 30 min of left renal warm ischemia. Basal arterial pressure and renal blood flow (RBF) were monitored in two kidneys before arterial occlusion and continuously thereafter throughout the experiment in one kidney using an electronic transducer and a flowmeter. From 60 to 120 min after the end of ischemia, urine output (µl/min), glomerular filtration rate (GFR, µl/min), measured by inulin clearance, and fractional reabsortion of sodium (FRNa) were determined every 20 min. Renal plasma flow (RPF, ml/min) and renal vascular resistance (VR, mm Hg/ml per min) were calculated. RPF was estimated as RBF (1−hematocrit). Before ischemia, the mean RPF and RBF were higher in EPA-fed than in olive oil-fed animals and after ischemia showed a significantly greater increase in EPA-fed animals than in olive oil-fed animals. Mean VR was lower in EPA-fed animals than in olive oil-fed animals, both before arterial occlusion and after ischemia. Mean urine output was similar in the OLI and EPA 20 groups, and significantly higher in the EPA 40 and EPA 80 groups than in the control group. GFR was significantly lower in the OLI and EPA 20 groups than in the control group. Finally, the EPA 40 group showed a similar and the EPA 80 group a slightly higher GFR than the control group. We conclude that EPA supplementation provides protection from renal ischemic-reperfusion injury, and this effect is more evident at higher EPA doses.

Key words Eicosapentaenoic acid supplementation · Renal ischemic · Reperfusion injury

Introduction

Increased dietary or parenteral intake of fish oils rich in n-3 fatty acids affects a large number of biochemical and functional parameters producing a beneficial effect on the course of some lipid, inflammatory and cardiovascular diseases [1]. Recently, n-3 fatty acids have been shown to have protective effects on renal hemodynam-

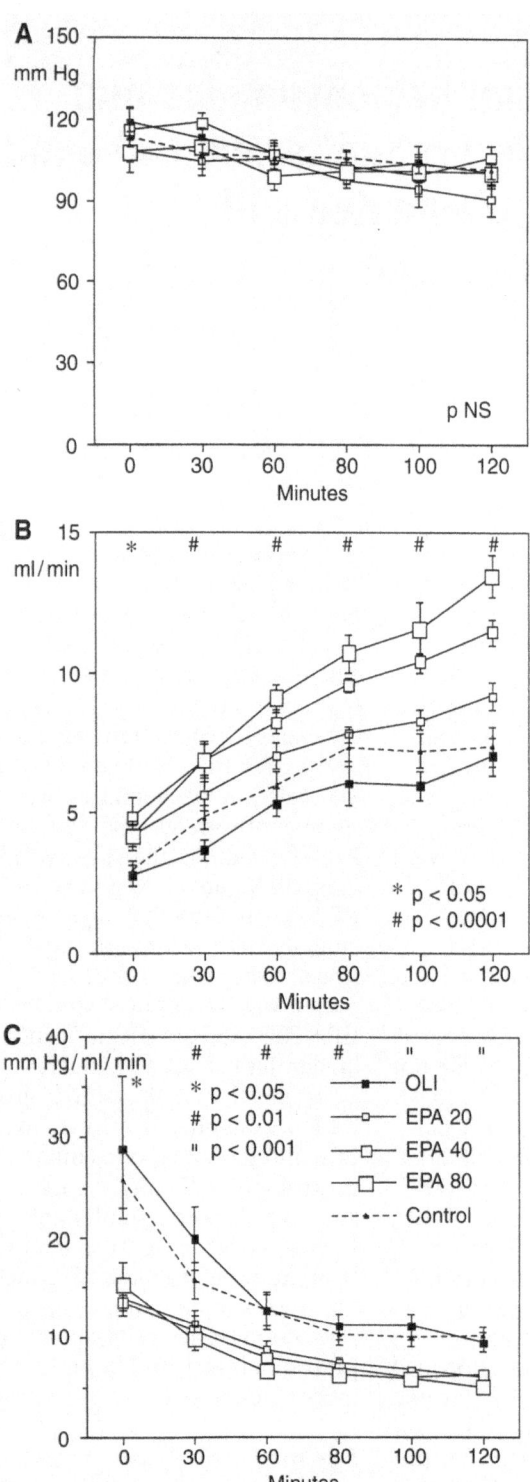

Fig. 1 A–C Effects of dietary supplementation with a lysine salt of eicosapentaenoic acid on arterial pressure (**A**), renal plasma flow (**B**), and renal vascular resistance (**C**) in rats with moderate acute renal failure (30 min)

ics and on blood pressure in renal transplant patients [2]. Also, n-3 fatty acids have been shown to be effective in ischemic experimental models [3–6]. Thus, in a stroke model, animals prefed with an n-3 fatty acid-enriched diet showed smaller infarcts than control animals [3]. In myocardial infarct models, it has been demonstrated that fish oils increase post-ischemic blood flow [4, 5]. However, there is a discrepancy in results concerning infarct size, a reduction being reported in some studies [4] and no modification in others [5].

To date, there are few studies on the effects of fish oils in renal ischemic models [6]. Warm or cold ischemia are present under various conditions in clinical nephrology and transplantation, for example in ischemic or atheromatous renal diseases, or during preservation in renal transplantation. So, the need to dispose of therapeutic or protective drugs in these situations is evident.

The aim of this study was to determine whether chronic animal supplementation with a purified salt of eicosapentaenoic acid (EPA), a fish-oil n-3 fatty acid, could modify the renal hemodynamics and physiology after normothermic ischemia of the kidney. In addition, we sought to determine if these effects were dose dependent.

Material and methods

Materials

A purified lysine salt of EPA (purity > 95%, bioavailability > 90%) soluble in water was obtained from Lasa Laboratories SAE (Barcelona, Spain).

Animal preparation and surgical technique

Young male Sprague-Dawley rats (6 weeks old; 100 g body weight) were obtained from our own animal facility. They were housed four per cage in a light-controlled room with a 12-h light/dark cycle and had access to food and water ad libitum.

EPA or olive oil were given by daily gavage. Animals were weighed twice a week and EPA or olive oil dose schedules adjusted as appropriate. Animals were randomly allocated to four dietary groups. These comprised a group supplemented with isovolumetric olive oil (2 ml/kg) plus α tocopherol 0.08 mg/ml (OLI group, n = 9), and three groups receiving EPA: 20 mg/kg per day (2 ml/kg) plus α tocopherol 0.04 mg/ml (EPA 20, n = 7), 40 mg/kg per day (2 ml/kg) plus α tocopherol 0.08 mg/ml (EPA 40, n = 7), and 80 mg/kg per day (2 ml/kg) plus α tocopherol 0.16 mg/ml (EPA 80, n = 8). Alpha tocopherol was added to retard autoxidation of EPA and to prevent cell membrane oxidation by EPA.

After 4 weeks on this diet, animals were anesthetized with ketamine hydrochloride (75 mg/kg), diazepam (5 mg/kg) and atropine (0.5 mg/kg) intramuscularly and placed on a heating pad to maintain body temperature at 37 °C. The abdominal cavity was opened, and vascular polyethylene catheters were implanted into the abdominal aorta and vena cava via the femoral vessels. The arterial catheter was used for continuous monitoring of arterial pressure using an electronic pressure transducer (Nihon Kohden Co., Germany) and blood sampling. The venous catheter was used throughout the experiment for the infusion of fluid (Ringer's lactate

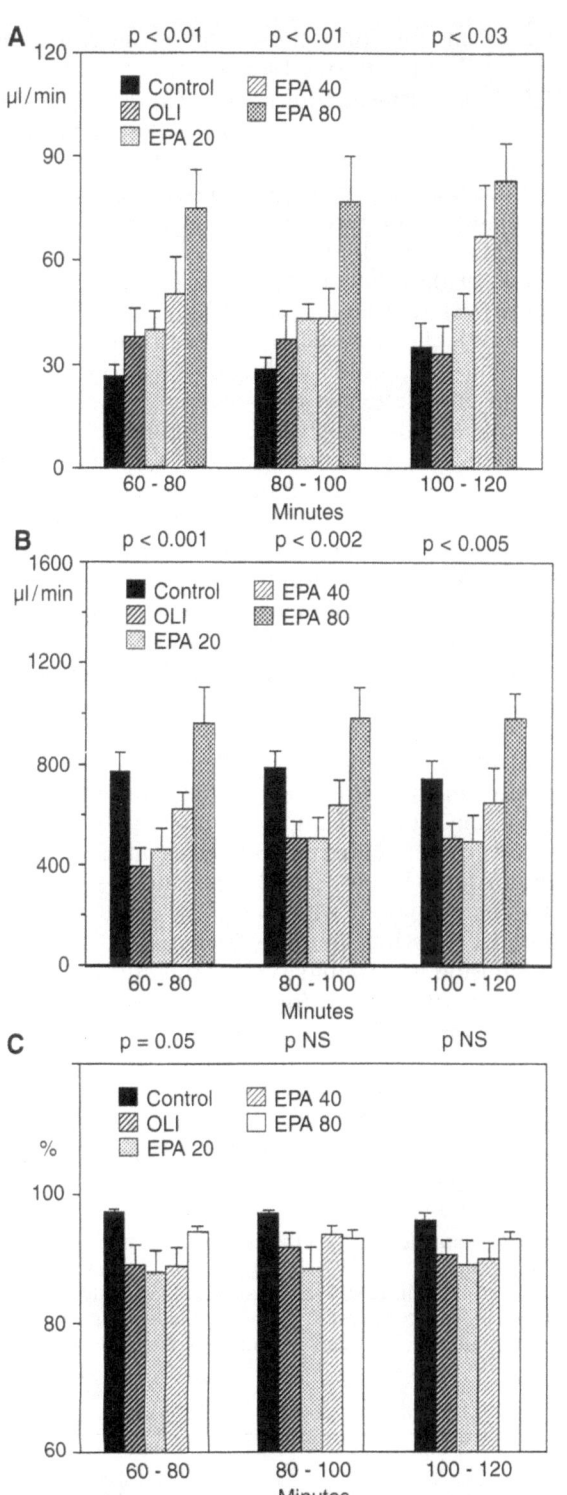

Fig. 2 A–C Effects of dietary supplementation with a lysine salt of eicosapentaenoic acid on urine output (**A**), GFR (**B**), and FRNa (**C**) in rats with moderate acute renal failure (30 min)

1.5 ml/h per 100 g) and inulin (0.65 mg/ml of serum) (Polyfructosan, Laevosan, Linz, Austria). The left ureter was cannulated for the collection of urine with polyethylene tubing.

The left renal artery was exposed and an electronic flow probe (Transonic Systems, USA) was placed around the vessel to measure basal renal blood flow (RBF) before arterial occlusion and continuously thereafter throughout the experiment. The left renal artery was occluded for 30 min with a nontraumatic clamp to induce a moderate acute renal failure [7] and, meanwhile, contralateral nephrectomy was performed. A 120-min reperfusion period was then monitored, allowing a 1-h equilibration for inulin, followed by three 20-min urine collections for inulin and electrolyte measurement. At the mid point of these 20-min periods, a blood sample (300 µl) was drawn for inulin and electrolyte measurement. Two additional blood samples (200 µl) were drawn just before ischemia and at the end of the experiment for hematocrit measurement. After every blood sample withdrawal, an equal volume of blood obtained from a pool of rats was reinfused.

A group of rats with a similar body weight (control group, n = 11) that had been fed neither olive oil nor EPA were used as controls. These animals were experimentally managed in the same way as the study groups but without warm ischemia.

Analytical methods and estimations

Glucose was measured enzymatically by the hexokinase/glucose-6-phosphate dehydrogenase method (Boehringer Mannheim, Germany), and polyfructosan was measured after acid hydrolysis by including glucose-6-phosphate isomerase in the assay [8]. Sodium levels were measured by flame photometry (Ciba Corning, Spain). Hematocrit was measured using an automated method (288 blood gas system, Ciba Corning).

Renal plasma flow (RPF, ml/min) was calculated from the formula RPF = RBF(1–hematocrit) and renal vascular resistance (VR, mm Hg/ml per min) from the formula VR = arterial pressure/RBF. Urine output was measured by collecting urine into preweighed tubes (µl/min). Glomerular filtration rate (GFR, µl/min) was evaluated from inulin clearance using the formula GFR = urine output × urine inulin/plasma inulin. Finally, fractional sodium reabsortion (FRNa) was calculated from the formula: FRNa = 100 × (1 – urine Na/perfusate Na × perfusate inulin/urine inulin).

Statistical analysis

For comparisons between more than two groups, one-way analysis of variance was performed followed by Fisher's procedure for multiple pairwise comparisons. When a nonparametric test was needed, the Kruskal Wallis analysis was used. All P-values were two tailed and a P-value of < 0.05 was considered statistically significant. Data are presented as mean ± SEM.

Results

Mean arterial pressure was similar in all groups throughout the experiment (Fig. 1 A). As shown in Figure 1 B, basal mean RPF was similar in the control and OLI groups, and both were significantly lower than mean RPF in the EPA groups, suggesting a state of chronic vasodilatation. After ischemia, the mean RPF increased progressively in all groups. The EPA groups

S 458

showed a significantly greater increase in mean RPF with time during the experiment than the OLI group. There was a dose-dependent effect in this increase in mean RPF. This increase was probably due to adaptive mechanisms to contralateral nephrectomy and to the high fluid infusion. RBF followed a similar pattern (data not shown). Concerning VR, EPA-fed animals showed lower mean values than olive oil-fed animals, both before arterial occlusion and after ischemia (Fig. 1 C).

Urine output showed similar mean values in the control, OLI and EPA 20 groups. The EPA 40 and EPA 80 groups showed significantly higher mean values than the other groups (Fig. 2 A). Concerning GFR (Fig. 2 B), the OLI and EPA 20 groups showed a significantly lower mean value than the control group, the EPA 40 group showed a mean value similar to the control group, and the EPA 80 group showed a slightly but not significantly higher mean value than control group. Mean FRNa showed no conclusive results (Fig. 2 C): in the 60–80-min period there was a significantly higher mean value in the control group than in the OLI, EPA 20 and EPA 40 groups but not compared to the EPA 80 group which showed similar values, but in the two other periods there were no significant differences between the groups.

Discussion

The results of this study demonstrated that chronic supplementation of rats with a purified lysine salt of EPA increased renal blood and plasma flow, and decreased renal vascular resistance in the basal state and after warm ischemia, compared with rats fed with olive oil. In addition, kidney function, evaluated as the GFR and the urine output, was also protected in rats supplemented with EPA. These protective effects of EPA on overall renal function were dose-dependent.

Our positive results are quite similar to those of other studies in animal models of cerebral or cardiac ischemia [3–5], suggesting the potential preventive role of fish oils rich in n-3 fatty acids in ischemic states. Our results also agree with those reported in a study in uninephric conscious dogs in which prefeeding with fish oils ameliorated the course of acute ischemic renal failure [6].

However, in this study there was no modification of RBF or VR either during feeding with fish oils or after ischemia, in contrast to our results. There are some possible mechanisms that could explain these beneficial effects [1, 5, 9]: decreased formation of vasoconstricting and proaggregatory prostaglandins from the endothelium (mainly thromboxane B_2); enhanced release of nitric oxide/endothelium-derived relaxing factor; decreased polymorphonuclear cell recruitment within the ischemic zone during reperfusion, due to reduced production of leukotriene B_4, platelet activating factor and interleukin-1; reduced production of PDGF-like protein; and modulation of the receptor characteristics of vasoactive substances [10]. Concerning the effects on the kidneys, it is well known that EPA exerts important effects on renal function in normal humans [11] and favorably influences renal function and prostanoid production in experimental animals and transplanted patients receiving cyclosporin [2, 12].

The use of fish oils is increasing in humans. There are currently some ongoing studies in cardiovascular diseases, in IgA nephropathy and in the prevention of rejection in renal transplantation [1]. Their use in clinical ischemic states or in preservation during solid organ transplantation has not been tested yet. There is a time limitation in their use since all reported studies used long feeding protocols. Short treatment periods to study the protective effects of n-3 fatty acids on renal ischemia might be done. In this regard, a promising study has recently been reported which used the rapid administration of EPA by infusion of a trieicosapentaenoyl-glycerol emulsion into rabbits [13]. In this study, 6 h following infusion, the ex vivo formation of leukotriene B_4 by polymorphonuclear alls was markedly suppressed compared with preinfusion values, suggesting that the administered EPA had reached physiologically relevant levels. The use of EPA in ischemic states or preservation is therefore potentially possible and deserves further consideration.

Acknowledgements This work was supported in part by a grant from FISS (number 94/1296), by a grant from Sandoz SAE, Spain, and by a grant from LASA Laboratories. Marta Riera Oliva is a fellow of 'Fundació August Pi i Sunyer', Ciutat Sanitaria i Universitaria de Bellvitge. We thank Susana Miró for her technical help.

References

1. Endres S, De Caterina R, Schmid EB, Kristensen SD (1995) n-3 Polyunsaturated fatty acids: update 1995. Eur J Clin Invest (in press)

2. Homan van der Heide JJ, Bilo HJG, Donker JM, Wilmik JM, Tegzess AM (1993) Effect of dietary fish oil on renal function and rejection in cyclosporin-treated recipients of renal transplants. N Engl J Med 329: 769–773

3. Lai ML, Hsu CY, Liu TH, He YY, Xu J, Navidi M, Sun G, Hogan EL (1993) Effects of fish oil supplementation on acute ischemic brain injury in the rat. Neurology 43: 1227–1232

4. Hock CE, Holahan MA, Reibel DK (1987) Effect of dietary fish oil on myocardial phospholipids and myocardial ischemic damage. Am J Physiol 252: H554–H560

5. Force Th, Malis ChD, Guerrero JL, Varadarajan GS, Bonventre JV, Weber PC, Leaf A (1989) n-3 Fatty acids increase postischemic blood flow but do not reduce myocardial necrosis. Am J Physiol 257: H1204–H1210

6. Neumayer HH, Heinrich Schmissas M, Haller H, Wagner K, Luft CF (1992) Amelioration of ischemic acute renal failure by dietary fish oil administration in concious dogs. J Am Soc Nephrol 3: 1312–1320

7. Gellai M, Jugus M, Fletcher T, DeWolf R, Nambi P (1994) Reversal of postischemic acute renal failure with a selective endothellin A receptor antagonist in the rat. J Clin Invest 93: 900–906

8. Schmidt FH (1961) Die enzymatische Bestimmung von Glukose und Fruktose nebeneinander. Klin Wochenschr 39: 1244–1247

9. Leaf A, Weber PC (1988) Cardiovascular effects of n-3 fatty acids. N Engl J Med 318: 549–557

10. Awazu M, Yared A, Swift LL, Hoover RL, Ichikawa I (1992) Dietary fatty acids modulate glomerular atrial natriuretic peptide receptor. Kidney Int 42: 265–271

11. Dusing R, Struck a, Gobel BO, Weisser B, Vetter H (1990) Effects of n-3 fatty acids on renal function and renal prostaglandin E metabolism. Kidney Int 38: 315–319

12. Torras J, Valles J, Sanchez J, Sabate I, Seron D, Carrera M, Castelao AM, Herrero I, Puig Parellada P, Alsina J, Grinyo JM, Prevention of experimental cyclosporine nephrotoxicity by dietary supplementation with LSL 90202, a lisine salt of eicosapentaenoic acid. Role of thomboxane and prostacyclin in renal tissue.

13. Sawazaki S, Nakamura N, Hamazaki T, Yamazaki K, Urazake M Yano (1992) Intravenous infusion of trieicosapentaenoyl glycerol and LTB_4 and LTB_5 production by leukocytes of rabbits. Am J Physiol 262: H1711–H1718

Transpl Int (1996) 9 [Suppl 1]: S 460–S 463
© Springer-Verlag 1996

M. Cardillo
L. Mascaretti
C. Pizzi
G. Piccolo
L. Lecchi
A. Aniasi
G. Puglisi
M. Scalamogna
G. Sirchia

Donor organ procurement in the North Italy Transplant program (NITp) in 1994: the beginning of a promising trend?

M. Cardillo (✉) · C. Pizzi · G. Piccolo ·
L. Lecchi · A. Aniasi · G. Puglisi · G. Sirchia
Centro Trasfusionale e di Immunologia dei
Trapianti, Ospedale Maggiore Policlinico,
via F. Sforza 35, I-20122 Milano, Italy

L. Mascaretti · M. Scalamogna
Servizio Autonomo per il Prelievo e la
Conservazione di Parti da Cadavere,
Ospedale Maggiore Policlinico,
via F. Sforza 35, I-20122 Milano, Italy

Abstract Donor organ procurement is a world-wide problem. In Italy it is particularly so and the reasons for this are investigated. An overall increase in the number of donors has been noted in 1994 and the first 8 months of 1995, and ways of continuing this encouraging trend should be pursued by improvements in education, legislation, and hospital organization.

Key words Donor organ procurement · Education · Legislation · Brain death

Introduction

Italy has suffered in recent years from a chronic shortage of organs for transplantation. The problem was so well known that it even reached the foreign press. On 17 October 1994, Time magazine in an article concerning a young American boy killed in Italy and who became an organ donor, referred to Italy's donor rate as being "one of the lowest" in Europe [1]. Figure 1 shows that the donor rate per million population (pmp) per year in Italy and in the North Italy Transplant program (a transplant organization which has served an area with 18 million inhabitants since 1972) is much lower than the European mean [2]. Organ shortage leads to an accumulation of patients on the waiting list, long waiting times, and a high mortality rate for patients on the heart and liver waiting list who have no alternative treatment to transplantation.

Causes of scanty organ procurement

Public knowledge and its attitude toward transplantation

The health education of the Italian population is far from satisfactory and, in particular, information regarding transplantation is very poor. From a survey carried out by Centro Studi Investimenti Sociali (CENSIS) in the Lazio region in 1992, it emerged that 53.6 % of subjects had scarce knowledge concerning transplantation and 40 % had doubts about brain death [3]. Thus it is not surprising that opposition to organ retrieval by the next of kin is quite high; a study performed in 68 intensive care units (ICUs) in North Italy showed that out of 255 potential donors there was denial of consent from donor families in 74 cases (29 %).

Attitude of mass media in relation to transplantation

The general population's uneasiness concerning transplantation is reflected by the mass media which usually approaches transplantation in three different ways:
1. Events are presented objectively, highlighting technical and scientific content (information).

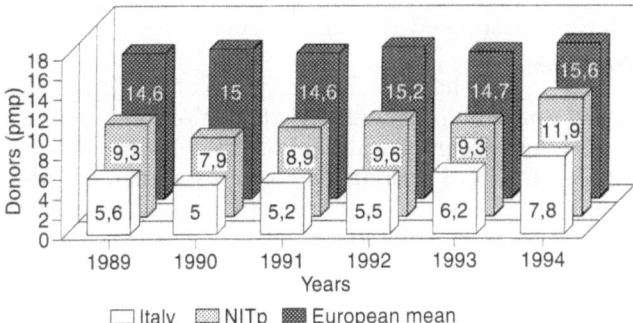

Fig. 1 Donors used (per million population) in Italy and in NITp compared with the European mean

Table 1 NITp. Organ procurement and transplantation activity. Comparison between 1993 and 1994

Donors/transplants	1993	1994	Percentage variation
Donors used	169	215	+ 27.2 %
Transplants			
Kidney	320	416	+ 30.0 %
Heart	182	208	+ 14.3 %
Liver	168	202	+ 20.2 %

2. Events (and surgeons) are "celebrated" or some aspects are reported incorrectly (misinformation).
3. Untrue and horrifying aspects are emphasized (disinformation).

The latter approach is that which shifts the spotlight to shocking news which is published in the chronicle section of newspapers. In recent years, the mass media have furnished a great amount of confused and contradictory news with particular regard to organ trafficking or the use of organs from patients who could have been saved, and the stories of criminal organizations which kidnap children or young adults to remove their organs. Many of these stories are "metropolitan legends" which contain some elements of modern living but the contents are emphasized and distorted [4]. It can be hypothesized that these stories are an expression of a "primal anxiety" of man regarding transplantation, a field which embraces such frontline topics as brain death and highly technological medical procedures which give patients who would die in the short term a longer life expectancy.

Attitude of health care workers toward transplantation

Misinformation is one of the problems of health workers, who often do not have the opportunity of going into different aspects of organ retrieval and transplantation during their professional life. From a survey carried out in 1994 among 1119 health workers from a large teaching hospital in Verona, with the aim of investigat-

ing how health workers perceived organ donation and transplantation [5], 22.5 % of subjects ignored the meaning of brain death and 35 % believed in the possibility of organ trafficking in Italy.

Attitude of hospitals

For many years, Italian public hospitals run by the National Health System have been financed independently of the services they produced, few pursued efficiency, and most did not have a modern approach to the management of human resources, including the use of incentives for those who make a special effort as is the case for donor organ procurement. It is no surprise that few hospitals were committed to organ procurement, and those which have been active in such programs have done so on a voluntary basis, often facing several organizational problems, such as a low number of ICU beds, a lack of subintensive units, and no doctor present in the ICU ward during night hours. Other organizational difficulties include establishing the medical/legal commission for ascertaining brain death, the absence of a professional figure in charge of managing the organ donor and of coordinating organ retrieval procedures, and the difficulties of access to diagnostic facilities such as computerized tomography and electroencephalography.

Organ procurement and transplantation activity in NITp in 1994 and in the first 8 months of 1995: a turning point?

Compared with 1993, there was a significant increase in the number of donors used in NITp in 1994 (+ 27.2 %) (Table 1), with some fluctuations in the monthly donor rate (Fig. 2). A reduction in the summer months can be seen as opposed to a consistent increase in the last 3 months of the year. News related to transplantation has constantly been in the papers and on television prior to October 1995. In June, during a television talkshow a patient declared that he payed a large amount of money to obtain a transplant, giving the impression that in Italy there is an "organ market". At the end of the summer, the Minister for the Family declared that some children born in South America were adopted in Italy only to be sold to organ trafficking organizations. There was no proof to support these declarations; nonetheless, the scandal was very harmful for the image of the transplant community and organ procurement dropped dramatically.

At the beginning of October, Nicholas, a young American boy on holiday with his parents in South Italy, was killed by criminals and became an organ donor. This news was widely covered by the media and the whole nation was touched by the family's decision. The increase in the donor rate following this event has been

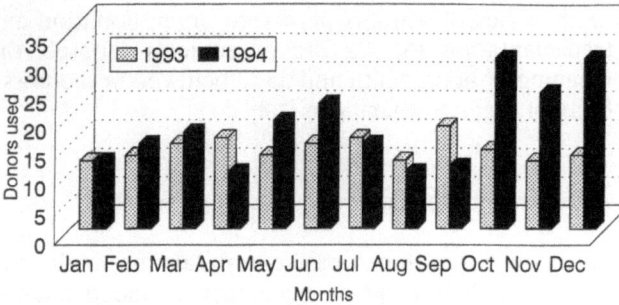

Fig. 2 NITp. Organ procurement, comparison between 1993 and 1994

Table 2 NITp. Organ procurement and transplantation activity. Comparison between the first 8 months of 1994 and 1995

Donors/Transplants	Jan–Aug 1994	Jan–Aug 1995	Percentage variation
Donors used	120	181	+ 50.8 %
Transplants			
Kidney	229	345	+ 50.6 %
Heart	114	174	+ 52.6 %
Liver	113	151	+ 33.6 %

called the "Nicholas effect". We believe that positive and negative news on the mass media only partly explain the 1994 data. Certainly, the brain death law issued in the autumn and the initiatives taken by NITp focusing on organ procurement have played an important role in reversing the trend of organ procurement in our area. In the first 8 months of 1995 the trend in donor rate has been satisfactory (Table 2).

Measures adopted to improve transplantation

Measures adopted at a national level

In December 1993, a law establishing the criteria for brain death was issued (law n. 578 dated 29 December 1993). This is a good law since it unequivocally states that there is only one type of death, which occurs when the brain is totally and irreversibly damaged. The main feature of this law is that the diagnostic criteria are fixed by a decree (DM 582 effective from 19 October 1994) which can be modified more easily than a law. The time period for diagnosis of death in adults is reduced from 12 h (law 644 dated December 1975) to 6 h (for children aged 1–5 years the diagnosis period is 12 h whereas for babies under 1 year it is 24 h); brain death criteria are also applied in the case of brain death secondary to anoxia, which is different from that foreseen by the previous legislation. Finally, the law clearly states that the presence of spinal reflexes has no influence on the diagnosis of brain death.

Measures adopted at a regional level

NITp regions have lately been very active in promoting organ procurement and transplantation. The measures taken have been educational programs in hospitals, the appointment of regional and local transplant coordinators, and the Veneto region has recently approved a law which foresees reimbursement for organ procurement activity.

Measures adopted in NITp

In the past few years, NITp has endeavoured to improve organ donation in three ways. Firstly, much effort has been put into promoting organ procurement in its ICUs. An itinerant commission made up of an ICU doctor and a representative of the Interregional Reference Center has visited the most important ICUs in our area to become acquainted with the local problems which could hinder organ procurement. Where possible, a solution was looked for together with ICU doctors and the hospital's medical director. Secondly an Italian version of the European Donor Hospital Educational Program (EDHEP) has been prepared and implemented in some of our hospitals. Thirdly, a psychology unit has been established with two objectives: on the one hand to assist donor families in overcoming psychological problems related to a "complicated grieving process" and on the other hand, to help intensive care workers with asking families for consent [6, 7].

Discussion

It seems clear that a new and more effective system for health education must be devised. The university together with the schooling system and the relevant scientific societies should coordinate their efforts and come up with clear information about organ donation and transplantation, and this should be transmitted to the public in proper ways; this, however, is a difficult and expensive task out of our reach.

Educational programs should continually address health workers which deal with transplantation, and in this regard there are many models which one can choose from, such as the already mentioned EDHEP program, the Transplant Coordinator Management courses organized by Organizacion Nacional de Transplantes, or the training program for neurosurgeons and for medical and nursing students of the North American United Network of Organ Sharing. All of the above-mentioned educational programs use effective instruments such as videos, interactive computer programs, and simulations of real situations encountered in the hospital setting.

To improve the efficiency and quality of Italian hospitals, laws n. 502 and 517 issued in 1992 and 1993, respectively, foresee the introduction in public hospitals of mechanisms resembling those of private management. From 1 January 1995 hospitals should be financed with a limited fixed amount by the region and for the rest they should be financed according to the services rendered. It is unclear whether these measures will be successful, since the Italian hospitals have become corporations but have not been given the necessary instruments to act as such; for instance, decisions such as the number of staff assigned to each ward are still taken by the Central Health Authority.

So it is our belief that for the future, two very important points must be solved; firstly, the hospital corporations must be allowed to become real enterprises and, secondly, organ procurement procedures must be reimbursed and assigned a high value so as to encourage hospitals and the personnel involved to identify all possible cadaver organ donors. When these two aspects are overcome, hospitals will be able to reorganize their ICUs as they deem necessary, implement effective training for its personnel, and nominate local transplant coordinators (LTC) which have been recognized by Spain [8, 9] and other countries as being the real "engine" of organ procurement programs. The LTC's job should be that of stimulating organ procurement, devising education programs in the hospital and, whenever a donor becomes available, the LTC should be in charge of organizing the donor operation. To be effective, it is mandatory that LTCs be officially recognized by the health authorities and backed up by a budget which covers some expenses and provides incentives to the teams more closely involved in organ procurement.

Acknowledgements This study was in part financed by Ricerca Finalizzata 1993 "Nuove caratteristiche fisiopatologiche del donatore cadavere di organi".

References

1. Time Magazine (1994) Gift from the grave. A grieving family's generosity stirs hearts
2. Council of Europe 1994 Transplant 6: 271–278
3. Centro Studi Investimenti Sociali 1992 La donazione degli organi nel Lazio. February
4. Comazzi AM, Clerici CA (1996) La trapiantologia attraverso i mass media (in press)
5. Boschiero L, Licata C, Procaccio F (1996) Indagine sulla percezione della morte cerebrale e donazione degli organi tra il personale sanitario degli Ospedali di Verona (in press)
6. Comazzi AM, La Spina F (1994) Umanità e scienza in aiuto ai parenti del donatore. Not Brevi Policlinico 5: 4–6
7. Matesanz R, Miranda B, Felipe C (1994) Organ procurement in Spain: Impact of transplant coordination. Clin Transplant 8: 281–286
8. Matesanz R (1993) Organ procurement in Spain: The importance of a transplant coordinating network. Transplant Proc 25: 3132–3135
9. Matesanz R, Miranda B (1995) Coordinacion y Trasplantes. El modelo espanol. Grupo Aula medica S. A., Madrid

Transpl Int (1996) 9 [Suppl 1]: S 464–S 468
© Springer-Verlag 1996

K. T. E. Beckurts
K. W. Jauch
A. H. Hölscher
M. Anthuber
C.-D. Heidecke
M. Stangl
W.-D. Illner
C. Schulz
W. Land

Regionalization of donor organ procurement: first experiences in southern Bavaria and results of a regional donor hospital survey

K. T. E. Beckurts (✉) · A. H. Hölscher ·
C.-D. Heidecke
Chirurgische Klinik und Poliklinik,
Technische Universität München,
Klinikum Rechts der Isar,
Ismaninger Strasse 22,
D-81675 München, Germany
Tel. +49 89 41 40 20 11;
Fax +49 89 41 40 48 84

K. W. Jauch · M. Anthuber · M. Stangl
Department of Surgery,
Klinikum Großhadern der Ludwig-
Maximilians-Universität, München,
Germany

W.-D. Illner · C. Schulz · W. Land
Division of Transplant Surgery,
Klinikum Großhadern der Ludwig-
Maximilians-Universität, Munich,
Germany

Abstract In order to improve organizational, qualitative, and economic aspects of organ procurement, a model of regionalization was established in the local area of southern Bavaria, as from September 1993, with the following characteristics. A collaborative 24 h-duty schedule with surgeons from all active regional transplant programs. Surgeons are grouped according to their operative qualification level: (1) Group I, capable of retrieving all abdominal organs (liver, pancreas, kidney), (2) Group II, capable of removing kidneys, and (3) Group III, surgical assistance in procurement procedures. All donor organs in the local region are explanted by the local team and foreign recipient centers are supplied with the organs removed by a standardized technique. Only three times during the first, and not once during the second year, did a foreign team insist on traveling to our region to perform a liver retrieval. A survey clearly documented univocal acceptance of this model by donor hospital executives. Simplified organization and less disturbance in operating theaters were among the most frequent arguments in favor, and the familiarity of explant teams in donor hospitals was considered advantageous. Most donor hospitals do not expect to profit in terms of financial savings. When asked for further possible measures to improve organ donation, a clearer legal situation, but also the need for more information and education programs, including better media representation of transplant issues, were cited most frequently. An improvement in financial reimbursements for the donor hospitals as an instrument to enhance willingness for organ donation was not considered essential. In conclusion, our model of regionalization of organ procurement proved to be effective in achieving a high quality of organ retrieval and a reduction in personnel requirements for the transplant centers. In addition, the response from donor hospitals was unequivocally positive and may, thus, positively influence donor activity. Relevant financial savings can result from reduced on-call duties and minimized traveling costs. Further attempts to rationalize organ procurement could possibly include heart(-/lung)surgeons in the regionalized teams.

Key words Donor organ procurement · Abdominal organs · Local procurement teams

Introduction

Transplant programs, as a part of the general trend in health care, are increasingly experiencing pressure on budgets and limitations of personnel and organizational resources. On the contrary, there is a constant challenge to improve the results of clinical organ transplantation and the procedures involved, one of them being the standards of organ procurement and, thus, the quality and quantity of organs retrieved.

In an attempt to enhance the performance of our local program, we decided to reorganize the practice of abdominal organ procurement in the region of southern Bavaria. Until September 1993, only a team of surgeons for the retrieval of donor kidneys in the region had been established and organized by the transplant head office in Munich. When multiple organ donors were reported, the procurement of other abdominal organs (liver, pancreas) was carried out by the retrieval team of the transplant program to which the respective organ had been allocated by Eurotransplant, Leiden (ET). As a consequence, all three departments with active transplant programs for liver and/or pancreas were forced to run an individual "on-call" schedule for the procurement of organs potentially offered to them by ET, and so, at any given time, up to nine surgeons and perfusion technicians were on-call simultaneously. When organs from the southern Bavarian region had been allocated to recipients of remote transplant programs, the respective centers had to organize for their own procurement teams to travel to the donor hospital in southern Bavaria. For the donor hospital, this could lead to the following typical scenario: A 27-year-old male is confirmed dead from brain trauma. The next of kin (wife and parents) agree to multiple organ donation and the donor is reported via the transplant office in Munich to ET. The liver is allocated to a high-urgency recipient in Berlin, the pancreas is accepted by a team from Brussels, and the heart/lung is accepted by a center in Munich. Procurement commences after all the teams have organized and confirmed their participation. The local kidney team (two surgeons, and a perfusion technician) begin with the removal of the kidney. The heart-lung team arrives (two surgeons and two technicians), perform a bronchoscopy, and then open the chest and inspect the lung and heart. The liver team then arrives (two surgeons, one technician, and one visiting doctor from abroad), the surgeons scrub, and inspect the liver anatomy and quality. Finally, the pancreas team arrives (two surgeons and one technician), the surgeons scrub, and inspect the pancreas. Discussions on preferred means of cannulation, techniques of retrieval, anatomical variations, length of desired vascular structures, and who will do what and when follow. The Theater nurse is confronted with a variety of different requests for material and instruments and the anesthetist is confronted with a variety of (redundant) questions on donor condition, plus various requests for blood samples, specific drug applications, etc. Technicians and organizing personnel from each team require (repeated!) telephone contact to their own centers. It is obvious, that such a complex procurement scenario is highly demanding for the resources of the donor hospital, aside from the problems of cost and timing of transportation for each individual team. In addition, even with optimal cooperation of teams, a prolongation of the procedure is inevitable.

Thus, it was planned to establish a collaborative procurement team for all abdominal organs in the region of southern Bavaria. This team was to be centrally organized by the transplant head office in Munich and was to be responsible for the retrieval of organs both for regional use and for "export" to other ET centers.

Material and methods

In order to realize a regionalized procurement, a 24-hour, on-call schedule was designed as follows: (1) one surgeon "group I" (= qualified to remove all abdominal organs), (2) one surgeon "group II" (= qualified to remove kidneys only), (3) one surgeon "group III" (= qualified to assist in above operations), and (4) one perfusion technician. The surgeons were derived from the teams of all three active transplant centers in the region and were stratified according to their surgical skills into Groups I–III to participate in the on-call duties in weekly rotations. Reimbursement and insurance were standardized and taken care of by the transplant head office. In any given donor situation, a team of normally two surgeons and the perfusion technician would be transfered to the donor hospital to perform the necessary procurement. If desired, technical requirements could be discussed with the recipient hospitals in advance. Timing of the procurement and shipping of the organs was also organized by the transplant head office and the details of all procurement activities were documented there prospectively.

In order to be able to assess the opinions of the executives of the regional donor hospitals, as well as to inform them about the new concept of regionalized organ procurement, a survey was performed. A personal letter of information accompanied by a questionnaire was mailed to the clinic directors and heads of intensive care units in 46 representative donor hospitals in the region of southern Bavaria. The questionnaire allowed the candidates to: (1) express their approval/disapproval of the new concept on a scale of 1 to 5 ("very favorable … indifferent … unfavorable), (2) to express in more detail what they considered to be the main advantages of the new concept by checking appropriate boxes, (3) to choose one or multiple items from a list of factors that might help to improve donor activity in their domain of responsibility, and (4) to make individual comments or requests. The questionnaires were anonymous unless the candidates wished to identify themselves.

Table 1 Abdominal organ procurement in the region of southern Bavaria from September 1993 to August 1995 (*MOD* multiple organ donors)

Time period	Kidneys	Livers	Pancreata[a]	MOD
9/93–8/94	167	35	11	46/87 = 53 %
9/94–8/95	174	47	14	62/92 = 67 %
Total	341	82	25	108/179 = 60 %

[a] Only pancreata for solid organ transplantation listed

Results

In the two years following the introduction of the new retrieval concept, a total of 179 organ donors were reported to the transplant office from 30 different hospitals. The figures for the time periods September 1993 to August 1994 and September 1994 to August 1995 are given in Table 1.

In addition to these regional procurement activities, the retrieval team had to travel to remote regions in order to explant livers allocated to one of the regional centers (Klinikum Großhadern der LMU/Klinikum Rechts der Isar der TU) on 35 occasions in the 2-year period. When the activities of the year 1994 were analyzed, the procurement teams had to perform, on average, slightly more than two operations per week, but the distribution of activities was rather wide. It ranged from no procurements in 7 out of 52 weeks, to four to seven procedures in 10 out of 52 weeks, with an intermediate pensum of one to three procurements in 35 out of 52 weeks.

In the period between September 1993 and August 1994, 20 locally procured livers were shipped to other centers in the ET region to which the organs had been allocated. On three occasions, remote transplant teams insisted on traveling to the southern Bavarian region to perform the judgement of organ suitability and retrieval themselves (in two of these occasions, the organs were rejected for medical reasons). In the period between September 1994 and August 1995, 47 livers were procured locally by our team and of these, 29 (62 %) were shipped to other destinations, and in no case did foreign teams express reluctance to rely on our judgement of organ viability or our technique of organ retrieval.

From the questionnaires mailed to the regional donor hospitals, 26/46 (57 %) were returned within 8 weeks and formed the basis of this evaluation. Concerning the general approval of regionalization, 26/26 (100 %) chose grades 4 and 5 of the answering scale and, thus, expressed a high level of appreciation of the new concept. The results of the evaluation of the detailed questions are as follows. What are, in your opinion, the main (potential) advantages of the proposed new concept of regionalization of organ procurement (multiple answers possible):

1. Organizational simplification	89 %
2. Operating theater relief	69 %
3. Less disturbance in donor hospital	52 %
4. Procurement teams familiar to donor hospitals	58 %
5. Possible cost reduction for donor hospital	23 %

Which measures could, in your opinion, help to further increase donor availability in the future (multiple answers possible):

1. More information/educational activities	42 %
2. Transplant law /clearer legislation	81 %
3. Better media representation	46 %
4. Higher reimbursements for donor hospitals	4 %

In addition, 7/26 (27 %) of the hospital executives who answered the questionnaire took the opportunity of making individual remarks and comments. These were as follows:

1. General practitioners need more information on transplantation and organ donation.
2. More information material must be distributed to the public.
3. Young doctors need better education on donor conditioning.
4. The potential donor's relatives are frequently hesitant to agree to organ donation.
5. Failure to define a clear transplantation law discourages doctors from asking for permission for organ retrieval.
6. Disasterous media coverage on questions of brain death and organ trade raises doubts.
7. Sometimes there is a lack of respect toward the deceased donor by the procurement teams.

The actual overall cost savings that could be achieved after the implementation of the regionalized procurement concept were not evaluated in this study, but the significant reduction in the number of surgeons and technicians on call, as well as the fact that numerous transplants exported to other regions were shipped by regular airline services, suggests that significant savings could be made.

Discussion

Until very recently, the procurement of multiorgan donors lacked characteristics of rationalization, in that, for the retrieval of abdominal organs alone, up to three teams with three or four members each traveled to the donor hospital. This is not only a great strain on material resources (transport costs, costs for the procurement team labor, etc.), but in addition often proved to be a serious source of disturbance for the local donor hospital. On the other hand, techniques of organ preservation and retrieval have progressed [1–4], and results of recent publications [5–7] as well as personal communications on various occasions indicated a growing tendency of centers to agree on common standards of judgement on organ quality and procurement techniques not only for the kidney, but also for the liver and pancreas. This lead to our new concept of regionalization of organ procurement, which was implemented in the region of southern Bavaria in September 1993 and has been in effect since then. Its main characteristics are a collaborative "on-call" schedule with participants of all active transplant programs in the region, stratified according to their level of surgical skill. This team should be responsible for virtually any procurement of abdominal organs in the region and would make it unneccessary for foreign teams to have to travel to the region of southern Bavaria to procure organs allocated to them. Instead, organs would be procured locally by a standardized technique and shipped to their final destination, preferably by regular airline services. The possible advantages of this concept are mainly: (1) simplification of organization and timing of procurements, (2) a significant reduction in personnel resources by avoiding redundant on-call schedules and an unnecessary multitude of transplant surgeons participating in the procurement procedure, (3) advantages from the viewpoint of donor hospitals by simplifying the event of multiorgan donation, and (4) additional financial savings by the preferred use of regular airline carriers for the shipment of organs, rather than chartered aircrafts for the whole procurement team [8].

The experiences with our concept of regionalized organ procurement have been positive throughout. There were no serious complaints from remote centers about the quality of imported organs, and the fact that, in the second year, no foreign team insisted on participating in the procurement of livers or pancreata allocated to them is a good indicator of agreement on retrieval standards. As a further measure of quality control, a follow-up form has been designed for liver grafts and this is shipped along with every organ; the results of this prospective assessment will be published in the near future. The response of (potential) donor hospitals in our region has been very positive, as can be concluded from the results of the survey: organizational simplification, relief of operating theaters, and avoidance of disturbance in the hospital are all considered important

points. In addition, it seems to be of advantage to the donor hospitals to know the teams (and the transplant centers in charge) personally. For the donor hospitals, the argument of cost reduction seems to play a less important role, as indicated by only 29 % of positive answers in this regard. On the other hand, it was very informative to learn about the attitude toward other measures with potential positive effect on organ donation. The urgent need for a comprehensive and clear transplant law in Germany is expressed by 81 % of those responding to our questionnaire and is in good agreement with previous reports [9–11]. Further efforts in education of both the public and of medical professionals, and a better media representation were cited by 42 % and 46 % of candidates, respectively, and this underlines the necessity of ongoing activities in this regard. Nevertheless, the discrepancy between the declared support of organ donation and actual consent rates is a known phenomenon [12, 13]. Again, the improvement in financial reimbursements of donor hospitals seems to be of subordinate importance and was mentioned in only 4 % of forms and, thus, does not reflect the situation in the USA [14].

In conclusion, our new concept of regionalization of organ procurement proved to be effective in achieving a high quality of organ retrieval with, at the same time, a reduction of personnel requirements for the transplant centers. In addition, the response of donor hospitals was positive and may, thus, positively influence donor activity in the future. The evaluation of the survey helped to identify problems and give directions for possible improvements in the cooperation of transplant centers and donor hospitals, and future activities. Also, it informed the donor hospitals about the new concept. Relevant financial savings can result from reduced on-call duties and minimized traveling costs; this will be evaluated in more detail in the future. Further attempts to rationalize organ procurement could possibly include heart(-/lung)surgeons in the regionalized teams or even the delegation of thoracic organ retrieval into the responsibility of one multiorgan retrieval team.

Acknowledgements The authors wish to thank all participating donor hospitals as well as the numerous members of the local procurement team and the team of the local transplant office.

References

1. Dunn DL, Morel P, Schlumpf R, Mayoral JL, Gillingham KJ, Moudry-Munns KC, Krom RA, Gruessner RW, Payne WD, Sutherland DE, et al (1991) Evidence that combined procurement of pancreas and liver grafts does not affect transplant outcome. Transplantation 51 (1): 150–157

2. D'Alessandro AM, Sollinger HW, Hoffmann RW, Kalayoglu M, Melzer JS, Reed A, Knechtle SJ, Pirsch JD, Belzer FO (1990) Experience with combined hepatic, pancreaticoduodenal, and renal procurement with UW solution. Transplant Proc 22 (4): 2076–2076

3. Gubernatis G (1989) Techniques of organ procurement and preservation of liver and pancreas. Baillieres Clin Gastroenterol 3 (4): 799–811

4. Marsh CL, Perkins JD, Sutherland DE, Corry RJ, Sterioff S (1989) Combined hepatic and pancreaticoduodenal procurement for transplantation. Surg Gynecol Obstet 168 (3): 254–258

5. Miller CM, Teodorescu V, Harrington M, Harrington EB, Schwartz ME, Ambrosina G, Kadian M, Sampson J (1990) Regional procurement and export of hepatic allografts for transplantation. M Sinai J Med NY 57 (2): 93–96

6. Langnas AN, Duckworth RM, Stratta RJ, Wood RP, Rikkers LF, Marujo W, Grazi GL, Pillen TJ, Shaw BW Jr (1990) Imported hepatic allografts: a single center experience. Transplant Proc 22 (2): 414–415

7. Jonas S, Bechstein WO, Keck H, Blumhardt G, Lemmens HP, Neuhaus P (1993) Transplantation of shipped donor livers. Transplant Int 6 (4): 206–208

8. Langnas AN, Stratta RJ, Marujo WC, Wood RP, Duckworth RM, Shaw BW Jr (1991) Imported hepatic allografts: use of commercial airlines for transport. Transplant Proc 23 (5): 2319

9. Gnant MF, Wamser P, Goetzinger P, Sautner T, Steininger R, Muehlbacher F (1991) The impact of the presumed consent law and a decentralized organ procurement system on organ donation: quadruplication in the number of organ donors. Transplant Proc 23 (5): 2685–2686

10. Roels L, Coosemans W, Christiaens M-R, Waer M, Vanrenterghem Y (1995) The relative impact of legislative incentives on multi-organ donation rates in Europe. Transplant Proc 27 (1): 795–796

11. Bauer H (1992) Organ donation to hospitals not specializing in transplantation. Langenbecks Arch Chir Suppl Kongressbd pp 238–242

12. Schütt GR, Smit H, Duncker G (1995) Huge discrepancy between declared support of organ donation and actual rate of consent for organ retrieval. Transplant Proc 27 (1): 1450–1451

13. Wakeford RE, Stepney R (1989) Obstacles to organ donation. Br J Surg 76 (5): 436–439

14. Evans RW (1993) Organ procurement expenditures and the role of financial incentives. J Am Med Assoc 269 (24): 3113–3118, 3155–3156

Transpl Int (1996) 9 [Suppl 1]: S 469–S 471
© Springer-Verlag 1996

S. Agnes
A. W. Avolio
S. C. Magalini
G. Grieco
M. Castagneto

Marginal donors for patients on regular waiting lists for liver transplantation

S. Agnes (✉) · A. W. Avolio · S. C. Magalini
G. Grieco · M. Castagneto
Department of Surgery – Division of Organ
Transplantation, Catholic University,
Policlinico Gemelli, Largo Gemelli 8,
00168, Rome, Italy

Abstract The use of marginal donors is well accepted by most centers for emergency situations, but there is debate on their use for patients on regular waiting lists. We report our experience of the 1-year survival for patients on waiting lists ($n = 147$, 1-year survival = 32 %), patients transplanted from good donors ($n = 60$, 1-year survival = 84 %), and patients transplanted from marginal donors ($n = 15$, 1-year survival = 56 %). We concluded that liver transplantation from marginal donors (a) is a safe procedure (b) has a 1-year survival that is significantly better than that on a waiting list (c) is ethically justified especially in countries with donor shortages, and (d) may allow transplantation of "special" high risk and poor long-term outcome patients.

Key words Liver waiting list · Marginal donor · Donor shortage · Donor selection criteria · Liver transplantation

Introduction

Worldwide the waiting lists for solid organ transplants are steadily but constantly lengthening because of the enlarging spectrum of indications and the increasing number of patients with end-stage organ failure. Unfortunately, the number of donors does not match that of recipients, and a large number of patients awaiting transplantation die while on a waiting list [1]. This has lead to a broadening of donor acceptance criteria, and in the 1990s the term "marginal donor" entered the transplant terminology. Originally, the term was used to indicate only donors over 55 years of age [2, 3], but it is now used to indicate all donors with relevant alterations to one or more data relative to "classical" acceptance criteria [4–6]. Results from large series in terms of graft and patient survival after transplantation with these organs seem encouraging [7, 8], and it seems probable that in the future these organs will be used to transplant patients on regular waiting lists. In a retrospective study we analyzed data from 75 consecutive donor-recipient pairs transplanted in our center in an effort to identify the relations between donor quality and recipient outcome.

Patients and methods

Data from 75 consecutive donor-recipient liver pairs were analyzed to define if and how donor conditions influence 1-year graft survival after liver transplantation. Organs were allocated by the Nord Italia Transplant Program (NITp) on the basis of a national liver transplant waiting list. The policy of the transplant center of the Catholic University of Rome in the past excluded the possibility of accepting donors over 55 years of age, non-heart-beating donors, or overweight donors, so no donors with these characteristics are present in the donor group. The donor parameters we chose to analyze to discriminate "good" and "marginal" donors were the following: systolic pressure, urinary output, bilirubin levels, ALT/AST levels, prothrombin time, serum sodium level, PaO_2, and intensive care unit stay (Table 1). According to these criteria two groups were defined: Group I, good donors (GD: $n = 60$), in which all hemodynamic parameters and chemistry data were within the normal range or that presented a single minor alteration in one (i. e., < 2 times the standard deviation from the normal range) and group II, marginal donors (MD: $n = 15$), that presented one single major alteration (i. e., > 2 times the standard deviation from the normal range of the parameter studied) or multiple minor alterations.

The outcome of recipients was compared in relation to donor status (good donors group vs marginal donors group) by Kaplan Meier life table analysis at 1–12 months. For the statistical evaluation the Cox Mantel test and the log rank test were used.

S 470

Table 1 Donor parameters used to discriminate good and marginal donors

	Minor alteration	Major alteration
Systolic blood pressure (mmHg)	< 70 for 1 h	< 50 for 1 h
Urinary output	Oliguria	Anuria
Bilirubin (mg/dl)	Up to 2	> 2
ALT and/or AST (IU/dl)	Up to 150	> 150
Prothrombin time (%)	Down to 50 %	< 50 %
Na + (mEq/l)	Up to 160	> 160
PaO$_2$ (mmHg)	< 80	< 60
ICU stay (days)	3–7	> 7

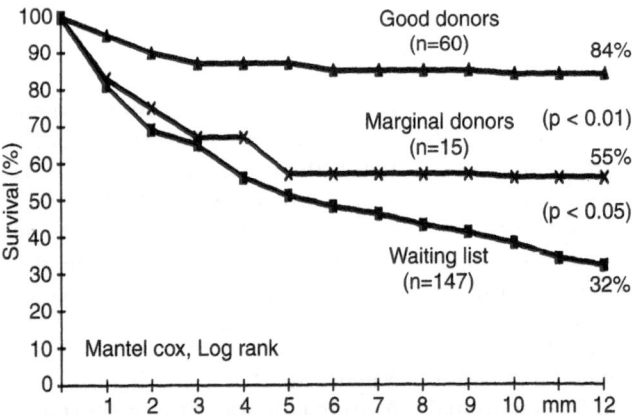

Fig. 1 One to 12-months survival by Kaplan-Meier life table analysis for patients transplanted with good donors *(triangle)*, marginal donors *(cross)*, and on the waiting list *(square)*

Results

One-year survival was 32 % for patients on the waiting list (*n* = 147) and 76 % for patients who underwent liver transplantation (*n* = 75). The difference in the 1-year survival rate was significant (*P* < 0.01). The difference in 1-year graft survival between patients who received livers from good donors (84 %, *n* = 60) and patients who received livers from marginal donors (56 %, *n* = 15) was also significant. The *P* values were: Cox Mantel *P* = 0.038, log rank *p* = 0.047 (Fig. 1).

Discussion

Liver transplantation is the current therapeutic choice for end-stage liver failure, but the number of donors available does not match number of patients on the waiting lists. In Italy, among European countries, the problem is more critical because of the lower number of donors per million inhabitants (7 vs 15 in France, vs 17 in the United Kingdom, vs 25 in Spain, vs 14 in Eurotransplant, and vs 17 in Northern Europe).

The use of marginal donors is well accepted by most centers for emergency situations (i. e., fulminant liver failure or retransplantation), but there is still debate on their use for patients on regular waiting lists. This is understandable when one considers that the 1-year survival figures of 70–80 % (with variability due to center effect, patient age, disease pattern and immunosuppressive protocols) for regular donors are 10–20 % less for marginal donors (older age, alterations in liver tests, overweight, prolonged ischemia time). It must be kept in mind, however, that in Italy the 1-year mortality on the waiting list reaches almost 70 %.

In a recent analysis of donor acceptance policies conducted in 80 centers registered with the European Liver Transplant Group [5] 38 % of marginal donors were accepted (33–50 % in relation to different countries) for patients on regular waiting lists, 20 % were accepted only with additional information (e. g., histological reports), 17 % were accepted only for emergencies, and 23 % were refused.

The definition of "marginal donors" in our series was very restrictive since donors over 55 years of age and those who were overweight were not accepted. The indexes used to define the two groups were chosen on the basis of previous reports on the quantification of liver damage and prediction of survival after transplantation, showing these parameters to be precisely discriminative among survival curves [9, 10]. It is possible that the donors that we defined as marginal may not be so classified by others with even less strict selection criteria [8]. However, the strict criteria we used made the difference in the 1-year patient survival between recipients of good or marginal donors even more evident. This difference can only be amplified even further when the acceptance criteria are widened.

The systematic use of marginal or nonoptimal donors could present three main effects: (a) the donor pool will be enlarged at least by 15–25 %; (b) the overall survival after liver transplantation will probably decrease more or less by 5–10 %; (c) a 10–15 % difference in the 1-year survival will be evident between transplants from regular and marginal donors. On the other hand, current survival data of patients transplanted from marginal donors are much better than those observed in selected groups of patients who are transplanted over the age of 65 years, who have hepatic tumors, or who have multiple organ failure. These patients are considered by most transplant centers to be at higher risk, as are also patients who are likely to present with a recurrence of pre-existing disease (hepatitis or liver cancer). Marginal donors could be used to transplant these patients considering the odds of an already biased survival rate.

In conclusion, our data demonstrated an advantage in the enlargement of the donor pool by using marginal donors, but the specific decision on who should be assigned a nonoptimal liver remains an open question.

References

1. 1993 Annual Report of the US Scientific Registry of Transplant Recipients and the Organ Procurement and Transplantation Network (1993) Transplant data 1988–91. Appendix H: Deaths on the waiting list. H2
2. Roels L, Vabrenterghem Y, Waer M, et al (1990) The aging kidney donor: another answer to organ shortage? Transplant Proc 22: 368
3. Pettersen G, Berglin E, Berggren WO, et al (1990) Are older donors acceptable for heart transplantation? Transplant Proc 22: 247
4. Alexander JW, Vaughn WK (1991) The use of marginal donors for organ transplantation: the influence of donor age on outcome. Transplantation 51: 135
5. Mirza DF, Gunson BK, Da Silva R, et al (1994) Policies in Europe on "marginal quality" donor livers. Lancet 344: 1480
6. Pruim H, Klompmaker IJ, Haagsma EB, et al (1993) Selection criteria for liver donation: a review. Transplant Int 6: 226–35
7. Temperman L, Podesta L, Mieles L, et al (1989) The successful use of older donors for liver transplantation. JAMA 262: 2837
8. Mor E, Klintman GB, Gonwa TA, et al (1992) The use of marginal donors for liver transplantation: a retrospective study of 365 liver donors. Transplantation 53: 383–386
9. Avolio AW, Agnes S, Magalini SC, Nanni G, Castagneto M (1992) "Recovery index" a useful tool for quantification of liver injury after liver transplantation and prediction of one year survival. Transplant Proc 24: 2707–2708
10. Avolio AW, Agnes S, Magalini SC, Nanni G, Castagneto M (1993) Quantification of liver damage and prediction of one-year survival after liver transplantation by a multifactorial "recovery score". Transplant Proc 25: 1868–1869

Transpl Int (1996) 9 [Suppl 1]: S472–S476
© Springer-Verlag 1996

R. Lange
J. Erhard
U. Rauen
A. Hellinger
H. de Groot
F. W. Eigler

Injury to hepatocytes and non-parenchymal cells during the preservation of human livers with UW or HTK solution: a determination of hepatocellular enzymes in the effluent perfusate for preoperative evaluation of the transplant quality

R. Lange (✉) · J. Erhard · A. Hellinger ·
F. W. Eigler
Department of General Surgery,
University Clinic of Essen,
Hufelandstrasse 55, 45122 Essen, Germany

U. Rauen · H. de Groot
Institute of Physiological Chemistry,
University Clinic of Essen,
Hufelandstrasse 55, 45122 Essen, Germany

Abstract In 50 livers harvested for transplantation, injury was assessed by determination of the enzymes in the effluent perfusate after cold ischemia. The results were compared to the histology and the clinical course after transplantation. Whereas the release of the markers of endothelial cell injury did neither correlate with the history of the graft nor with the postoperative course, the release of hepatocellular enzymes in the perfusate did indicate preexisting damage of the liver even when the biopsy showed normal liver tissue. Of 12 livers with high activity of hepatocellular enzymes in the effluent (activity of more than twice the median), 7 showed delayed onset of function or a primary non-function. In the other 38 livers with an enzyme activity below this borderline no delayed function or primary non-function was observed. Because of additional influences a prognosis of the function after transplantation was not possible, but the determination of the enzymes in the effluent of marginal livers probably allows the preoperative recognition of organs which will do well.

Key words Graft preservation · Cell injury · Graft function

Introduction

For pre- and perioperative prognostic evaluation of transplant function, there are only investigations describing statistical probabilities deduced from different single factors. These evaluations are not able to predict satisfactory or good function in the individual case [5, 8, 16]. Postoperative graft function is primarily influenced by the quality of the donor organ and preexisting injury. The extent of preservation injury has until now only been shown in experimental studies [1, 15]. In rat livers, which were preserved with Euro-Collins and University of Wisconsin organ preservation (UW) solutions, a predominant injury to the endothelium was found after cold ischemia [4]. This result was confirmed for the human liver by examination of 21 UW- or HTK-perfused grafts [12].

The results of this study suggested it may be possible to estimate the "quality" of the transplant and predict the graft function by the activity of hepatocellular enzymes in the effluent of the preserved organ at the end of the cold ischemia time. To evaluate this parameter we looked for a correlation between enzyme activity at the end of the cold ischemia time and the postoperative graft function in 50 livers, which were harvested and preserved for transplantation.

Materials and methods

For this retrospective study, 50 livers were examined in a 10-month period. The livers were harvested for transplantation in the transplant center of Essen. The interval of cold ischemia times enclosed a period from 6 to 16 hours with a mean value of 13.2 hours. Thirty-nine livers were perfused with UW solution and 11 with HTK solution. Depending on the preservation solution primarily used, the livers were rinsed again at the beginning of the back table preparation with 500 ml UW or HTK solution. The perfusion was performed via a balloon catheter placed in the portal vein [7, 9]. During perfusion, the infrahepatic vena cava was clamped. From the first 100 ml of effluent from the liver veins, three 10 ml portions (P 1–3) were collected. The collected samples were stored at 4 °C and centrifuged as soon as possible (900 × g for 10 min at 4 °C). In the supernatant, the enzymes lactate dehydrogenase (LDH), aspartate transaminase (AST), alanine transaminase (ALT), glutamate dehydrogenase (GLDH) and creatine kinase (CK) were measured by standard methods [2]. Thrombomodulin was determined by ELISA (Diagnostica Stago, Asnières sur Seine, France). An aliquot of the supernatant was deproteinised and used for the measurement of glucose [2]. The relative release of the endothelial and hepatocellular enzymes was measured as described in [12].

The back table preparation was done simultaneously to the hepatectomy of the recipient. Thus, the period between the collection of the effluent samples and the beginning of warm ischemia (start of the implantation of the graft) was no longer than 40–80 min. The warm ischemia time was 60 min on average (40–70 min.) During the warm ischemia time another perfusion was performed with 500 ml Ringer's solution (2 %, 20 °C) in the case of UW-perfused organs. The HTK-perfused grafts were rinsed with 500 ml of cold HTK solution.

All 50 livers were biopsied after reperfusion (0-biopsy) for histological examination. The tissue was studied for preexisting damage and for alterations resulting from the harvesting procedure and the preservation. In addition, the determination of LDH and the transaminases was performed 24 h after reperfusion.

For the estimation of graft function, the parameters of liver synthesis (thromboplastin time, partial thrombin time, thrombin time, and fibrinogen) and the clinical course were documented for the first five postoperative days. An initial non-function (INF) was defined as the need for intensive care treatment with ventilation, increasing circulatory instability, and the necessity of substitution of the coagulation factors. Delayed graft function was said to be present if the stabilization of the patient and the normalization of the biochemical parameters was not observed earlier than 48 h after transplantation [6, 7]. The statistical evaluation was done using Student's t-test, the significance being fixed at $P < 0.05$.

Results

The highest activities of the enzymes LDH, AST, ALT, CK, and GLDH can be measured in the first three 10 ml samples (P 1–3), as shown in the former study [12]. Here, the averages of these three samples were determined (Table 1). The median of enzyme activity in the effluent of HTK-perfused organs was twice the activity of UW-perfused. The correlation between LDH as a marker of the global injury and AST and ALT as markers of hepatocellular damage was high ($r = 0.984$ for AST, $r = 0.927$ for ALT), but there was no correlation between the hepatocellular enzymes and GLDH. GLDH activity varied in the different organs between 0 and 1142 U/l.

There was no significant correlation between the length of cold ischemia time and the activity of the hepatocellular enzymes (the median for the grafts with high LDH activity was 13.3 h (Table 2), the median of the grafts with moderate enzyme activity was 12 h. Two grafts with good postoperative function had a phase of circulatory instability and depression in the donor his-

Table 1 Enzyme activity in the effluent while rinsing during back table preparation. UW-preserved livers were rinsed with 500 ml UW solution, HTK-preserved livers with 500 ml HTK solution. The samples were collected from the liver veins. The median values of the first 30 ml were presented (with minima and maxima)

	UW	HTK
LDH (U/l)	1635 (183–23250)	3070 (223–21250)
AST (U/l)	403 (9–6050)	880 (45–5505)
ALT (U/l)	324 (7–5434)	712 (38–4907)
GLDH (U/l)	18 (0–1142)	58 (6–148)
CK (U/l)	120 (9–461)	233 (100–446)
Thrombomodulin (ng/ml)	67 (0–2286)	142 (44–440)

tory (liver: PA, GR). These organs had high activity of the markers of hepatocellular damage as a sign of an additional ischemic reaction. Another reason for high enzyme activity in the effluent was the splitting of the organ in the cold ischemia time (liver: ME) (Table 2).

All livers with abnormalities concerning histology, perfusate enzyme activity (LDH > 3300 U/l for UW-preserved organs and > 6100 U/l for HTK-preserved organs), or function (delayed function or primary nonfunction) are summarized in Table 2. An LDH activity of 3300 U/l in UW-preserved organs and 6100 U/l in HTK-preserved organs is double the activity of the median of LDH activity in the total number of preserved organs. Out of 12 livers with LDH values above this borderline, 5 showed an initial non-function after transplantation and 2 developed a delayed function. The other 38 livers with LDH activities below the borderline did not show a functional disorder (Fig. 1). Two out of 6 livers with histological changes in the 0-biopsy had an initial non-function, but 3 of 44 livers with a normal biopsy also had an initial non-function. In 2 organs classified as normal, the function was delayed. The markers of endothelial damage, creatine kinase and thrombomodulin, showed a different course to the hepatocellular enzymes. They were neither increased in the case of preexisting damage of the organ nor did they show a correlation to the postoperative function. Although in the majority of the livers the relative release of creatine kinase was higher than the relative release of the hepatocellular enzymes, the activity of creatine kinase did not correlate to the period of cold ischemia.

In the effluent of all livers we measured high concentrations of glucose. Glucose concentrations were significantly higher in the UW-preserved organs (median for glucose concentration in UW-preserved organs: 23.3 mM, in HTK-preserved organs 11.7 mM, $P = 0.0085$).

Table 2 Liver enzyme activity in back table rinse correlated to histology and to postoperative graft function. Presented are all organs with peculiarities in effluent, histology, or function. Of three HTK-preserved livers with LDH activities over 6100 U/l and nine UW-preserved livers with LDH activities over 3300 U/l, five showed an initial non-function and two a delayed function. Two out of 5 livers with a pathological histology in 0-biopsy developed an initial non-function (*CIT* cold ischemia time, *INF* initial non-function, *o. k.* satisfactory)

Liver	Preservation solution	CIT (h)	LDH (U/l) (P 1–3)	Anamnesis of the donor	Histology	LDH (U/l) (24 h)	Function
KO	HTK	13	2670	32 years, CCT, o. k.	**Severe harvesting lesion**	746	o. k.
SL	UW	12	1526	52 years, ICB	**50 % fatty degeneration**	673	o. k.
OM	UW	14.5	**5317**	35 years, CCT, o. k.	Fatty degeneration < 5 %, o. B.	761	o. k.
PA	UW	13.5	**9150**	18 years, cerebral tumor AST 85 U/l, ALT 195 U/l, resuscitation	o. k.	1464	o. k.
ME	UW	16	**27650**	21 years, CO$_2$ intoxication, split liver	o. k.	857	o. k.
GR	HTK	16	**21125**	48 years, Carotis occlusion, noradrenaline	**Exogenous toxic liver damage, fatty, degeneration 15 %**	1275	o. k.
LY	UW	12.5	**5628**	25 years, CCT, o. k.	**Harvesting lesion °II, fatty degeneration < 10 %**	926	o. k.
SM	UW	10	**25925**	45 years, ICB, resuscitation	o. k.	3650	**Delayed**
CO	UW	7	**16183**	53 years, CCT, AST 700 U/l, alcohol anamnesis, bleeding, shock	< 15 % fatty degeneration	2510	**Delayed**
KL	UW	13	**5140**	20 years, CCT, o. k.	o. k.	3879	Arterial occlusion, INF
FE	HTK	14.5	**16200**	57 years, ICB resuscitation, alcohol anamnesis	o. k.	9276	**INF**
MS	UW	6	**3618**	48 years, ICB, o. k.	Parenchyma o. k., conspicuous vascularization	4870	**INF**
BE	HTK	14	**7377**	23 years, CCT, AST 95 U/l	**Exogenous toxic liver damage, fatty degeneration 5 %**	9250	**INF**
WO	UW	7	**4277**	69 years, ICB, LDH 4200 U/l, sod 163 mval/l	**30 % hepatocyte necrosis**	5055	**INF**

Discussion

The enzyme activity in the effluent samples can comprise the injury of a preserved liver until the end of cold ischemia, i.e. the damages occurring during the cold ischemia time, but also preexisting injury can aggravate the ischemic injury. The effluent of HTK-preserved livers shows a significantly higher level of enzyme activity than the effluent of UW-preserved organs. This might be the result of the different viscosities of the two solutions giving better rinsing of the liver with HTK solution [12]. Preexisting damage, for example, instability of circulation [liver: GR, PA, FE], as well as damage acquired during the cold ischemia time [liver: ME], gives rise to a clear increase in the activity of LDH, AST, and ALT in the effluent. The release of GLDH is delayed because of the intramitochondrial localization of this enzyme. This delay in release might account for the lack of correlation of GLDH activity with the other enzyme activity.

Comparing the findings of the histology and of the effluent samples with the graft function, it was remarkable that in all cases of initial non-function and delayed function the effluent samples showed high enzyme activity. On the contrary, the histological examination only yielded pathological results in two out of seven livers (graft: CO, SM, FE, KL, and MS). So the sensivity of the effluent samples in the prediction of poor function was higher than the prediction based on the histology (100 % : 29 %). This might result from the delay with which insults lead to morphological alterations of the tissue.

As shown in Table 2, high enzyme activity in the effluent samples does not necessarily induce a malfunc-

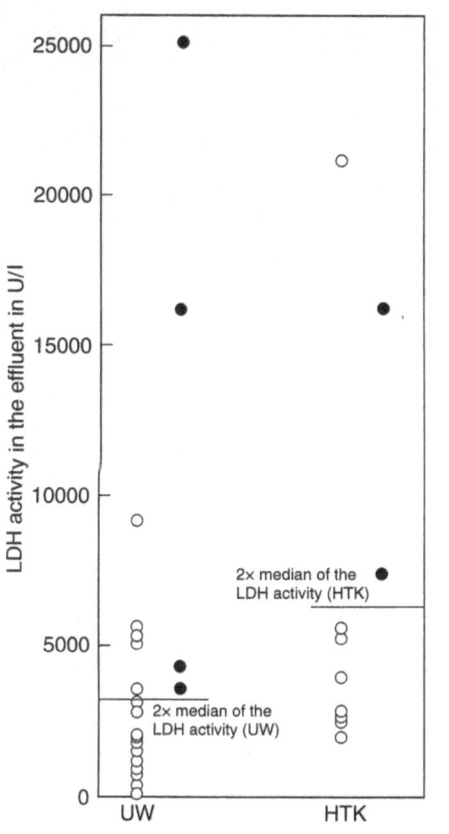

Fig. 1 LDH activities in the effluent in comparison to graft function, the values for UW- (*n* = 39) and HTK-preserved organs (*n* = 11) are presented separately. The borderline between normal LDH activity and increased liberation was set at twice the median of all activity (for UW 3300 U/l, for HTK 6100 U/l). The borderlines are indicated by *lines*. (*INF* initial non-function)

time, circulatory insufficiency, infection, and rejection [16]. Unfortunately, a "good" liver may slide into nonfunction for such reasons. Conversely, a transplantation without any problems may develop successfully even with a graft that had a history of damage [5].

All earlier investigations, which wanted to predict graft function by donor criteria, recipient risks, or function tests, were unsuccessful in predicting the outcome for the individual case [5, 6, 14, 16]. Similarly, it is not possible to exclude errors in prediction based on the effluent samples, but low LDH, AST, and ALT activity indicates a high probability that sufficient graft function will follow a transplantation without major complications.

As reported earlier [11, 12], in the effluent of preserved livers, high levels of activity of CK-BB and thrombomodulin can be demonstrated, showing significant damage to endothelial cells [3, 10, 13, 17, 18]. Surprisingly, this damage to endothelial cells, which in the majority of the livers is greater than the hepatocellular damage, does not correlate to graft function [13, 14]. This suggests that the hepatocellular damage is the limiting factor for graft function [11].

In conclusion, the effluent samples were a sensible marker for preexisting damage or damage acquired during cold ischemia. Additionally, the effluent samples give a helpful parameter for the decision to transplant a marginal organ. The test can be performed during back table preparation before the recipient hepatectomy is started. In our study, when there was low enzyme activity in the effluent samples an initial non-function was not seen. In our opinion, low effluent enzyme activity therefore suggests that the risk of graft failure due to donor problems can be excluded. Nevertheless, the prognosis for the transplant finally depends on the course of the operation and the condition of the recipient.

Acknowledgements The study was supported by the Deutsche Forschungsgemeinschaft, (Gr 815/6-1).

tion of the graft (liver: ME, PA, GR), but the danger of a dysfunction is increased significantly (42 %). Specifity is relatively low in comparison to sensivity (42 % : 100 %). This is probably caused by the high influence of additional factors that might affect the organ after determination of the effluent samples, e.g., warm ischemia

References

1. Aminalai A, Kehrer G, Großmann F, Richter J, Bretschneider HJ (1992) Morphological investigations of porcine liver directly following preservation with Euro-Collins, University of Wisconsin and Bretschneider's HTK-solution. Langenbecks Arch Chir 377: 81–88
2. Bergmeyer HU (1974) Methoden der enzymatischen Analyse. Verlag Chemie, Weinheim

3. Boffa MC, Karochkine M, Bérard M (1991) Plasma thrombomodulin as a marker of endothelium damage. Nouv Rev Hematol 33: 529–530
4. Caldwell-Kenkel JC, Currin RT, Tanaka Y, Thurman RG, Lemasters JJ (1991) Kupffer cell activation and endothelial cell damage after storage of rat livers: effect of reperfusion. Hepatology 13: 83–95

5. Doyle HR, Marino IR, Jabbour N, Zetti G, McMichael J, Mitchell S, Fung J, Starzl TE (1994) Early death or retransplantation in adults after orthotopic liver transplantation. Transplantation 57: 1028–1036
6. Erhard J, Lange R, Gersing E, Scherer R, Gebhard MM, Sanchez P, Bretschneider HJ (1993) Die Impedanzmessung zur Beurteilung von Ischämieschäden der humanen Leber in der Vorbereitung zur Transplantation. Langenbecks Arch Chir 378: 233–238

7. Erhard J, Lange R, Scherer R, Kox WJ, Bretschneider HJ, Gebhard MM, Eigler FW (1994) Comparison of histidine-tryptophan-ketoglutarate (HTK) solution versus University of Wisconsin (UW) solution for organ preservation in human liver transplantation – a prospective, randomized study. Transplant Int 7: 177:181

8. Fukusazawa K, Schwartz ME, Acarli K, Katz E, Gabrielson G, Gettes M, Jakobs E, Miller CM (1994) Flushing with autologous blood improves intraoperative hemodynamic stability and early graft function in clinical hepatic transplantation. Am J Surg 178: 541–547

9. Gubernatis G, Pichlmayr R, Lamesch P, Grosse H, Bornscheuer A, Meyer H-J, Ringe B, Farle M, Bretschneider HJ (1990) HTK solution (Bretschneider) for human liver transplantation. Langenbecks Arch Chir 375: 66–70

10. Ishii H, Uchiyama H, Kazama M (1991) Soluble thrombomodulin antigen in conditioned medium is increased by damage of endothelial cells. Thromb Haemostas 65: 618–623

11. Karayalcin K, Harrison JD, Attard A, Gunson BK, Jones S, Mayer D, Buckels JAC, McMaster P (1993) Can effluent hyaluronic acid or creatine kinase predict sinusoidal injury severity after cold ischemia? Transplantation 56: 1336–1339

12. Rauen U, Erhard J, Kühnhenrich P, Lange R, Moissidis M, Eigler FW, Groot H de (1994) Nonparenchymal cell and hepatocellular injury to human liver grafts assessed by enzyme-release into the perfusate. Langenbecks Arch Chir 379: 241–247

13. Sawada K, Yamamoto H, Suehiro S (1992) A simple assay to detect endothelial cell injury: measurement of released thrombomodulin from cells. Exp Mol Pathol 57: 116–123

14. Schön R, Eisenberg JU, Lemmens HP, Blumhardt G, Schulz E, Neuhaus P (1994) The correlation of serum hyaluronan of liver donors with posttransplant liver functions. Transplant Int 7: 128–133

15. Shimada M, Yanaga K, Kishikawa K, Kakizoe S, Itasaka H, Ikeda T, Suehiro T, Sugimachi K (1993) Prediction of hepatic graft viability before reperfusion: an analysis of effluent from porcine allografts. Transplant Int 6: 4–7

16. Strasberg S, Howard T, Molmenti E, Hertl M (1994) Selecting the donor liver: risk factors for poor function after orthotopic liver transplantation. Hepatology 20: 829–838

17. Takahashi H, Ito S, Hanano M, Wada K, Niwano H, Seki Y, Shibata A (1992) Circulating thrombomodulin as a novel endothelial cell marker: comparison of its behavior with von Willebrand factor and tissue-type plasminogen activator. Am J Hematol 41: 32–39

18. Vaubourdolle M, Chazouilleres O, Poupon R, Ballet F, Braunwald J, Legendre C, Baudin B, Kirn A, Giboudeau J (1993) Creatine kinase-BB: a marker of liver sinusoidal damage in ischemia reperfusion. Hepatology 17: 423–428

Transpl Int (1996) 9 [Suppl 1]: S 477–S 478
© Springer-Verlag 1996

M. Schilling
C. Redaelli
H. Friess
M. W. Büchler

Pharmacokinetics of rinse solutions at 4° celsius

M. Schilling (✉) · C. Redaelli · H. Friess · M. W. Büchler
Department of Visceral and Transplant Surgery,
University of Bern, Inselspital, CH-3010 Bern, Switzerland

Introduction

With the introduction of University of Wisconsin (UW) solution in liver preservation, rinsing of the graft before reperfusion with either blood or synthetic solutions has become a standard procedure [1, 2]. Synthetic rinse solutions were developed not only to rinse out potassium and metabolites from the liver graft, but also to apply protective substances during the rinse-out phase [2–4]. In this study, we investigated the uptake of radiolabelled adenosine as an example of the uptake of low molecular protective substances during a rinse with a high viscosity solution at 4 °C.

Materials and methods

Experiments were carried out according to the guidelines of the local animal ethics committee. Male Wistar rats (270–320 g) were used in all experiments. After intraperitoneal anaesthesia with pentobarbital, livers and kidneys were flushed out through the aorta (10 ml solution at 2 ml/min) and the portal vein (5 ml at 1 ml/min) with 4 °C cold UW solution. Livers and kidneys (en bloc) were excised and stored at 4 °C with a portal and an aortic catheter ligated in the respective vessel. Microdialysis membranes were placed in livers (10-mm membrane) and kidneys (5-mm membrane) and perfused at 10 μl/min with a Krebs-Henseleit buffer in a similar set-up as described by Van Wylen et al [5]. After 2 h of storage, livers and kidneys were rinsed at 4 °C or 37 °C with UW supplemented with ^{3}H-adenosine. Effluent from the microdialysis membranes was collected and counted in a beta counter. Also, random samples were taken from livers and kidneys and minced in scintillation liquid also to be counted. Results are given as mean counts per minute for the microdialysis effluent and the mean ± SE for the fraction of the recovered radioactivity divided by the total applied radioactivity.

Results

Results are given in Figs. 1 and 2. At 4 °C 12 ± 3 % of the total applied ^{3}H-adenosine was taken up by the liver centre, 6.7 ± 1.6 % by the liver periphery, and 2.0 ± 1.4 % and 1.9 ± 1.1 % by the renal cortex and medulla, respectively. At 37 °C the uptake was considerably higher: 20.7 ± 5.5 % for the liver centre, 12.3 ± 4.1 % for the liver periphery, and 3.0 ± 1.8 % and 2.9 ± 1.7 % for the renal cortex and the medulla, respectively. Diffusion of labelled adenosine from the portal system into the microdialysis membranes was much higher than diffusion of labelled adenosine from the arterial system to the membranes. Diffusion of labelled adenosin from the vascular system in livers to the luminal space of the microdialysis membranes decreased rapidly after appliciation of the rinse.

Discussion

Rinsing livers before reperfusion is implemented to rinse out potassium and/or adenosine in order to avoid cardiac arrythmias [1]. Furthermore, the rinsing of or-

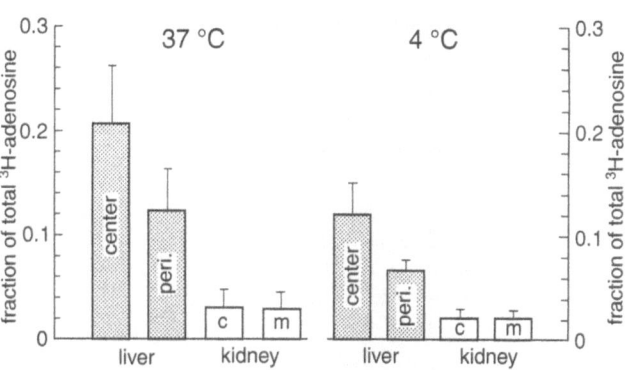

Fig. 1 Uptake of ^{3}H-adenosine by the liver and kidney at 37 °C and at 4 °C (*peri.* Periphery, *c* cortex, *m* medulla)

S 478

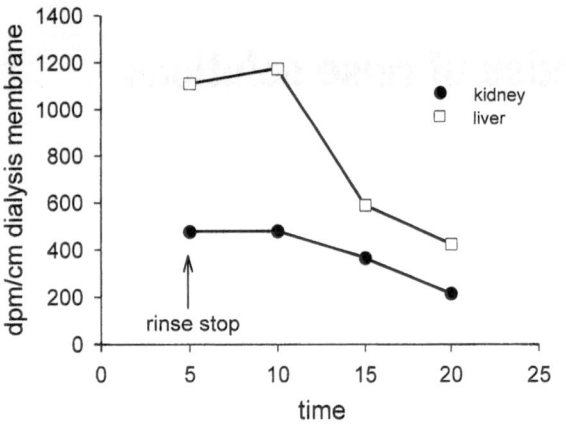

Fig. 2 Diffusion of labelled adenosine from the portal and arterial systems into the microdialysis membranes

gans has improved graft survival by rinsing inflammatory mediators [6] and thus decreasing leucocyte-endothelial and Kupffer cell interaction [7]. Adenosine itself [4] and the rinse temperature have been found to be important factors that improve graft function in experimental liver transplantation [8, 9]. In this study we demonstrated that at 37 °C the amount of adenosine being taken up by the graft from the rinse solution was significantly higher than at 4 °C. At temperatures below the transition temperature of membranes most active transport processes stop and intracellular uptake of protective substances is facilitated by diffusion only or along a pressure gradient. If cytoprotective substances are to be applied during a rinse or a flush-out, temperatures above the transition temperature of cell membranes facilitate that uptake.

References

1. Belzer FO (1990) Correct use of University of Wisconsin preservation solution (letter). Lancet 335 (8685): 362
2. Sanchez-Urdazpal L, Gores GJ, Lemasters JJ, Thurman RG, Steers JL, Wahlstrom HE, Hay EI, Porayko MK, Wiesner RH, Krom RA (1993) Carolina rinse solution decreases liver injury during clinical liver transplantation. Transplant Proc 25 (1 Pt 2): 1574–1575
3. Gao W, Takei Y, Marzi I, Lindert KA, Caldwell-Kenkel JC, Currin RT, Tanaka Y, Lemaster JJ, Thurman RG (1991) Carolina rinse solution – a new strategy to increase survival time after orthotopic liver transplantation in the rat. Transplantation 52: 417–424
4. Gao W, Hijioka T, Lindert KA, Caldwell-Kenkel JC, Lemaster JJ, Thurman RG (1991) Evidence that adenosine is a key component in Carolina rinse reducing graft failure after orthotopic liver transplantation in the rat. Transplantation 52: 992–998
5. Van Wylen DG, Schmit TJ, Lasley RD, Gingell RL, Mentzer RM Jr (1992) Cardiac microdialysis in isolated rat hearts: interstitial purine metabolites during ischemia. Am J Physiol 262 (6 Pt 2): H1934–1938
6. Schilling M, Tilton B, Storck M, Hammer C, Abendroth D (1993) Mediator clearing effects of rinse solution in lung preservation. Transplant Proc 25: 3212
7. Post S, Palma P, Rentsch M, Gonzalez AP, Menger MD (1993) Differential impact of Carolina rinse and University of Wisconsin solutions on microcirculation, leucocyte adhesion, Kupffer cell activity and biliary excretion after liver transplantation. Hepatology 18: 1490–1497
8. Bachmann S, Caldwell-Kenkel JC, Oleksy I, Steffen R, Lemaster JJ, Thurman RG (1992) Warm Carolina rinse solution prevents graft failure from storage injury after orthotopic rat liver transplantation with arterialization. Transplant Int 5: 108–114
9. Takei Y, Gao WS, Hijioka T, Savier E, Lindert KA, Lemasters JJ, Thurman RG (1991) Increase in survival of liver grafts after rinsing with warm Ringer's solution due to improvement of hepatic microcirculation. Transplantation 52: 225–230

Transpl Int (1996) 9 [Suppl 1]: S 479–S 482
© Springer-Verlag 1996

Assessment of oxygen radicals during kidney transplantation – effect of radical scavenger

R. Hower
Th. Minor
H. Schneeberger
J. Theodorakis
S. Rembold
W.-D. Illner
G. O. Hofmann
P. Fraunberger
W. Isselhard
W. Land

R. Hower (✉) · H. Schneeberger ·
J. Theodorakis · S. Rembold · W.-D. Illner ·
G. O. Hofmann · P. Fraunberger · W. Land
Division of Transplant Surgery,
Department of Surgery,
University of Munich,
Klinikum Großhadern, Marchioninistr. 15,
D-81377 Munich, Germany,
Fax: + 49/89/700 41 60

Th. Minor · W. Isselhard
Department of Experimental Surgery,
University of Cologne, Germany

Abstract In the present study, levels of free oxygen radicals, generated in the very early period of reperfusion during human kidney transplantation, were assessed by determination of malondialdehyde (MDA) levels using a high-pressure liquid chromatography (HPLC) method. Renal blood samples were obtained during reperfusion by intraoperative cannulation of the renal vein. Simultaneously, systemic MDA levels were determined. Furthermore, local and systemic levels of interleukin 6 (IL-6), tumor necrosis factor (TNF) receptors, p55 and p75, and vitamin E were measured. In a second group of patients, 500 mg of ascorbic acid were given prior to reperfusion. Renal MDA levels in the control group were always higher compared to systemic levels. IL-6 showed a marked increase shortly after reperfusion in the renal blood. In the scavenger group there was a diminution of these effects. TNF receptor levels and vitamin E remained largely unchanged. The results of this pilot study demonstrated clinically the moderate production of reactive oxygen species and the liberation of IL-6 shortly after reperfusion of human transplanted kidneys. Furthermore, the modulating effect of a radical scavenger on these effects was shown.

Key words Oxygen free radicals · Kidney transplantation · IL-6 · TNF receptors · Vitamin E · Radical scavenger

Introduction

The mechanisms of ischemia-reperfusion injury in the context of organ transplantation are of increasing importance, apart from immunological considerations [1, 2]. Ischemia of the donor organ after harvesting and during conservation, as well as the subsequent reperfusion may lead to endothelial injury [3]. Membrane lipids are peroxidated by the generation of free oxygen radicals, and these lipidperoxidate products can be measured as conjugated dienes or malondialdehyde (MDA) [4]. Furthermore, there is an expression of adhesion molecules and cytokine release with systemic inflammatory reactions. Recently, the question of whether these early local damages of the transplanted organ may lead to an increased immunogenicity and subsequently to an increased rate of rejection has been discussed [5]. In the present pilot study, indirect measurements of free oxygen radicals, cytokines, and vitamin E levels were done intraoperatively in the very early reperfusion period during human kidney transplantation. Furthermore, the effect of vitamin C as a radical scavenger was tested.

Patients and methods

The patients involved in this study consisted of 17 patients undergoing kidney transplantation at our center. They were randomly assigned to a control group ($n = 8$) or a vitamin C group ($n = 9$), receiving 500 mg ascorbic acid (Ascorvit) intraoperatively prior to reperfusion. Both groups received a standard immunosuppressive protocol with triple-drug induction therapy (cyclosporin A, azathioprine, steroids).

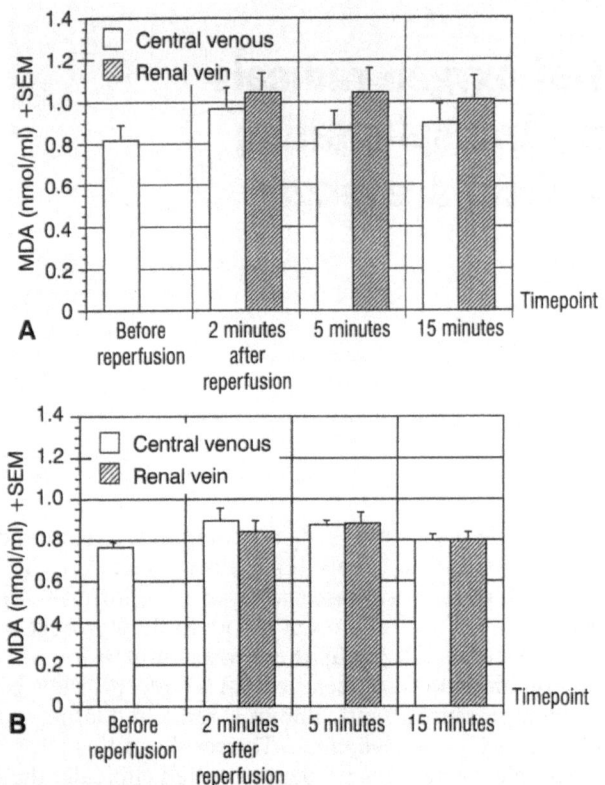

Fig. 1 Malondialdehyde (MDA) levels in **A** control group and **B** vitamin C group intraoperatively after kidney transplantation. Renal blood samples were obtained by cannulating the renal vein

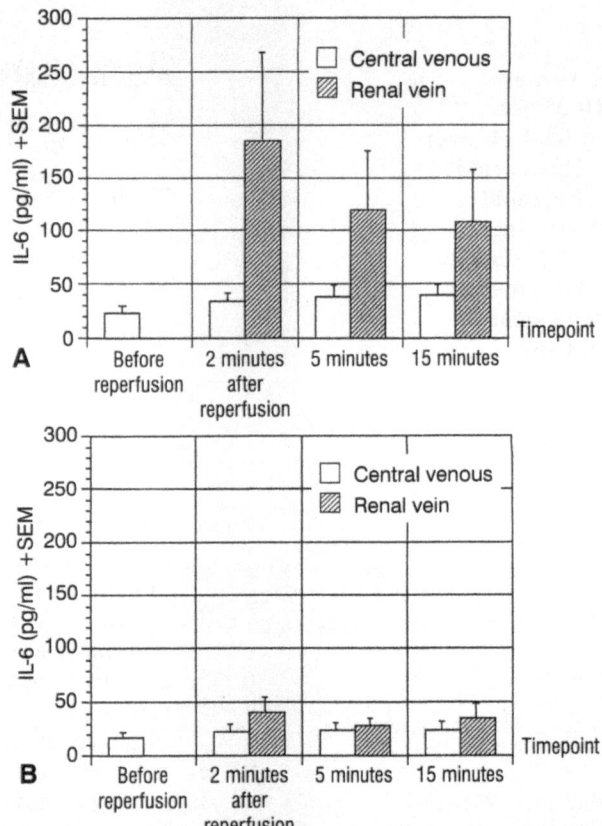

Fig. 2 Interleukin 6 (IL-6) levels in **A** control group and **B** vitamin C group intraoperatively after kidney transplantation

Table 1 Demographic data of the donors and recipients included in the pilot study. There were no significant differences between the groups (*ATG* antilymphocyte globulin, *HD* hemodialysis, *TX* transplant, *ATN* acute tubular necrosis)

	Control group ($n = 9$)	Vitamin C group ($n = 8$)
Donor data		
Age (years) 48 ± 5	37 ± 8	
Sex	4M/5F	5M/3F
Last creatinin level	0.8 ± 0.1 mg/dl	1.0 ± 0.2 mg/dl
Recipient data		
HLA-A mismatch	88 %	62.5 %
– B	77 %	62.5 %
– DR	44 %	25 %
Antibodies	0 %	0 %
ATG treatment	5	4
Cold ischemia time (h)	20.8 ± 3	27.1 ± 3
Early function parameters		
Amount of HD until TX function	7	2
Days until drop in creatinin	14	7
ATN	55 %	25 %

Concerning demographic data, there was no significant difference in donor age, last creatinin level or systolic blood pressure. Cold ischemia time was also comparable in both groups (Table 1). Using the amount of hemodialysis required till transplant function and days up to the first drop in creatinin as early indicators of transplant function, there was a trend for earlier function in the vitamin C group (Table 1).

The renal vein of the donor organ was cannulated intraoperatively and blood samples were taken at 2, 5, and 15 min after the onset of reperfusion of the transplanted kidney. Concomitantly, blood samples were taken from the central line before reperfusion and at the same timepoints following reperfusion. The plasma was seperated by centrifugation and immediately stored at – 70 °C until analysis.

Lipid peroxidation was assessed by measuring MDA levels. MDA-thiobarbituric acid adducts were determined by high-pressure liquid chromatography (HPLC), according to Wong et al. [6]. Levels of interleukin-6 (IL-6) and tumor necrosis factor (TNF) receptors, p55 and p75, were measured by ELISA. Vitamin E was measured by HPLC. Statistical analysis was performed by the nonparametric Mann-Whitney U test.

Results

Systemic and renal MDA levels in the control group showed an increase shortly after reperfusion (Fig. 1 A). MDA levels in the renal vein, as a marker of lipid per-

Table 2 Intraoperative values of tumor necrosis factor (TNF) receptors, p55 and p75, and of vitamin E (mean ± SEM)

	Baseline	2	5	15
TNF receptor p55 (ng/ml)				
Control central venous	25.5 ± 2.5	26.1 ± 2.5	26.3 ± 2.5	22.9 ± 1.4
Vitamin C central venous	24.5 ± 3.6	23.2 ± 3.5	22.8 ± 3	19.7 ± 3.3
Control renal vein		24.4 ± 2.7	28.0 ± 2.8	25.9 ± 2.5
Vitamin C renal vein		21.2 ± 2.3	20.5 ± 2.7	16.8 ± 3.1
TNF receptor p75 (ng/ml)				
Control central venous	17.7 ± 2.0	15.9 ± 1.6	17.4 ± 2.1	18.0 ± 2.0
Vitamin C central venous	18.0 ± 1.5	16.8 ± 1.5	17.0 ± 1.2	18.3 ± 0.9
Control renal vein		17.3 ± 1.3	17.4 ± 0.9	18.4 ± 0.7
Vitamin C renal vein		16.4 ± 1.6	17.3 ± 1.9	17.4 ± 1.7
Vitamin E (µg/mg chol.)				
Control central venous	5.27 ± 1.3	6.09 ± 0.2	5.31 ± 0.6	5.77 ± 0.8
Vitamin C central venous	6.11 ± 0.9	5.52 ± 0.8	6.04 ± 0.8	5.82 ± 0.7
Control renal vein		7.10 ± 1.2	5.87 ± 0.3	6.19 ± 0.4
Vitamin C renal vein		6.31 ± 1.0	5.10 ± 0.9	5.98 ± 0.7

oxidation, showed, for example, after 2 min of reperfusion an increase of 30 % compared with the systemic baseline value. MDA levels in the renal vein were always higher than systemic values, but without definite significance. Treatment with vitamin C prior to reperfusion resulted in a slight increase in MDA levels mainly in renal venous blood samples (Fig. 1 B). IL-6 values peaked in the renal blood of the control group 2 min after reperfusion. This peak was not seen in the treatment group (Fig. 2). There were no differences in the levels of the two TNF receptors, p55 and p75, in either group (Table 2). The levels of α-tocopherol (vitamin E), as a marker of endogenous scavenger pool, also showed no significant difference in either group (Table 2).

Discussion

Transplantation of a solid organ is linked regulary with processes of ischemia-reperfusion, resulting in a so-called reperfusion injury [7]. Free oxygen radicals, generated during reperfusion [8], may damage the microvascular endothelium, leading to increased immunogenicity and finally to an increased incidence of acute and chronic rejection, as discussed earlier by Land et al. [5].

The production of free oxygen radicals, indirectly measured by MDA levels, as the key event of reperfusion injury [9] was shown by our group clinically for the first time in transplanted kidneys intraoperatively. Renal MDA levels in the control group were always higher compared to systemic levels, indicating local release at the site of reperfusion. The peak in IL-6 2 min after reperfusion in the venous renal blood may be caused by local injury following reperfusion, thus IL-6 is a marker after trauma or injury [10].

The nonresponse of TNF receptors in this very early phase of reperfusion could be explained by the time course of production of this cytokine. In other settings of reperfusion, levels are measurable about 30–60 min after the onset of reperfusion [11].

Vitamin E, as a lipophil vitamin and an indicator for endogenous antioxidative capacity [12], may be a parameter that is too weak for this early phase of reperfusion injury. Application of the radical scavenger, vitamin C, resulted mainly in a moderate reduction in locally measured MDA and IL-6 levels at the transplanted kidney site. These statistically nonsignificant but measurable differences showed a slight trend for a diminution in acute injury in the very early period of kidney transplantation. Application of a multivitamin mixture and measurement of MDA levels in the later time course after kidney transplantation have shown similar results [13].

Thus, our data confirmed clinically earlier observations concerning the possible role of antioxidants in the elimination of reperfusion injury after transplantation [14]. Further studies may be indicated for the registration of microvascular injury and its prevention.

References

1. Koyama I, Bulkley GB, Williams GM, Im MJ (1985) The role of oxygen free radicals in mediating the reperfusion injury of cold-preserved ischemic kidneys. Transplantation 40: 590–595
2. Schneeberger H, Schleibner S, Illner WD, Messmer K, Land W (1993) The impact of free radical-mediated reperfusion injury on acute and chronic rejection events following cadaveric renal transplantation. Clin Transplant 219–232
3. Andreoli SP, McAteer JA (1990) Reactive oxygen molecule-mediated injury in endothelial and renal tubular epithelial cells in vitro. Kidney Int 38: 785–794
4. Paller MS, Hoidal JR, Ferris TF (1984) Oxygen free radicals in ischemic acute renal failure in the rat. J Clin Invest 74: 1156–1164
5. Land W, Schneeberger H, Schleibner S, Illner WD, Abendroth D, Rutili G, Arfors KE, Messmer K (1994) The beneficial effect of human recombinant superoxide dismutase on acute and chronic rejection events in recipients of cadaveric renal transplants. Transplantation 57: 211–217
6. Wong SHY, Knight JA, Hopfer SM, Zaharia O, Leach CN, Sunderman FW (1987) Lipoperoxides in plasma as measured by liquid-chromatographic seperation of malondialdehyde-thiobarbituric acid adduct. Clin Chem 33: 214–220
7. Parks DA, Bulkley GB, Granger DN (1983) Role of oxygen free radicals in shock, ischemia, and organ preservation. Surgery 94: 407–411
8. Granger DN, Höllwarth ME, Parks DA (1986) Ischemia-reperfusion injury: role of oxygen derived free radicals. Acta Physiol Scand 548: 47–63
9. Parks DA, Granger DN (1988) Ischemia-reperfusion injury: a radical view. Hepatology 8: 680
10. Schlüter B, König B, Bergmann U, Müller FE, König W (1991) Interleukin 6 – a potential mediator of lethal sepsis after major thermal trauma: evidence for increased IL-6 production by peripheral blood mononuclear cells. J Trauma 31: 1663–1670
11. Bittermann H, Lazarovich H, Kinarty A, Cohen L, Lahat N (1990) The profile of cytokines and cytokine inhibition during splanchnic artery occlussion (SAO) shock. Circ Shock 31: 25
12. Defraigne JO, Pincemail J, Franssen C, Meurisse D, Defechereux T, Philippart C, Serteyn D, Lamy M, Deby C, Limet R (1993) In vivo free radical production after cross-clamping and reperfusion of the renal artery in the rabbit. Cardiovasc Surg 1: 343–349
13. Rabl H, Khoschsorur G, Colombo T, Petritsch P, Rauchenwald M, Költringer P, Tatzber F, Esterbauer H (1993) A multi-vitamin infusion prevents lipid peroxidation and improves performance of transplanted kidneys in humans. Kidney Int 43: 912–917
14. Rangan U, Bulkley GB (1993) Prospects for treatment of free radical-mediated tissue injury. Br Med Bull 49: 700–718

Tissue

Transpl Int (1996) 9 [Suppl 1]: S485–S491
© Springer-Verlag 1996

TISSUE

Juan J. López-Lozano
Gonzalo Bravo
Javier Abascal
Begoña Brera
M. Luisa Pascual
Roberto Martínez
Carolina de la Torre
Raquel Moreno

Clinical experience with cotransplantation of peripheral nerve and adrenal medulla in patients with Parkinson's disease

J. J. López-Lozano (✉) · G. Bravo ·
J. Abascal · B. Brera · M. L. Pascual ·
R. Martínez · C. de la Torre · R. Moreno
CPH Neural Transplantation Group
(Departments of Neurology, Neurosurgery,
Surgery and Laboratory Neurobiology),
Clínica Puerta de Hierro,
San Martín de Porres, 4, E-28035 Madrid,
Spain
Tel. +34/316 30 40 (ext. 474);
Fax +34/373 76 67

Abstract Coimplants of adrenal medulla (AM) and peripheral nerve (PN) in animal models of Parkinson's disease (PD) have shown that AM cells survive longer, tend to show neuronal phenotype, and enhance sprouting of host fibers. Since 1987, our implants of perfused AM and fetal ventral mesencephalon (FVM) in PD patients have achieved varying degrees of clinical improvement. If the donor tissue determines the improvement, different types of implants should result in qualitatively and quantitatively different degrees of improvement. The purpose of this study is to determine whether or not the clinical course, improvement slope, and reduction of medication observed in PD patients who undergo tissue transplantation (Tx) depend on the donor tissue type. In a pilot study, four grade IV–V PD patients received implants of precoincubated autologous AM and intercostal nerve in the caudate nucleus (open surgery). Clinical assessment was based on international scales (UPD)

as reported for Tx of FVM and perfused AM. There were no systemic or neurologic complications. Four years post-Tx, longer On phases and improved PD symptoms (ADL and motor-UPD) in On and Off persist in four cases, with reduced dyskinesias. Progress appears to be stepwise, starting within weeks of Tx (similar to AM and sooner than our FVM implants), followed by a period of stability and, after a second wave of improvement 12–18 months post-Tx (similar to FVM implants), continues to date. L-dopa medication has been reduced by more than 60 % and dopamine agonist use has not resumed. We conclude that our recipients continue to be clinically better than prior to Tx. The course of recovery after co-Tx of AM and PN differs from that of FVM or AM implants. This fact may be related to the etiological factors that produce the improvement.

Key words Parkinson's disease · Grafts · Dopamine · Adrenal medulla · Neurotrophic

Introduction

In view of the results obtained in animal models involving substantia nigra or adrenal medulla transplants, together with the fact that many parkinsonian patients do not respond to medication, Parkinson's disease has, in recent years, become one of the most widely studied neurological disorders by workers in the field of neural

transplants. Clinical trials with adrenal medulla and embryonic tissue have been carried out in several research centers around the world, especially in Europe and America [for review see 8, 17, 18, 30]. The reported clinical results have not been homogeneous, ranging from minor or non-significant clinical changes to moderate or marked alleviation of the motor symptoms, generally accompanied by a greater or lesser reduction in the

L-dopa intake. In most cases, the published results have been more modest than expected.

In 1987, we undertook a controlled study to determine whether the implantation of neural tissue into an open cavity in the caudate nucleus was capable of producing an improvement in severely affected parkinsonian patients, and whether this improvement depended on the type of tissue implanted or was the consequence of surgical trauma and the implantation site. The results obtained in the first two series of graft recipients have shown that the implantation of perfused adrenal medulla [21, 22] or fetal ventral mesencephalon [23, 25] into the caudate nucleus by open surgery can improve the clinical symptomatology of severely impaired parkinsonian patients, and that this recovery is accompanied by a reduction in the L-dopa intake of more than 50 %. However, the duration of the clinical improvement observed and the moment of onset differ depending on the tissue implanted; that observed with fetal tissue graft occurred later and lasted longer than that resulting from implantation of adrenal medulla which occurred earlier and followed a stormier course.

As a continuation of our research into the relationship between the type of tissue implanted and the clinical improvement observed, we present our third series of patients. This report describes the overall clinical course of four grade IV–V Parkinson's disease patients 3 years after coimplantation of adrenal medulla and peripheral nerve (AM+PN) into the caudate nucleus. The incubation and implantation of peripheral nerve together with the adrenal medulla is justified by animal experiments showing that coimplants of adrenal medulla and peripheral nerve or implantation of adrenal medulla plus chronic nerve growth factor infusion increases the survival of the chromaffin cells of the adrenal medulla, favors the tendency of these cells to be of neuronal phenotype, and enhances the sprouting of host fibers [4–6, 14, 31].

Patients and methods

Between May and July of 1990, four parkinsonian patients in our center received coimplants of autologous adrenal medulla and intercostal nerve. The patients consented to participate in the study after being informed of the clinical and surgical risks, the possible lack of improvement, and the fact that the study focused more on clinical research than on the therapeutic measure. The use of the donor tissue and the experimental procedure were approved by the human research ethics committees of the center, with the consent of the Spanish National Institute of Health, and followed the guidelines of the pertinant Spanish law.

Patient selection and preoperative clinical features

The selection criteria for the patients were those used in our previous series of recipients of perfused adrenal medulla [21, 22] or fetal ventral mesencephalon [23, 25] transplanted into the caudate nucleus: parkinsonian patients in an advanced stage of the disease, with a history of Parkinson's disease of several years' duration, with no pharmaceutical control, and who presented normal daily fluctuations and dyskinesias. All the patients had responded to L-dopa administration at the onset of their disease. The mean age at surgery was 60 ± 6.78 years (range 52–67 years), the mean duration of their disease course was 10.87 ± 1.75 years (range 9–13 years), and they had been receiving L-dopa/inhibitor for 10.25 ± 1.26 years (range 9–12 years). They had participated in other clinicopharmaceutical trials with no appreciable control of their symptomatology. All the patients had received dopaminergic agonists. Disease severity ranged between grades IV and V of the Hoehn-Yahr scale, with one grade IV patient and three in grade IV–V.

Evaluation of the patients (clinical monitoring)

The subjects were assessed pre- and postoperatively, during On and Off stages under their usual medication and during predefined Off and On periods, and their status was determined on the basis of internationally accepted rating scales (CAPIT protocol) [16]. Predefined Off was considered to be the clinical situation of a patient examined between 10 and 11 am, 2–2.5 h after waking, before breakfast and 12–14 h after the last L-dopa dose. Predefined On was established as the clinical situation of a patient at the time of maximal therapeutic benefit, 1–1.5 h after the first regular morning L-dopa dose. Patient disability was classified as Hoehn-Yahr stages I–V on the basis of the Hoehn-Yahr scale. Motor function and normal daily activities were rated according to the Unified Parkinson's Disease Scale (UPDS, v. 3.0.1) and the North Western University Disability Scale (NWDS). Magnetic resonance imaging of the brain was performed prior to surgery and 1, 6 and 12 months after.

Pharmaceutical management

As in our first two series of implant recipients, the subjects of this trial were maintained on optimal doses of medication (L-dopa, agonists, and anticholinergics) until 1–2 weeks before surgery, at which time the dopaminergic agonists and/or amantadine were gradually tapered off, to be discontinued 1 day before implantation. Immediately after surgery, all the patients received dexamethasone (4 mg four times daily) and phenytoin at the standard postoperative dose. In this series of patients, it was also necessary to reduce L-dopa intake during the initial postoperative weeks, due mainly to motor complications. During the period of analysis (3 years), the dose was reduced whenever an increase in the dyskinesias or onset of psychiatric symptoms was observed.

Surgical procedure

The methods employed in the implantation procedure did not differ from those used for perfused adrenal medulla implants [21, 22], with the exception of the procurement and dissection of a peripheral nerve and its incubation with the pieces of adrenal medulla. The right adrenal gland was removed retroperitoneally using a superior subcostal approach. The gland was cut into slices about

5 mm thick and the adrenal medulla was dissected and incubated first in calcium- and magnesium-free buffer, and later in minimum essential medium (MEM), as previously described [19]. The viability of the chromaffin cells was over 70 %. The 12th intercostal nerve was dissected, freed of fat and the surrounding connective tissue, and then minced and incubated with the adrenal medulla in enriched Dulbecco's modified Eagle medium (DMEM) for approximately 1 h. The time between tissue preparation and implantation was less than 3 h. The donor tissue (a cohesive mass made up of 15–20 pieces of adrenal medulla and peripheral nerve measuring 2–3 mm each) was implanted into a cavity created in the right caudate nucleus (in direct contact with the cerebrospinal fluid of the lateral ventricle) after right frontal cariectomy and a transcortical (F2) approach to the lateral ventricle. The tissue was secured within the cavity with Surgical and clips.

Statistical study

The means and standard deviations of the clinical values were determined and the changes occurring over the entire course of the study were compared using non-parametric analysis of variance (Friedman's test) and Wilcoxon's paired test.

Results

Postoperative course, clinical symptoms, and medication

Thirty-six months after implantation, all four patients presented a sustained improvement in their parkinsonian symptomatology in On and Off (Fig. 1) and an increment in the percentage of their waking hours spent in On phase (Table 1), with decreased duration and reduced intensity of dyskinesias (Table 2). The improvement or increment in the number of waking hours spent in On appears to commence in month 2 and progresses steadily thereafter until the end of the follow-up (36 months after surgery). At the same time, the increase in time spent in On is accompanied by a reduction in the L-dopa administered; thus, not only did the patients spend most of the day in On stage, but they also took 69.5 % less medication (Table 3). Moreover, the quality of the time the patients spent in On was better (with respect to both routine daily activities and social life), since the improvement in motor function in the patients was also accompanied by a marked reduction in the duration (75 % less) and intensity of the dyskinesias (Table 2). The most notable decrease in the time spent with dyskinesias in On appeared to commence in months 2 to 3 when a reduction was observed in all four patients. At the end of the follow-up, the four patients had reduced the amount of On time spent with dyskinesias by 100 % to 54.5 % of the preoperative values.

Figure 1 shows the overall clinical course of the symptoms in predefined On and Off phases from the preoperative period to 36 months after implantation. As shown, the improvement in the clinical symptoms in

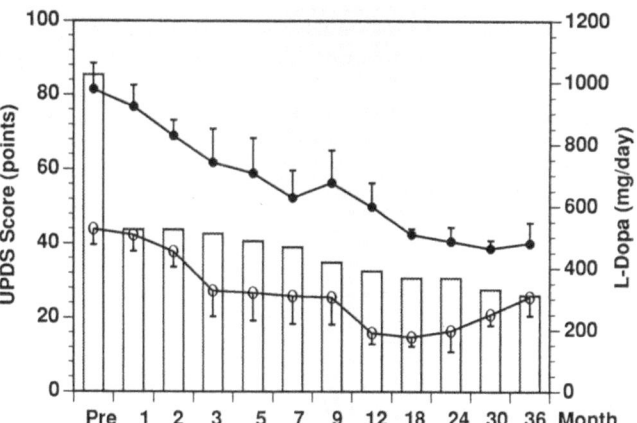

Fig. 1 Overall progress in the parkinsonian symptomatology from presurgery to 36 months postsurgery, assessed according to the Unified Parkinson's Disability Scale (UPDS), during practically defined Off and On periods as compared to L-dopa/inhibitor treatment course. Values are mean scores ± SD. Presurgery values represent the means ± SD of the evaluation performed over the 6 months prior to implantation

Off followed two separate waves, one commencing in the first month of follow-up and persisting until months 7–9, and the second occurring 12–18 months postsurgery, with progression until the end of the follow-up period. In the initial postoperative weeks, as in our other implant series [21–23, 25], there was a slight deterioration in the symptoms, probably as a consequence of the withdrawal of dopamine agonists and the reduction in medication secondary to the onset of the motor and psychiatric complications. The clinical improvement involved all the symptoms analyzed in Off phase, although the degree and period of onset varied for each one (Table 4) and differed from those observed in the group of patients who received fetal tissue implants [25]. Facies and rigidity were the symptoms associated with the earliest (1 month after surgery) and the most notable recovery in the four patients, while postural stability, gait, and body bradykinesia improved later (5th month) and to a slightly lesser degree. Tremor was was the symptom that presented the least recovery.

Complications

There were no apparent systemic or general neurologic complications, but three of the four patients presented psychiatric complications in the form of personality changes (in one patient), confusion (in two), hallucinations (in three), delusions (in one), and vivid dreams (in two), while dyskinesias increased in all the recipients. From the experience gained in the first two series of patients [21–23, 25], L-dopa/inhibitor was gradually reduced from 1025 ± 210.59 mg/day presurgery to 525 ± 178.78 mg/day by the second month; this reduc-

Table 1 Mean percentage waking hours spent in On/day from month 1 to 36 months after surgery, as compared to mean percentage presurgery On time

Time of assessment	Percentage time spent in On/day
Presurgery	46.2 ± 10.4
Months after surgery	
2	63.75 ± 14.88
7	71.06 ± 10.90
18	73.21 ± 12.44
24	76.84 ± 7.78
36	87.5 ± 10.4

Table 2 Mean percentage On time spent with dyskinesias ± SD from 1 to 36 months after surgery as compared to mean percentage presurgery On time with dyskinesias

Time of assessment	% On time with dyskinesias
Presurgery	67.10 ± 9.18
Months after surgery	
2	45.11 ± 13.05
3	18.72 ± 37.63
9	10.55 ± 9.08
12	11.0 ± 10.36
24	15.9 ± 7.0
36	17.08 ± 13.76

Table 3 Mean L-dopa/carbidopa dose from 1 to 36 months after surgery as compared to mean presurgery dose

Time of assessment	L-dopa/inhibitor (mg/day)
Presurgery	1025.00 ± 210.59
Months after surgery	
2	525.00 ± 170.78
7	468.75 ± 177.12
12	391.25 ± 320.16
18	368.75 ± 189.66
24	368.75 ± 124.79
30	331.25 ± 87.50
36	312.50 ± 180.97

tion was associated with an improvement in the motor complications and the disappearance of hallucinations and delusions.

Discussion

The results of this pilot study demonstrate that parkinsonian patients improve after the cografting of AM + PN implants. This recovery changes the daily living activities of the patients, allowing them to perform routine activities with increasing ease. This improvement is evident in the decrease in severity of all the parkinsonian symptoms, although to different degrees and with different rates of onset. To the physicians that have been fol-

lowing these patients for years, the reduction in the dosage of medication (L-dopa), the parallel increase in the length of time throughout the day in which the patient is in On, with alleviation of the secondary motor complications (mainly dyskinesias) and the lowering of the disease grade is suggestive of a return to an earlier and more benign stage of the disease, as though time had been turned back.

As we have mentioned in earlier publications, the difference in the study design makes it difficult to compare our results with those of other groups, whether they employed stereotactic techniques [1, 2, 9, 11, 13] or open surgery [26, 27]. If in the former case, the main differences lie in the implantation site and the surgical technique employed, in the latter which is more comparable given the similarity in the surgical technique, they lie in the type of patients undergoing implantation (younger and with a shorter history of chronic medication), in the clinical follow-up, and in the fact that none of the research teams has performed implantation using adrenal medulla and peripheral nerve as donor tissue.

Having arrived at this point, the reader may ask how can it be that the results of so many of the studies documented in the literature show the improvement of implant recipients when these reports generally disagree with respect to the site of implantation (caudate or putamen or both), the type of tissue (adrenal medulla or fetal tissue), the amount of tissue implanted (tissue from one or more fetuses), the severity of the disease in the implant recipients (grade III–V), and the protocol for clinical follow-up. Reading these articles creates the impression that some degree of improvement can be obtained in transplant recipients regardless of the donor tissue employed. From our point of view, this consideration is misleading. A critical reader of this article who is familiar with our work may arrive at the conclusion that, in the paradigma employed by us, consisting of "implantation, using an open surgery technique, of tissue grafts from different sources into the caudate nucleus of severely disabled parkinsonian patients", the patients in each study series (perfused adrenal medulla, fetal tissue, and AM + PN coimplants) [20–25] improve postoperatively and return to a certain degree of disability, regardless of the tissue implanted. In agreement with this rationale, the response would be that the recipients of implants in the caudate nucleus do indeed improve regardless of the tissue employed. However, the degree of recovery and its time of onset and clinical course are different for each tissue type. In implants of perfused adrenal medulla [20–22], the improvement has an early but stormy commencement, starting in the first month and progressing stepwise until months 9–12. From then on, the gains stabilize in most of the patients, with no further progress. In contrast, when fetal ventral mesencephalon is implanted, the onset of clinical recovery and the improvement in symptoms occurs later and is less

Table 4 Effects of implantation on individual symptoms of Parkinson's disease

Symptoms of Parkinson's disease Off	First significant change (months)	Peak change	Peak month	Mean (range) at end of follow-up of 36 months
Facies	1	70 %	30	70 % (100–33.3)
Rigidity	1	57.91 %	18	50 % (66.67–33.3)
Postural stability	5	57 %	18	43.75 % (100–0)
Rising sitting position	2	66.67 %	24	64.5 % (100–0)
Speech	2	64.58 %	24	41.67 % (75–0)
Bradykinesia	5	50 %	36	50 % (83.3–0)
Gait	5	50 %	30–36	50 % (83.3–0)
Tremor	24	35.65 %	24	35.6 % (50–12.5)

pronounced during the first year than when adrenal medulla grafts or coimplants are used. Although after fetal transplantation, [23, 25] clinical progress is detected 3–4 months after surgery in some of the patients, overall, it is not until the 5th month that recovery is statistically significant, becoming qualitatively and quantitatively more marked in the 7th month. Although the clinical improvement is moderate over the first 7 months, later on, in contrast to our perfused adrenal medulla transplant recipients [22], these Parkinson's patients continue to recover, with improvement peaks at postoperative months 12–18 and progressive gains until months 30–42. The recipients of AM + PN implants represent a mixed situation [24] since they improve earlier than those receiving fetal tissue [23, 25], as do the recipients of perfused adrenal medulla [20–22]. However, they differ from the latter in that they exhibit a second wave of recovery after the first postimplantation year, similar to that observed in fetal implant recipients.

The causes of improvement still remain a matter of hypothesis. Two separate but complementary sets of causes or mechanisms have been proposed for this recovery: on the one hand, those related to the viability and integration of the implanted cells and, on the other, those secondary to the enhancement of the striatal cells of the host and/or to the activation-repair-modification process of the basal ganglia circuits of the recipient. The comparison of the clinical course of the patients in this pilot study with that of our earlier series of perfused adrenal medulla and fetal ventral mesencephalon recipients [20–25] allows us to theorize as to the causes or factors governing this improvement in our model.

How can we explain the early gains observed in recipients of adrenal medulla implants (whether consisting of perfused adrenal medulla or coimplants) given the later progress observed in our series of fetal tissue recipient? What differentiates the adrenal medulla implants from the AM + PN coimplants, making the course of improvement in the cografts an intermediate situation between adrenal medulla implants and fetal grafts? The improvement observed in the early postimplantation months may be a consequence of a number of causes or factors. The reduction in medication and the motor and psychiatric complications observed in our patients in the early weeks may be due, firstly to the release of dopamine and/or other factors by the cells injured during tissue preparation and, secondly, to surgical trauma. The edema surrounding the needle track and/or the minor hemorrhage in the operative field may act as traumatic factors. The inflammatory-immunological response of the host tissue and the presence, initially, of debris and injured cells and, subsequently, of the implanted adrenal medulla and peripheral nerve tissues may trigger a cascade of events in the host caudate cells, in which secondarily activated glial cells may play the major role.

If the clinical differences among the three implant series lie in the type of tissue implanted, it appears obvious that the grafted cells (and cell injury) may play different roles in the recovery produced by each type of implant. Theoretically, the adrenal medulla tissue would exert its effect, either through direct (secretory?) action of the cells on the host fibers or through indirect action involving the striatal cells [3, 14, 29] or the fenestrated vessels that it contains. However, there are few data on the survival of the adrenal medulla cells. The few autopsies performed [7, 10, 12, 14, 28, 33] have not helped to clarify this issue since only a few surviving tyrosine hydroxylase positive (TH+) cells have been detected in one case [15]. The subject, a parkinsonian patient, had received an adrenal medulla implant 30 months prior to death and had presented clinical improvement during the first 18 months. The pathological study disclosed that the graft site was necrotic and filled with macrophages; among these cells only a few surviving TH(+) cells could be observed. Surrounding the implant, especially on its ventral aspect, there was a dense network of TH-immunoreactive terminals and processes. The authors suggest, and we agree, that this response might represent sprouting by residual host dopaminergic cells secondary to injury. We should also mention that the possibility that the sprouting may have been mediated by the implanted cells can not be ruled out since, when the pathological study was performed, the patient had returned to his preoperative clinical situation and, by then, the chromaffin cells may have been dead. To our knowledge, there are no data from autopsies carried out in patients who, at death, were in better clinical condition than prior to implantation.

Although we have stated [21–23, 25] that the cause of the improvement during the first postimplantation months may be related to indirect or direct effects of the implanted cells or of the traumatic injury to the host and that this progress becomes stable during the first year, how can it be explained that recipients of AM + PN implants continue to improve during the second postoperative year? The only possible conclusion is that the incubation of PN with AM and its subsequent implantation has an impact either on the survival of the adrenal medulla cells (and supposedly on their phenotype as well), [4, 14, 31] maintaining the tropic-trophic influence on the host cells or, perhaps, the peripheral nerve (consisting of fibroblasts, schwann cells, etc.) provokes a direct mediator effect on the growth of the host fibers [6, 32] or an indirect effect through the recipient striate cells. To date, there are no pathological data from parkinsonian patients to support any of these hypotheses. Only animal studies are available [4–6, 14, 31, 34], showing that implantation of peripheral nerve in combination with adrenal medulla increases the survival of chromaffin cells and enhances the recovery of the surviving host nigrostriatal dopaminergic cells.

Thus, we conclude that, in our implant model, there appears to be more than one cause for the improvement. The surgical lesion, caudotomy and a frontal transcortical approach to the lateral ventricle, could partly explain the recovery observed in the third series. However, the differences among the respective courses following implantation of perfused adrenal medulla, fetal tissue, and coimplants suggests that, while in adrenal medulla implants, the major factor may be related to injury to the host cells and that, in fetal tissue implants, the primary factor influencing the improvement in the 2nd and 3rd years may be the implanted dopaminergic cells, in the case of AM + PN implants, we have to suppose that the fact that the recovery continues to progress during the second postoperative year is mainly due to the peripheral nerve or to its maintenance of the adrenal medulla cells. The results of this pilot study are sufficiently encouraging to induce us to carry out a broader clinical trial.

Acknowledgements We thank Martha Messman for her editorial assistance. This work was supported by research grants from the Fondo de Investigaciones Sanitarias (FIS 90/197 and 93/493) and by a Fundación Areces award to JJLL.

References

1. Backlund EO, Grandberg PO, Hamberger B, Kuntsson E, Martensson A, Goran S, Seiger A, Olson L (1985) Transplantation of adrenal medullary tissue to striatum in Parkinsonism: First clinical trials. J Neurosurg 62: 169–173

2. Bakay RAE, Allen GS, Apuzzo M, Borges LF, Bullard DE, Ojemann GA, Olfield EH, Penn R, Purvis JT, Tindall GT (1990) Preliminary report on adrenal medullary grafting from the American Association of Neurological Surgeons GRAFT project. Prog Brain Res 82: 603–610

3. Bohn MC, Cupit L, Marciano F, Gash DM (1987) Adrenal medulla grafts enhance recovery of striatal dopaminergic fibers. Science 237: 913–916

4. Date I, Felten SY, Felten DL (1990) Cografts of adrenal medulla with peripheral nerve enhance the survivability of transplanted adrenal chromaffin cells and recovery of the host nigrostriatal dopaminergic system in MPTP-treated young adult mice. Brain Res 537: 33–39

5. Date I, Yoshimoto Y, Imaoka T, Miyoshi Y, Furuta T, Asari S, Ohmoto T (1994) Effect of host age upon the degree of nigrostriatal dopaminergic system recovery following cografts of adrenal medulla and pretransected peripheral nerve. Brain Res 21: 50–56

6. Doering LC (1992) Peripheral nerve segments promote consistent long term survival of adrenal medulla transplants in the brain. Exp Neurol 118: 253–260

7. Foimo LS, Langston JW (1992) Unfavorable outcome of adrenal medullary transplant for Parkinson's disease. Acta Neuropathol 81: 691–694

8. Freed WJ (1993) Neural Transplantation: prospects for clinical use. Cell Transplant 2: 13–31

9. Goetz CG, Stebbins GT, Klawans HL, Koller WC, Grossman RG, Bakay RAE, Penn RD (1991) United Parkinson-Foundation Neurotransplantation Registry. Multicenter United States and Canadian data Base, presurgical and 12 months follow-up. Neurology 41: 1719–1722

10. Hirsch EC, Duyckaerts C, Javoy-Agid F, Hauw JJ, Agid Y (1990) Does adrenal graft enhance recovery of dopaminergic neurons in Parkinson's disease? Ann Neurol 27: 676–682

11. Hitchcock ER, Clugh CG, Hughes RC, Kenny BG (1989) Transplantation in Parkinson's diseae: stereotactic implantation of adrenal medulla and foetal mesencephalon. Acta Neurochir (Suppl) 46: 48–50

12. Hurtig H, Joyce J, Sladek JR, Trojanowski JQ (1989) Post-mortem analysis of adrenal medulla to caudate autografts in a patient with Parkinson's disease. Ann Neurol 25: 607–614

13. Jiao SS, Ding YJ, Zhang WC, Cao JK, Zhang GF, Zhang ZM, Ding MC, Zhang Z, Meng JM (1989) Adrenal medullary autografts in patients with Parkinson's disease. N Engl J Med 321: 324–325

14. Kordower JH, Fiandaca MS, Notter MFD, Hansen JT, Gash DM (1990) Peripheral nerve provides NGF-like trophic support for grafted Rhesus adrenal chromaffin cells. J Neurosurg 73: 418–428

15. Kordower JH, Cochran E, Penn RD, Goetz CG (1991) Putative chromaffin cell survival and enhanced host-derived TH-fiber innervation following a functional adrenal medulla autograft for Parkinson's disease. Ann Neurol 29: 405–412

16. Langston WJ, Widner H, Goetz OG (1992) Core assessment program for intracerebral transplantation (CAPIT). Mov Discard 7: 2–13

17. Lindvall O, Björklund A, Widner H (1991) Experimental basis and clinical experiences. In: Lindvall O, Björklund A, Widner H (eds) Intracerebral transplantation in movement disorders. Elsevier, Amsterdam, Restor Neurol 4: 69–131

18. López-Lozano JJ, Brera B (1993) Neural transplants in Parkinson's disease. Transplant Proc 25: 1005–1011

19. López-Lozano JJ, Brera B, Abascal J, Bravo G (1989) Preparation of adrenal medullary tissue for transplantation in Parkinson's patients: A new procedure. J Neurosurg 71: 552–555

20. López-Lozano JJ, Abascal J, Bravo G, CPH Neural Transplantation Group (1990) A year follow-up of autoimplants of perfused adrenal medulla into parkinsonian patients. Prog Brain Res 82: 657–663

21. López-Lozano JJ, Bravo G, Abascal J, CPH Neural Transplantation Group (1990) A long-term study of Parkinson's patients subjected to autoimplants of perfused adrenal medulla into the caudate nucleus. Transplant Proc 22: 2243–2246

22. López-Lozano JJ, Bravo G, Abascal J, The Clínica Puerta de Hierro Neural Transplantation Group (1991) Grafting of perfused adrenal medullary tissue into the caudate nucleus of patients with Parkinson's disease. J Neurosurg 75: 234–243

23. López-Lozano JJ, Bravo G, Brera B, Uría J, Dargallo J, Salmeán J, Insausti J, Cerrolaza J, CPH Neural Transplantation Group (1991) Can an analogy be drawn between the clinical evolution of Parkinson's patients who undergo auto-implantation of adrenal medulla and those of fetal ventral mesencephalon recipients? In: Lindvall O, Björklung A, Widner H (eds) Intracerebral transplantation in movement disorders. Elsevier, Amsterdam, Restor Neurol 4: 83–94

24. López-Lozano JJ, Bravo G, Abascal Brea B, Santos H, Gómez-Angulo JC, CPH Neural Transplantation Group (1992) Co-transplantation of peripheral nerve and adrenal medulla in Parkinson's disease. Lancet 339: 430

25. López-Lozano JJ, Bravo G, Brera B, Dargallo J, Salmean J, Uria J, Insausti J, CPH Neural Transplantation group (1995) Long term follow-up in 10 Parkinsons's patients subjected to fetal grafting into a cavity in caudate nucleus: The Clinica Puerta de Hierro Experience. Transplant Proc 27: 1395–1400

26. Madrazo I, Drucker-Collin R, Díaz V, Martínez-Mata J, Torres C, Becerril JJ (1987) Open microsurgical autograft of adrenal medulla to the right caudate nucleus in two patients with intractable Parkinson's disease. N Engl J Med 316: 831–834

27. Molina H, Galarraga J, Quiñones R, Figueredo R, Estrada R, Alvarez L, Hernandez R, Rachid M, Oduardo H, Coutin P, Diaz G, Duque A, Hernandez H, Basco E (1988) El Neurotransplante en la Enfermedad de Parkinson. Experiencia Cubana. Reporte Preliminary. Ciudad Habana: Centro de Transplante y Regeneración del Sistema Nervioso, 18 pp

28. Peterson DI, Price L, Small CS (1989) Autopsy findings in a patient who had an adrenal-to-brain transplant for Parkinson's disease. Neurology 39: 235–238

29. Plunkett RJ, Bankiewicz KS, Cummins A, Miletich RS, Schwartz JP, Oldfield EH (1990) Long-term evaluation of hemiparkinsonian monkeys after adrenal autografting or cavitation alone. J Neurosurg 73: 918–926

30. Stoddard SL (1994) The adrenal medulla and Parkinson's disease. Rev Neurosci 5: 293–307

31. Stromberg I, Herrera-Marschitz M, Ungerstendt U, Ebendal T, Olson L (1985) Chronic implants of chromaffin tissue into dopamine-denervated striatum. Effects of NGF on graft survival, fiber growth and rotational behavior. Exp Brain Res 60: 335–349

32. Tello F (1911) La influencia del neurotropismo en la regeneración de los centros nerviosos. Trab Lab Invest Biol 9: 123–159

33. Waters C, Itabashi HH, Apuzzo ML, Weiner LP (1990) Adrenal to caudate transplantation-postmortem study. Mov Disord 5: 248–250

34. Watts RL, Mandir AS, Bakay RA (1995) Intrastriatal of autologous adrenal medulla and sural nerve in MPTP-induced parkinsonian macaques: behavioural and anatomical assessment. Cell Transplant 4: 27–38

Transpl Int (1996) 9 [Suppl 1]: S492–S496
© Springer-Verlag 1996

B. Lukomska
M. Durlik
E. Cybulska
W. L. Olszewski

Comparative analysis of immunological reconstitution induced by vascularized bone marrow versus bone marrow cell transplantation

B. Lukomska (✉) · M. Durlik ·
E. Cybulska · W. L. Olszewski
Department for Surgical Research and
Transplantology, Medical Research Center
Institute, Polish Academy of Sciences,
5, Chalubinskiego Street, 02 004 Warsaw,
Poland

Abstract We have reported previously that vascularized bone marrow transplantation (VBMT) in an orthotopic hind limb graft brings about complete repopulation of bone marrow cavities in lethally irradiated syngeneic recipients within 10 days. Intravenous infusion of an equivalent volume of bone marrow cell suspension was evidently less effective. The purpose of this study was to investigate the reconstitution of immunocompetent compartments of lethally irradiated syngeneic rats after VBMT. Lewis rat hind limbs were transplanted orthotopically into irradiated recipients. Ten days after irradiation and bone marrow transplantation, bone marrow, mesenteric lymph nodes, and sera from rats were harvested. Mesenteric lymph node lymphocytes were analyzed. The responsiveness fo mesenteric lymph node lymphocytes (MLNL) to mitogens and cell proliferation in the presence of sera and bone marrow cell (BMC) culture supernatants were measured. Our studies have shown that vascularized bone marrow transplantation brings about rapid replenishment of lymphoid organs of lethally irradiated syngeneic recipients. The repopulating subsets are fully responsive to mitogens. Sera from reconstituting rats had no effect on the proliferation of mature lymphocytes. Intravenous infusion of a number of BMC in suspension equivalent to that grafted in hind limb transplant was less efficient in reconstitution of lymphoid tissue.

Key words Lymphopoiesis · Bone marrow transplantation · Mitogenic response · Stromal cells

Introduction

Immunodeficiency after bone marrow transplantation (BMT) is one of the major problems encountered in bone marrow recipients. The chemoradiotherapy used to prepare marrow graft recipients ablates immune cells to permit engraftment of hematopoietic elements. Although the immunodeficiency is created under controlled circumstances, bone marrow transplanted patients can experience life-threatening infection with bacterial, viral, and fungal antigens, especially in terms of the first 3 months postgrafting. Deppresion in the generation of the immunological response against different pathogens has been shown to correlate with impaired myelopoiesis. Recent observations provide evidence that the immune system regulates hemopoiesis. Lymphocytes seem to be required for the optimal growth of bone marrow progenitor cells [7, 8, 14]. Therefore the study of the recovery process of the immune system in such bone marrow graft recipients is of great interest.

We have reported previously that vascularized bone marrow transplantation (VBMT) in an orthotopic hind limb graft brings about complete repopulation of bone marrow cavities in lethally irradiated syngeneic recipients within 10 days [5]. Intravenous infusion of an equivalent volume of bone marrow cells (BMC) was evidently less effective. The question arises whether

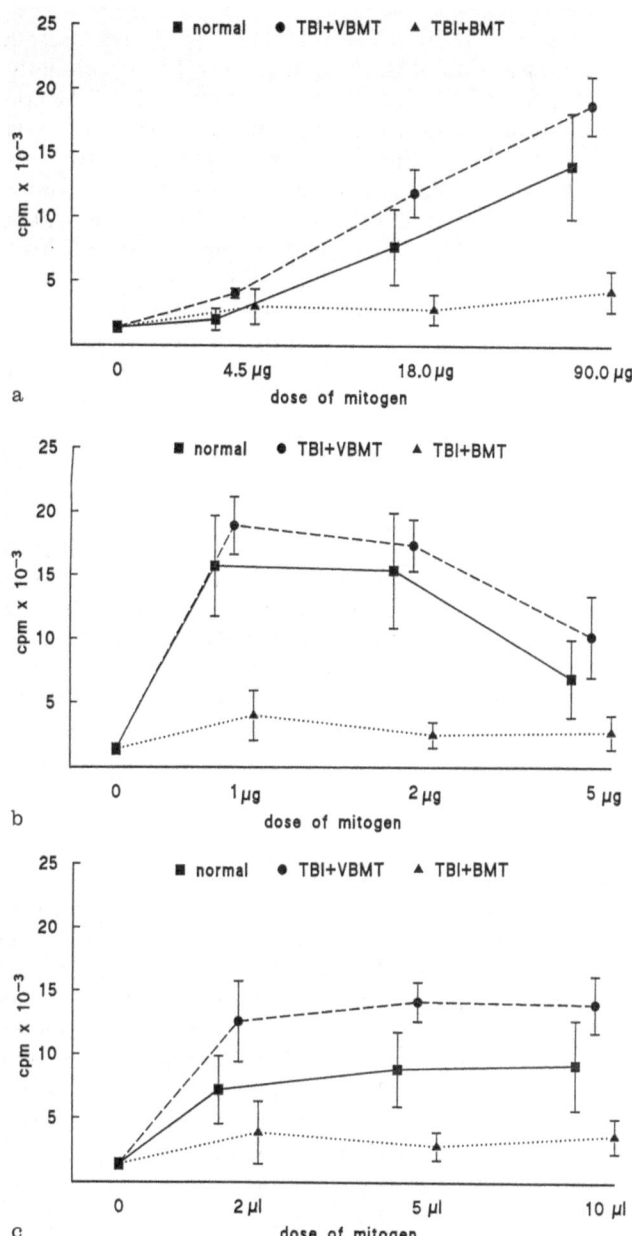

Fig. 1 Responsiveness of mesenteric lymph node lymphocytes (MLNL) to different doses of mitogens: **(a)** phytohemagglutinin (PHA); **(b)** concanavalin A; **(c)** pokeweed mitogen (mean values ± SD, $n = 6$), *TBI* total body irradiation, *VBMT* vascularized bone marrow transplantation, *BMT* bone marrow transplantation)

VBMT also promotes rapid replenishment of lymphoid organs.

The aim of the study was to investigate the reconstitution of immunocompetent compartments of lethally irradiated syngeneic rats after VBMT.

Materials and methods

Animals

Three-month-old male Lewis rats (RT1l) bred and maintained in our own animal facility, were used throughout this study. Recipients were exposed to 8 Gy of τ irradiation from a ^{60}Co source (Theratron) at a dose rate of 150 cGy/min.

Hind limb transplantation

The donor hind limb was amputated at the groin level with a long vascular stump. The hind limb of the recipient was amputated at the mid-thigh level. End-to-end anastomoses of the graft and recipient vessels were performed with the use of 10-0 monofilament sutures. The stumps of sciatic nerves were stiched. Femurs were anastomosed with an intramedullary metallic stent.

Experimental design

Group I: Total body irradiation (TBI) was followed by transplantation of a syngeneic hind limb. Group II: TBI was followed by i. v. infusion of syngeneic BMC ($6 \times 10_7$). Group III: TBI without subsequent treatment. Normal non-treated rats served as a control.

Cell collection

Ten days after irradiation and transplantation, BMC, mesenteric lymph node lymphocytes (MLNL), and peripheral blood were harvested.

Condition supernatants

Bone marrow cells were grown for 24 h in D-MEM medium supplemented with 15 % fetal calf serum and antibiotics. Supernatants were passed through a 0.2-μm filter and stored at – 70 °C.

Proliferation assay

Responsiveness of MLNL isolated from different experimental groups to the mitogens phytohemagglutinin (PHA), concanavalin A (Con A), and pokeweed mitogen (PWM) was measured in 72-h cultures. The effect of sera and BMC supernatants on normal MLNL responsiveness to PHA (90 μg/ml) was studied in a 72-h assay. Incorporation of methyl [^{3}H]-thymidine, added 18 h before cell harvesting, was measured in a Beckman liquid-scintillation radiation counter.

Results

Histological analysis

Group I. Ten days after TBI and hind limb transplantation, the normal cellular pattern was observed in mesenteric lymph nodes (MLN). The cortex contained lymphoid follicles with active germinal centers. Group II. After BMC infusion, MLN remained largely depleted of lymphocytes. Dilated sinuses filled with erythrocytes

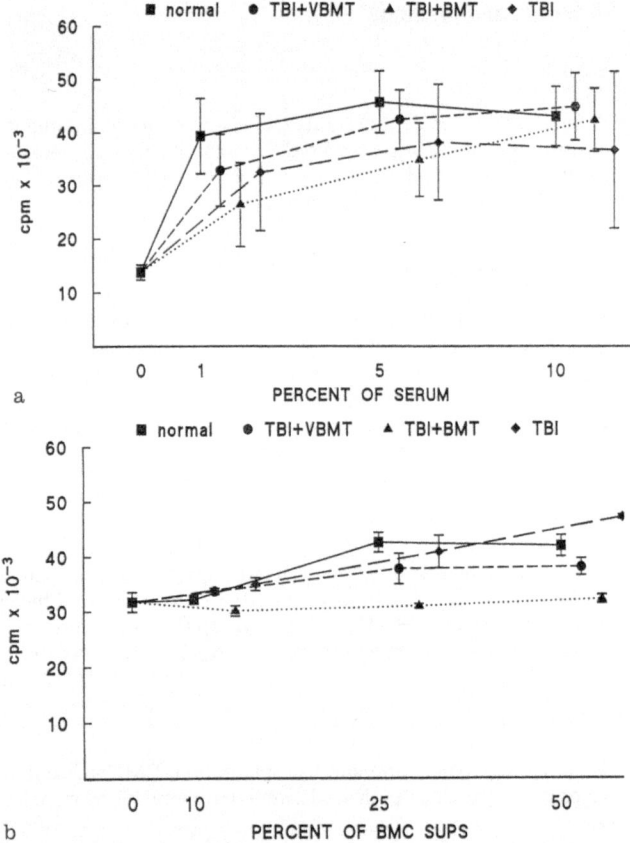

Fig. 2 Responsiveness of normal MLNL to PHA (90 µg/ml), **(a)** in the presence of sera from graft recipients; **(b)** in the presence of bone marrow cell *(BMC)* culture supernatants from graft recipients (mean values ± SD, $n = 6$)

and macrophages were observed. Group III: TBI rats left without any treatment presented a picture of total lymphoid depletion in MLN. No signs of regeneration were observed 10 days after TBI.

Cell yield

The MLNL yield of TBI rats with VBMT was $37.0 \pm 3.6 \times 10^7$/g of tissue on day 10 compared with $76.5 \pm 16.1 \times 10^7$/g in normal non-irradiated rats. In group II, the MLNL yield was found to be 80 % lower $(12.8 \pm 2.6 \times 10^7$/g of tissue). Total body irradiation in non-transplanted rats brought about a decrease of lymphocyte number to $1.4 \pm 1.2 \times 10^7$/g of the MLN.

Responsiveness to mitogens

Ten days after VBMT, the responsiveness of MLNL to PHA (4.5; 18.0; 90.0 µg) was comparable with control values (2026 ± 321 vs 2016 ± 840; 11 871 ± 1867 vs

7665 ± 2958; 18 767 ± 2280 vs 14 011 ± 4134 cpm, respectively). Infusion of BMC revealed low PHA stimulation of MLNL (3020 ± 1367; 2806 ± 1168; 4256 ± 1580 cpm, at the different doses of mitogen) (Fig. 2 a). Concanavalin A and PWM stimulation showed similar patterns of MLNL responsiveness to that of PHA. Proliferation of MLNL in the presence of Con A (1.0; 2.0; 5.0 µg) 10 days after VBMT reached normal rat MLNL levels (18 895 ± 2280 vs 15 708 ± 3973; 17 322 ± 2028 vs 15 350 ± 4549; 10 150 ± 6878 vs 6878 ± 3030 cpm, respectively). Transplanted BMC suspensions gave lower values of MLNL responsiveness to 1.0, 2.0, and 5.0 µg of Con A (3995 ± 1929; 2503 ± 983; 2708 ± 13 030 cpm, respectively). The responsiveness of MLNL from VBMT recipients to different doses of PWM (2.0; 5.0; 10.0 µl) was above that of control rats (12 594 ± 3174 vs 7204 ± 2666; 14 172 ± 1554 vs 8850 ± 2942; 13 991 ± 2246 vs 9186 ± 3531 cpm, respectively). An infusion of BMC did not restore proliferation levels of MLNL to normal rat values (3878 ± 2431; 2836 ± 1095; 3665 ± 1367 cpm in the presence of 2.0, 5.0, and 10.0 µl of PWM, respectively) (Fig. 1).

Proliferation assay in the presence of sera and BMC culture supernatants

Sera and supernatants from cultured BMC of VBMT or BMT recipients had no effect on third-party MLNL cultured with PHA. The responsiveness of normal MLNL to PHA (90 µg/ml) in the presence of sera (10 v/v) isolated from VBMT, BMT, and TBI recipients did not differ from that of normal rat serum (44 920 ± 14 786; 42 437 ± 5931; 36 789 ± 14 786 vs 43 053 ± 5640 cpm, respectively). The presence of BMC culture supernatants (50 v/v) from VBMT, BMT, and TBI did not change the responsiveness of third-party MLNL to PHA (90 µg) in comparison to the effect of normal BMC culture supernatants (38 106 ± 1541; 32 249 ± 790; 47 185 ± 385 vs 41 930 ± 1946 cpm, respectively) (Fig. 2).

Discussion

The survival of patients undergoing BMT is critically dependent on the nature and rate of reconstitution of the immune system. Immunological recovery requires both a quantitative and a qualitative repopulation of lymphocytes.

Multipotential stem cells differentiate into hemopoietic or lymphoid progenitors [2, 4, 19]. Specialized microenvironments and specific cytokines direct the fate of these multipotent progenitor cells [3, 13]. In contrast to other hematopoietic cells, lymphocyte development and differentiation occurs nor only within bone marrow cavities but also within peripheral lymphoid compartments such as lymph nodes. The significance of extrathymic T-cell differentiation is underscored by the fact that BMT results in recovery of T-cell function in the absence of thymus [16]. Terminal differentiation for T-lymphocytes is linked to L-selectin expression allowing migration to lymph node compartments [20]. The finding that stem cells express L-selectin raises the possibility that, following BMT, early T-cells may directly migrate to lymph nodes [18]. The results of our previous studies revealed that a large proportion of BMC transplanted in suspension or, in bone, as a vascularized bone marrow graft into lethally irradiated rats accumulates in the lymph nodes, spleen, and gut [12].

Our experiments described here showed that the ability of lymphocytes to localize into lymph nodes was significantly different in VBMT and BMT recipients. The fast repopulation of lymphoid compartments from hind limb graft remains in sharp contrast to the results obtained in rats infused with BMC suspension. It seems that transplantation of stromal cells present in the bone promoted lymphopoiesis. There is evidence that stromal cells support expansion of lymphoid cells by cytokine production [1, 11, 15]. Growth factors released into the circulation can exert an effect on lymphocyte replenishment and maturation. Clinically, BMC are frequently transplanted into recipients with functional insufficiency of stromal cells. The preparatory regimens for BMT such as radio- and chemotherapy damage the host stroma and bring about loss of synthesis of different regulatory molecules [9, 10]. Bone marrow cell inoculum transplanted intravenously contains only hematopoietic and not stromal cells. This could be reflected in

scanty replenishment of lymphoid organs in irradiated recipients repopulated with BMC suspension. Bone marrow transplantation has been shown to be associated not only with a decline in lymphoid cell number but also with a deficit in various T-cell mediating functions [6, 17, 21]. The results of our studies revealed more rapid reconstitution of function of the immune system after VBMT than after BMT. The repopulating subsets of MLNL isolated from hind limb recipients were fully responsive to mitogen stimulation whereas a low MLNL proliferation rate was seen in rats receiving BMC suspension.

Cell proliferation assays are useful for estimating cytokine production. For that purpose, the effect of sera or BMC culture supernatants from transplanted rats on PHA-induced proliferation of MLNL isolated from normal rats was measured. Our studies have shown that sera and supernatants of reconstituted bone marrow cells had no effect on the proliferation of normal third-party lymphocytes. However, they could contain factors required for the mobilization of lymphoid progenitors and their accelerated differentiation.

The results of our studies clearly indicate that bone marrow cell transplantation in hind limb graft is highly effective in the replenishment of lymphoid compartments of lethally irradiated rats. Two mechanisms may be responsible for the fast repopulation of lymph nodes. One would be immediate seeding of lymphoid precursors from the transplanted bone marrow in the hind limb graft, the other, the release of cytokines from transplanted stromal cells, facilitating local proliferation of lymphocytes in the secondary lymphoid compartments.

References

1. Deryugina EI, Ratnikow BI, Bourdon MA, Muller-Sieburg ChE (1994) Clonal analysis of primary marrow stroma: functional homogeneity in support of lymphoid and myeloid cell lines and identification of positive and negative regulators. Exp Hematol 22: 910–918
2. Ho AD, Maruyama M, Maghazachi A, Mason JR, Gluck S, Corringham ET (1994) Soluble CD4, soluble CD8, soluble CD25, lymphopoietic recovery, and endogenous cytokines after high-dose chemotherapy and blood stem cell transplantation. Blood 84: 3550–3557
3. Ikuta K, Uchida N, Friedman J, Weissman IL (1992) Lymphocyte development from stem cells. Annu Rev Immunol 10: 759–783
4. Kollmann TR, Kim A, Zhuang X, Hachamovitch M, Goldstein H (1994) Reconstitution of SCID mice with human lymphoid and myeloid cells after transplantation with human fetal bone marrow without the requirement for exogenous human cytokines. Proc Natl Acad Sci USA 91: 8032–8036
5. Lukomska B, Durlik M, Morzycka-Michalik M, Olszewski WL (1991) Transplantation of vascularized bone marrow. Transplant Proc 23: 887–888
6. Lum LG (1987) The kinetics of immune reconstitution after human marrow transplantation. Blood 69: 369–380
7. Maciejewski JP, Hibbs JR, Anderson S, Katevas P, Young NS (1994) Bone marrow and peripheral blood lymphocyte phenotype in patients with bone marrow failure. Exp Hematol 22: 1102–1110
8. Martin PJ (1995) Influence of alloreactive T-cells on initial hematopoietic reconstitution after marrow transplantation. Exp Hematol 23: 174–179
9. Mauch P, Rosenblatt M, Hellmann S (1988) Permanent loss of stem cell self renewal capacity following stress to the marrow. Blood 72: 1193–1199
10. McGlave PB, Beatty P, Ash R, Hows JM (1990) Therapy for chronic myelogenous leukemia with unrelated donor bone marrow transplantation. Blood 75: 1728–1735
11. Medlock ES, Kenna SD, Goldschneider I (1993) A selective culture system for generating terminal deoxynucleotidyl transferase-positive lymphoid cells in vitro. III. Structure of the bone marrow microenvironment for early lymphopoiesis. Lab Invest 69: 616–628
12. Olszewski WL, Lukomska B, Durlik M, Namyslowski A, Cybulska E (1994) Bone marrow cells transplanted in suspension or in vascularized bone marrow graft repopulate not only bone marrow but also lymphoid organs. Transplant Proc 26: 3319–3320

13. Palacios R, Samaridis J (1993) Bone marrow clones representing an intermediate stage of development between hematopoietic stem cells and pro-T-lymphocyte or pro-B-lymphocyte progenitors. Blood 81: 1222–1238

14. Pantel K, Nakeff A (1993) The role of lymphoid cells in hematopoietic regulation. Exp Hematol 21: 738–742

15. Pietrangeli CE, Hayashi SI, Kincade PW (1988) Stromal cell lines which support lymphocyte growth: characterization, sensitivity to radiation and responsiveness to growth factors. Eur J Immunol 18: 863–872

16. Sackstein R (1993) Physiologic migration of lymphocytes to lymph nodes following bone marrow transplantation: role in immune recovery. Semin Oncol 20: 34–39

17. Samlowski WE, Johnson HM, Hammond EH, Robertson BA, Daynes RA (1987) Marrow ablative doses of gamma-irradiation and protracted changes in peripheral lymph node microvasculature of murine and human bone marrow transplant recipients. Lab Invest 56: 85–95

18. Terstappen LWMM, Huang S, Picker LJ (1992) Flow cytometric assessment of human T-cell differentiation in thymus and bone marrow. Blood 79: 666–677

19. Tjonnfjord GE, Steen R, Veiby OP, Friedrich W, Egeland T (1994) Evidence for engraftment of donor-type multipotent CD34$^+$ cells in a patient with selective T-lymphocyte reconstitution after bone marrow transplantation for BSCID. Blood 84: 3584–3589

20. Wilson A, Scollay R, Reichert RA (1987) The correlation of lectin-stimulated proliferation and cytotoxicity in murine thymocytes with expression of the Mel-14-defined homing receptor. J Immunol 138: 352–357

21. Witherspoon RP, Lum LG, Storb R (1984) Immunologic reconstitution after human marrow grafting. Semin Hematol 21: 2–11

Transplant International

1. General

Diskettes are very welcome, but should be submitted only after the reviewing process has been completed. Authors are requested to follow the technical instructions printed in each issue. Manuscripts should be submitted to the Editor-in-Chief:

Gauke Kootstra, M. D.
Department of Surgery
University Hospital
P. Debyelaan 25
P. O. Box 5800
6202 AZ Maastricht
The Netherlands
Fax: + 31 43 3875473

Papers must be written in English, and authors are urged to aim for clarity, brevity and accuracy of information and language. Non-English-speaking authors should have their papers checked for linguistic accuracy by a native English speaker.

Manuscripts must contain a statement to the effect that all human studies have been reviewed by the appropriate ethics committee and have therefore been performed in accordance with the ethical standards laid down in an appropriate version of the 1964 Declaration of Helsinki. It should also be stated clearly in the text that all persons gave their informed consent prior to their inclusion in the study. Details that might disclose the identity of the subjects under study should be omitted.

Reports of animal experiments must state that the "Principles of laboratory animal care" (NIH publication No. 86–23, revised 1985) were followed, as well as specific national laws (e.g. the current version of the German Law on the Protection of Animals) where applicable. The Editor-in-Chief reserves the right to reject manuscripts that do not comply with the above-mentioned requirements. The author will be held responsible for false statements or for failure to fulfill the above-mentioned requirements.

To accelerate publication, *only one set of proofs* is sent to the authors. It is therefore essential that manuscripts be submitted in their final form and that the positions of figures and tables be indicated in the margins.

To facilitate communication between the authors, editors and publisher, the author should furnish a telex or fax number on the title page of the manuscript.

2. Format

Authors must submit 3 copies of a manuscript (original manuscript typed on one side of the paper plus 2 copies photocopied on both sides) and 3 sets of illustrations (one set of original figures and two sets of photocopies). Manuscripts should be typed double-spaced with wide margins.

They should follow the format: *title page* listing the title, names of all authors, institutions with full address, and address of author to whom correspondence should be sent; *Abstract* of not more than 150 words, stating the main problem, methods, results, and conclusions; *Key words* (up to 6); *text*, arranged in the order: Introduction, Materials and methods, Results, Discussion, Acknowledgements; *References; tables; legends* for all figures listed together on a separate page; *figures*.

Footnotes should be avoided whenever possible. Essential footnotes should be numbered consecutively and placed at the bottom of the page to which they refer.

3. References

The author is responsible for the accuracy of the references. Citations in the text should be identified by numbers in brackets, and the list of references at the end of the paper should be both alphabetized under the first author's name and numbered. Works by two authors are in alphabetical order by coauthor and those by more than two authors in chronological order. Only works referred to in the text and already accepted for publication can be included:

a) *Articles from journals:* name(s) and initials of all author(s), year in parentheses, full title, journal name as abbreviated in *Index Medicus*, volume followed by a colon, first and last page numbers.

Bock HP, Sombolos V, Lucas PA, Bardin F (1987) Complications of gastric surgery in transplanted patients. J Transplant Surg 38: 213–216

b) *Books*: name(s) and initials of all author(s), year in parentheses, title, edition, publisher, place of publication.

Kay PJ (1978) Graft versus host disease. Springer, Berlin Heidelberg New York

c) *Multiauthor books:* name(s) and initials of all author(s), year in parentheses, title of the paper. In: name(s) and initials of all editor(s), title of the book, publisher, place of publication, first and last page numbers.

Feldman SP (1974) The role of leucocytes in rejection. In: Dragon S, Curius P, Velasques RC (eds) The process of rejection. Nijhof, The Hague, pp 38–46

4. Tables

Each table should be typed on a separate sheet and numbered consecutively with Arabic numerals. Footnotes to tables should be indicated by lower-case superscript letters.

5. Illustrations

Illustrations should be limited to those essential for the text. The same results should be presented as either graphs or tables, not as both.

Color illustrations will be accepted; however, the authors will be expected to make a contribution (DM 1,200.00 for the first page and DM 600.00 for each additional page) towards the extra costs.

All figures, whether photographs, graphs, or diagrams, should be numbered consecutively and kept separate from the text. Photo- or micrographs should be mounted together to save space without necessarily taking into consideration their numerical order. Line drawings should be supplied as clear black-and-white drawings suitable for reproduction. All lines should be of uniform thickness. Letters and numbers should be of professional quality and proper dimensions. Computer drawings are acceptable if the quality is comparable to line drawings. Computer-drawn curves and lines must be smooth. All illustrations should be of a size permitting direct printing (with no reduction): up to 8.6 cm column width, up to 17.6 cm page width, not higher than 22.4 cm. The publisher reserves the right to reduce or enlarge illustrations. Photographs and electron micrographs should be submitted as sharp high-contrast prints on glossy paper, trimmed at right angles. Arrows, letters, and numbers should be inserted with template rub-on letters. If this is not possible, inscriptions should be made on a transparent overlay (not on the actual photograph). Micrographs should have an internal magnification marker; the magnification should also be stated in the caption. Legends must be brief, self-sufficient explanations of the illustrations in no more than four or five lines. Remarks such as "For explanation, see text" should be avoided. The legends should be typed on a separate page.

6. Offprints

Offprints can be ordered at cost price provided the order is received with the corrected proofs.

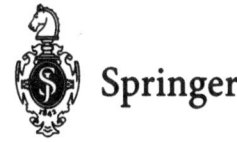

Springer